Cyclic Nucleotide Signaling and the Cardiovascular System

Cyclic Nucleotide Signaling and the Cardiovascular System

Special Issue Editors

Thomas Brand
Enno Klussmann

MDPI • Basel • Beijing • Wuhan • Barcelona • Belgrade

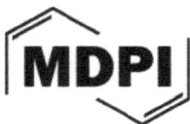

MDPI

Special Issue Editors

Thomas Brand
Imperial College London
UK

Enno Klussmann
Max Delbrück Center Berlin for
Molecular Medicine (MDC)
Germany

Editorial Office
MDPI
St. Alban-Anlage 66
Basel, Switzerland

This is a reprint of articles from the Special Issue published online in the open access journal *Journal of Cardiovascular Development and Disease* (ISSN 2308-3425) from 2017 to 2018 (available at: http://www.mdpi.com/jcdd/special_issues/cyclic_nucleotide)

For citation purposes, cite each article independently as indicated on the article page online and as indicated below:

LastName, A.A.; LastName, B.B.; LastName, C.C. Article Title. *Journal Name* **Year**, *Article Number*, Page Range.

ISBN 978-3-03842-989-0 (Pbk)
ISBN 978-3-03842-990-6 (PDF)

Cover image courtesy of Prof. Thomas Brand and Dr. Subreena Simrick, Imperial College London.

Contents

About the Special Issue Editors

Thomas Brand, Professor and Chair in Developmental Dynamics, studied Biology and received his Diploma in 1987 and his Ph.D. in 1991 from the University of Bielefeld. Currently, he is a Full Professor and Chair in Developmental Dynamics at Imperial College London. He was a Postdoctoral Researcher (1991) at Baylor College in Houston, U.S.A and (1994) at the Technical University in Braunschweig, Germany. In 2004 he became Professor of Molecular Developmental Biology at the University of Würzburg, Germany until he took his current position in London in 2009. His main research interest is to characterize the molecular functions of the Popeye domain-containing proteins, a novel class of cAMP effector proteins in skeletal muscle and the heart.

Enno Klussmann, PD Dr., studied Genetics in London, UK (BSc, 1988) and Biology at the University of Marburg, Germany (Diploma, 1992). He received his doctoral degree from the University of Marburg (1996). After postdoctoral positions at the Free University Berlin and the Leibniz-Forschungsinstitut für Molekulare Pharmakologie Berlin (FMP) in addition to a residency in pharmacology and toxicology at the Charité-University Medicine Berlin (2005), he became group leader at the FMP. Currently, he is the leader of the Anchored Signaling group at the Max Delbrück Center for Molecular Medicine Berlin in the Helmholtz Association (MDC). His main research interest is to elucidate functions of the cardiovascular system through the analysis of compartmentalized cAMP signaling and to devise novel pharmacological strategies for the treatment of cardiovascular diseases.

Preface to "Cyclic Nucleotide Signaling and the Cardiovascular System"

Cyclic nucleotide signaling is one of the most important signaling pathways in the heart and control vital functions such as excitation-contraction coupling, pacemaking, relaxation, and speed of conduction [1]. Recent insights revealed that the different elements of this signaling pathway interact and form protein complexes, which control the size and subcellular localization of cAMP nanodomains and ensure the signal-specific activation of different effector proteins [2].

Adenylate cyclases (AC) produce cAMP and nine different membrane-bound isoforms exist in the mammalian heart. This Special Issue starts with a review by Baldwin and Dessauer on the role of AC isoforms in cardiac myocytes [3]. A single soluble AC isoform is present in cardiac myocytes and the review by Pozdniakova and Ladilov discuss the functional importance of this isoform and the different mechanisms of its activation in the heart and other tissues [4].

The compartmentation of cyclic nucleotide signaling is determined to a large extent by phosphodiesterases (PDEs), of which there are 11 different families and approximately 50 different isoforms. This enormous complexity is dealt with by several reviews in this issue. Movsesian and colleagues give an overview of the functional role of PDE3 isoforms in the heart and therapeutic opportunities to modulate their function [5]. The role of PDE4 isoforms in the heart are reviewed by Fertig and Baillie [6], followed by a review article by Chen et al. on PDE1 isoforms and their roles in pathological remodeling and cardiac dysfunction [7]. While PDEs are also important for cardiac pacemaking, the individual functions of PDE3 and 4 isoforms are less clear St. Clair et al. report on their experiments to elucidate the impact of PDE3 and PFDE4 isoforms on the funny current (If) in the murine sinoatrial node [8].

A kinase anchor proteins (AKAPs) are a large and diverse family of proteins which primarily interact with protein kinase A (PKA) but are also responsible for the assembly of cAMP nanodomains by binding PDEs, ACs, and other signaling proteins. Two reviews in this book discuss the various AKAPS found in the heart [9] and the role of a specific AKAP, AKAP-LBC, in the adaptive response to stress of the heart [10].

Four classes of cAMP effector proteins are known to date, including PKA, exchange protein directly activated by cAMP (EPAC), cyclic nucleotide-gated (CNG) channels, and the Popeye domain-containing (POPDC) genes. A review of the pulmonary and cardiac functions of EPAC by Laudette et al. [11] is followed by a review of the newly discovered cAMP effector protein family encoded by the POPDC genes [12].

The visualization of small molecules such as cAMP was a challenging problem until recently. However, the development of sensors on the basis of cAMP-binding domains and the use of live-cell imaging of Foerster resonance energy transfer (FRET) activity made it possible to detect cAMP nanodomains. Schleicher and Zaccolo outline the current utilization of cAMP sensors to analyze cAMP nanodomains and to detect stimulus-dependent differences in cAMP signal amplitude and kinetics [13]. Pavlaki and Nikolaev describe the use of EPAC-derived FRET sensors to analyze the cAMP-cGMP-mediated cross-talk, which is mediated by PDE2 and PDE3 [14]. Bhogal et al. then review the currently available data on cAMP compartmentation in atrial and ventricular myocytes [15].

Given the importance of cAMP for the heart, relatively little is known about the disease association of proteins of the cAMP signaling pathway. In their article, Suryavanshi et al. review the available literature on knockout phenotypes in mice and mutations in genes encoding AKAP proteins [16]. Holland et al. discuss the importance of cyclic nucleotide kinases in cardiovascular inflammation and growth [17]. Lehners et al. address the function of cGMP signaling in the control of vascular smooth muscle cell plasticity [18].

Attempts to translate the accumulated knowledge into clinical practice will probably involve the identification of small molecules or peptides that are able to activate or inhibit a particular protein involved in cAMP signaling. Barker et al. report on their attempt to generate a novel class of EPAC1-seective agonists, which might be able to block cardiovascular inflammation [19].

Many articles in this issue point out where we currently stand and what we do not know. Often, technological advances generate novel insight but also spark the curious minds of a new generation of researchers.

1. Perera, R.K.; Nikolaev, V.O. Compartmentation of cAMP signaling in cardiomyocytes in health and disease. Acta Physiol. (Oxf.) 2013, 207, 650-662.

2. Lefkimmiatis, K.; Zaccolo, M. cAMP signaling in subcellular compartments. Pharmacol. Ther. 2014, 143, 295-304.

3. Baldwin, T.A.; Dessauer, C.W. Function of adenylyl cyclase in heart: The AKAP connection. J. Cardiovasc. Dev. Dis. 2018, 5, 2.

4. Pozdniakova, S.; Ladilov, Y. Functional significance of the ADCY10-dependent intracellular cAMP compartments. J. Cardiovasc. Dev. Dis. 2018, 5, 29.

5. Movsesian, M.; Ahmad, F.; Hirsch, E. Functions of PDE3 isoforms in cardiac muscle. J. Cardiovasc. Dev. Dis. 2018, 5, 10.

6. Fertig, B.A.; Baillie, G.S. PDE4-mediated cAMP signaling. J. Cardiovasc. Dev. Dis. 2018, 5, 8.

7. Chen, S.; Knight, W.E.; Yan, C. Roles of PDE1 in pathological cardiac remodeling and dysfunction. J. Cardiovasc. Dev. Dis. 2018, 5, 22.

8. St Clair, J.R.; Larson, E.D.; Sharpe, E.J.; Liao, Z.; Proenza, C. Phosphodiesterases 3 and 4 differentially regulate the funny current, if, in mouse sinoatrial node myocytes. J. Cardiovasc. Dev. Dis. 2017, 4, 10.

9. Ercu, M.; Klussmann, E. Roles of A-kinase anchoring proteins and phosphodiesterases in the cardiovascular system. J. Cardiovasc. Dev. Dis. 2018, 5, 14.

10. Diviani, D.; Osman, H.; Reggi, E. A-kinase anchoring protein-Lbc: A molecular scaffold involved in cardiac protection. J. Cardiovasc. Dev. Dis. 2018, 5, 12.

11. Laudette, M.; Zuo, H.; Lezoualc'h, F.; Schmidt, M. Epac function and cAMP scaffolds in the heart and lung. J. Cardiovasc. Dev. Dis. 2018, 5, 9.

12. Brand, T. The popeye domain containing genes and their function as cAMP effector proteins in striated muscle. J. Cardiovasc. Dev. Dis. 2018, 5, 18.

13. Schleicher, K.; Zaccolo, M. Using cAMP sensors to study cardiac nanodomains. J. Cardiovasc. Dev. Dis. 2018, 5,17.

14. Pavlaki, N.; Nikolaev, V.O. Imaging of PDE2- and PDE3-mediated cGMP-to-cAMP cross-talk in cardiomyocytes. J. Cardiovasc. Dev. Dis. 2018, 5, 4.

15. Bhogal, N.K.; Hasa, A.; Gorelik, J. The development of compartmentation of camp signaling in cardiomyocytes: The role of t-tubules and caveolae microdomains. J. Cardiovasc. Dev. Dis. 2018, 5, 25.

16. Suryavanshi, S.V.; Jadhav, S.M.; McConnell, B.K. Polymorphisms/mutations in a-kinase anchoring proteins (AKAPs): Role in the cardiovascular system. J. Cardiovasc. Dev. Dis. 2018, 5, 7.

17.   Holland, N.A.; Francisco, J.T.; Johnson, S.C.; Morgan, J.S.; Dennis, T.J.; Gadireddy, N.R.; Tulis, D.A. Cyclic nucleotide-directed protein kinases in cardiovascular inflammation and growth.   J. Cardiovasc. Dev. Dis. 2018, 5, 6.

18.   Lehners, M.; Dobrowinski, H.; Feil, S.; Feil, R. cGMP signaling and vascular smooth muscle cell plasticity. J. Cardiovasc. Dev. Dis. 2018, 5, 20.

19.   Barker, R.; Parnell, E.; van Basten, B.; Buist, H.; Adams, D.R.; Yarwood, S.Y. The potential of a novel class of EPAC-selective agonists to combat cardiovascular inflammation. J. Cardiovasc. Dev. Dis. 2018, 4, 22.

Thomas Brand, Enno Klussmann
Special Issue Editors

Journal of
*Cardiovascular
Development and Disease*

MDPI

Review

Function of Adenylyl Cyclase in Heart: the AKAP Connection

Tanya A. Baldwin [ID] **and Carmen W. Dessauer *** [ID]

Department of Integrative Biology and Pharmacology, McGovern Medical School,
University of Texas Health Science Center, Houston, TX 77030, USA; Tanya.Baldwin@uth.tmc.edu
* Correspondence: Carmen.W.Dessauer@uth.tmc.edu; Tel.: +1-713-500-6308

Received: 19 December 2017; Accepted: 11 January 2018; Published: 16 January 2018

Abstract: Cyclic adenosine monophosphate (cAMP), synthesized by adenylyl cyclase (AC), is a universal second messenger that regulates various aspects of cardiac physiology from contraction rate to the initiation of cardioprotective stress response pathways. Local pools of cAMP are maintained by macromolecular complexes formed by A-kinase anchoring proteins (AKAPs). AKAPs facilitate control by bringing together regulators of the cAMP pathway including G-protein-coupled receptors, ACs, and downstream effectors of cAMP to finely tune signaling. This review will summarize the distinct roles of AC isoforms in cardiac function and how interactions with AKAPs facilitate AC function, highlighting newly appreciated roles for lesser abundant AC isoforms.

Keywords: adenylyl cyclase; A-kinase anchoring proteins; cyclic AMP; cardiomyocytes

1. Introduction

The heart continuously balances the interplay of various signaling mechanisms in order to maintain homeostasis and respond to stress. One pathway that contributes to cardiac physiology and stress is the cyclic adenosine monophosphate (cAMP) pathway. cAMP is a universal second messenger that integrates input from G-protein-coupled receptors to coordinate subsequent intracellular signaling. Synthesis of cAMP from adenosine triphosphate (ATP) is controlled by the enzyme adenylyl cyclase (AC). In the heart, cAMP acts downstream on a variety of effectors including protein kinase A (PKA), hyperpolarization-activated cyclic nucleotide-gated channels (HCN), exchange protein directly activated by cAMP (EPAC), Popdc proteins, and a fraction of phosphodiesterases (PDEs). PKA is the most well-known and studied cAMP effector. PKA phosphorylation of intracellular targets coordinates a number of physiological outputs including contraction [1,2] and relaxation [3]. HCN channel regulation by cAMP maintains basal heart rate [4] while EPAC facilitates calcium handling and cardiac hypertrophy [5]. PDEs degrade cAMP, further defining the temporal regulation of the signal. The most recently discovered cAMP effector, Popdc, is important for heart rate dynamics through regulation of the potassium channel TREK1 [6].

The AC family is composed of nine membrane-bound isoforms (AC 1–9) and one soluble isoform (sAC). All of the isoforms can be found in the heart with the exception of AC8 [7,8]. Cardiac fibroblasts express AC 2–7 [9], while in adult cardiac myocytes AC5 and AC6 are considered the major isoforms [10,11]. Lower levels of AC2, AC4, and AC9 are reported in myocytes [12,13].

2. Adenylyl Cyclases (ACs) and Their Role in Cardiac Function: Knockout Phenotypes

AC5 and AC6 are closely related isoforms that share similar regulatory mechanisms, including inhibition by $G\alpha i$ as the hallmark of this group; however, physiologically they appear to play distinct roles in cardiac function [8,14]. Additional modes of regulation for AC5/6 are extensively reviewed elsewhere [15]. AC5 and AC6 are differentially expressed in development, with age, and in a pressure overload model of cardiac hypertrophy where an increase in AC5 protein is observed in neonatal heart and models of heart disease [16,17]. Another potential distinction between these two isoforms is subcellular localization [18].

Several overexpression and deletion studies have focused on roles of these isoforms in cardiac function. Two independent AC5-deletion (AC5$^{-/-}$) mouse lines have been generated. Overall, deletion of AC5 decreases total cAMP activity in cardiac membranes and isolated myocytes (~35–40%) under basal and stimulated (isoproterenol and forskolin) conditions [19,20]. The two studies reported varying results for changes in cardiac function. Okumura et al. [19] observed a decrease in isoproterenol-stimulated left ventricular (LV) ejection fraction (LVEF) but no alterations in basal cardiac function (with intravenous isoproterenol). Conversely, Tang et al. [20] noted basal changes in the contractile function of perfused isolated hearts in addition to a decreased sensitivity to β_1-adrenergic receptor agonist. The most notable finding of AC5$^{-/-}$ mice was the effect on parasympathetic regulation of cAMP. Inhibition of cAMP production by Gi-coupled acetylcholine treatment is ablated and Ca^{2+}-mediated inhibition is significantly reduced upon AC5 deletion [19]. Physiologically, this corresponds to a reduction in LVEF and heart rate in response to muscarinic agonists and an attenuation of baroreflexes [19,20]. Similarly, AC6 deletion results in a significant reduction of cAMP production in stimulated LV homogenates or cardiac myocytes (60–70%), with no changes to basal cAMP production [21]. AC6 deletion revealed a number of unique contributions not observed in AC5$^{-/-}$ including impaired calcium handling, which results in depressed LV function [21]. In addition, levels of AC6, but not AC5, limit β-adrenergic receptor (βAR) signaling in heart [22,23].

In addition to cardiac contractility, AC5 and AC6 play important roles with regard to cardiac stress. Deletion of AC5 is protective in a number of models of cardiac stress, including transverse aorta constriction, chronic isoproterenol infusion, age-related cardiomyopathy, and high-fat diet, but not overexpression of Gq [19,24–26]. While knockout of AC5 can be beneficial to heart, overexpression of AC6 in heart infers protection in response to myocardial ischemia or dilated cardiomyopathy [27–29], but not chronic pressure overload using transverse aorta constriction [30]. However, the protection provided upon AC6 overexpression is independent of its catalytic activity as expression of catalytically inactive AC6 is also cardioprotective [31], but requires proper localization via the N-terminus of AC6 [32]. In fact, the expression of AC6 using adenoviral vectors for the treatment of heart disease is currently in clinical trials [33]. Therefore, it is tempting to simplify the system and suggest that AC5 is largely associated with stress responses while AC6 is necessary for calcium handling and contractility. For these reasons, there has been considerable interest in AC5-selective inhibitors for the treatment of heart disease. However, deletion of AC6 can also be protective from chronic pressure overload in female but not male mice [34]; therefore, roles for AC isoforms may depend on the type of heart disease model. AC inhibitors such as Ara-A (Vidarabine) do have benefits for the treatment of myocardial ischemia when delivered after coronary artery reperfusion in mice [35]. However, Ara-A and related AC inhibitors are not selective for AC5 over AC6, although they show considerable selectivity over other AC isoforms [36,37]. Therefore, any benefits of Ara-A likely arise from inhibition of both AC isoforms. However, this could prove risky as AC6 deletion increases mortality during sustained catecholamine stress [38].

Surprisingly, no polymorphisms that give rise to cardiovascular disease are known to occur in ACs [39]. However, mutations in AC5 are linked to familial dyskinesia with facial myokymia (FDFM), a disease characterized by uncontrolled movement of limb and facial muscles [40,41]. These patients may also have a predisposition to congestive heart failure [41]. Two FDFM mutations occur in a newly appreciated region of AC5, a helical domain that is present immediately after the transmembrane domain and precedes the catalytic cyclase domain (Figure 1). In other nucleotidyl cyclases, this domain forms a tight hairpin to induce an active dimeric conformation of the catalytic domains [42]. Thus, the helical domain may play a role in the stability of the catalytic core or direct regulation of activity.

Roles for additional AC isoforms in cardiac function have been largely overlooked. AC1 was proposed to function as the calcium-stimulated AC in the sinoatrial node that modulates the I(f) pacemaker current [43,44]. However, AC1 knockout mice are not reported to have a heart rate defect and RNA sequencing detects higher expression of AC1 in the right atrium versus the sinoatrial node [45]. Roles for AC2 and/or AC4 are unknown. Currently, a knockout of AC4 is unavailable and AC2 knockout mice display no cardiac phenotype, although RNA for AC2 is elevated in pediatric dilated cardiomyopathy subjects [46]. Cardiac functions for AC9 are discussed below.

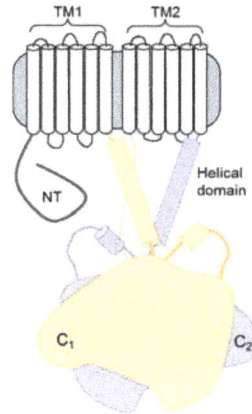

Figure 1. Topology of adenylyl cyclase (AC) isoforms. The structural topology of mammalian membranous ACs consists of an N-terminal (NT) domain followed by a repeating set of transmembrane, helical dimerization, and cytoplasmic domains. The two cytoplasmic domains (C1 and C2) make up the catalytic core and the binding site for many regulatory proteins.

3. The AKAP Connection: Generating Specificity for AC Function

Tissue distribution and regulation provide one mode for how the AC isoforms contribute to distinct physiological functions [8,15]. Another mode of signal specificity comes from the formation of AC macromolecular complexes through the scaffolding family of A-kinase anchoring proteins (AKAPs). AKAPs not only facilitate cellular localization of ACs but they also enhance temporal regulation of cAMP signaling. A number of AKAPs exist in heart including AKAP15/18, AKAP79/150, Yotiao, mAKAP, AKAP-Lbc, and Gravin [47] (Figure 2). In the heart, the spatial and temporal regulation by AKAPs provide an important mechanism to facilitate stress response. The associations of ACs with AKAPs facilitate regulation of PKA, downstream effectors, and ACs. This was shown in the dorsal root ganglion where the activation of the transient receptor potential vanilloid 1 (TRPV1) channel by forskolin or prostaglandin E2 is facilitated by AKAP79-AC5-PKA-TRPV1 complex formation and shifts the response to lower concentrations of forskolin by ~100 fold. Disruption of this complex attenuates sensitization of the channel, as anchoring of both PKA and AC5 were required to elicit the maximal effect on TRPV1 current [48]. Anchoring of PKA and ACs to AKAPs can also regulate AC activity. Association of AC5/6 with AKAP79/150 creates a negative feedback loop where cAMP production is inhibited by PKA phosphorylation of AC5/6 [49]. Although this complex feedback mechanism was defined in the nervous system, modulation of TRPV1 in heart is suggested to influence cardiovascular response to disease and injury [50]. Fine tuning of the signal is important for modulating a number of effectors contributing to physiological function.

AC localization is assessed primarily through functional roles of associated complex members enriched at various cardiomyocytes substructures (Figure 2). Association of both AC5 and AC6 with AKAP5 suggests localization at the t-tubule based upon functional association with calcium-induced calcium release [51]. However, with respect to β adrenergic signaling, AC5 is enriched with β2AR in t-tubules whereas AC6 localizes outside the t-tubule [18,52]. Disruption of cAMP compartmentalization is potentially an underlying mechanism of heart failure [52]. AC9 association with Yotiao and KCNQ1 suggests localization at intercalated discs, the sarcolemma, and t-tubules [53]. These AC–AKAP complexes are discussed below.

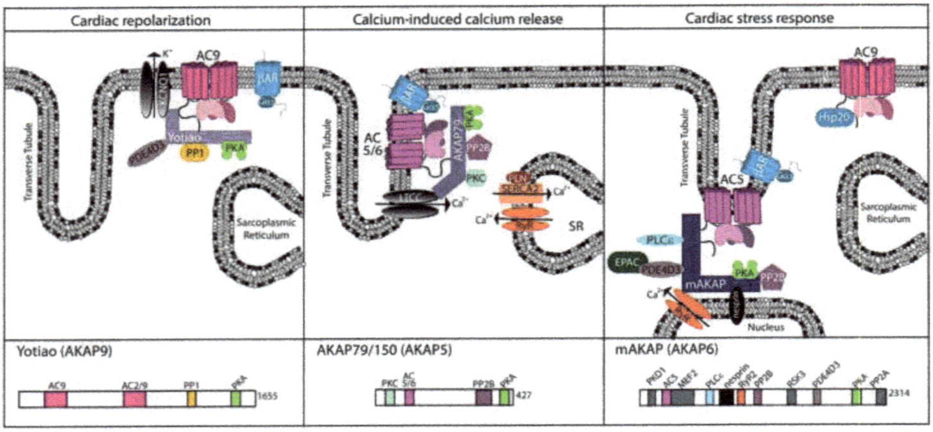

Figure 2. Cardiac AC complexes. AC-associated A-kinase anchoring protein (AKAP) complexes localize to distinct locations within the cardiomyocyte to facilitate physiological function. For each AKAP, a subset of known binding partners and their interaction sites are represented. The model is based upon functional localization of the AC complexes.

3.1. AKAP5

The AKAP5 family of orthologs are named for their size on SDS-PAGE and for different species—for example, human AKAP79, mouse AKAP150, and bovine AKAP75. AKAP79/150 can associate with AC 2, 3, 5, 6, 8, and 9 as evaluated in tissue culture models [49,54]. In heart, AKAP79 primarily interacts with AC5/6 [51]. The interaction site is located on the N-terminus of AC and in the second and third polybasic domain on AKAP79 (aa 77–153). In cells, AKAP79-scaffolded PKA phosphorylates AC5/6 to inhibit cAMP production [49,54]. This feedback loop allows for precisely timed activation and inactivation of the cAMP signal. Although AKAP79-anchored AC5/6 is inhibited by associated PKA, it is unclear how AKAP79 regulates AC2 activity in isolated plasma membranes.

Physiologically, AKAP79/150 has been studied in isolated cardiomyocytes from wild-type and AKAP150 knockouts. Deletion of AKAP150 significantly reduced stimulated calcium transients and calcium sparks in response to isoproterenol. Additionally, phosphorylation of the ryanodine receptor (RyR) and phospholamban (PLN) was eliminated in cardiomyocytes from knockout mice. It was further shown that AKAP150 forms a complex with AC5/6, PKA, protein phosphatase type 2 (PP2B or calcineurin), $Ca_v1.2$, and caveolin 3 (CAV3). This complex is found on t-tubules, while disruption of complex formation upon AKAP150 deletion alters CAV3 and AC6 localization [51].

AKAP150 has additional roles that are independent of AC and PKA. AKAP150 localizes protein kinase C (PKC) and L-type calcium channels to the sub-sarcolemma in atrial myocytes enabling regulation of calcium sparklets [55]. TRPV4 sparklets are also modulated by the AKAP150–PKC complex in a distance-dependent manner; a distance less than 200 nM between the TRPV4 and AKAP150–PKC is ideal for proper regulation [56]. AKAP150 is also implicated in β_1AR recycling. Knockdown or knockout of AKAP150 in isolated myocytes inhibits recycling of β_1AR back to the membrane after isoproterenol stimulation, but not internalization. Isolated $AKAP150^{-/-}$ cardiomyocytes have an enhanced contraction rate in response to isoproterenol and an increased cell size at basal and stimulated conditions. Based on these results it was postulated that AKAP150 is cardioprotective because the hypertrophy phenotype was enhanced in AKAP150$^{-/-}$ [57].

AKAP150 has been examined in a number of pathology models including myocardial infarction and pressure overload. AKAP150$^{-/-}$ mice were subjected to transverse aortic constriction surgery (TAC) to induce pressure overload; AKAP150 expression significantly decreased in conjunction with a significant increase in hypertrophy, fibrosis, and cell death. Physiologically, deletion of AKAP150 increased left ventricular end diastolic size and impaired fractional shortening after TAC compared to sham animals. Physiological changes were mirrored by alterations in calcium signaling, as AKAP150 creates a complex between the PLN, RyR, and the sarcoplasmic endoplasmic reticulum calcium ATPase 2 (SERCA2). Phosphorylation of RyR and PLN in addition to calcium transients were impaired in response to isoproterenol [58]. A model of myocardial infarction (MI) was also examined in AKAP150$^{-/-}$ mice. Alteration in cardiac signaling that occurs after MI is well documented. MI causes an increase in NFATc3 activation and associated K_V channel downregulation. AKAP150$^{-/-}$ cardiomyocytes displayed impaired NFAT translocation in response to phenylephrine, which was dependent on calcineurin activity, preventing downregulation of K_V channel currents [59]. Cardiovascular disease is a co-morbidity associated with diabetes [60]. Unlike the other models, in a model of diabetes mellitus, knockdown of AKAP150 ameliorates glucotoxicity-induced diastolic dysfunction in mice. In rat cardiomyocytes from diabetic animals or treated with high glucose, AKAP150 expression is enhanced combined with increased active PKC at the plasma membrane. This, in turn, promotes activation of NFκB and Nox [61], players in the reactive oxygen species pathway that underlie diabetes-induced cardiovascular injury [60]. Thus, while AKAP150 may play a cardioprotective role in some pathology models, this is not always the case.

3.2. mAKAP (AKAP6)

Anchored to the nuclear envelope, the cardiac splice variant of muscle AKAP (mAKAPβ) interacts with AC5 to facilitate cardiac signaling [62,63]. mAKAP is localized to the nuclear envelope through its interaction with nesprin [64] while much lower levels of mAKAP are found at the sarcoplasmic reticulum (SR) [65]. While mAKAP is intracellularly located primarily at the nuclear envelope and AC5 is membrane-bound, it is thought that localization of AC5 to the t-tubules allows for this interaction due to the close proximity of the nucleus and t-tubules at sites within the cardiomyocyte [66,67]. AC5 interacts with mAKAP through a unique binding site on the N-terminus (245–340). Similar to AKAP79, PKA binding to the mAKAP complex creates a negative feedback loop to inhibit AC5 activity [63].

A number of molecules implicated in hypertrophy are anchored by mAKAP, including protein phosphatases 2A and 2B (PP2A/2B), PDE4D3, hypoxia-inducible factor 1α (HIF1α), phospholipase Cε (PLCε), myocyte enhancer factor-2 (MEF2) [68], and p90 ribosomal S6 kinase 3 (RSK3) [69–73]. Other proteins are associated indirectly with mAKAP complexes, including EPAC1 and the ERK5 and MEK5 mitogen-activated protein kinases via interactions with PDE4D3 [74]. The interaction of mAKAP and the RyR at the SR promotes phosphorylation and enhances calcium release [75], while RyR located within the nucleus promotes hypertrophy as discussed below.

A role for mAKAP in pathological hypertrophy was first described in mAKAP knockdown myocytes [76] and subsequently shown in mAKAP knockout mice where knockout mice subjected to TAC had reduced hypertrophy, cell death, and did not display TAC-inducible gene expression [77]. Further characterization of the mAKAP macromolecular complex highlights how multiple pathways converge on mAKAP to integrate hypertrophic signaling. The cAMP pathway is integrated through AC5–mAKAP–PDE4D3–EPAC binding to utilize and maintain local cAMP pools [63,69,71,74]. Activated calcineurin is recruited to the complex and is required for nuclear translocation of NFAT [78]. PLCε binds to a complex containing mAKAP, EPAC, protein kinase D (PKD), and RyR2 contributing to PKD activity and nuclear calcium levels [72,79].

3.3. Yotiao (AKAP9)

Yotiao is a 250 kDa splice variant of AKAP9 that is present in heart. Yotiao interacts with the alpha subunit (KCNQ1) of the slowly activating delayed rectifier K^+ current (I_{Ks}), a critical component for the late phase repolarization of the cardiac action potential in humans [80]. I_{Ks} is made up of four alpha subunits and accessory beta subunits, KCNE1. Beta-adrenergic control of I_{Ks} by PKA phosphorylation of KCNQ1 increases channel current to shorten the action potential and maintain diastolic intervals in response to an increase in heart rate. Mutations in KCNQ1 are associated with long QT syndrome type 1 (LQT1), a potentially lethal hereditary arrhythmia. Not only do mutations in the KCNQ1 lead to this disease, but mutations within Yotiao (LQT11) and KCNE1 (LQT5) can also give rise to LQT syndrome [81,82]. A subset of these mutations in either Yotiao (S1570L) or KCNQ1 (G589D) disrupts the KCNQ1–Yotiao interaction, resulting in altered regulation of the I_{Ks} channel [81].

Yotiao creates a macromolecular complex between KCNQ1 and important regulators of KCNQ1 phosphorylation. Yotiao scaffolds both positive (PKA) and negative regulators, protein phosphatase 1 (PP1) and phosphodiesterase 4DE3 (PDE4D3), of KCNQ1 phosphorylation [80,83–85]. Loss of this scaffold decreases cAMP-dependent PKA phosphorylation of KCNQ1, eliminates the functional response by I_{Ks}, and prolongs the action potential [85]. Yotiao is the key to maintaining a tightly regulated feedback loop for I_{Ks}-dependent cardiac repolarization and heart rate. Although Yotiao facilitates cardiac repolarization, it cannot overcome channel mutations that alter the capacity for phosphorylation. For example, an A341V mutation in KCNQ1 acts as a dominant negative that reduces basal channel activity and KCNQ1 phosphorylation with no alteration in Yotiao binding [86].

Of the AC isoforms that Yotiao scaffolds (AC 1, 2, 3, and 9) [87], AC9 is the only one present in cardiomyocytes. Unlike the other AKAPs that interact with AC in heart, Yotiao does not scaffold the major cardiac isoforms AC5/6. While Yotiao binds to the N-terminus of AC9, there appear to be multiple sites of interaction of AC9 on Yotiao with the primary site located within the first 808 amino acids and a second, weaker site that overlaps with the AC2 binding site on Yotiao (amino acids 808–956). The interaction of AC9 with Yotiao and KCNQ1 was shown by immunoprecipitation of the complex from cells co-expressing all three proteins, a transgenic mouse line with cardiac expression of KCNQ1–KCNE1, and from guinea pig hearts, which endogenously express the complex. Co-expression of AC9 and Yotiao in CHO cells stably expressing KCNQ1–KCNE1 sensitize PKA phosphorylation of KCNQ1 in response to isoproterenol compared to AC9 or Yotiao expression alone [13]. Yotiao inhibits AC2 and AC3 activity but the mechanism of inhibition is unknown; no inhibition of AC9 activity is observed [87]. Based on these results we would postulate that the AC9–Yotiao–PKA–KCNQ1 macromolecular complex generates a local pool of cAMP that is critical for cardiac repolarization in humans.

4. Newly Appreciated ACs in Heart

4.1. AC9 Knockout Phenotype

An in-depth look at the role of AC9 in cardiomyocytes has long been overlooked. This is likely due to the low level of expression of AC9 in cardiomyocytes, the fact that AC5/6 accounts for nearly all of the total cAMP production [8], and observations from Antoni showing deletion of AC9 through conventional targeting was embryonically lethal [88]. Interaction of AC9 with the Yotiao–I_{Ks} complex sparked renewed interest in examining its role in cardiac physiology [13]. Meanwhile, the Mutant Mouse Regional Resource Center, an NIH funded strain repository, generated a viable AC9 deletion mouse utilizing a gene trapping cassette. Examination of this AC9 deletion strain resulted in two distinct physiological phenotypes, bradycardia and diastolic dysfunction with preserved ejection fraction; no structural abnormalities were observed in AC9$^{-/-}$ mice using echocardiograms [89]. In addition, Yotiao-anchored AC9 activity is present in the sinoatrial node, supporting a role for AC9 in heart rate. These findings, while intriguing, require further validation. Bradycardia measurements were made while under anesthesia, which has reported effects on heart rate; it will be of interest to see whether the bradycardia phenotype is recapitulated in a conscious mouse model [90].

4.2. Complexes and Signaling Alterations in $AC9^{-/-}$ Heart

Deletion of either AC5 or AC6, the major cardiac AC isoforms, results in a significant reduction in total cAMP activity, whereas deletion of AC9 is estimated to contribute to less than three percent of total cardiac membrane AC activity (Gαs stimulated). To try and reveal the low AC9 activity in cardiac membranes from WT and $AC9^{-/-}$ hearts, adenylyl cyclase activity was stimulated with Gαs in the presence of the P-site inhibitor, SQ 22,536, which displays >100 fold selectivity for AC5/6 over AC9 [36,89]. This estimate provides only an upper limit to which AC9 contributes to total AC activity in heart. Although the global contribution of AC9 is negligible, it is required for maintaining local cAMP levels in macromolecular complexes. AC9 can interact with two cardiac AKAPs: AKAP79/150 and Yotiao. Yotiao-associated AC activity, as determined by immunoprecipitation-adenylyl cyclase assay [49,63,87], was completely abolished in AC9 knockout hearts, confirming AC9 as the only cardiac isoform associated with Yotiao [87]. Conversely, local cAMP pools associated with AKAP150 were unchanged in $AC9^{-/-}$; AC5 and AC6 are the largest contributors to the AKAP79/150 local pool [51,54].

Similarly, AC9 deletion has a limited impact on global PKA signaling but is important for targeted downstream signaling in local complexes. Although AC9 association with Yotiao sensitizes I_{Ks} phosphorylation in cells [13], it could not be evaluated in the $AC9^{-/-}$ mouse as adult mice do not express a functional I_{Ks} channel [80,89,91,92]. Nonetheless, AC9 deletion reduces basal phosphorylation of the small heat shock protein 20 (Hsp20). Hsp20 and AC9 interact independently of Yotiao as demonstrated by immunoprecipitation and proximity ligation assays. Disruption of this complex by expression of a catalytically inactive AC9 in rat neonatal cardiomyocytes significantly impaired isoproterenol stimulated phosphorylation of Hsp20 [89]. Taken together, this suggests that cardioprotection is yet another role for AC9, by controlling baseline PKA-mediated phosphorylation of Hsp20. Hsp20's role in cardioprotection is well documented against a variety of insults: prolonged beta-agonist induced hypertrophy, ischemia/reperfusion injury, and doxorubicin cardiotoxicity [93–95]. Although AC9 is a binding partner with Hsp20, it is likely that other ACs also bind Hsp20. Deletion of AC9 reduced Hsp20-associated AC activity by only 30%, indicating that other AC(s) interact with Hsp20 in heart [89].

The deletion of AC9 emphasizes the importance of localized cAMP signaling and complex formation, as AC9 contributes to different aspects of cardiac physiology, despite its very low level of activity in heart. AC9 association with the Yotiao–I_{Ks} complex contributes to cardiac repolarization in humans, while an AC9–Hsp20 complex is potentially important for cardioprotection. Further support for an AC9 cardioprotective role in heart comes from an observed upregulation of the micro RNA that regulates AC9 expression (miR-142-3p) in patients with non-ischemic dilated cardiomyopathy and in mouse models of hypertrophic cardiomyopathy [96–99]. Additional investigations into the role of AC9 regulation of Hsp20 phosphorylation are needed to understand how this complex functions under stress and whether there are other proteins associated with this complex.

4.3. AC9 Regulation

Of the AC isoforms, AC9 is the most divergent in sequence and has been the least studied. Expression analysis shows that AC9 is widely expressed in the central nervous system, heart, and other tissues [100–103]. While the regulatory mechanisms of the other isoforms have been well studied, studies of AC9 regulation have yielded conflicting results. Potential modes of AC9 regulation include stimulation by Gαs, protein kinase C βII (PKCβII) [104], or calcium–calmodulin kinase II (CaMKII) [105] and inhibition by Gαi/o [106], novel PKC isoforms [106], or calcium/calcineurin (CaN) [101]. Determining the regulatory modalities for various AC isoforms is crucial for understanding how the individual isoforms function physiologically. Ideally, the regulation of AC9 would be

J. Cardiovasc. Dev. Dis. **2018**, *5*, 2

examined in biochemical and tissue culture models and then confirmed in cardiomyocytes; however, due to the low levels of expression, examining AC9 regulation will prove difficult in this system.

4.3.1. G-Protein Regulation

Every membrane-bound AC isoform is stimulated by Gαs [8]. Compared to AC6, AC9 has a right-shifted Gαs dose-response curve in Sf9 cells, showing a reduced sensitivity to Gαs (TA Baldwin, unpublished observations). This would potentially impact signaling, where a decreased sensitivity to Gαs would reduce downstream signaling outputs, making AC9 even more dependent on complex formation to facilitate local pools of cAMP. Interestingly, all of the alterations in cardiac physiology observed in AC9$^{-/-}$ mice were at basal levels, suggesting that AC9 may be more important for setting the basal tone in cardiac signaling [89]. However, in cells AC9 requires Yotiao anchoring to sensitize the phosphorylation of KCNQ1 in response to isoproterenol [13], emphasizing again the need for complex-dependent signaling.

The original cloning and characterization of human AC9 examined Gαi/o regulation of AC9 in HEK293 cells but did not detect inhibition of AC9 by endogenously expressed somatostatin receptors [101]. Subsequently, Gαi/o regulation of AC9 was reexamined in HEK293 cells upon transient expression of the dopamine receptor (D2L); cells treated with a D2L selective agonist had a significant reduction in AC activity. Thus, the researchers concluded that Gαi/o could inhibit AC9 [106]. It is unclear whether the discrepancy between these two studies is due to the type of Gαi/o-coupled receptor, receptor preference for Gαi versus Gαo, or background activity of endogenously expressed AC6. Interestingly, AC9 does not contain the important residues that are required for Gαi binding and inhibition of AC5 [107]. Further studies are needed to determine whether Gαi is a direct regulator of AC9.

Gβγ is another common regulator of AC activity, inhibiting AC1, AC3, and AC8 or stimulating AC2, AC4, and AC5–7 [8,15]. AC9 regulation by Gβγ had been postulated based on neutrophil chemotaxis studies but never tested in cells [108]. Gβγ does not regulate basal or Gαs-stimulated AC9 activity when assaying membranes from Sf9 cells overexpressing AC9 (TA Baldwin, unpublished observations). Despite not having a direct regulatory role, Gβγ binds the N-terminus of AC9 [89,109].

4.3.2. Kinase and Phosphatase Regulation

Gq regulation of AC9 through CaMKII and PKC was examined in HEK293 cells expressing AC9 stably with transient transfection of either the muscarinic receptor M_5 or the serotonin receptor $5HT_{2A}$. Treatment of cells with the receptor agonists (M5, carbachol or $5HT_{2A}$, 5HT) potentiated AC9 activity in the presence of isoproterenol; expression of the constitutively active Gαq mutant (Q209L) showed similar results. Co-treatment with receptor agonists and the PKC inhibitor, bisindolylmaleimide, further potentiated activity suggesting that PKC acted as an inhibitor of AC9 activity. The authors also examined potentiation of AC9 activity by calcium/calmodulin (CaM) kinase (CaMK) through the M_5 receptor, by treating cells with carbachol in the presence of a CaM (W-7) or CaMKII (KN-93) inhibitor; both inhibitors reduced AC9 activity. Thus, Gq potentiation of AC activity occurs through activation of CaMKII. However, the authors could not determine whether AC9 is directly phosphorylated by these kinases or whether regulation was via an indirect mechanism [105].

AC9 is also important for neutrophil chemotaxis through activation of AC9 by PKCβII. Neutrophils express high levels of AC9 and have also been used to examine AC9 regulation. Knockdown of AC9 in a neutrophil cell line was shown to inhibit chemotaxis in response to fMLP caused by a decrease in cAMP in extending pseudopods [108]. This mechanism was further dissected to show that PKCβII knockdown recapitulated the AC9 knockdown phenotype. It was proposed that AC9 phosphorylation by PKCβII was the mechanism for increased cAMP in neutrophils leading to chemotaxis [104].

AC9 was originally cloned from a mouse as a calcineurin-inhibited isoform [110]. In HEK293 cells expressing mouse AC9, activity was inhibited by calcium in a concentration-dependent manner but was restored by increasing treatments with the calcineurin inhibitors FK506 or cyclosporin A [100,110]. Subsequent characterizations of human AC9 show conflicting results for calcineurin inhibition [101,102]. The discrepancy is suggested to occur due to differences in variants of AC9 mRNA. Overall, it is unclear whether regulator differences reported for AC9 are due to different expression systems, species differences, or interaction with cell-specific proteins (including AKAPs).

5. Conclusions

Multiple distinct AC complexes exist in heart and are important regulators of cardiac physiology. While great strides have been made to understand the composition and roles of these complexes, there are still many questions left to answer. Pharmacological targeting of AC isoforms has been actively pursued but obtaining isoform specificity is difficult, especially for AC5 and AC6. An alternative and widely considered approach is the targeting of specific protein–protein interactions within the cardiac AC complexes. Targeting components of a complex could provide specificity, unlike pan enzyme inhibitors, as these complexes frequently contain only a small percentage of the total protein in the cell. This was the idea behind disrupting the AC5–mAKAP complex as mAKAP-localized cAMP signaling is involved in cardiac hypertrophy [63]. While disruption of this complex was proposed to have a beneficial effect on hypertrophy, the opposite effect was observed. In cardiomyocytes, disruption of AC5–mAKAP binding leads to cellular hypertrophy through an increase in cAMP levels. As previously discussed, AC5 binding to the mAKAP complex creates multiple feedback loops to inhibit cAMP production. These data show how important the fine-tuning of cAMP signaling is and emphasizes the need for extensive studies when designing AKAP complex disruptors for therapeutic use. Finally, many ACs interact with up and or downstream effectors through AKAP-facilitated interactions. However, there is still the possibility that other AC–AKAP complexes have yet to be identified. Currently, an AKAP is not known to interact with the AC9–Hsp20 complex. Moving forward, the possibility of AC complexes independent of AKAPs should also be considered.

Acknowledgments: This work was supported by NIGMS T32 GM089657 (TAB) and GM60419 (CWD).

Author Contributions: Both authors, T.A.B. and C.W.D., contributed to the writing of this manuscript.

Conflicts of Interest: The authors declare no conflict of interest.

References

1. Antos, C.L.; Frey, N.; Marx, S.O.; Reiken, S.; Gaburjakova, M.; Richardson, J.A.; Marks, A.R.; Olson, E.N. Dilated cardiomyopathy and sudden death resulting from constitutive activation of protein kinase A. *Circ. Res.* **2001**, *89*, 997–1004. [CrossRef] [PubMed]
2. Fink, M.A.; Zakhary, D.R.; Mackey, J.A.; Desnoyer, R.W.; Apperson-Hansen, C.; Damron, D.S.; Bond, M. AKAP-mediated targeting of protein kinase A regulates contractility in cardiac myocytes. *Circ. Res.* **2001**, *88*, 291–297. [CrossRef] [PubMed]
3. Zhang, R.; Zhao, J.; Mandveno, A.; Potter, J.D. Cardiac troponin i phosphorylation increases the rate of cardiac muscle relaxation. *Circ. Res.* **1995**, *76*, 1028–1035. [CrossRef] [PubMed]
4. Alig, J.; Marger, L.; Mesirca, P.; Ehmke, H.; Mangoni, M.E.; Isbrandt, D. Control of heart rate by cAMP sensitivity of hcn channels. *Proc. Natl. Acad. Sci. USA* **2009**, *106*, 12189–12194. [CrossRef] [PubMed]
5. Metrich, M.; Laurent, A.C.; Breckler, M.; Duquesnes, N.; Hmitou, I.; Courillau, D ; Blondeau, J.P.; Crozatier, B.; Lezoualc'h, F.; Morel, E. Epac activation induces histone deacetylase nuclear export via a ras-dependent signalling pathway. *Cell Signal* **2010**, *22*, 1459–1468. [CrossRef] [PubMed]
6. Schindler, R.F.; Brand, T. The popeye domain containing protein family—A novel class of cAMP effectors with important functions in multiple tissues. *Prog. Biophys. Mol. Biol.* **2016**, *120*, 28–36. [CrossRef] [PubMed]
7. Willoughby, D.; Cooper, D.M. Organization and Ca^{2+} regulation of adenylyl cyclases in cAMP microdomains. *Physiol. Rev.* **2007**, *87*, 965–1010. [CrossRef] [PubMed]
8. Sadana, R.; Dessauer, C.W. Physiological roles for g protein-regulated adenylyl cyclase isoforms: Insights from knockout and overexpression studies. *Neurosignals* **2009**, *17*, 5–22. [CrossRef] [PubMed]

9. Ostrom, R.S.; Naugle, J.E.; Hase, M.; Gregorian, C.; Swaney, J.S.; Insel, P.A.; Brunton, L.L.; Meszaros, J.G. Angiotensin ii enhances adenylyl cyclase signaling via Ca^{2+}/calmodulin. Gq-Gs cross-talk regulates collagen production in cardiac fibroblasts. *J. Biol. Chem.* **2003**, *278*, 24461–24468. [CrossRef] [PubMed]

10. Okumura, S.; Kawabe, J.; Yatani, A.; Takagi, G.; Lee, M.C.; Hong, C.; Liu, J.; Takagi, I.; Sadoshima, J.; Vatner, D.E.; et al. Type 5 adenylyl cyclase disruption alters not only sympathetic but also parasympathetic and calcium-mediated cardiac regulation. *Circ. Res.* **2003**, *93*, 364–371. [CrossRef] [PubMed]

11. Iwatsubo, K.; Minamisawa, S.; Tsunematsu, T.; Nakagome, M.; Toya, Y.; Tomlinson, J.E.; Umemura, S.; Scarborough, R.M.; Levy, D.E.; Ishikawa, Y. Direct inhibition of type 5 adenylyl cyclase prevents myocardial apoptosis without functional deterioration. *J. Biol. Chem.* **2004**, *279*, 40938–40945. [CrossRef] [PubMed]

12. Ping, P.; Anzai, T.; Gao, M.; Hammond, H.K. Adenylyl cyclase and g protein receptor kinase expression during development of heart failure. *Am. J. Physiol. Heart Circ. Physiol.* **1997**, *273*, H707–H717. [CrossRef] [PubMed]

13. Li, Y.; Chen, L.; Kass, R.S.; Dessauer, C.W. The A-kinase anchoring protein Yotiao facilitates complex formation between type 9 adenylyl cyclase and the IKs potassium channel in heart. *J. Biol. Chem.* **2012**, *287*, 29815–29824. [CrossRef] [PubMed]

14. Efendiev, R.; Dessauer, C.W. A kinase-anchoring proteins and adenylyl cyclase in cardiovascular physiology and pathology. *J. Cardiovasc. Pharmacol.* **2011**, *58*, 339–344. [CrossRef] [PubMed]

15. Dessauer, C.W.; Watts, V.J.; Ostrom, R.S.; Conti, M.; Dove, S.; Seifert, R. International union of basic and clinical pharmacology. Ci. Structures and small molecule modulators of mammalian adenylyl cyclases. *Pharmacol. Rev.* **2017**, *69*, 93–139. [CrossRef] [PubMed]

16. Scarpace, P.J.; Matheny, M.; Tumer, N. Myocardial adenylyl cyclase type V and Vi mRNA: Differential regulation with age. *J. Cardiovasc. Pharmacol.* **1996**, *27*, 86–90. [CrossRef] [PubMed]

17. Hu, C.L.; Chandra, R.; Ge, H.; Pain, J.; Yan, L.; Babu, G.; Depre, C.; Iwatsubo, K.; Ishikawa, Y.; Sadoshima, J.; et al. Adenylyl cyclase type 5 protein expression during cardiac development and stress. *Am. J. Physiol. Heart Circ. Physiol.* **2009**, *297*, H1776–H1782. [CrossRef] [PubMed]

18. Timofeyev, V.; Myers, R.E.; Kim, H.J.; Woltz, R.L.; Sirish, P.; Heiserman, J.P.; Li, N.; Singapuri, A.; Tang, T.; Yarov-Yarovoy, V.; et al. Adenylyl cyclase subtype-specific compartmentalization: Differential regulation of l-type Ca^{2+} current in ventricular myocytes. *Circ. Res.* **2013**, *112*, 1567–1576. [CrossRef] [PubMed]

19. Okumura, S.; Takagi, G.; Kawabe, J.; Yang, G.; Lee, M.C.; Hong, C.; Liu, J.; Vatner, D.E.; Sadoshima, J.; Vatner, S.F.; et al. Disruption of type 5 adenylyl cyclase gene preserves cardiac function against pressure overload. *Proc. Natl. Acad. Sci. USA* **2003**, *100*, 9986–9990. [CrossRef] [PubMed]

20. Tang, T.; Lai, N.C.; Roth, D.M.; Drumm, J.; Guo, T.; Lee, K.W.; Han, P.L.; Dalton, N.; Gao, M.H. Adenylyl cyclase type V deletion increases basal left ventricular function and reduces left ventricular contractile responsiveness to β-adrenergic stimulation. *Basic Res. Cardiol.* **2006**, *101*, 117–126. [CrossRef] [PubMed]

21. Tang, T.; Gao, M.H.; Lai, N.C.; Firth, A.L.; Takahashi, T.; Guo, T.; Yuan, J.X.; Roth, D.M.; Hammond, H.K. Adenylyl cyclase type 6 deletion decreases left ventricular function via impaired calcium handling. *Circulation* **2008**, *117*, 61–69. [CrossRef] [PubMed]

22. Gao, M.; Ping, P.; Post, S.; Insel, P.A.; Tang, R.; Hammond, H.K. Increased expression of adenylylcyclase type vi proportionately increases beta-adrenergic receptor-stimulated production of cAMP in neonatal rat cardiac myocytes. *Proc. Natl. Acad. Sci. USA* **1998**, *95*, 1038–1043. [CrossRef] [PubMed]

23. Tepe, N.M.; Lorenz, J.N.; Yatani, A.; Dash, R.; Kranias, E.G.; Dorn, G.W., II; Liggett, S.B. Altering the receptor-effector ratio by transgenic overexpression of type V adenylyl cyclase: Enhanced basal catalytic activity and function without increased cardiomyocyte β-adrenergic signalling. *Biochemistry* **1999**, *38*, 16706–16713. [CrossRef] [PubMed]

24. Okumura, S.; Vatner, D.E.; Kurotani, R.; Bai, Y.; Gao, S.; Yuan, Z.; Iwatsubo, K.; Ulucan, C.; Kawabe, J.; Ghosh, K.; et al. Disruption of type 5 adenylyl cyclase enhances desensitization of cyclic adenosine monophosphate signal and increases akt signal with chronic catecholamine stress. *Circulation* **2007**, *116*, 1776–1783. [CrossRef] [PubMed]

25. Yan, L.; Vatner, D.E.; O'Connor, J.P.; Ivessa, A.; Ge, H.; Chen, W.; Hirotani, S.; Ishikawa, Y.; Sadoshima, J.; Vatner, S.F. Type 5 adenylyl cyclase disruption increases longevity and protects against stress. *Cell* **2007**, *130*, 247–258. [CrossRef] [PubMed]

26. Timofeyev, V.; Porter, C.A.; Tuteja, D.; Qiu, H.; Li, N.; Tang, T.; Singapuri, A.; Han, P.L.; Lopez, J.E.; Hammond, H.K.; et al. Disruption of adenylyl cyclase type v does not rescue the phenotype of cardiac-specific overexpression of galphaq protein-induced cardiomyopathy. *Am. J. Physiol. Heart Circ. Physiol.* **2010**, *299*, H1459–H1467. [CrossRef] [PubMed]
27. Lai, N.C.; Tang, T.; Gao, M.H.; Saito, M.; Takahashi, T.; Roth, D.M.; Hammond, H.K. Activation of cardiac adenylyl cyclase expression increases function of the failing ischemic heart in mice. *J. Am. Coll. Cardiol.* **2008**, *51*, 1490–1497. [CrossRef] [PubMed]
28. Roth, D.M.; Bayat, H.; Drumm, J.D.; Gao, M.H.; Swaney, J.S.; Ander, A.; Hammond, H.K. Adenylyl cyclase increases survival in cardiomyopathy. *Circulation* **2002**, *105*, 1989–1994. [CrossRef] [PubMed]
29. Roth, D.M.; Gao, M.H.; Lai, N.C.; Drumm, J.; Dalton, N.; Zhou, J.Y.; Zhu, J.; Entrikin, D.; Hammond, H.K. Cardiac-directed adenylyl cyclase expression improves heart function in murine cardiomyopathy. *Circulation* **1999**, *99*, 3099–3102. [CrossRef] [PubMed]
30. Guellich, A.; Gao, S.; Hong, C.; Yan, L.; Wagner, T.E.; Dhar, S.K.; Ghaleh, B.; Hittinger, L.; Iwatsubo, K.; Ishikawa, Y.; et al. Effects of cardiac overexpression of type 6 adenylyl cyclase affects on the response to chronic pressure overload. *Am. J. Physiol. Heart Circ. Physiol.* **2010**, *299*, H707–H712. [CrossRef] [PubMed]
31. Gao, M.H.; Lai, N.C.; Giamouridis, D.; Kim, Y.C.; Guo, T.; Hammond, H.K. Cardiac-directed expression of a catalytically inactive adenylyl cyclase 6 protects the heart from sustained beta-adrenergic stimulation. *PLoS ONE* **2017**, *12*, e0181282. [CrossRef] [PubMed]
32. Wu, Y.S.; Chen, C.C.; Chien, C.L.; Lai, H.L.; Jiang, S.T.; Chen, Y.C.; Lai, L.P.; Hsiao, W.F.; Chen, W.P.; Chern, Y. The type VI adenylyl cyclase protects cardiomyocytes from β-adrenergic stress by a PKA/STAT3-dependent pathway. *J. Biomed. Sci.* **2017**, *24*, 68. [CrossRef] [PubMed]
33. Hammond, H.K.; Penny, W.F.; Traverse, J.H.; Henry, T.D.; Watkins, M.W.; Yancy, C.W.; Sweis, R.N.; Adler, E.D.; Patel, A.N.; Murray, D.R.; et al. Intracoronary gene transfer of adenylyl cyclase 6 in patients with heart failure: A randomized clinical trial. *JAMA Cardiol.* **2016**, *1*, 163–171. [CrossRef] [PubMed]
34. Tang, M.; Zhang, X.; Li, Y.; Guan, Y.; Ai, X.; Szeto, C.; Nakayama, H.; Zhang, H.; Ge, S.; Molkentin, J.D.; et al. Enhanced basal contractility but reduced excitation-contraction coupling efficiency and β-adrenergic reserve of hearts with increased Cav1.2 activity. *Am. J. Physiol. Heart Circ. Physiol.* **2010**, *299*, H519–H528. [CrossRef] [PubMed]
35. Bravo, C.A.; Vatner, D.E.; Pachon, R.; Zhang, J.; Vatner, S.F. A food and drug administration-approved antiviral agent that inhibits adenylyl cyclase type 5 protects the ischemic heart even when administered after reperfusion. *J. Pharmacol. Exp. Ther.* **2016**, *357*, 331–336. [CrossRef] [PubMed]
36. Brand, C.S.; Hocker, H.J.; Gorfe, A.A.; Cavasotto, C.N.; Dessauer, C.W. Isoform selectivity of adenylyl cyclase inhibitors: Characterization of known and novel compounds. *J. Pharmacol. Exp. Ther.* **2013**, *347*, 265–275. [CrossRef] [PubMed]
37. Braeunig, J.H.; Schweda, F.; Han, P.L.; Seifert, R. Similarly potent inhibition of adenylyl cyclase by p-site inhibitors in hearts from wild type and ac5 knockout mice. *PLoS ONE* **2013**, *8*, e68009. [CrossRef] [PubMed]
38. Tang, T.; Lai, N.C.; Wright, A.T.; Gao, M.H.; Lee, P.; Guo, T.; Tang, R.; McCulloch, A.D.; Hammond, H.K. Adenylyl cyclase 6 deletion increases mortality during sustained β-adrenergic receptor stimulation. *J. Mol. Cell. Cardiol.* **2013**, *60*, 60–67. [CrossRef] [PubMed]
39. Ikoma, E.; Tsunematsu, T.; Nakazawa, I.; Shiwa, T.; Hibi, K.; Ebina, T.; Mochida, Y.; Toya, Y.; Hori, H.; Uchino, K.; et al. Polymorphism of the type 6 adenylyl cyclase gene and cardiac hypertrophy. *J. Cardiovasc. Pharmacol.* **2003**, *42* (Suppl. 1), S27–S32. [CrossRef] [PubMed]
40. Chen, Y.Z.; Friedman, J.R.; Chen, D.H.; Chan, G.C.; Bloss, C.S.; Hisama, F.M.; Topol, S.E.; Carson, A.R.; Pham, P.H.; Bonkowski, E.S.; et al. Gain-of-function adcy5 mutations in familial dyskinesia with facial myokymia. *Ann. Neurol.* **2014**, *75*, 542–549. [CrossRef] [PubMed]
41. Chen, Y.Z.; Matsushita, M.M.; Robertson, P.; Rieder, M.; Girirajan, S.; Antonacci, F.; Lipe, H.; Eichler, E.E.; Nickerson, D.A.; Bird, T.D.; et al. Autosomal dominant familial dyskinesia and facial myokymia: Single exome sequencing identifies a mutation in adenylyl cyclase 5. *Arch. Neurol.* **2012**, *69*, 630–635. [CrossRef] [PubMed]
42. Vercellino, I.; Rezabkova, L.; Olieric, V.; Polyhach, Y.; Weinert, T.; Kammerer, R.A.; Jeschke, G.; Korkhov, V.M. Role of the nucleotidyl cyclase helical domain in catalytically active dimer formation. *Proc. Natl. Acad. Sci. USA* **2017**, *114*, E9821–E9828. [CrossRef] [PubMed]

43. Mattick, P.; Parrington, J.; Odia, E.; Simpson, A.; Collins, T.; Terrar, D. Ca^{2+}-stimulated adenylyl cyclase isoform AC1 is preferentially expressed in guinea-pig sino-atrial node cells and modulates the i(f) pacemaker current. *J. Physiol.* **2007**, *582*, 1195–1203. [CrossRef] [PubMed]

44. Younes, A.; Lyashkov, A.E.; Graham, D.; Sheydina, A.; Volkova, M.V.; Mitsak, M.; Vinogradova, T.M.; Lukyanenko, Y.O.; Li, Y.; Ruknudin, A.M.; et al. Ca(2+) -stimulated basal adenylyl cyclase activity localization in membrane lipid microdomains of cardiac sinoatrial nodal pacemaker cells. *J. Biol. Chem.* **2008**, *283*, 14461–14468. [CrossRef] [PubMed]

45. Vedantham, V.; Galang, G.; Evangelista, M.; Deo, R.C.; Srivastava, D. Rna sequencing of mouse sinoatrial node reveals an upstream regulatory role for islet-1 in cardiac pacemaker cells. *Circ. Res.* **2015**, *116*, 797–803. [CrossRef] [PubMed]

46. Nakano, S.J.; Sucharov, J.; van Dusen, R.; Cecil, M.; Nunley, K.; Wickers, S.; Karimpur-Fard, A.; Stauffer, B.L.; Miyamoto, S.D.; Sucharov, C.C. Cardiac adenylyl cyclase and phosphodiesterase expression profiles vary by age, disease, and chronic phosphodiesterase inhibitor treatment. *J. Card. Fail.* **2017**, *23*, 72–80. [CrossRef] [PubMed]

47. Scott, J.D.; Dessauer, C.W.; Tasken, K. Creating order from chaos: Cellular regulation by kinase anchoring. *Annu. Rev. Pharmacol. Toxicol.* **2013**, *53*, 187–210. [CrossRef] [PubMed]

48. Efendiev, R.; Bavencoffe, A.; Hu, H.; Zhu, M.X.; Dessauer, C.W. Scaffolding by A-kinase anchoring protein enhances functional coupling between adenylyl cyclase and TRPV1 channel. *J. Biol. Chem.* **2013**, *288*, 3929–3937. [CrossRef] [PubMed]

49. Bauman, A.L.; Soughayer, J.; Nguyen, B.T.; Willoughby, D.; Carnegie, G.K.; Wong, W.; Hoshi, N.; Langeberg, L.K.; Cooper, D.M.; Dessauer, C.W.; et al. Dynamic regulation of cAMP synthesis through anchored pka-adenylyl cyclase v/vi complexes. *Mol. Cell* **2006**, *23*, 925–931. [CrossRef] [PubMed]

50. Randhawa, P.K.; Jaggi, A.S. Trpv1 channels in cardiovascular system: A double edged sword? *Int. J. Cardiol.* **2017**, *228*, 103–113. [CrossRef] [PubMed]

51. Nichols, C.B.; Rossow, C.F.; Navedo, M.F.; Westenbroek, R.E.; Catterall, W.A.; Santana, L.F.; McKnight, G.S. Sympathetic stimulation of adult cardiomyocytes requires association of akap5 with a subpopulation of L-type calcium channels. *Circ. Res.* **2010**, *107*, 747–756. [CrossRef] [PubMed]

52. Nikolaev, V.O.; Moshkov, A.; Lyon, A.R.; Miragoli, M.; Novak, P.; Paur, H.; Lohse, M.J.; Korchev, Y.E.; Harding, S.E.; Gorelik, J. β2-adrenergic receptor redistribution in heart failure changes cAMP compartmentation. *Science* **2010**, *327*, 1653–1657. [CrossRef] [PubMed]

53. Kurokawa, J.; Motoike, H.K.; Rao, J.; Kass, R.S. Regulatory actions of the A-kinase anchoring protein yotiao on a heart potassium channel downstream of pka phosphorylation (vol 101, pg 16374, 2004). *Proc. Natl. Acad. Sci. USA* **2004**, *101*, 16374–16378. [CrossRef] [PubMed]

54. Efendiev, R.; Samelson, B.K.; Nguyen, B.T.; Phatarpekar, P.V.; Baameur, F.; Scott, J.D.; Dessauer, C.W. AKAP79 interacts with multiple adenylyl cyclase (Ac) isoforms and scaffolds AC5 and -6 to alpha-amino-3-hydroxyl-5-methyl-4-isoxazole-propionate (AMPA) receptors. *J. Biol. Chem.* **2010**, *285*, 14450–14458. [CrossRef] [PubMed]

55. Navedo, M.F.; Nieves-Cintron, M.; Amberg, G.C.; Yuan, C.; Votaw, V.S.; Lederer, W.J.; McKnight, G.S.; Santana, L.F. Akap150 is required for stuttering persistent Ca^{2+} sparklets and angiotensin ii-induced hypertension. *Circ. Res.* **2008**, *102*, e1–e11. [CrossRef] [PubMed]

56. Tajada, S.; Moreno, C.M.; O'Dwyer, S.; Woods, S.; Sato, D.; Navedo, M.F.; Santana, L.F. Distance constraints on activation of trpv4 channels by akap150-bound pkcalpha in arterial myocytes. *J. Gen. Physiol.* **2017**, *149*, 639–659. [CrossRef] [PubMed]

57. Li, X.; Nooh, M.M.; Bahouth, S.W. Role of AKAP79/150 protein in β1-adrenergic receptor trafficking and signaling in mammalian cells. *J. Biol. Chem.* **2013**, *288*, 33797–33812. [CrossRef] [PubMed]

58. Li, L.; Li, J.; Drum, B.M.; Chen, Y.; Yin, H.; Guo, X.; Luckey, S.W.; Gilbert, M.L.; McKnight, G.S.; Scott, J.D.; et al. Loss of akap150 promotes pathological remodelling and heart failure propensity by disrupting calcium cycling and contractile reserve. *Cardiovasc. Res.* **2017**, *113*, 147–159. [CrossRef] [PubMed]

59. Nieves-Cintron, M.; Hirenallur-Shanthappa, D.; Nygren, P.J.; Hinke, S.A.; Dell'Acqua, M.L.; Langeberg, L.K.; Navedo, M.; Santana, L.F.; Scott, J.D. Akap150 participates in calcineurin/nfat activation during the down-regulation of voltage-gated k(+) currents in ventricular myocytes following myocardial infarction. *Cell Signal* **2016**, *28*, 733–740. [CrossRef] [PubMed]

60. Matheus, A.S.; Tannus, L.R.; Cobas, R.A.; Palma, C.C.; Negrato, C.A.; Gomes, M.B. Impact of diabetes on cardiovascular disease: An update. *Int. J. Hypertens.* **2013**, *2013*. [CrossRef] [PubMed]

61. Zeng, C.; Wang, J.; Li, N.; Shen, M.; Wang, D.; Yu, Q.; Wang, H. Akap150 mobilizes cpkc-dependent cardiac glucotoxicity. *Am. J. Physiol. Endocrinol. Metab.* **2014**, *307*, E384–E397. [CrossRef] [PubMed]

62. Kapiloff, M.S.; Schillace, R.V.; Westphal, A.M.; Scott, J.D. Makap: An A-kinase anchoring protein targeted to the nuclear membrane of differentiated myocytes. *J. Cell Sci.* **1999**, *112*, 2725–2736. [PubMed]

63. Kapiloff, M.S.; Piggott, L.A.; Sadana, R.; Li, J.; Heredia, L.A.; Henson, E.; Efendiev, R.; Dessauer, C.W. An adenylyl cyclase-makapbeta signaling complex regulates cAMP levels in cardiac myocytes. *J. Biol. Chem.* **2009**, *284*, 23540–23546. [CrossRef] [PubMed]

64. Pare, G.C.; Easlick, J.L.; Mislow, J.M.; McNally, E.M.; Kapiloff, M.S. Nesprin-1α contributes to the targeting of makap to the cardiac myocyte nuclear envelope. *Exp. Cell Res.* **2005**, *303*, 388–399. [CrossRef] [PubMed]

65. Ruehr, M.L.; Russell, M.A.; Bond, M. A-kinase anchoring protein targeting of protein kinase A in the heart. *J. Mol. Cell. Cardiol.* **2004**, *37*, 653–665. [CrossRef] [PubMed]

66. Gao, T.; Puri, T.S.; Gerhardstein, B.L.; Chien, A.J.; Green, R.D.; Hosey, M.M. Identification and subcellular localization of the subunits of l-type calcium channels and adenylyl cyclase in cardiac myocytes. *J. Biol. Chem.* **1997**, *272*, 19401–19407. [CrossRef] [PubMed]

67. Escobar, M.; Cardenas, C.; Colavita, K.; Petrenko, N.B.; Franzini-Armstrong, C. Structural evidence for perinuclear calcium microdomains in cardiac myocytes. *J. Mol. Cell. Cardiol.* **2011**, *50*, 451–459. [CrossRef] [PubMed]

68. Vargas, M.A.; Tirnauer, J.S.; Glidden, N.; Kapiloff, M.S.; Dodge-Kafka, K.L. Myocyte enhancer factor 2 (mef2) tethering to muscle selective a-kinase anchoring protein (makap) is necessary for myogenic differentiation. *Cell Signal* **2012**, *24*, 1496–1503. [CrossRef] [PubMed]

69. Dodge, K.L.; Khouangsathiene, S.; Kapiloff, M.S.; Mouton, R.; Hill, E.V.; Houslay, M.D.; Langeberg, L.K.; Scott, J.D. Makap assembles a protein kinase a/pde4 phosphodiesterase cAMP signaling module. *EMBO J.* **2001**, *20*, 1921–1930. [CrossRef] [PubMed]

70. Wong, W.; Goehring, A.S.; Kapiloff, M.S.; Langeberg, L.K.; Scott, J.D. Makap compartmentalizes oxygen-dependent control of HIF-1α. *Sci. Signal* **2008**, *1*, ra18. [CrossRef] [PubMed]

71. Dodge-Kafka, K.L.; Bauman, A.; Mayer, N.; Henson, E.; Heredia, L.; Ahn, J.; McAvoy, T.; Nairn, A.C.; Kapiloff, M.S. cAMP-stimulated protein phosphatase 2a activity associated with muscle a kinase-anchoring protein (makap) signaling complexes inhibits the phosphorylation and activity of the cAMP-specific phosphodiesterase pde4d3. *J. Biol. Chem.* **2010**, *285*, 11078–11086. [CrossRef] [PubMed]

72. Zhang, L.; Malik, S.; Pang, J.; Wang, H.; Park, K.M.; Yule, D.I.; Blaxall, B.C.; Smrcka, A.V. Phospholipase cepsilon hydrolyzes perinuclear phosphatidylinositol 4-phosphate to regulate cardiac hypertrophy. *Cell* **2013**, *153*, 216–227. [CrossRef] [PubMed]

73. Li, J.; Kritzer, M.D.; Michel, J.J.; Le, A.; Thakur, H.; Gayanilo, M.; Passariello, C.L.; Negro, A.; Danial, J.B.; Oskouei, B.; et al. Anchored p90 ribosomal s6 kinase 3 is required for cardiac myocyte hypertrophy. *Circ. Res.* **2013**, *112*, 128–139. [CrossRef] [PubMed]

74. Dodge-Kafka, K.L.; Soughayer, J.; Pare, G.C.; Carlisle Michel, J.J.; Langeberg, L.K.; Kapiloff, M.S.; Scott, J.D. The protein kinase A anchoring protein makap coordinates two integrated cAMP effector pathways. *Nature* **2005**, *437*, 574–578. [CrossRef] [PubMed]

75. Ruehr, M.L.; Russell, M.A.; Ferguson, D.G.; Bhat, M.; Ma, J.J.; Damron, D.S.; Scott, J.D.; Bond, M. Targeting of protein kinase A by muscle a kinase-anchoring protein (makap) regulates phosphorylation and function of the skeletal muscle ryanodine receptor. *J. Biol. Chem.* **2003**, *278*, 24831–24836. [CrossRef] [PubMed]

76. Pare, G.C.; Bauman, A.L.; McHenry, M.; Michel, J.J.; Dodge-Kafka, K.L.; Kapiloff, M.S. The makap complex participates in the induction of cardiac myocyte hypertrophy by adrenergic receptor signaling. *J. Cell Sci.* **2005**, *118*, 5637–5646. [CrossRef] [PubMed]

77. Kritzer, M.D.; Li, J.; Passariello, C.L.; Gayanilo, M.; Thakur, H.; Dayan, J.; Dodge-Kafka, K.; Kapiloff, M.S. The scaffold protein muscle A-kinase anchoring protein beta orchestrates cardiac myocyte hypertrophic signaling required for the development of heart failure. *Circ. Heart Fail.* **2014**, *7*, 663–672. [CrossRef] [PubMed]

78. Li, J.; Negro, A.; Lopez, J.; Bauman, A.L.; Henson, E.; Dodge-Kafka, K.; Kapiloff, M.S. The makapbeta scaffold regulates cardiac myocyte hypertrophy via recruitment of activated calcineurin. *J. Mol. Cell. Cardiol.* **2010**, *48*, 387–394. [CrossRef] [PubMed]

79. Zhang, L.; Malik, S.; Kelley, G.G.; Kapiloff, M.S.; Smrcka, A.V. Phospholipase c epsilon scaffolds to muscle-specific a kinase anchoring protein (makapbeta) and integrates multiple hypertrophic stimuli in cardiac myocytes. *J. Biol. Chem.* **2011**, *286*, 23012–23021. [CrossRef] [PubMed]

80. Marx, S.O.; Kurokawa, J.; Reiken, S.; Motoike, H.; D'Armiento, J.; Marks, A.R.; Kass, R.S. Requirement of a macromolecular signaling complex for β adrenergic receptor modulation of the KCNQ1-KCNE1 potassium channel. *Science* **2002**, *295*, 496–499. [CrossRef] [PubMed]

81. Chen, L.; Marquardt, M.L.; Tester, D.J.; Sampson, K.J.; Ackerman, M.J.; Kass, R.S. Mutation of an A-kinase-anchoring protein causes long-QT syndrome. *Proc. Natl. Acad. Sci. USA* **2007**, *104*, 20990–20995. [CrossRef] [PubMed]

82. Duggal, P.; Vesely, M.R.; Wattanasirichaigoon, D.; Villafane, J.; Kaushik, V.; Beggs, A.H. Mutation of the gene for isk associated with both jervell and lange-nielsen and romano-ward forms of long-QT syndrome. *Circulation* **1998**, *97*, 142–146. [CrossRef] [PubMed]

83. Westphal, R.S.; Tavalin, S.J.; Lin, J.W.; Alto, N.M.; Fraser, I.D.; Langeberg, L.K.; Sheng, M.; Scott, J.D. Regulation of NMDA receptors by an associated phosphatase-kinase signaling complex. *Science* **1999**, *285*, 93–96. [CrossRef] [PubMed]

84. Lin, J.W.; Wyszynski, M.; Madhavan, R.; Sealock, R.; Kim, J.U.; Sheng, M. Yotiao, a novel protein of neuromuscular junction and brain that interacts with specific splice variants of NMDA receptor subunit nr1. *J. Neurosci.* **1998**, *18*, 2017–2027. [PubMed]

85. Terrenoire, C.; Houslay, M.D.; Baillie, G.S.; Kass, R.S. The cardiac IKs potassium channel macromolecular complex includes the phosphodiesterase PDE4D3. *J. Biol. Chem.* **2009**, *284*, 9140–9146. [CrossRef] [PubMed]

86. Heijman, J.; Spatjens, R.L.; Seyen, S.R.; Lentink, V.; Kuijpers, H.J.; Boulet, I.R.; de Windt, L.J.; David, M.; Volders, P.G. Dominant-negative control of cAMP-dependent IKs upregulation in human long-QT syndrome type 1. *Circ. Res.* **2012**, *110*, 211–219. [CrossRef] [PubMed]

87. Piggott, L.A.; Bauman, A.L.; Scott, J.D.; Dessauer, C.W. The A-kinase anchoring protein Yotiao binds and regulates adenylyl cyclase in brain. *Proc. Natl. Acad. Sci. USA* **2008**, *105*, 13835–13840. [CrossRef] [PubMed]

88. Antoni, F.A. Adenylyl cyclase type 9. *UCSD Nat. Mol. Pages* **2006**. [CrossRef]

89. Li, Y.; Baldwin, T.A.; Wang, Y.; Subramaniam, J.; Carbajal, A.G.; Brand, C.S.; Cunha, S.R.; Dessauer, C.W. Loss of type 9 adenylyl cyclase triggers reduced phosphorylation of hsp20 and diastolic dysfunction. *Sci. Rep.* **2017**, *7*, 5522. [CrossRef] [PubMed]

90. Ho, D.; Zhao, X.; Gao, S.; Hong, C.; Vatner, D.E.; Vatner, S.F. Heart rate and electrocardiography monitoring in mice. *Curr. Protoc. Mouse Biol.* **2011**, *1*, 123–139. [PubMed]

91. Honore, E.; Attali, B.; Romey, G.; Heurteaux, C.; Ricard, P.; Lesage, F.; Lazdunski, M.; Barhanin, J. Cloning, expression, pharmacology and regulation of a delayed rectifier k+ channel in mouse heart. *EMBO J.* **1991**, *10*, 2805–2811. [PubMed]

92. Salama, G.; Baker, L.; Wolk, R.; Barhanin, J.; London, B. Arrhythmia phenotype in mouse models of human long QT. *J. Interv. Card. Electrophysiol.* **2009**, *24*, 77–87. [CrossRef] [PubMed]

93. Fan, G.C.; Yuan, Q.; Song, G.; Wang, Y.; Chen, G.; Qian, J.; Zhou, X.; Lee, Y.J.; Ashraf, M.; Kranias, E.G. Small heat-shock protein hsp20 attenuates β-agonist-mediated cardiac remodeling through apoptosis signal-regulating kinase 1. *Circ. Res.* **2006**, *99*, 1233–1242. [CrossRef] [PubMed]

94. Fan, G.C.; Zhou, X.; Wang, X.; Song, G.; Qian, J.; Nicolaou, P.; Chen, G.; Ren, X.; Kranias, E.G. Heat shock protein 20 interacting with phosphorylated akt reduces doxorubicin-triggered oxidative stress and cardiotoxicity. *Circ. Res.* **2008**, *103*, 1270–1279. [CrossRef] [PubMed]

95. Martin, T.P.; Hortigon-Vinagre, M.P.; Findlay, J.E.; Elliott, C.; Currie, S.; Baillie, G.S. Targeted disruption of the heat shock protein 20-phosphodiesterase 4D (PDE4D) interaction protects against pathological cardiac remodelling in a mouse model of hypertrophy. *FEBS Open Bio* **2014**, *4*, 923–927. [CrossRef] [PubMed]

96. Baskerville, S.; Bartel, D.P. Microarray profiling of micrornas reveals frequent coexpression with neighboring mirnas and host genes. *RNA* **2005**, *11*, 241–247. [CrossRef] [PubMed]

97. Voellenkle, C.; van Rooij, J.; Cappuzzello, C.; Greco, S.; Arcelli, D.; Di Vito, L.; Melillo, G.; Rigolini, R.; Costa, E.; Crea, F.; et al. Microrna signatures in peripheral blood mononuclear cells of chronic heart failure patients. *Physiol. Genom.* **2010**, *42*, 420–426. [CrossRef] [PubMed]

98. Bagnall, R.D.; Tsoutsman, T.; Shephard, R.E.; Ritchie, W.; Semsarian, C. Global microrna profiling of the mouse ventricles during development of severe hypertrophic cardiomyopathy and heart failure. *PLoS ONE* **2012**, *7*, e44744. [CrossRef] [PubMed]

99. Tijsen, A.J.; Pinto, Y.M.; Creemers, E.E. Circulating micrornas as diagnostic biomarkers for cardiovascular diseases. *Am. J. Physiol. Heart Circ. Physiol.* **2012**, *303*, H1085–H1095. [CrossRef] [PubMed]

100. Antoni, F.A.; Barnard, R.J.O.; Shipston, M.J.; Smith, S.M.; Simpson, J.; Paterson, J.M. Calcineurin feedback inhibition of agonist-evoked cAMP formation. *J. Biol. Chem.* **1995**, *270*, 28055–28061. [PubMed]

101. Hacker, B.M.; Tomlinson, J.E.; Wayman, G.A.; Sultana, R.; Chan, G.; Villacres, E.; Disteche, C.; Storm, D.R. Cloning, chromosomal mapping, and regulatory properties of the human type 9 adenylyl cyclase (ADCY9). *Genomics* **1998**, *50*, 97–104. [CrossRef] [PubMed]

102. Paterson, J.M.; Smith, S.M.; Simpson, J.; Grace, O.C.; Sosunov, A.A.; Bell, J.E.; Antoni, F.A. Characterisation of human adenylyl cyclase ix reveals inhibition by Ca^{2+}/calcineurin and differential mRNA plyadenylation. *J. Neurochem.* **2000**, *75*, 1358–1367. [CrossRef] [PubMed]

103. Sosunov, S.A.; Kemaikin, S.P.; Kurnikova, I.A.; Antoni, F.A.; Sosunov, A.A. Expression of adenylyl cyclase type ix and calcineurin in synapses of the central nervous system. *Bull. Exp. Biol. Med.* **2001**, *131*, 172–175. [CrossRef] [PubMed]

104. Liu, L.; Gritz, D.; Parent, C.A. PkcβII acts downstream of chemoattractant receptors and MTORC2 to regulate cAMP production and myosin ii activity in neutrophils. *Mol. Biol. Cell.* **2014**, *25*, 1446–1457. [CrossRef] [PubMed]

105. Cumbay, M.G.; Watts, V.J. Galphaq potentiation of adenylate cyclase type 9 activity through a Ca^{2+}/calmodulin-dependent pathway. *Biochem. Pharmacol.* **2005**, *69*, 1247–1256. [CrossRef] [PubMed]

106. Cumbay, M.G.; Watts, V.J. Novel regulatory properties of human type 9 adenylate cyclase. *J. Pharmacol. Exp. Ther.* **2004**, *310*, 108–115. [CrossRef] [PubMed]

107. Dessauer, C.W.; Tesmer, J.J.; Sprang, S.R.; Gilman, A.G. Identification of a gialpha binding site on type v adenylyl cyclase. *J. Biol. Chem.* **1998**, *273*, 25831–25839. [CrossRef] [PubMed]

108. Liu, L.; Das, S.; Losert, W.; Parent, C.A. mTORC2 regulates neutrophil chemotaxis in a cAMP- and RhoA-dependent fashion. *Dev. Cell* **2010**, *19*, 845–857. [CrossRef] [PubMed]

109. Brand, C.S.; Sadana, R.; Malik, S.; Smrcka, A.V.; Dessauer, C.W. Adenylyl cyclase 5 regulation by gbetagamma involves isoform-specific use of multiple interaction sites. *Mol. Pharmacol.* **2015**, *88*, 758–767. [CrossRef] [PubMed]

110. Paterson, J.M.; Smith, S.M.; Harmar, A.J.; Antoni, F.A. Control of a novel adenylyl cyclase by calcineurin. *Biochem. Biophys. Res. Commun.* **1995**, *214*, 1000–1008. [CrossRef] [PubMed]

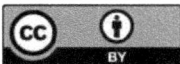

Journal of
Cardiovascular
Development and Disease

MDPI

Review

Functional Significance of the Adcy10-Dependent Intracellular cAMP Compartments

Sofya Pozdniakova [1,2,*] and Yury Ladilov [1,2]

[1] Institute of Gender in Medicine, Center for Cardiovascular Research, Charite, 10115 Berlin, Germany; yury.ladilov@charite.de

[2] DZHK (German Center for Cardiovascular Research), Berlin Partner Site, 10115 Berlin, Germany

* Correspondence: sofyapozdniakova@gmail.com

Received: 5 March 2018; Accepted: 9 May 2018; Published: 11 May 2018

Abstract: Mounting evidence confirms the compartmentalized structure of evolutionarily conserved $3'$–$5'$-cyclic adenosine monophosphate (cAMP) signaling, which allows for simultaneous participation in a wide variety of physiological functions and ensures specificity, selectivity and signal strength. One important player in cAMP signaling is soluble adenylyl cyclase (sAC). The intracellular localization of sAC allows for the formation of unique intracellular cAMP microdomains that control various physiological and pathological processes. This review is focused on the functional role of sAC-produced cAMP. In particular, we examine the role of sAC-cAMP in different cellular compartments, such as cytosol, nucleus and mitochondria.

Keywords: adcy10; cAMP; phosphodiesterase; compartmentalization

---

1. Introduction

Even though $3'$–$5'$-cyclic adenosine monophosphate (cAMP) was discovered more than half a century ago, it still remains an object of scientific interest. cAMP signaling plays an important role in a wide variety of physiological processes: transcription regulation [1,2], metabolism [3,4], cell migration [5,6], mitochondrial homeostasis [7–11] (reviewed in Reference [12]), as well as cell proliferation [13] (reviewed in Reference [14]) and cell death [15] (reviewed in Reference [16]). The importance of cAMP signaling is underlined by the fact that this pathway is evolutionarily conserved and can be found in all species from microorganisms to mammals [17–19].

There are two main sources of cAMP in the cell: Transmembrane (tmAC) and intracellularly localized soluble adenylyl cyclases (sAC). In mammalian cells, nine genes encode tmAC and one gene encodes sAC. The structural organization of tmAC is common for all members of this subfamily (9 tmAC) and the activity of tmAC is controlled by hormones and neurotransmitters [20,21]. Two important properties characterize the principal difference between tmAC and sAC: First, Gs, Gi, Gαi/o, Gßγ and Gq proteins regulate tmAC activity [22,23], whereas sAC activity is regulated by bicarbonate [24]; second, tmAC's localization is restricted to the plasma membrane, while sAC is widely distributed within the cell and organelles [25]. The distinct spatial distribution of the two main cAMP sources leads to the formation of multiple intracellular cAMP compartments, thereby enabling the specificity and selectivity of cAMP signaling.

The specificity of cAMP signaling is further achieved through the restriction of cAMP diffusion due to physical barriers, i.e., mitochondria [26], and phosphodiesterases (PDEs) [27–29]. Therefore, with the exception of a rare internalization of tmAC [30], cAMP produced by tmAC under physiological conditions is mainly localized close to the plasma membrane. In contrast, sAC builds cAMP pools within various cellular compartments, e.g., cytosol, mitochondria, nucleus or the subplasmalemmal compartment [31–33]. In this review, we focus on sAC-dependent cAMP signaling, with a particular focus on its role in mitochondrial biology.

2. Structure and Regulation of sAC Activity

2.1. Structure

Mammalian sAC shows structural and functional similarities with cyanobacterial sAC [24], which argues for a bacterial origin of mammalian sAC that has been strongly conserved throughout the process of evolution [34]. The structure of the sAC catalytic core has a typical Class III pseudo-heterodimer arrangement of structurally similar C_1 (residues 34–219) and C_2 (residues 288–463) domains positioned at the N-terminus and connected by a linker [35]. The C-terminal region of sAC starts with a small motive, mediating auto-inhibitory effect [36], that most likely acts together with the neighboring putative NTPase domain [37]. Additionally, the C-terminal region contains a heme-binding domain that can bind nitric oxide (NO), carbon monoxide, and other potential gaseous signaling molecules [38]. Active cyclase is a heterodimer of two catalytic domains [19]. sAC is encoded by a single functional sAC gene in the human genome (*ADCY10*), comprising of 33 exons covering approximately 104 kb of genomic DNA [39,40]. sAC mRNA undergoes extensive alternative splicing which leads to smaller splice variants [41]. In mammalian cells the predominant isoform is a 50 kDa truncated sAC (sAC_t) which is categorized as a splice variant of the full-length enzyme. sAC_t is restricted to the N-terminal part of the full-length protein covering C_1 and C_2 [42]. sAC_t shows a higher activity than the full-length enzyme, as the activity of the latter is suppressed by the small auto-inhibitory module at the C-terminal [36]. More splice sAC variants have also been identified in human somatic tissue. These isoforms predominantly consist of C_2 domain and require a partner protein to become active due to a missing or incomplete C_1 domain [19,43].

2.2. Posttranslational Regulation of sAC

sAC is insensitive to heterotrimeric G-protein regulation due to a missing or modified $G_{s\alpha}$ and $G_{\beta\gamma}$ binding region, which is important for the activation of tmAC [44]. A recent study performed by Hebert-Chatelain et al., however, challenged this paradigm of sAC insensitivity to G proteins. The authors demonstrated that the activation of mitochondrial $G_{\alpha i}$ proteins through cannabinoid receptors inhibits mitochondrial sAC [45]. However, the authors investigated the role of sAC applying the sAC inhibitor KH7, which may have also led to sAC-independent effects on the mitochondria [9,46]. The results could also be explained by an indirect downregulation of sAC activity.

sAC activity requires divalent metal cations in the catalytic active site of the enzyme in order to coordinate the binding and cyclizing of ATP. sAC is most active in the presence of Mn^{2+}, however it is not clear whether the physiological intracellular Mn^{2+} concentration would support sAC activity [47]. Mg^{2+} and Ca^{2+} concentrations within the expected intracellular range 1–10 mmol/L for Mg^{2+} and 2–1200 nmol/L for Ca^{2+} make significant contributions to the regulation of sAC activity [43]. Furthermore, sAC serves as an intracellular ATP sensor because its activity is dependent on physiological changes in ATP concentrations. When the ATP level is reduced, sAC shows decreased activity due to substrate limitation [48].

A unique property of sAC is its activation through bicarbonate binding, which makes sAC the only protein with enzymatic activity regulated by bicarbonate. Bicarbonate directly binds to and activates sAC in a pH-independent manner [24]. The EC_{50} for the bicarbonate stimulation of mammalian sAC is within the 10–25 mmol/L range, which is appropriate for sensing physiological bicarbonate levels of 2–25 mmol/L [24]. It is also worth mentioning that sAC activity increases synergistically in the presence of bicarbonate and Ca^{2+} [43,49].

2.3. Pharmacological Regulation of sAC

sAC is involved in a wide variety of physiological processes, including metabolism, proliferation, apoptosis, differentiation, migration development, ion transport, pH regulation and gene expression (reviewed in [16,47]). It is also involved in different pathologies such as hyperproliferative skin disease, hypercalciuria, type 2 diabetes glaucoma and prostate cancer [40,50–55]. Therefore, the pharmacological inhibition or activation of sAC may be considered for the treatment of the pathologies and the maintenance of the physiological processes mentioned above. Although the search for potential sAC activators remains unsuccessful, several inhibitors have been discovered. Catechol estrogens (CEs) are physiologically occurring steroid derivatives that can inhibit mammalian AC enzymes. 2-hydroxy estradiol (2-CE) and 4-hydroxy estradiol (4-CE) inhibit purified mammalian sAC (IC$_{50}$ 2–8 µmol/L) as well as some purified tmAC isoforms with comparable potency [44,56]. CEs are postulated to be non-competitive inhibitors of AC that bind to a pocket near the enzyme's active site [57].

Another potent sAC inhibitor is (E)-2-(1H-Benzo[d]imidazol-2-ylthio)-N'-(5-bromo-2-hydroxybenzylidene) propanehydrazide (KH7) (IC$_{50}$~3 µmol/L) [58]. KH7 shows good membrane permeability and has no significant effect on tmACs, GC or PDEs up to a concentration of 100 µmol/L [56]. KH7 has been used as a pharmacological tool in a large number of studies and seems to be a promising compound for drug development. Unfortunately, KH7 exhibits an intrinsic fluorescence and is therefore of limited use when studies involve fluorescence-based live cell cAMP sensors, according to our own observations and research [9]. In addition, KH7 leads to mitochondrial uncoupling in a sAC-independent manner [9,46]. Therefore, KH7 use should be restricted to short-term assays and the results should be interpreted carefully.

Recently, LRE1—an improved sAC-specific inhibitor—has been identified [46]. LRE1 inhibits sAC by occupying the bicarbonate binding site. LRE1 neither exhibits cell toxicity nor results in uncoupling of isolated brain mitochondria [46]. In our experiments, we have not observed any interference between LRE1 and fluorescence, which allows the compound to be used in live cell imaging.

3. Functional Role of sAC in Different Cellular Compartments

sAC-generated cAMP is involved in the regulation of multiple cellular functions as it is generated locally within particular microdomains containing cAMP effectors (PKA, EPAC, cyclic nucleotide-gated ion channels and Popeye domain-containing proteins [59–62]), scaffolding proteins (A-kinase anchoring proteins, AKAPs) and a subset of PDEs, that degrade cAMP, and thus suppress cAMP diffusion [28,29,63]. AKAPs form the complexes of cAMP and its downstream targets, and bind these complexes to particular subcellular compartments [22]. Tight spatiotemporal regulation of cAMP dynamics inside discrete signaling compartments provides specific responses to diverse stimuli at certain locations and avoids unregulated cross-communication between microdomains.

Mammalian sAC is distributed over different compartments throughout the cell: the cytosol, nucleus, plasma membrane and mitochondria [25,64–68]. Although numerous cellular functions have been attributed to the activity of sAC, the functional significance of sAC in particular compartments is still in need of clarification. Therefore, in this review, the functional significance of different sAC domains will be described according to the sAC subcellular localization (Figure 1).

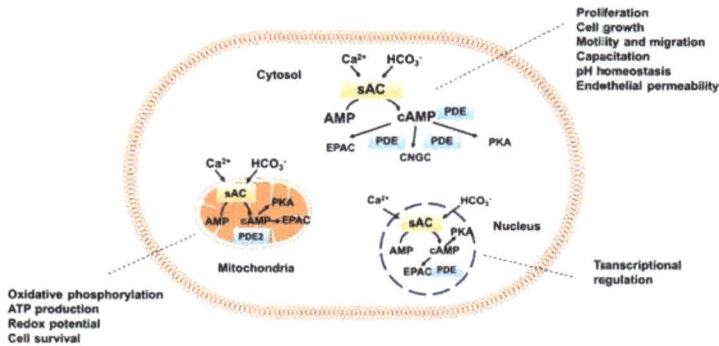

Figure 1. Intracellular distribution of sAC-dependent cAMP pool. sAC, soluble adenylyl cyclase; PKA, protein kinase A, EPAC, exchange protein directly activated by cAMP; CNGC, cyclic nucleotide gated channels; PDE, phosphodiesterase.

3.1. Role of sAC-Dependent cAMP Signaling in Microtubules and Centrioles

It has been suggested that sAC both co-localizes with microtubules and centrioles, while also playing a role in mitosis and cytokinesis [25]. During prophase, sAC is dispersed from the nucleus. In metaphase and anaphase, it accumulates at the mitotic poles and spindle fibers. During cytokinesis, sAC is localized in the midbody. In the centrioles, the main pathway that promotes the phosphorylation cascade is PKA-dependent, whereas in the microtubules it is EPAC-dependent [25].

3.2. Role of Cytosolic/Nuclear sAC-Dependent cAMP Signaling

3.2.1. Proliferation and Cell Growth

Cytosolic sAC makes a significant contribution to the regulation of cell growth, particularly in hyperplasia [16]. In prostate carcinoma tissue and cells (LNCaP, PC3), sAC was shown to be overexpressed and the suppression of sAC activity significantly reduced the proliferation rate [53]. A subsequent analysis of the underlying cellular mechanisms revealed the role of the EPAC/Rap1/B-Raf axis in the sAC-dependent regulation of cell growth. Inhibiting sAC down regulates cyclin B_1 and cyclin-dependent kinase 1, which are the key proteins involved in the G2/M transition. Thus, sAC suppression causes cell cycle arrest in the G2 phase [53]. In another tumor cell line (PC12), nerve growth factor stimulation via sAC was shown to induce cAMP elevation, which, in turn, promoted the activation of Rap1 [69]. This mechanism is considered to be implicated in the process of brain-derived neurotrophic factor-mediated axonal guidance. A study performed in breast cancer cells postulated that sAC in the EPAC-Rap1 dependent mechanism is involved in a metabolic switch, thereby favoring the development of malignant progression [70].

sAC also plays a role in non-proliferative cell growth, i.e., hypertrophy. It is expressed in embryonic neurons and generates cAMP in response to netrin-1, a member of the laminin-related secreted proteins family, thus affecting axon outgrowth [71]. Moreover, retinal ganglion cell survival and axon growth is regulated by Ca^{2+}-dependent cAMP-PKA signaling [64]. Our recent study revealed a novel role for sAC in cardiac hypertrophy induced by either β-adrenergic stimulation or pressure overload [72]. B-Raf's involvement in sAC-dependent hypertrophy was also demonstrated in that study.

3.2.2. Motility

sAC plays a central role in sperm physiology [58,73]. During one of the first definable events in capacitation, Ca^{2+} and bicarbonate enter into sperm and activate sAC to produce cAMP. This promotes an asymmetrical flagellar beat frequency and results in vigorous forward sperm motility [47]. In keeping with this role of sAC in sperm motility, male sAC knockout mice show an infertility phenotype [74]. Though sAC's role in cell motility was initially exclusively considered for sperm, a recent report suggested that sAC is also involved in the regulation of leukocyte trans-endothelial migration through the CD99 [75]. CD99 and sAC are co-localized in a signaling complex with ezrin and PKA. The stimulation of CD99 promotes the sAC-PKA pathway that activates membrane trafficking from the lateral border recycling compartment to sites of trans-endothelial migration, facilitating the passage of leukocytes across the endothelium [75].

3.2.3. pH Homeostasis

sAC plays an important role in the regulation of pH homeostasis [76,77]. In epididymal clear cells and in kidney intercalated cells, sAC-produced cAMP promotes the translocation of the vacuolar proton pumping ATPase (V-ATPase) to the acid-secreting surface in a PKA-dependent manner [78,79]. The apical translocation of V-ATPase, associated with the protein activation, plays an important role in the regulation of pH homeostasis and extracellular acidification/alkalinization. The maintenance of acid/base balance is important for the regulation of acids in the body. V-ATPase dysfunction is one of the factor that leads to renal distal tubular acidosis, the formation of kidney stones and proteinuria [80].

Recently, sAC's control of the endosomal-lysosomal acidification has been shown to function in a PKA-dependent manner. The absence of sAC disrupts V-ATPase localization at the lysosomal membrane which is rescued by treatment with membrane-permeable cAMP [81]. It is interesting to note that a disturbance in lysosomal acidification through sAC knockout leads to an impaired autophagic degradative system.

3.2.4. Transcriptional Regulation

An increasing number of reports argue for the essential role of sAC in regulating the transcriptional activity of the cell. Indeed, sAC has been identified as a unique source of cAMP in the nucleus that in PKA-dependent manner regulates CREB activity [68]. sAC, in a PKA-dependent manner, is especially involved in corticotropin-releasing hormone-mediated CREB phosphorylation and c-fos (endogenous CREB target) induction in hippocampal neuronal cells [82]. A recent study demonstrated that sAC contributes to the regulation of CREB-mediated Na^+/K^+-ATPase expression in the vascular endothelium and is an important regulator of endothelial stiffness [83,84]. Besides promoting CREB activity, sAC also regulates several other transcription factors. For example, sAC supports hypercapnia-accelerated adipogenesis via the activation of pro-adipogenic transcription factors, such as CREB, CCAAT/enhancer binding protein ß and proliferator-activated receptor γ [85]. Similarly, sAC-PKA-dependent phosphorylation, and thus the activation of transcription factor 4, is required for brain development [86].

3.2.5. CFTR Regulation

The Cystic Fibrosis Transmembrane Conductance Regulator (CFTR) is a chloride channel, primarily localized in the apical membrane of secretory epithelial cells. Mutations in the CFTR lead to the development of cystic fibrosis [87]. In cultured human airway epithelial cells, it has been found that sAC, activated by bicarbonate, modulates CFTR function in a PKA-dependent manner. The inhibition of sAC attenuated bicarbonate-stimulated CFTR activity [88]. Further studies have demonstrated that CFTR is involved in bicarbonate entry into granulosa cells, which further promotes the nuclear cAMP-PKA-CREB axis [89]. CFTR is involved in triggering sperm capacitation, as CFTR promotes bicarbonate secretion by the endometrium [90] which, in turn, activates sAC in sperm, increases cAMP production, and then activates PKA and the cyclic nucleotide gate cation channels [91,92]. Moreover, CFTR via the sAC-cAMP-PKA pathway has been shown to promote embryo development through the suppression of p53-dependent development arrest [93]. Taken together, the CFTR-sAC axis seems to play an important role in reproductive processes [94].

3.2.6. Na$^+$/K$^+$-ATPas Endocytosis

In alveolar epithelial cells, a high CO_2 concentration promotes the sAC-cAMP axis, which in turn induces a PKA-dependent phosphorylation of α-adducin, a component of the actin cytoskeleton, resulting in Na$^+$/K$^+$-ATPase endocytosis [95]. In the vascular endothelium, the role that the sAC-cAMP axis plays in Na$^+$/K$^+$-ATPase regulation has been demonstrated, as the inhibition of sAC (KH7 and interfering RNA) significantly decreases the mRNA and protein levels of Na$^+$/K$^+$-ATPase [84]. A recent study confirmed that the sAC-dependent regulation of Na$^+$/K$^+$-ATPase in the vascular endothelium plays an important role in endothelial stiffness [83].

3.2.7. Endothelial Permeability

The importance of the intracellular distribution of cAMP for endothelial barrier function has been demonstrated, because the stimulation of plasma membrane and cytosolic cAMP pools exerts the opposite effects [96,97].

A recent study suggested that sAC has a protective effect on endothelial barrier function under inflammatory and hypoxic conditions [98]. In this study, the bicarbonate-mediated activation of sAC elevated cellular cAMP levels was followed by PKA and EPAC activation, which led to the inhibition of RhoA/Rock signaling and the translocation of VE-cadherin at cell–cell junctions. Moreover, sAC activation abrogated thrombin and hypoxia/reoxygenation-induced endothelial cells hyperpermeability. Pharmacological inhibition or knockdown of sAC worsened the thrombin-induced endothelial hyperpermeability suggesting that basal sAC activity is required for the maintenance of the endothelial barrier function under inflammatory conditions.

3.3. Role of Mitochondrial sAC-Dependent cAMP Signaling

3.3.1. Extra-Mitochondrial sAC

According to the current view on mitochondrial cAMP signaling, two main cores that contain distinct cAMP signaling pathways—the extra-mitochondrial sAC (outer mitochondrial membrane (OMM)) and intra-mitochondrial (the mitochondrial matrix)—can be distinguished [99]. The specificity of cAMP in OMM is mainly achieved through PKA tethering to OMM by several AKAPs, which allows multiple processes to be carried out, including mitochondrial protein import, autophagy, mitophagy, mitochondrial fission and fusion, and apoptosis [99]. Our recent study defined the role that sAC plays in regulating mitochondrial biogenesis and mitophagy [100].

It has been demonstrated that the cytosolic pool of cAMP generated by sAC is also involved in controlling mitochondrial apoptosis. Under stress conditions, the translocation of cytosolic sAC to the mitochondria leads to a selective activation of PKA, followed by phosphorylation and binding of the pro-apoptotic protein Bax to mitochondria and the release of cytochrome c in coronary endothelial cells, cardiomyocytes and aortic smooth muscle cells [15,101,102]. Furthermore, the overexpression of cytosolic sAC, but not intra-mitochondrial sAC, promotes the activation of the mitochondrial pathway of apoptosis under oxysterol treatment [102].

3.3.2. Intra-Mitochondrial sAC

An increasing amount of evidence suggests that intra-mitochondrial cAMP/PKA signaling is present in mammals [8,45,103] and yeast [104]. Although transmembrane adenylyl cyclase was initially assumed to be a source of mitochondrial cAMP [105], a recent study [9] reconsidered this paradigm and demonstrated that cytosolic cAMP cannot permeate the inner mitochondrial membrane and a mitochondria-localized cAMP source, i.e., sAC, is required [99]. In a recent study [106] we confirmed the previously published findings [9] that activating plasmalemmal adenylyl cyclase with forskolin leads to a rapid elevation of cytosolic cAMP, but does not affect cAMP concentration in mitochondria. It is worth noting that we [106], as well as other authors [9,107,108], have all observed a rapid increase in intra-mitochondrial cAMP under sAC stimulation with bicarbonate.

Bicarbonate and Ca^{2+} stimulation of mitochondrial sAC may couple the activity of the TCA cycle—the main source of CO_2/bicarbonate in the cell—and alterations in the intra-mitochondrial Ca^{2+} concentration to the OXPHOS activity [9]. Indeed, the seminal studies of Acin-Perez et al. demonstrated that cAMP produced in the mitochondrial matrix promotes cytochrome c oxidase activity via a PKA-dependent phosphorylation of cytochrome c oxidase subunit IV [8,109]. Knockout of sAC in fibroblasts causes a decline in OXPHOS activity that is compensated with elevated OXPHOS expression, whereas restoring sAC expression in the mitochondrial matrix rescues OXPHOS activity [110]. Similar results (regulation of OXPHOS activity via cAMP-PKA axis) were obtained in yeast, where the inhibition of sAC caused a decline in respiration and OXPHOS activity [104]. Furthermore, in a study on human fibroblasts, the inhibition of sAC depressed complex I activity was rescued by adding a membrane-permeable cAMP analog [111].

The role of intra-mitochondrial sAC in the regulation of memory processing was recently demonstrated [45]. The authors suggested that the activation of mitochondrial localized type-1 cannabinoid receptors ($mtCB_1$) decreases mitochondrial cAMP, complex I activity, mitochondrial respiration and cellular ATP content in hippocampal cell culture. In their study bicarbonate stimulation fully reversed the effect of $mtCB_1$-receptor activation and eliminated the cannabinoid-induced reduction in respiration. The study also confirmed that the modulation of brain mitochondrial respiration occurs through the PKA-dependent phosphorylation of complex I subunit NDUFS2 [45].

In addition to the post-translational regulation of OXPHOS activity via PKA-dependent phosphorylation, [8] it has also been suggested that sAC has an effect on the turnover of OXPHOS proteins. Indeed, intra-mitochondrial cAMP prevents the digestion of nuclear-encoded subunits of complex I by mitochondrial proteases and supports its NADH-ubiquinone oxidoreductase activity [111].

Aside from the above-mentioned studies, several other reports have demonstrated the presence of functional PKA in the mitochondrial matrix [112,113]. In a notable study that applied a PKA-sensing system with a robust dynamic range, Agnes et al. [113] characterized the compartmentalized location of PKA activity as being in bovine heart mitochondria. The experimentally determined PKA activity ratio—79:8:13 in mitochondrial matrix/intermembrane space/outer membrane respectively—provided evidence that the major PKA activity is located in the mitochondrial matrix. In agreement with that study, Sardanelli et al. [112], applying densitometric immunoblot analysis and activity assays, concluded that the majority (~90%) of mitochondrial PKA is localized in the inner mitochondrial compartment. Nevertheless, this issue of PKA localization is still a matter of debate [114]. Indeed, applying FRET-based analysis of PKA activity Lefkimmiatis et al. found no evidence of PKA activity in the mitochondrial matrix [115]. In addition, it was demonstrated that calcium-induced cardiac mitochondrial respiration is PKA independent [116]. This obvious discrepancy may be due to differences in the methods used in the analysis of PKA activity or cell models (reviewed in Valsecchi et al. [114]). In fact, the absence of PKA activity in Lefkimmiatis's study may be due to the use of predominantly glycolytic cell lines, i.e., HeLa and HEK cells. In addition, in many studies PKA activity was examined through treatment with H89, which is an unspecific PKA inhibitor and may lead to numerous side effects.

Though PKA has long been considered the most active kinase in the matrix and the main effector of intra-mitochondrial cAMP [12], another cAMP downstream target involved in the regulation of mitochondrial function—EPAC—has also been described [117]. The mitochondrial sAC-cAMP-EPAC pathway regulates coupling efficiency and the structural organization of F_0F_1ATP synthase in mammalian mitochondria [118]. In a recent study, Wang et al. [107] demonstrated a down-regulation of sAC in an animal model of heart failure, which was accompanied by a reduced resistance to Ca^{2+} overload in cardiac mitochondria. The authors underlined the inhibitory effect of the sAC/cAMP/Epac1 axis on the Ca^{2+} overload-induced opening of mitochondrial permeability pore transition [107]. In contrast, a study by Fazal et al. [119] postulated that activation of the mitochondrial sAC-cAMP-EPAC axis stimulates the mitochondrial Ca^{2+} entry, the opening of mitochondrial permeability pore transition and cell death.

3.3.3. Intra-Mitochondrial PDE2

In addition to the sAC, PDEs also contribute to the intra-mitochondrial cAMP level. PDE2A has been found to be a predominant intra-mitochondrial isoform [103]. This PDE is activated by cGMP that enables a negative cGMP-cAMP cross-talk [103,120]. A study performed with mitochondria isolated from mouse brains suggested that PDE2A, and the PDE2A2 isoform in particular, is localized in the mitochondrial matrix—due to the mitochondrial targeted sequence at N terminus of PDE2A2—where it regulates the activity of the mitochondrial respiratory chain [103]. Applying the super-resolution stimulated emission depletion microscopy in neonatal rat ventricular myocytes, Monterisi et al. revealed the localization of PDE2A outside of the mitochondrial matrix, particularly at the outer or inner mitochondrial membrane, where it regulates mitochondrial morphology, mitochondrial membrane potential and cell death via sAC-independent mechanisms [121]. Further investigation is required to clarify the localization and activity of PDE2 in mitochondria.

Since the PDE2 is activated by cGMP, it is tempting to speculate that an activation of NO signaling may lead to the activation of mitochondrial PDE2. In fact, our new report demonstrated a decline in mitochondrial cAMP concentration after NO signaling activation, either by NO donor or estradiol, in a PDE2- and sGC-dependent manner [106]. It is worth nothing that the localization of sGC in mitochondria was confirmed by western blot analysis. The reduction of mitochondrial cAMP level was accompanied by a decline in mitochondrial COX activity in a PDE2-dependent manner [106]. These data are in agreement with a previous report that demonstrated that the inhibition of PDE2A with BAY60-7550 increases oxygen consumption and ATP production in isolated mitochondria [103].

To prove whether the beneficial effect of PDE2 inhibition may be translated to cardiac pathology, adult rat cardiomyocytes were challenged metabolically with cyanide followed by a recovery phase. Inhibition of PDE2A with BAY60-7550 significantly improved cell viability [122]. In alignment with these results, a recent report suggested that PDE2 inhibition has a protective effect in a brain ischemia/reperfusion model, although it was delayed rather than acute effects of reperfusion that were analyzed [123]. Similarly, an inhibition of matrix localized PDE2A with BAY60-7550 reduced the uncoupled respiration rate and increased cytochrome c oxidase activity in septic mice [124].

3.4. Importance of sAC in the Cardiovascular System

The role of cAMP in the regulation of numerous physiological and pathological processes in the heart is well known [125–127]. Nevertheless, knowledge about the role of sAC in the cardiovascular system is limited. A seminal study by Sayner et al. [97] showed sAC's regulation of endothelial barrier function. We have also demonstrated that sAC plays a role in cardiovascular apoptosis [15,101]. The importance of sAC in cardiac pathology, like heart failure, has recently been suggested by Wang et al. [107]. The authors revealed a dramatic downregulation of sAC in mitochondrial fraction isolated from rat hearts at the late phase of cardiomyopathy and linked it to the reduced Ca^{2+} resistance of mitochondria. Our recent study presented further evidence of the importance of sAC in cardiac hypotrophy induced by isoprenaline (isolated cardiomyocytes) or pressure overload (sAC-knockout mice) [72].

4. Conclusions

cAMP signaling plays a fundamental role in controlling numerous cellular functions. The system is complex and has a well-organized spatiotemporal structure. Different mechanisms are involved in the compartmentalized structure of cAMP within the cell, including phosphodiesterases, tmAC- and sAC-dependent cAMP sources. The discovery of sAC as an alternative, intracellular source of cAMP significantly expands our knowledge of the spatial compartmentalization of cAMP signaling. The multifunctional role of sAC in the regulation of mitochondrial function and transcriptional activity in the cells, together with other functions described in this review, shows how important this cyclase is for cellular and organismal homeostasis and health. In this light, an in-depth understanding of sAC biology may contribute significantly to the prevention, prediction and treatment of several pathologies. The appearance of recent data describing the role of sAC in cardiovascular physiology [9] and pathology [11,15,72,102,107,119,124] is not surprising, especially considering the fundamental role that cAMP signaling plays in the regulation of heart function.

Author Contributions: S.P. and Y.L. wrote the manuscript.

Acknowledgments: This study was supported by DZHK (German Centre for Cardiovascular Research) partner site Berlin (Project DZHK TP BER 3.2 HF).

Conflicts of Interest: The authors declare no conflict of interest.

Abbreviations

cAMP	3′–5′-cyclic adenosine monophosphate
sAC	soluble adenylyl cyclase
tmAC	transmembrane adenylyl cyclase
PDEs	phosphodiesterases
PKA	protein kinase A
EPAC	exchange protein directly activated by cAMP
CREB	cAMP-response element binding protein
CE	Catechol estrogens
GC	guanylyl cyclase
AKAP	A-kinase anchoring proteins
CFTR	cystic fibrosis transmembrane conductance regulator
V-ATPase	vacuolar H^+-ATPase
IMS	intra-mitochondrial space
OMM	outer mitochondrial membrane
IMM	inner mitochondrial membrane
NTPase	nucleoside-triphosphatase
OXPHOS	oxidative phosphorylation

References

1. Wu, Z.; Huang, X.; Feng, Y.; Handschin, C.; Feng, Y.; Gullicksen, P.S.; Bare, O.; Labow, M.; Spiegelman, B.; Stevenson, S.C. Transducer of regulated CREB-binding proteins (TORCs) induce PGC-1α transcription and mitochondrial biogenesis in muscle cells. *Proc. Natl. Acad. Sci. USA* **2006**, *103*, 14379–14384. [CrossRef] [PubMed]

2. Chowanadisai, W.; Bauerly, K.A.; Tchaparian, E.; Wong, A.; Cortopassi, G.A.; Rucker, R.B. Pyrroloquinoline quinone stimulates mitochondrial biogenesis through cAMP response element-binding protein phosphorylation and increased PGC-1α expression. *J. Biol. Chem.* **2010**, *285*, 142–152. [CrossRef] [PubMed]

3. Catterall, W.A. Regulation of cardiac calcium channels in the fight-or-flight response. *Curr. Mol. Pharmacol.* **2015**, *8*, 12–21. [CrossRef] [PubMed]

4. Kashina, A.S.; Semenova, I.V.; Ivanov, P.A.; Potekhina, E.S.; Zaliapin, I.; Rodionov, V.I. Protein kinase A, which regulates intracellular transport, forms complexes with molecular motors on organelles. *Curr. Biol.* **2004**, *14*, 1877–1881. [CrossRef] [PubMed]

5. Burdyga, A.; Conant, A.; Haynes, L.; Zhang, J.; Jalink, K.; Sutton, R.; Neoptolemos, J.; Costello, E.; Tepikin, A. cAMP inhibits migration, ruffling and paxillin accumulation in focal adhesions of pancreatic ductal adenocarcinoma cells: Effects of PKA and EPAC. *Biochim. Biophys. Acta* **2013**, *1833*, 2664–2672. [CrossRef] [PubMed]

6. Zimmerman, N.P.; Roy, I.; Hauser, A.D.; Wilson, J.M.; Williams, C.L.; Dwinell, M.B. Cyclic AMP regulates the migration and invasion potential of human pancreatic cancer cells. *Mol. Carcinog.* **2015**, *54*, 203–215. [CrossRef] [PubMed]

7. Acin-Perez, R.; Salazar, E.; Brosel, S.; Yang, H.; Schon, E.A.; Manfredi, G. Modulation of mitochondrial protein phosphorylation by soluble adenylyl cyclase ameliorates cytochrome oxidase defects. *EMBO Mol. Med.* **2009**, *1*, 392–406. [CrossRef] [PubMed]

8. Acin-Perez, R.; Salazar, E.; Kamenetsky, M.; Buck, J.; Levin, L.R.; Manfredi, G. Cyclic AMP produced inside mitochondria regulates oxidative phosphorylation. *Cell Metab.* **2009**, *9*, 265–276. [CrossRef] [PubMed]

9. Di Benedetto, G.; Scalzotto, E.; Mongillo, M.; Pozzan, T. Mitochondrial Ca^{2+} uptake induces cyclic AMP generation in the matrix and modulates organelle ATP levels. *Cell Metab.* **2013**, *17*, 965–975. [CrossRef] [PubMed]

10. Valsecchi, F.; Ramos-Espiritu, L.S.; Buck, J.; Levin, L.R.; Manfredi, G. cAMP and mitochondria. *Physiology* **2013**, *28*, 199–209. [CrossRef] [PubMed]

11. Signorile, A.; Santeramo, A.; Tamma, G.; Pellegrino, T.; D'Oria, S.; Lattanzio, P.; De Rasmo, D. Mitochondrial cAMP prevents apoptosis modulating Sirt3 protein level and OPA1 processing in cardiac myoblast cells. *Biochim. Biophys. Acta* **2017**, *1864*, 355–366. [CrossRef] [PubMed]

12. Zhang, F.; Zhang, L.; Qi, Y.; Xu, H. Mitochondrial cAMP signaling. *Cell. Mol. Life Sci.* **2016**, *73*, 4577–4590. [CrossRef] [PubMed]

13. Bacallao, K.; Monje, P.V. Opposing roles of PKA and EPAC in the cAMP-dependent regulation of schwann cell proliferation and differentiation [corrected]. *PLoS ONE* **2013**, *8*, e82354. [CrossRef] [PubMed]

14. Stork, P.J.; Schmitt, J.M. Crosstalk between cAMP and MAP kinase signaling in the regulation of cell proliferation. *Trends Cell Biol.* **2002**, *12*, 258–266. [CrossRef]

15. Appukuttan, A.; Kasseckert, S.A.; Micoogullari, M.; Flacke, J.P.; Kumar, S.; Woste, A.; Abdallah, Y.; Pott, L.; Reusch, H.P.; Ladilov, Y. Type 10 adenylyl cyclase mediates mitochondrial bax translocation and apoptosis of adult rat cardiomyocytes under simulated ischaemia/reperfusion. *Cardiovasc. Res.* **2012**, *93*, 340–349. [CrossRef] [PubMed]

16. Ladilov, Y.; Appukuttan, A. Role of soluble adenylyl cyclase in cell death and growth. *Biochim. Biophys. Acta* **2014**, *1842*, 2646–2655. [CrossRef] [PubMed]

17. Ohmori, M.; Okamoto, S. Photoresponsive cAMP signal transduction in cyanobacteria. *Photochem. Photobiol. Sci.* **2004**, *3*, 503–511. [CrossRef] [PubMed]

18. Knapp, G.S.; McDonough, K.A. Cyclic amp signaling in mycobacteria. In *Molecular Genetics of Mycobacteria*, 2nd ed.; American Society of Microbiology: Washington, DC, USA, 2014; pp. 281–295.

19. Kamenetsky, M.; Middelhaufe, S.; Bank, E.M.; Levin, L.R.; Buck, J.; Steegborn, C. Molecular details of cAMP generation in mammalian cells: A tale of two systems. *J. Mol. Biol.* **2006**, *362*, 623–639. [CrossRef] [PubMed]

20. Federman, A.D.; Conklin, B.R.; Schrader, K.A.; Reed, R.R.; Bourne, H.R. Hormonal stimulation of adenylyl cyclase through Gi-protein βγ subunits. *Nature* **1992**, *356*, 159–161. [CrossRef] [PubMed]

21. Dessauer, C.W.; Watts, V.J.; Ostrom, R.S.; Conti, M.; Dove, S.; Seifert, R. International union of basic and clinical pharmacology. Ci. Structures and small molecule modulators of mammalian adenylyl cyclases. *Pharmacol. Rev.* **2017**, *69*, 93–139. [CrossRef] [PubMed]

22. Baldwin, T.A.; Dessauer, C.W. Function of adenylyl cyclase in heart: The AKAP connection. *J. Cardiovasc. Dev. Dis.* **2018**, *5*, 2. [CrossRef] [PubMed]

23. Ostrom, R.S.; Naugle, J.E.; Hase, M.; Gregorian, C.; Swaney, J.S.; Insel, P.A.; Brunton, L.L.; Meszaros, J.G. Angiotensin ii enhances adenylyl cyclase signaling via Ca^{2+}/calmodulin. Gq-Gs cross-talk regulates collagen production in cardiac fibroblasts. *J. Biol. Chem.* **2003**, *278*, 24461–24468. [CrossRef] [PubMed]

24. Chen, Y.; Cann, M.J.; Litvin, T.N.; Iourgenko, V.; Sinclair, M.L.; Levin, L.R.; Buck, J. Soluble adenylyl cyclase as an evolutionarily conserved bicarbonate sensor. *Science* **2000**, *289*, 625–628. [CrossRef] [PubMed]

25. Zippin, J.H.; Chen, Y.; Nahirney, P.; Kamenetsky, M.; Wuttke, M.S.; Fischman, D.A.; Levin, L.R.; Buck, J. Compartmentalization of bicarbonate-sensitive adenylyl cyclase in distinct signaling microdomains. *FASEB J.* **2003**, *17*, 82–84. [CrossRef] [PubMed]

26. Richards, M.; Lomas, O.; Jalink, K.; Ford, K.L.; Vaughan-Jones, R.D.; Lefkimmiatis, K.; Swietach, P. Intracellular tortuosity underlies slow cAMP diffusion in adult ventricular myocytes. *Cardiovasc. Res.* **2016**, *110*, 395–407. [CrossRef] [PubMed]

27. Mika, D.; Leroy, J.; Vandecasteele, G.; Fischmeister, R. Pdes create local domains of cAMP signaling. *J. Mol. Cell. Cardiol.* **2012**, *52*, 323–329. [CrossRef] [PubMed]

28. Agarwal, S.R.; Clancy, C.E.; Harvey, R.D. Mechanisms restricting diffusion of intracellular cAMP. *Sci. Rep.* **2016**, *6*, 19577. [CrossRef] [PubMed]

29. Fischmeister, R.; Castro, L.R.; Abi-Gerges, A.; Rochais, F.; Jurevicius, J.; Leroy, J.; Vandecasteele, G. Compartmentation of cyclic nucleotide signaling in the heart: The role of cyclic nucleotide phosphodiesterases. *Circ. Res.* **2006**, *99*, 816–828. [CrossRef] [PubMed]

30. Godbole, A.; Lyga, S.; Lohse, M.J.; Calebiro, D. Internalized tsh receptors en route to the tgn induce local Gs-protein signaling and gene transcription. *Nat. Commun.* **2017**, *8*, 443. [CrossRef] [PubMed]

31. Calebiro, D.; Maiellaro, I. CAMP signaling microdomains and their observation by optical methods. *Front. Cell. Neurosci.* **2014**, *8*, 350. [CrossRef] [PubMed]

32. Musheshe, N.; Schmidt, M.; Zaccolo, M. cAMP: From long-range second messenger to nanodomain signalling. *Trends Pharmacol. Sci.* **2017**, *39*, 209–222. [CrossRef] [PubMed]

33. Lefkimmiatis, K.; Zaccolo, M. cAMP signaling in subcellular compartments. *Pharmacol. Ther.* **2014**, *143*, 295–304. [CrossRef] [PubMed]

34. Kobayashi, M.; Buck, J.; Levin, L.R. Conservation of functional domain structure in bicarbonate-regulated "soluble" adenylyl cyclases in bacteria and eukaryotes. *Dev. Genes Evol.* **2004**, *214*, 503–509. [CrossRef] [PubMed]

35. Kleinboelting, S.; Diaz, A.; Moniot, S.; van den Heuvel, J.; Weyand, M.; Levin, L.R.; Buck, J.; Steegborn, C. Crystal structures of human soluble adenylyl cyclase reveal mechanisms of catalysis and of its activation through bicarbonate. *Proc. Natl. Acad. Sci. USA* **2014**, *111*, 3727–3732. [CrossRef] [PubMed]

36. Chaloupka, J.A.; Bullock, S.A.; Iourgenko, V.; Levin, L.R.; Buck, J. Autoinhibitory regulation of soluble adenylyl cyclase. *Mol. Reprod. Dev.* **2006**, *73*, 361–368. [CrossRef] [PubMed]

37. Leipe, D.D.; Koonin, E.V.; Aravind, L. Stand, a class of p-loop ntpases including animal and plant regulators of programmed cell death: Multiple, complex domain architectures, unusual phyletic patterns, and evolution by horizontal gene transfer. *J. Mol. Biol.* **2004**, *343*, 1–28. [CrossRef] [PubMed]

38. Middelhaufe, S.; Leipelt, M.; Levin, L.R.; Buck, J.; Steegborn, C. Identification of a haem domain in human soluble adenylate cyclase. *Biosci. Rep.* **2012**, *32*, 491–499. [CrossRef] [PubMed]

39. Farrell, J.; Ramos, L.; Tresguerres, M.; Kamenetsky, M.; Levin, L.R.; Buck, J. Somatic 'soluble' adenylyl cyclase isoforms are unaffected in Sacy^{tm1lex}/Sacy^{tm1lex} 'knockout' mice. *PLoS ONE* **2008**, *3*, e3251. [CrossRef] [PubMed]

40. Reed, B.Y.; Gitomer, W.L.; Heller, H.J.; Hsu, M.C.; Lemke, M.; Padalino, P.; Pak, C.Y. Identification and characterization of a gene with base substitutions associated with the absorptive hypercalciuria phenotype and low spinal bone density. *J. Clin. Endocrinol. Metab.* **2002**, *87*, 1476–1485. [CrossRef] [PubMed]

41. Chen, X.; Baumlin, N.; Buck, J.; Levin, L.R.; Fregien, N.; Salathe, M. A soluble adenylyl cyclase form targets to axonemes and rescues beat regulation in soluble adenylyl cyclase knockout mice. *Am. J. Respir. Cell Mol. Biol.* **2014**, *51*, 750–760. [CrossRef] [PubMed]

42. Buck, J.; Sinclair, M.L.; Schapal, L.; Cann, M.J.; Levin, L.R. Cytosolic adenylyl cyclase defines a unique signaling molecule in mammals. *Proc. Natl. Acad. Sci. USA* **1999**, *96*, 79–84. [CrossRef] [PubMed]

43. Geng, W.; Wang, Z.; Zhang, J.; Reed, B.Y.; Pak, C.Y.; Moe, O.W. Cloning and characterization of the human soluble adenylyl cyclase. *Am. J. Physiol. Cell Physiol.* **2005**, *288*, C1305–C1316. [CrossRef] [PubMed]

44. Steegborn, C. Structure, mechanism, and regulation of soluble adenylyl cyclases—Similarities and differences to transmembrane adenylyl cyclases. *Biochim. Biophys. Acta* **2014**, *1842*, 2535–2547. [CrossRef] [PubMed]

45. Hebert-Chatelain, E.; Desprez, T.; Serrat, R.; Bellocchio, L.; Soria-Gomez, E.; Busquets-Garcia, A.; Pagano Zottola, A.C.; Delamarre, A.; Cannich, A.; Vincent, P.; et al. A cannabinoid link between mitochondria and memory. *Nature* **2016**, *539*, 555–559. [CrossRef] [PubMed]

46. Ramos-Espiritu, L.; Kleinboelting, S.; Navarrete, F.A.; Alvau, A.; Visconti, P.E.; Valsecchi, F.; Starkov, A.; Manfredi, G.; Buck, H.; Adura, C.; et al. Discovery of LRE1 as a specific and allosteric inhibitor of soluble adenylyl cyclase. *Nat. Chem. Biol.* **2016**, *12*, 838–844. [CrossRef] [PubMed]

47. Tresguerres, M.; Levin, L.R.; Buck, J. Intracellular cAMP signaling by soluble adenylyl cyclase. *Kidney Int.* **2011**, *79*, 1277–1288. [CrossRef] [PubMed]

48. Zippin, J.H.; Chen, Y.; Straub, S.G.; Hess, K.C.; Diaz, A.; Lee, D.; Tso, P.; Holz, G.G.; Sharp, G.W.; Levin, L.R.; et al. CO_2/HCO_3^-- and calcium-regulated soluble adenylyl cyclase as a physiological ATP sensor. *J. Biol. Chem.* **2013**, *288*, 33283–33291. [CrossRef] [PubMed]

49. Litvin, T.N.; Kamenetsky, M.; Zarifyan, A.; Buck, J.; Levin, L.R. Kinetic properties of "soluble" adenylyl cyclase. Synergism between calcium and bicarbonate. *J. Biol. Chem.* **2003**, *278*, 15922–15926. [CrossRef] [PubMed]

50. Magro, C.M.; Yang, S.E.; Zippin, J.H.; Zembowicz, A. Expression of soluble adenylyl cyclase in lentigo maligna: Use of immunohistochemistry with anti-soluble adenylyl cyclase antibody (R21) in diagnosis of lentigo maligna and assessment of margins. *Arch. Pathol. Lab. Med.* **2012**, *136*, 1558–1564. [CrossRef] [PubMed]

51. Magro, C.M.; Crowson, A.N.; Desman, G.; Zippin, J.H. Soluble adenylyl cyclase antibody profile as a diagnostic adjunct in the assessment of pigmented lesions. *Arch. Dermatol.* **2012**, *148*, 335–344. [CrossRef] [PubMed]

52. Ramos, L.S.; Zippin, J.H.; Kamenetsky, M.; Buck, J.; Levin, L.R. Glucose and GLP-1 stimulate cAMP production via distinct adenylyl cyclases in INS-1E insulinoma cells. *J. Gen. Physiol.* **2008**, *132*, 329–338. [CrossRef] [PubMed]

53. Flacke, J.P.; Flacke, H.; Appukuttan, A.; Palisaar, R.J.; Noldus, J.; Robinson, B.D.; Reusch, H.P.; Zippin, J.H.; Ladilov, Y. Type 10 soluble adenylyl cyclase is overexpressed in prostate carcinoma and controls proliferation of prostate cancer cells. *J. Biol. Chem.* **2013**, *288*, 3126–3135. [CrossRef] [PubMed]

54. Pierre, S.; Eschenhagen, T.; Geisslinger, G.; Scholich, K. Capturing adenylyl cyclases as potential drug targets. *Nat. Rev. Drug Discov.* **2009**, *8*, 321–335. [CrossRef] [PubMed]

55. Lee, Y.S.; Tresguerres, M.; Hess, K.; Marmorstein, L.Y.; Levin, L.R.; Buck, J.; Marmorstein, A.D. Regulation of anterior chamber drainage by bicarbonate-sensitive soluble adenylyl cyclase in the ciliary body. *J. Biol. Chem.* **2011**, *286*, 41353–41358. [CrossRef] [PubMed]

56. Bitterman, J.L.; Ramos-Espiritu, L.; Diaz, A.; Levin, L.R.; Buck, J. Pharmacological distinction between soluble and transmembrane adenylyl cyclases. *J. Pharmacol. Exp. Ther.* **2013**, *347*, 589–598. [CrossRef] [PubMed]

57. Steegborn, C.; Litvin, T.N.; Hess, K.C.; Capper, A.B.; Taussig, R.; Buck, J.; Levin, L.R.; Wu, H. A novel mechanism for adenylyl cyclase inhibition from the crystal structure of its complex with catechol estrogen. *J. Biol. Chem.* **2005**, *280*, 31754–31759. [CrossRef] [PubMed]

58. Hess, K.C.; Jones, B.H.; Marquez, B.; Chen, Y.; Ord, T.S.; Kamenetsky, M.; Miyamoto, C.; Zippin, J.H.; Kopf, G.S.; Suarez, S.S.; et al. The "soluble" adenylyl cyclase in sperm mediates multiple signaling events required for fertilization. *Dev. Cell* **2005**, *9*, 249–259. [CrossRef] [PubMed]

59. Kaupp, U.B.; Seifert, R. Cyclic nucleotide-gated ion channels. *Physiol. Rev.* **2002**, *82*, 769–824. [CrossRef] [PubMed]

60. Froese, A.; Breher, S.S.; Waldeyer, C.; Schindler, R.F.; Nikolaev, V.O.; Rinne, S.; Wischmeyer, E.; Schlueter, J.; Becher, J.; Simrick, S.; et al. Popeye domain containing proteins are essential for stress-mediated modulation of cardiac pacemaking in mice. *J. Clin. Investig.* **2012**, *122*, 1119–1130. [CrossRef] [PubMed]

61. Simrick, S.; Schindler, R.F.; Poon, K.L.; Brand, T. Popeye domain-containing proteins and stress-mediated modulation of cardiac pacemaking. *Trends Cardiovasc. Med.* **2013**, *23*, 257–263. [CrossRef] [PubMed]

62. Schmidt, M.; Dekker, F.J.; Maarsingh, H. Exchange protein directly activated by cAMP (EPAC): A multidomain cAMP mediator in the regulation of diverse biological functions. *Pharmacol. Rev.* **2013**, *65*, 670–709. [CrossRef] [PubMed]

63. Lomas, O.; Zaccolo, M. Phosphodiesterases maintain signaling fidelity via compartmentalization of cyclic nucleotides. *Physiology* **2014**, *29*, 141–149. [CrossRef] [PubMed]

64. Corredor, R.G.; Trakhtenberg, E.F.; Pita-Thomas, W.; Jin, X.; Hu, Y.; Goldberg, J.L. Soluble adenylyl cyclase activity is necessary for retinal ganglion cell survival and axon growth. *J. Neurosci.* **2012**, *32*, 7734–7744. [CrossRef] [PubMed]

65. Han, H.; Stessin, A.; Roberts, J.; Hess, K.; Gautam, N.; Kamenetsky, M.; Lou, O.; Hyde, E.; Nathan, N.; Muller, W.A.; et al. Calcium-sensing soluble adenylyl cyclase mediates tnf signal transduction in human neutrophils. *J. Exp. Med.* **2005**, *202*, 353–361. [CrossRef] [PubMed]

66. Stowe, D.F.; Gadicherla, A.K.; Zhou, Y.; Aldakkak, M.; Cheng, Q.; Kwok, W.M.; Jiang, M.T.; Heisner, J.S.; Yang, M.; Camara, A.K. Protection against cardiac injury by small Ca^{2+}-sensitive K^+ channels identified in guinea pig cardiac inner mitochondrial membrane. *Biochim. Biophys. Acta* **2013**, *1828*, 427–442. [CrossRef] [PubMed]

67. Monterisi, S.; Zaccolo, M. Components of the mitochondrial cAMP signalosome. *Biochem. Soc. Trans.* **2017**, *45*, 269–274. [CrossRef] [PubMed]

68. Zippin, J.H.; Farrell, J.; Huron, D.; Kamenetsky, M.; Hess, K.C.; Fischman, D.A.; Levin, L.R.; Buck, J. Bicarbonate-responsive "soluble" adenylyl cyclase defines a nuclear cAMP microdomain. *J. Cell Biol.* **2004**, *164*, 527–534. [CrossRef] [PubMed]

69. Stessin, A.M.; Zippin, J.H.; Kamenetsky, M.; Hess, K.C.; Buck, J.; Levin, L.R. Soluble adenylyl cyclase mediates nerve growth factor-induced activation of Rap1. *J. Biol. Chem.* **2006**, *281*, 17253–17258. [CrossRef] [PubMed]

70. Onodera, Y.; Nam, J.M.; Bissell, M.J. Increased sugar uptake promotes oncogenesis via EPAC/Rap1 and o-glcnac pathways. *J. Clin. Investig.* **2014**, *124*, 367–384. [CrossRef] [PubMed]

71. Wu, K.Y.; Zippin, J.H.; Huron, D.R.; Kamenetsky, M.; Hengst, U.; Buck, J.; Levin, L.R.; Jaffrey, S.R. Soluble adenylyl cyclase is required for netrin-1 signaling in nerve growth cones. *Nat. Neurosci.* **2006**, *9*, 1257–1264. [CrossRef] [PubMed]

72. Schirmer, I.; Bualeong, T.; Budde, H.; Cimiotti, D.; Appukuttan, A.; Klein, N.; Steinwascher, P.; Reusch, P.; Mugge, A.; Meyer, R.; et al. Soluble adenylyl cyclase: A novel player in cardiac hypertrophy induced by isoprenaline or pressure overload. *PLoS ONE* **2018**, *13*, e0192322. [CrossRef] [PubMed]

73. Buffone, M.G.; Wertheimer, E.V.; Visconti, P.E.; Krapf, D. Central role of soluble adenylyl cyclase and cAMP in sperm physiology. *Biochim. Biophys. Acta* **2014**, *1842*, 2610–2620. [CrossRef] [PubMed]

74. Esposito, G.; Jaiswal, B.S.; Xie, F.; Krajnc-Franken, M.A.; Robben, T.J.; Strik, A.M.; Kuil, C.; Philipsen, R.L.; van Duin, M.; Conti, M.; et al. Mice deficient for soluble adenylyl cyclase are infertile because of a severe sperm-motility defect. *Proc. Natl. Acad. Sci. USA* **2004**, *101*, 2993–2998. [CrossRef] [PubMed]

75. Watson, R.L.; Buck, J.; Levin, L.R.; Winger, R.C.; Wang, J.; Arase, H.; Muller, W.A. Endothelial cd99 signals through soluble adenylyl cyclase and PKA to regulate leukocyte transendothelial migration. *J. Exp. Med.* **2015**, *212*, 1021–1041. [CrossRef] [PubMed]

76. Chang, J.C.; Oude-Elferink, R.P. Role of the bicarbonate-responsive soluble adenylyl cyclase in pH sensing and metabolic regulation. *Front. Physiol.* **2014**, *5*, 42. [CrossRef] [PubMed]

77. Brown, D.; Bouley, R.; Paunescu, T.G.; Breton, S.; Lu, H.A. New insights into the dynamic regulation of water and acid-base balance by renal epithelial cells. *Am. J. Physiol. Cell Physiol.* **2012**, *302*, C1421–C1433. [CrossRef] [PubMed]

78. Pastor-Soler, N.M.; Hallows, K.R.; Smolak, C.; Gong, F.; Brown, D.; Breton, S. Alkaline ph- and cAMP-induced v-ATPase membrane accumulation is mediated by protein kinase a in epididymal clear cells. *Am. J. Physiol. Cell Physiol.* **2008**, *294*, C488–C494. [CrossRef] [PubMed]

79. Gong, F.; Alzamora, R.; Smolak, C.; Li, H.; Naveed, S.; Neumann, D.; Hallows, K.R.; Pastor-Soler, N.M. Vacuolar h+-atpase apical accumulation in kidney intercalated cells is regulated by PKA and AMP-activated protein kinase. *Am. J. Physiol.-Renal Physiol.* **2010**, *298*, F1162–F1169. [CrossRef] [PubMed]

80. Breton, S.; Brown, D. Regulation of luminal acidification by the v-atpase. *Physiology* **2013**, *28*, 318–329. [CrossRef] [PubMed]

81. Rahman, N.; Ramos-Espiritu, L.; Milner, T.A.; Buck, J.; Levin, L.R. Soluble adenylyl cyclase is essential for proper lysosomal acidification. *J. Gen. Physiol.* **2016**, *148*, 325–339. [CrossRef] [PubMed]

82. Inda, C.; Bonfiglio, J.J.; Dos Santos Claro, P.A.; Senin, S.A.; Armando, N.G.; Deussing, J.M.; Silberstein, S. cAMP-dependent cell differentiation triggered by activated crhr1 in hippocampal neuronal cells. *Sci. Rep.* **2017**, *7*, 1944. [CrossRef] [PubMed]

83. Mewes, M.; Nedele, J.; Schelleckes, K.; Bondareva, O.; Lenders, M.; Kusche-Vihrog, K.; Schnittler, H.J.; Brand, S.M.; Schmitz, B.; Brand, E. Salt-induced Na^+/K^+-atpase-alpha/beta expression involves soluble adenylyl cyclase in endothelial cells. *Pflugers Arch. Eur. J. Physiol.* **2017**, *469*, 1401–1412. [CrossRef] [PubMed]

84. Schmitz, B.; Nedele, J.; Guske, K.; Maase, M.; Lenders, M.; Schelleckes, M.; Kusche-Vihrog, K.; Brand, S.M.; Brand, E. Soluble adenylyl cyclase in vascular endothelium: Gene expression control of epithelial sodium channel-alpha, Na^+/K^+-ATPase-α/β, and mineralocorticoid receptor. *Hypertension* **2014**, *63*, 753–761. [CrossRef] [PubMed]

85. Kikuchi, R.; Tsuji, T.; Watanabe, O.; Yamaguchi, K.; Furukawa, K.; Nakamura, H.; Aoshiba, K. Hypercapnia accelerates adipogenesis: A novel role of high CO_2 in exacerbating obesity. *Am. J. Respir. Cell Mol. Biol.* **2017**, *57*, 570–580. [CrossRef] [PubMed]

86. Sepp, M.; Vihma, H.; Nurm, K.; Urb, M.; Page, S.C.; Roots, K.; Hark, A.; Maher, B.J.; Pruunsild, P.; Timmusk, T. The intellectual disability and schizophrenia associated transcription factor tcf4 is regulated by neuronal activity and protein kinase a. *J. Neurosci.* **2017**, *37*, 10516–10527. [CrossRef] [PubMed]

87. Lim, S.H.; Legere, E.A.; Snider, J.; Stagljar, I. Recent progress in cftr interactome mapping and its importance for cystic fibrosis. *Front. Pharmacol.* **2017**, *8*, 997. [CrossRef] [PubMed]

88. Wang, Y.; Lam, C.S.; Wu, F.; Wang, W.; Duan, Y.; Huang, P. Regulation of cftr channels by HCO_3—Sensitive soluble adenylyl cyclase in human airway epithelial cells. *Am. J. Physiol. Cell Physiol.* **2005**, *289*, C1145–C1151. [CrossRef] [PubMed]

89. Chen, H.; Guo, J.H.; Lu, Y.C.; Ding, G.L.; Yu, M.K.; Tsang, L.L.; Fok, K.L.; Liu, X.M.; Zhang, X.H.; Chung, Y.W.; et al. Impaired cftr-dependent amplification of fsh-stimulated estrogen production in cystic fibrosis and pcos. *J. Clin. Endocrinol. Metab.* **2012**, *97*, 923–932. [CrossRef] [PubMed]

90. Wang, X.F.; Zhou, C.X.; Shi, Q.X.; Yuan, Y.Y.; Yu, M.K.; Ajonuma, L.C.; He, L.S.; Lo, P.S.; Tsang, L.L.; Liu, Y.; et al. Involvement of cftr in uterine bicarbonate secretion and the fertilizing capacity of sperm. *Nat. Cell Biol.* **2003**, *5*, 902–906. [CrossRef] [PubMed]

91. Xu, W.M.; Shi, Q.X.; Chen, W.Y.; Zhou, C.X.; Ni, Y.; Rowlands, D.K.; Yi Liu, G.; Zhu, H.; Ma, Z.G.; Wang, X.F.; et al. Cystic fibrosis transmembrane conductance regulator is vital to sperm fertilizing capacity and male fertility. *Proc. Natl. Acad. Sci. USA* **2007**, *104*, 9816–9821. [CrossRef] [PubMed]

92. Chen, W.Y.; Xu, W.M.; Chen, Z.H.; Ni, Y.; Yuan, Y.Y.; Zhou, S.C.; Zhou, W.W.; Tsang, L.L.; Chung, Y.W.; Hoglund, P.; et al. Cl- is required for HCO_3^- entry necessary for sperm capacitation in guinea pig: Involvement of a Cl-/HCO_3^- exchanger (slc26a3) and cftr. *Biol. Reprod.* **2009**, *80*, 115–123. [CrossRef] [PubMed]

93. Lu, Y.C.; Chen, H.; Fok, K.L.; Tsang, L.L.; Yu, M.K.; Zhang, X.H.; Chen, J.; Jiang, X.; Chung, Y.W.; Ma, A.C.; et al. Cftr mediates bicarbonate-dependent activation of mir-125b in preimplantation embryo development. *Cell Res.* **2012**, *22*, 1453–1466. [CrossRef] [PubMed]

94. Chen, H.; Chan, H.C. Amplification of fsh signalling by cftr and nuclear soluble adenylyl cyclase in the ovary. *Clin. Exp. Pharmacol. Physiol.* **2017**, *44* (Suppl. S1), 78–85. [CrossRef] [PubMed]

95. Lecuona, E.; Sun, H.; Chen, J.; Trejo, H.E.; Baker, M.A.; Sznajder, J.I. Protein kinase a-ialpha regulates na,k-atpase endocytosis in alveolar epithelial cells exposed to high CO_2 concentrations. *Am. J. Respir. Cell Mol. Biol.* **2013**, *48*, 626–634. [CrossRef] [PubMed]

96. Sayner, S.L.; Frank, D.W.; King, J.; Chen, H.; VandeWaa, J.; Stevens, T. Paradoxical cAMP-induced lung endothelial hyperpermeability revealed by pseudomonas aeruginosa exoy. *Circ. Res.* **2004**, *95*, 196–203. [CrossRef] [PubMed]

97. Sayner, S.L.; Alexeyev, M.; Dessauer, C.W.; Stevens, T. Soluble adenylyl cyclase reveals the significance of cAMP compartmentation on pulmonary microvascular endothelial cell barrier *Circ. Res.* **2006**, *98*, 675–681. [CrossRef] [PubMed]

98. Das, A.; Härtel, F.; Ihle, K.; Ladilov, Y.; Noll, T. Role of soluble adenylyl cyclase on barrier function of human umbilical vein endothelial monolayers: P21–13. *Acta Physiol.* **2016**, *216*, 216.

99. Di Benedetto, G.; Gerbino, A.; Lefkimmiatis, K. Shaping mitochondrial dynamics: The role of cAMP signalling. *Biochem. Biophys. Res. Commun.* **2017**, *500*, 65–74. [CrossRef] [PubMed]

100. Jayarajan, V.; Appukuttan, A.; Reusch, P.; Ladilov, Y.; Regitz-Zagrosek, V. Soluble adenylyl cyclase controls AMPK activity, mitochondrial function and biogensis and may play a role in estradiol-dependent protection against oxidative stress. In Proceedings of the 42nd FEBS Congress on Molecules to Cells and back, Jerusalim, Israel, 10–14 September 2017.

101. Kumar, S.; Kostin, S.; Flacke, J.P.; Reusch, H.P.; Ladilov, Y. Soluble adenylyl cyclase controls mitochondria-dependent apoptosis in coronary endothelial cells. *J. Biol. Chem.* **2009**, *284*, 14760–14768. [CrossRef] [PubMed]

102. Appukuttan, A.; Kasseckert, S.A.; Kumar, S.; Reusch, H.P.; Ladilov, Y. Oxysterol-induced apoptosis of smooth muscle cells is under the control of a soluble adenylyl cyclase. *Cardiovasc. Res.* **2013**, *99*, 734–742. [CrossRef] [PubMed]

103. Acin-Perez, R.; Russwurm, M.; Gunnewig, K.; Gertz, M.; Zoidl, G.; Ramos, L.; Buck, J.; Levin, L.R.; Rassow, J.; Manfredi, G.; et al. A phosphodiesterase 2a isoform localized to mitochondria regulates respiration. *J. Biol. Chem.* **2011**, *286*, 30423–30432. [CrossRef] [PubMed]

104. Hess, K.C.; Liu, J.; Manfredi, G.; Muhlschlegel, F.A.; Buck, J.; Levin, L.R.; Barrientos, A. A mitochondrial CO_2-adenylyl cyclase-cAMP signalosome controls yeast normoxic cytochrome c oxidase activity. *FASEB J.* **2014**, *28*, 4369–4380. [CrossRef] [PubMed]

105. DiPilato, L.M.; Cheng, X.; Zhang, J. Fluorescent indicators of cAMP and EPAC activation reveal differential dynamics of cAMP signaling within discrete subcellular compartments. *Proc. Natl. Acad. Sci. USA* **2004**, *101*, 16513–16518. [CrossRef] [PubMed]

106. Pozdniakova, S.; Guitart-Mampel, M.; Garrabou, G.; Di Benedetto, G.; Ladilov, Y.; Regitz-Zagrosek, V. 17ß-estradiol reduces mitochondrial cAMP content and cytochrome oxidase activity in a phosphodiesterase 2-dependent manner. In Proceedings of the 42nd FEBS Congress on Molecules to Cells and back, Jerusalem, Israel, 10–14 September 2017.

107. Wang, Z.; Liu, D.; Varin, A.; Nicolas, V.; Courilleau, D.; Mateo, P.; Caubere, C.; Rouet, P.; Gomez, A.M.; Vandecasteele, G.; et al. A cardiac mitochondrial cAMP signaling pathway regulates calcium accumulation, permeability transition and cell death. *Cell Death Dis.* **2016**, *7*, e2198. [CrossRef] [PubMed]

108. Mukherjee, S.; Jansen, V.; Jikeli, J.F.; Hamzeh, H.; Alvarez, L.; Dombrowski, M.; Balbach, M.; Strunker, T.; Seifert, R.; Kaupp, U.B.; et al. A novel biosensor to study cAMP dynamics in cilia and flagella. *eLife* **2016**, *5*, e14052. [CrossRef] [PubMed]

109. Acin-Perez, R.; Gatti, D.L.; Bai, Y.; Manfredi, G. Protein phosphorylation and prevention of cytochrome oxidase inhibition by atp: Coupled mechanisms of energy metabolism regulation. *Cell Metab.* **2011**, *13*, 712–719. [CrossRef] [PubMed]

110. Valsecchi, F.; Konrad, C.; D'Aurelio, M.; Ramos-Espiritu, L.S.; Stepanova, A.; Burstein, S.R.; Galkin, A.; Magrane, J.; Starkov, A.; Buck, J.; et al. Distinct intracellular sac-cAMP domains regulate er Ca^{2+} signaling and oxphos function. *J. Cell Sci.* **2017**, *130*, 3713–3727. [CrossRef]

111. De Rasmo, D.; Signorile, A.; Santeramo, A.; Larizza, M.; Lattanzio, P.; Capitanio, G.; Papa, S. Intramitochondrial adenylyl cyclase controls the turnover of nuclear-encoded subunits and activity of mammalian complex i of the respiratory chain. *Biochim. Biophys. Acta* **2015**, *1853*, 183–191. [CrossRef] [PubMed]

112. Sardanelli, A.M.; Signorile, A.; Nuzzi, R.; Rasmo, D.D.; Technikova-Dobrova, Z.; Drahota, Z.; Occhiello, A.; Pica, A.; Papa, S. Occurrence of a-kinase anchor protein and associated cAMP-dependent protein kinase in the inner compartment of mammalian mitochondria. *FEBS Lett.* **2006**, *580*, 5690–5696. [CrossRef] [PubMed]

113. Agnes, R.S.; Jernigan, F.; Shell, J.R.; Sharma, V.; Lawrence, D.S. Suborganelle sensing of mitochondrial cAMP-dependent protein kinase activity. *J. Am. Chem. Soc.* **2010**, *132*, 6075–6080. [CrossRef] [PubMed]

114. Valsecchi, F.; Konrad, C.; Manfredi, G. Role of soluble adenylyl cyclase in mitochondria. *Biochim. Biophys. Acta* **2014**, *1842*, 2555–2560. [CrossRef] [PubMed]

115. Lefkimmiatis, K.; Leronni, D.; Hofer, A.M. The inner and outer compartments of mitochondria are sites of distinct cAMP/PKA signaling dynamics. *J. Cell Biol.* **2013**, *202*, 453–462. [CrossRef] [PubMed]

116. Covian, R.; French, S.; Kusnetz, H.; Balaban, R.S. Stimulation of oxidative phosphorylation by calcium in cardiac mitochondria is not influenced by cAMP and PKA activity. *Biochim. Biophys. Acta* **2014**, *1837*, 1913–1921. [CrossRef] [PubMed]

117. Laudette, M.; Zuo, H.; Lezoualc'h, F.; Schmidt, M. EPAC function and cAMP scaffolds in the heart and lung. *J. Cardiovasc. Dev. Dis.* **2018**, *5*, 9. [CrossRef] [PubMed]

118. De Rasmo, D.; Micelli, L.; Santeramo, A.; Signorile, A.; Lattanzio, P.; Papa, S. CAMP regulates the functional activity, coupling efficiency and structural organization of mammalian fof1 atp synthase. *Biochim. Biophys. Acta* **2016**, *1857*, 350–358. [CrossRef] [PubMed]

119. Fazal, L.; Laudette, M.; Paula-Gomes, S.; Pons, S.; Conte, C.; Tortosa, F.; Sicard, P.; Sainte-Marie, Y.; Bisserier, M.; Lairez, O.; et al. Multifunctional mitochondrial EPAC1 controls myocardial cell death. *Circ. Res.* **2017**, *120*, 645–657. [CrossRef] [PubMed]

120. Pavlaki, N.; Nikolaev, V.O. Imaging of pde2- and pde3-mediated cgmp-to-cAMP cross-talk in cardiomyocytes. *J. Cardiovasc. Dev. Dis.* **2018**, *5*, 4. [CrossRef] [PubMed]

121. Monterisi, S.; Lobo, M.J.; Livie, C.; Castle, J.C.; Weinberger, M.; Baillie, G.; Surdo, N.C.; Musheshe, N.; Stangherlin, A.; Gottlieb, E.; et al. Pde2a2 regulates mitochondria morphology and apoptotic cell death via local modulation of cAMP/PKA signalling. *eLife* **2017**, *6*, e21374. [CrossRef] [PubMed]

122. Rinaldi, L.; Pozdniakova, S.; Jayarajan, V.; Troidl, C.; Abdallah, Y.; Muhammad, A.; Ladilov, Y. Role of Soluble adenylyl cyclase in reperfusion-induced injury of cardiac cells. *Clin. Res. Cardiol.* **2018**. [CrossRef]

123. Soares, L.M.; Meyer, E.; Milani, H.; Steinbusch, H.W.; Prickaerts, J.; de Oliveira, R.M. The phosphodiesterase type 2 inhibitor bay 60-7550 reverses functional impairments induced by brain ischemia by decreasing hippocampal neurodegeneration and enhancing hippocampal neuronal plasticity. *Eur. J. Neurosci.* **2017**, *45*, 510–520. [CrossRef] [PubMed]

124. Neviere, R.; Delguste, F.; Durand, A.; Inamo, J.; Boulanger, E.; Preau, S. Abnormal mitochondrial cAMP/PKA signaling is involved in sepsis-induced mitochondrial and myocardial dysfunction. *Int. J. Mol. Sci.* **2016**, *17*, 2075. [CrossRef] [PubMed]

125. Lezoualc'h, F.; Fazal, L.; Laudette, M.; Conte, C. Cyclic amp sensor EPAC proteins and their role in cardiovascular function and disease. *Circ. Res.* **2016**, *118*, 881–897. [CrossRef] [PubMed]

126. Khaliulin, I.; Bond, M.; James, A.F.; Dyar, Z.; Amini, R.; Johnson, J.L.; Suleiman, M.S. Functional and cardioprotective effects of simultaneous and individual activation of protein kinase a and EPAC. *Br. J. Pharmacol.* **2017**, *174*, 438–453. [CrossRef] [PubMed]

127. Zoccarato, A.; Surdo, N.C.; Aronsen, J.M.; Fields, L.A.; Mancuso, L.; Dodoni, G.; Stangherlin, A.; Livie, C.; Jiang, H.; Sin, Y.Y.; et al. Cardiac hypertrophy is inhibited by a local pool of cAMP regulated by phosphodiesterase 2. *Circ. Res.* **2015**, *117*, 707–719. [CrossRef] [PubMed]

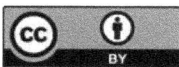

Journal of
*Cardiovascular
Development and Disease*

MDPI

Review

Functions of PDE3 Isoforms in Cardiac Muscle

Matthew Movsesian [1],*, Faiyaz Ahmad [2],† and Emilio Hirsch [3]

[1] Department of Internal Medicine/Division of Cardiovascular Medicine, University of Utah, Salt Lake City, UT 841132, USA
[2] Vascular Biology and Hypertension Branch, Division of Cardiovascular Sciences, National Heart, Lung and Blood Institute, Bethesda, MD 20892, USA; ahmadf@nhlbi.nih.gov
[3] Department of Molecular Biotechnology and Health Sciences, Center for Molecular Biotechnology, University of Turin, 10126 Turin, Italy; emilio.hirsch@unito.it
* Correspondence: matthew.movsesian@hsc.utah.edu; Tel.: +1-801-582-1565
† Beginning 18 February 2018: Sidra Medical Research Center, Doha, Qatar.

Received: 9 January 2018; Accepted: 1 February 2018; Published: 6 February 2018

Abstract: Isoforms in the PDE3 family of cyclic nucleotide phosphodiesterases have important roles in cyclic nucleotide-mediated signalling in cardiac myocytes. These enzymes are targeted by inhibitors used to increase contractility in patients with heart failure, with a combination of beneficial and adverse effects on clinical outcomes. This review covers relevant aspects of the molecular biology of the isoforms that have been identified in cardiac myocytes; the roles of these enzymes in modulating cAMP-mediated signalling and the processes mediated thereby; and the potential for targeting these enzymes to improve the profile of clinical responses.

Keywords: cyclic nucleotides; cAMP; cGMP; phosphodiesterase; PDE3; intracellular signalling; heart

1. Introduction

Cyclic nucleotide phosphodiesterases regulate intracellular signalling by hydrolysing cAMP and/or cGMP. Enzymes in the PDE3 family of phosphodiesterases are dual-specificity enzymes with high affinities for both cAMP and cGMP but much higher turnover rates for cAMP [1–3]. In cardiac muscle, these enzymes have been studied principally in the context of their role in regulating cAMP-mediated signalling, and this is the focus of our review.

Several isoforms of PDE3 are expressed in cardiac myocytes, and PDE3 inhibitors are used therapeutically to potentiate cAMP-mediated signalling in patients with heart failure. In the short term, these agents have the desired action of increasing myocardial contractility, but their long-term administration has been shown in several clinical trials to increase cardiovascular mortality [4–10]. This frustrating combination of beneficial and adverse effects of PDE3 inhibition presents a challenge that remains to be solved. Here we review the function of PDE3 isoforms in cardiac muscle and raise possibilities for targeting these isoforms so as to achieve more satisfying clinical outcomes.

2. The PDE3 Family of Cyclic Nucleotide Phosphodiesterases

Cyclic nucleotide phosphodiesterases comprise a superfamily of enzymes. As of now, more than 50 mammalian isoforms have been described and classified into eleven gene families (PDE1 through PDE11) defined on the basis of sensitivity to pharmacologic inhibitors, kinetic activity, and regulatory mechanisms [11]. PDE1, 2, 3, 10, and 11 hydrolyse both cAMP and cGMP; PDE4, PDE7, and PDE8 selectively hydrolyse cAMP; and PDE5, PDE6, and PDE9 selectively hydrolyse cGMP [11–13]. The N-terminal regulatory regions of phosphodiesterases contain sequences involved in post-translational modifications and protein–protein interactions that target the enzymes to specific functional compartments. Transcription start sites and alternative splicing lead to the generation of multiple different isoforms of the same family.

Enzymes in the PDE3 family are transcribed from two genes, PDE3A and PDE3B [14,15]. In the case of PDE3A, three isoforms (some prefer the term 'variants') are generated by transcription from alternative starts sites in the gene, yielding two mRNAs, as well as translation from alternative start sites in the smaller mRNA (Figure 1) [16]. As a result of these N-terminal 'deletions', the amino-acid sequences of these three isoforms differ only with respect to the lengths of their N-terminal sequences. PDE3A1 (length: 996 amino acids; MW: 109,980), which is transcribed from an upstream start site and translated from the second AUG in the PDE3A open reading frame—a possibly misleading term in this case, as no isoform translated from the first AUG has been described—has an N-terminal sequence containing hydrophobic loops that insert into intracellular membranes [17,18], as well as three sites of phosphorylation that regulate protein–protein interactions [19–21]. PDE3A2 (length: 842 amino acids; MW: 93,600) is transcribed from a downstream site in exon 1 and translated from the fourth AUG in the PDE3A open reading frame; it lacks the most N-terminal phosphorylation site and the transmembrane hydrophobic loops of PDE3A1. PDE3A3 (length: 659 amino acids; MW: 73,720) is translated from the same mRNA as PDE3A2 and lacks all of the hydrophobic loops and the upstream phosphorylation sites. These three isoforms are essentially indistinguishable with respect to their basal catalytic activity and their sensitivity to catalytic site inhibitors [22]. At this time, only one isoform of PDE3B (length: 1112 amino acids; MW: 124,333) has been described [15]. Like PDE3A1, its N-terminal sequence contains hydrophobic loops (six for PDE3B, as compared to four for PDE3A1) and phosphorylation sites, and its C-terminal sequence contains its catalytic region [23,24]. The sequence of the catalytic region of PDE3B is >80% identical to that of PDE3A (both contain a 44-amino-acid insert absent from other phosphodiesterase families), and its catalytic activity and inhibitor sensitivity are similar to those of PDE3A; the remainder of the PDE3B sequence is 20–30% identical to that of PDE3A [3].

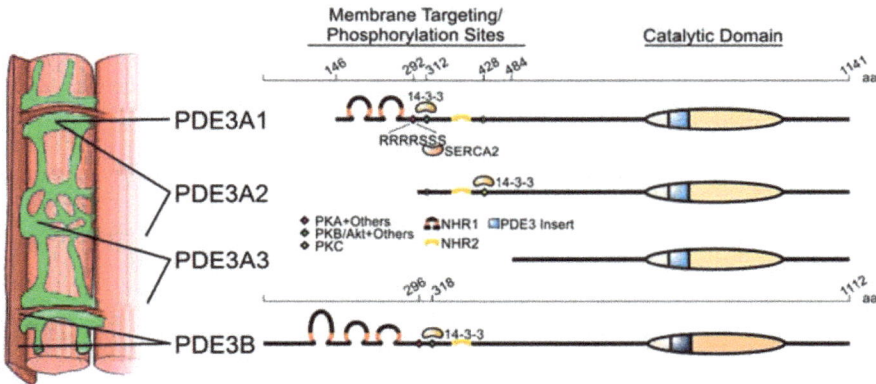

Figure 1. Structure and subcellular localisation of the PDE3 genes and their variants. Length in amino acids (aa) is provided at the top of the two PDE3 isoforms. PDE3A1 is translated from the second AUG codon of the open-reading frame found in the PDE3 mRNA. While the longest variant of PDE3A, PDE3A1, is mainly localised to the sarcoplasmic reticulum, PDE3A2 and PDE3A3 are found both in membranes and cytoplasm. PDE3B is mainly localised to plasma membrane invaginations known as T tubules. Coloured diamonds indicate phosphorylation sites. Selected PDE3-interacting proteins are listed where the precise binding sequences are known. Membrane-associated N-terminal hydrophobic regions 1 and 2 (NHR1 and 2) are depicted as loops. The catalytic domain, highly conserved between PDE3A and PDE3B, is indicated as a striped oval that includes the 44-amino-acid insert characteristic of PDE3 isoforms.

3. Intracellular Localisation of PDE3A and PDE3B in Cardiac Myocytes and Their Protein-Protein Interactions

Cyclic nucleotide-mediated signalling is highly compartmentalised in cardiac myocytes, and the roles of individual phosphodiesterases in regulating cAMP- and cGMP-mediated signalling depend upon their intracellular localisation. While PDE3A and PDE3B are both expressed in cardiac myocytes (PDE3A more abundantly [25]), their intracellular distributions are distinct, with PDE3A localised mainly to the sarcoplasmic reticulum and PDE3B to T tubules in proximity to mitochondria [26] (Figure 1). PDE3 activity is also associated with nuclear membranes in cardiac myocytes [27], though the specific isoforms have not been delineated. Furthermore, in subcellular preparations from cardiac muscle, PDE3A1 is recovered solely in microsomal fractions, while PDE3A2 and PDE3A3 are recovered in cytosolic as well as microsomal fractions [16]. This corresponds to studies in cells transfected with PDE3A1- and PDE3B-derived constructs that show that the N-terminal hydrophobic loops in these isoforms direct the insertion of these proteins into lipid membranes [17,18].

3.1. PDE3A

The precise intracellular localisation of PDE3 isoforms depends upon their interactions with anchoring, scaffold, and adaptor proteins that recruit the enzyme to multiprotein signalling complexes [28–33]. Localised A-kinase anchoring proteins (AKAPs) tether protein kinase A (PKA) and other signalling proteins—adenylyl cyclases, phosphatases, Epacs, PDEs and other effector molecules—to 'signalosomes' that allow selective phosphorylation of individual PKA substrates [31–34].

PDE3 has long been known to be associated with the sarcoplasmic reticulum of cardiac myocytes [35,36]. Confocal microscopy studies more recently demonstrated co-localisation of PDE3A with SERCA2, AKAP18, phospholamban, and desmin in the Z-bands of cardiac myocytes [37,38]. PDE3A was found to be a constituent of a multiprotein complex in the sarcoplasmic reticulum containing AKAP18, phospholamban, and SERCA2 [38,39]. Addition of cAMP to microsomes from human heart results in the phosphorylation of phospholamban by endogenous PKA; this leads to a dissociation of phospholamban from SERCA2 and an increase in SERCA2 activity, and this effect is potentiated by PDE3 inhibition [38] (Figure 2). Although PDE3 and PDE4 have both been found to co-immunoprecipitate with AKAP-based signalosomes from human and mouse myocardium and modulate effects of cAMP on L-type Ca^{2+} channels, ryanodine-sensitive Ca^{2+} channels, and SERCA2 [40–43], only PDE3 inhibition potentiates the PKA-mediated phosphorylation of phospholamban and the consequent stimulation of SERCA2 activity [37]. The role of PDE3A in modulating these effects is the likely explanation for the inotropic actions of PDE3 inhibition.

Furthermore, while PDE3 isoforms regulate the phosphorylation of other proteins through the cAMP/PKA pathway, they are themselves substrates for protein kinases that modulate their catalytic activity and protein–protein interactions [19,21,44–47]. The incorporation of PDE3A into the SERCA2 complex is an example. In co-immunoprecipitation experiments, phosphorylation of endogenous PDE3A by PKA increases its interactions with SERCA2, caveolin-3, PKA regulatory subunit (PKARII), PP2A, and AKAP18 [38]. Studies with recombinant proteins showed that phosphorylation of PDE3A by PKA increased its co-immunoprecipitation with SERCA2a and AKAP18, suggesting that PDE3A interacts directly with both proteins in a phosphorylation-dependent manner [38]. Deletion of the N-terminal region of PDE3A1/PDE3A2 blocked PKA-induced phosphorylation of PDE3A and its interaction with recombinant SERCA2. Of particular interest is the sequence RRRRSSS (amino acids 288–294 of the open reading frame, which are found only in PDE3A1), which provides three serines that can be phosphorylated in vitro by different kinases under different conditions [19]. The introduction of serine-to-alanine substitutions at S292-4 identified this sequence as the principal site responsible for regulating the interactions of PDE3A1 with SERCA2 (Figure 1).

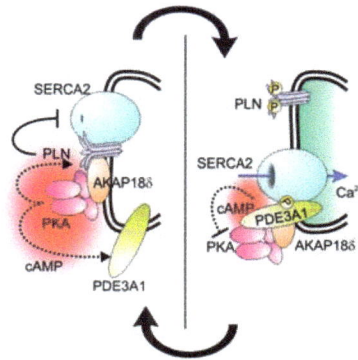

Figure 2. Control of SERCA2 activity by PDE3A. Left panel: Under resting conditions, phospholamban (PLN) binds to SERCA2, whose activity it inhibits, as well as AKAP18δ on the cytoplasmic surface of the sarcoplasmic reticulum (double black line). Upon β-adrenergic receptor-stimulated cAMP production, PKA associated with AKAP18δ is activated and phosphorylates PLN (upper dotted line) and PDE3A1 (lower dotted line). This leads to the condition shown in the right panel, where phosphorylated PLN detaches from SERCA2 and loses its inhibitory action. As a consequence, SERCA2-dependent Ca^{2+} uptake into the lumen of the sarcoplasmic reticulum is stimulated (encircled by the double black line). At the same time, phosphorylated PDE3A1 binds to SERCA2 and increases its cAMP-hydrolytic activity, which limits the extent to which β-adrenergic receptor-mediated signalling amplifies intracellular Ca^{2+} cycling.

The absence of the S292-4 site from PDE3A2 and PDE3A3 establishes a PDE3A1-specific mechanism for recruitment of PDE3A to the SERCA2 complex. The protein–protein interactions of PDE3 isoforms are distinct in other ways as well, as has been described for the phosphorylation-dependent interactions of PDE3A1, PDE3A2, and PDE3B with 14-3-3 [20,21,48–50]. The common sequence of PDE3A1 and PDE3A2 includes two 14-3-3-binding sites: S428, a PKC site; and S312, a PKA/PKB (alternatively referred to Akt) site that resembles S318, a 14-3-3-binding site in PDE3B [48,49] (Figure 1). In vitro, PDE3A1 is preferentially phosphorylated by PKA at S312, whereas PDE3A2 is preferentially phosphorylated by PKC at S428; in preparations from human hearts, PDE3A1 is phosphorylated primarily at S312, while PDE3A2 is phosphorylated primarily at S428 [50]. Furthermore, in transfected HEK293 cells, the phosphorylation-dependent interactomes of PDE3A1 and PDE3A2 are distinct [50]: PDE3A1 interacts with the $5\text{-HT}_{4(b)}$ receptor, for example, while PDE3A2, PDE3A3, and PDE3B do not [51]. These unique protein–protein interactions may provide opportunities for isoform-specific targeting of the protein–protein interactions of individual isoforms.

In cardiac myocytes, PDE3A is also part of a multiprotein complex containing the unconventional AKAP PI3Kγ [52]. While PI3Kγ directly binds the RII subunit of the PKA holoenzyme, how PDE3A contacts the complex is still unclear, though a likely intermediate is the PI3Kγ interactor p84/p87 [53]. Within this complex, PKA exerts a negative feedback regulation by phosphorylating and activating the different associated PDE isoforms, including PDE3A [39]. In line with the role of PDE3A (and PDE4A/B) in controlling SERCA2, loss of the scaffold function of PI3Kγ leads to cAMP elevation and PKA-mediated hyperphosphorylation of phospholamban and *L*-type Ca^{2+} channels [39,54] (Figure 3, left panel). In hearts lacking PI3Kγ and subjected to pressure overload, this effect causes cAMP elevation, contractile dysfunction, and increased mortality due to lethal arrhythmic events such as sustained ventricular tachycardia [39] (Figure 3, right panel). Interestingly, this abnormally increased cAMP accumulation appears to be selectively associated with signalling through β-adrenergic receptors localised to T tubules [55]. This would suggest that the PI3Kγ PKA/PDE complex is part of an 'insulating' system that blocks 'leakage' of cAMP from this compartment to the sarcoplasmic reticulum [39]. In heart failure, the expression of various elements of the PI3Kγ PKA/PDE3A-containing complex change their stoichiometric ratios, with reduced expression of p84/87 and coincident increased expression of PI3Kγ. This causes a dysfunctional cAMP regulation potentially contributing to the increase in ventricular arrhythmias associated with heart failure [52].

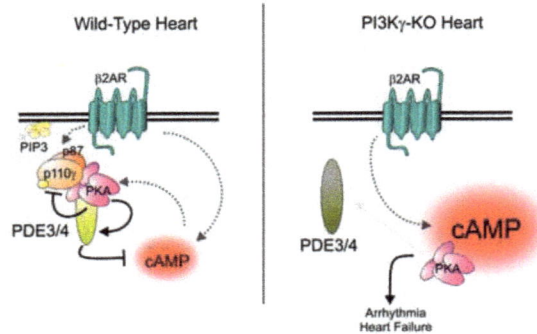

Figure 3. Regulation of PDE3 and PDE4 by the AKAP function of PI3Kγ. Left panel: Regulation of PI3Kγ and phosphodiesterase activity in healthy conditions. Upon stimulation of β-adrenergic receptors, cAMP production is promoted but simultaneously constrained by the activation of a negative feedback loop involving the scaffold function of PI3Kγ that directly binds the PKA holoenzyme containing the RII regulatory subunit as well as PDE3s and PDE4s. PKA activation leads to the phosphorylation of these phosphodiesterases and the consequent increase in their activity that, in turn, reduces cAMP levels. At the same time, PKA phosphorylates and inhibits PI3Kγ, thus blocking the classical PI3K pathway signalling. Right panel: In the absence of PI3Kγ, PKA is displaced from PDE3 and PDE4 enzymes and is unable to efficiently stimulate their activity. As a consequence, cAMP levels rise and cAMP diffuses to compartments that β-adrenergic receptor-mediated signalling does not usually affect.

3.2. PDE3B

In contrast to PDE3A, PDE3B is mainly located in caveolin-3-rich areas of the plasma membrane and, in cardiac myocytes, in the T tubules (Figure 1). This indicates that the two PDE3 genes are specifically involved in the regulation of spatially and functionally distinct pools of cAMP. In line with this view, while PDE3A is involved in the regulation of contractility, PDE3B appears more connected to the regulation of metabolism. PDE3B is also known to have a role in the liver, pancreatic β cells, and in the brown and white adipose tissue where it is involved in the control of the anti-lipolytic effect of insulin, generally in contrast to β-adrenergic signalling [56,57]. In the heart, the specific inactivation of PDE3A causes alterations in basal cardiac contractility, while genetic ablation of PDE3B has no major impact on contractility but protects the myocardium from ischemic damage [26,37]. Interestingly, the protective effect of PDE3 inhibitors in ischemic heart preconditioning had been known for several years, but the precise nature of the PDE3 isoform only emerged with studies in knockout mice that excluded a role of PDE3A. The specific localisation of PDE3B in T tubules, and particularly both in dyads and in close proximity to mitochondria, suggests that this particular phosphodiesterase plays a role in modulating energy metabolism. Elevation in cAMP concentration in this location might mediate cardioprotective signals that improve mitochondrial function and energy supply during ischaemia/reperfusion, where mitochondrial Ca^{2+} overload and consequent mitochondrial permeability transition (MPT) pore opening, oxidative stress, and apoptosis contribute to injury [58]. In hearts lacking PDE3B, mitochondria are enriched in Bcl-2, produce lower amounts of reactive oxygen species, and show more numerous contacts with T tubules. In response to ischaemia, mitochondria from PDE3B-deficient cardiac myocytes are more resistant to Ca^{2+}-induced opening of the MPT pore, and associate with caveolin-3-enriched membrane subfractions containing cardioprotective proteins. The recruitment of these cardioprotective proteins to these subfractions is PKA-dependent, and can be reproduced in wild-type mice by PDE3 inhibition [26].

The nature of the localization signal that keeps PDE3B in such spatially and functionally distinct cellular subdomains remains unknown. Various reports indicate that PDE3B can be recruited to different multiprotein complexes with distinct properties. In adipocytes, for example, treatment with insulin increases the phosphorylation of PDE3B associated with internal membranes, promoting its interactions with IRS-1 (insulin receptor substrate-1), IRS-2, PI3K p85 (p85-subunit of phosphoinositide 3-kinase), PKB (protein kinase B), HSP-90 (heat-shock protein 90), 14-3-3, and a 50 kD protein [46,47,56,59,60]. Conversely, treatment with β_3-adrenergic receptor agonists increases the phosphorylation of PDE3B associated with caveolin-1 in caveolae, promoting interactions with β_3-adrenergic receptors, PKA-RII (PKA regulatory subunit), and hormone-sensitive lipase [46,61]. Whether these associations also occur in cardiac myocytes is not yet clear. PDE3B has been reported to weakly associate in a complex containing the unconventional AKAP PI3Kγ, especially with overexpression in HEK293 cells [53,62]. Nonetheless, the significant effects on contractility and rhythm detected in mice lacking PI3Kγ indicate that the determinant of the cardiac phenotype is the ability of PI3Kγ to form more stable complexes with other phosphodiesterases, including PDE3A and PDE4A/B [39].

Of note, however, is that PDE3B can be phosphorylated not only by PKA but also by PKB, the main effector of the PI3K pathway. Although the weak interaction between PI3Kγ and PDE3B reported in the heart awaits further experimental confirmation, severe reduction of the G protein-coupled receptor-driven PI3K pathway by the concomitant loss of PI3Kγ and PI3K3 has been shown to lead to reduced PDE3B phosphorylation and activity in neurons [63]. Nonetheless, whereas the specific association of PI3Kγ with β-adrenergic signalling in T tubules supports at least a spatial co-localisation of both PI3K and PDE3B [39,53], experiments in knockout mice indicate that PI3Kγ and PDE3B might be part of different functional complexes. On the other hand, the association of PI3Kγ with PKA triggers a negative feedback loop where PKA phosphorylates and inhibits PI3Kγ itself. Interestingly, loss of PDE3B in the heart leads to an unexpectedly strong elevation of cAMP [26], which likely remains spatially confined due to the normal activity of the other phosphodiesterases. Whether this elevated cAMP and PKA activity influences PI3Kγ catalytic activity and, indirectly, the PKB signalling axis is yet to be determined. As enhanced PI3Kγ signalling is involved in the downregulation of β-adrenergic receptor density on the cell surface and, generally, in cardiac myocyte decompensation under stress, PDE3B inhibition could reduce a detrimental signal [64]. Inhibitors specifically distinguishing PDE3B from PDE3A are not currently available, but specific targeting of PDE3B may be therapeutically useful for ischaemia/reperfusion injury.

4. Inotropic Actions of PDE3A Inhibition

As discussed above, PDE3A is part of a multiprotein complex in the sarcoplasmic reticulum through which phospholamban phosphorylation and SERCA2 activity are regulated, and PDE3 inhibition potentiates the stimulatory effects of cAMP on SERCA2 activity in microsomes from cardiac muscle. These effects would be expected to increase contractility by increasing the amplitude of intracellular Ca^{2+} transients. Experiments in mice with selective ablation of PDE3A and PDE3B indicate that inotropic responses to PDE3 inhibition are attributable specifically to inhibition of PDE3A. Phospholamban phosphorylation, SERCA2 activity, intracellular Ca^{2+} cycling, and contractility are increased—and inotropic responses to PDE3 inhibition are eliminated—in *Pde3a*$^{-/-}$ mice; none of these effects are observed in *Pde3b*$^{-/-}$ mice [37]. Furthermore, myocardial contractility in mice is reduced when PDE3A1 is overexpressed [65]. Total intracellular cAMP levels are higher in *Pde3b*$^{-/-}$ mice than in *Pde3a*$^{-/-}$ mice [26], indicating that this is not simply a 'mass effect' reflecting the higher abundance of PDE3A relative to PDE3B in cardiac myocytes but is instead due to the specific functional consequences of the intracellular localisation of these isoforms. (A unique role of PDE3B in mitigating reperfusion injury, discussed below, is further evidence along these lines [26].)

5. Pro-Apoptotic Actions of PDE3A Inhibition

PDE3 inhibition in rats and *Pde3a* ablation in mice lead to increases in the phosphorylation of cAMP response element-binding protein (CREB) and consequent increases in the expression of inducible cAMP early repressors (ICER's), promoting apoptosis [66,67]. Inhibition of PDE3, and especially of PDE3A, by milrinone might involve a phospho-CREB-induced increase in the expression of ICER, with consequent apoptosis and myocardial pathological remodelling. Conversely, there is evidence that increased PDE3A activity, achieved by overexpression in mice, reduces ICER expression, increases Bcl-2 expression, and protects cardiac myocytes against apoptosis [65]. In fact, specific overexpression of myocardial PDE3A1 in transgenic mice confers protection during ischaemia/reperfusion by decreasing cAMP signalling and phosphorylation of CREB, resulting in decreased expression of ICER and reduced apoptosis [65]. PDE3 activity is associated with nuclear membranes in cardiac myocytes [27], and it is possible that the activity localised to this region is responsible for these pro-apoptotic changes in gene expression.

6. Pro-Hypertrophic Actions of PDE3A Inhibition

PDE3 inhibition has pro-hypertrophic actions in neonatal rat ventricular myocytes [68]. These effects are essentially reproduced by expression of a dominant-negative form of PDE3A2 induced by a single amino acid substitution in the C-terminal region that renders the protein catalytically inactive but otherwise intact [68]. This dominant-negative construct presumably functions as a competitive inhibitor of the localising protein–protein interactions of the native protein to disrupt its intracellular targeting; this is further evidence that the intracellular targeting of PDE3 isoforms is as important as their catalytic activity. The antihypertrophic effect is especially interesting in view of the description of a set of genetically unrelated missense mutations within a five-amino-acid sequence in PDE3A that increase catalytic activity and lead to a syndrome of brachydactyly and hypertension [69,70]. The hypertension is likely attributable to increased cGMP hydrolysis in vascular smooth muscle; the resulting decrease in intracellular cGMP content would lead to a combination of vasoconstriction and vessel wall hyperplasia. Despite the severe hypertension, however, patients with this syndrome have strikingly low levels of cardiac hypertrophy [71]. This suggests that an increase in PDE3A activity in cardiac myocytes may in fact be antihypertrophic, consistent with the benefits of PDE3A1 overexpression with respect to pathologic remodelling in animal models discussed above [65].

7. Clinical Experience with PDE3 Inhibition in the Treatment of Heart Disease

With respect to cardiac disease, PDE3 has been of interest principally as a target for increasing contractility in patients with heart failure, a condition in which decreases in β-adrenergic receptor density and increases in Gαi and β-adrenergic receptor kinase activity in cardiac myocytes attenuate cAMP generation lead to decreases in cAMP content, protein phosphorylation and the amplitude of intracellular Ca^{2+} transients [72–81]. Inhibiting PDE3 has the effect of compensating to some extent for these changes by blocking cAMP hydrolysis and potentiating cAMP-mediated signalling, leading to an increase in myocardial contractility [82–88].

This short-term benefit, unfortunately, is outweighed by an increase in mortality from sudden cardiac death of ~3% per year when these drugs are administered chronically [4–10]. The explanation for this increase is unclear (though it seems restricted to patients in whom PDE3 inhibition is used to treat contractile failure; no increase in mortality has been seen when the PDE3 inhibitor cilostazol has been used to treat intermittent claudication [89]). Overexpression of SERCA2 in animal models of ischaemia/reperfusion and chronic heart failure is anti-arrhythmic [90,91]. On the other hand, an increase in the phosphorylation of *L*-type and ryanodine-sensitive Ca^{2+} channels may be pro-arrhythmic [40–43]. It seems more probable, however, based on the fact that short-term administration of these agents is well tolerated, that mechanisms other than direct pro-arrhythmic actions are involved, and that the pro-apoptotic and pro-hypertrophic effects of PDE3 inhibition described above induce pathologic changes in the myocardium that increase the proclivity toward malignant arrhythmias.

8. Selective Targeting of PDE3 Isoforms

The fact that PDE3A and PDE3B have different roles in cardiac myocytes, with PDE3A controlling the pathways responsible for inotropic effects, raises the possibility that targeting PDE3A selectively—or, perhaps even better, selectively targeting one of its three known variants—might improve contractility without increasing sudden cardiac death (as noted above, PDE3A1 is restricted in its distribution to intracellular membranes, so that its inhibition may be less likely to elicit pro-apoptotic and pro-arrhythmic actions [16]). The catalytic activities, substrate affinities, and inhibitor sensitivities of PDE3A1, PDE3A2, and PDE3A3 are identical, making it impossible to selectively target the active sites of individual PDE3A variants [22]. The similarity of the PDE3B active site to the PDE3A active site suggested that selectivity between these two proteins would also prove challenging. Recently, however, investigators described a compound with a tenfold higher affinity for PDE3A relative to PDE3B [92], so this supposition needs to be reconsidered. It is not obvious how targeting all PDE3A isoforms without targeting PDE3B would confer a therapeutic advantage, however. To our knowledge, no compound with a significantly higher affinity for PDE3B relative to PDE3A has been reported.

Another possibility is that of targeting individual isoforms not through their active sites but through the protein–protein interactions by which they are localised intracellularly. As noted above, PDE3A1 and PDE3A2 are recruited, by phosphorylation within their N-terminal sequences, to a SERCA2/phospholamban/AKAP/PKA complex in the sarcoplasmic reticulum [37,93]. As a result of this recruitment, PDE3 inhibition has a particularly pronounced effect in potentiating phospholamban phosphorylation and increasing SERCA2 activity, leading to an increase in SERCA2 activity and intracellular Ca^{2+} [38]. Experiments using recombinant proteins have demonstrated direct interactions of PDE3A1 and PDE3A2 with both SERCA2 and AKAP18, and have shown that the interaction of PDE3A1 with SERCA2 is dependent upon its phosphorylation at serine 293, a site within its unique N-terminal extension (Figure 1) [38]. These findings indicate that the protein–protein interactions of the PDE3A isoforms responsible for inotropic responses are highly individualised, opening an avenue to isoform-selective targeting with a high degree of precision. In fact, this approach to isoform-selective targeting—displacing PDE3A from specific multiprotein complexes—has the added benefit of compartment selectivity, which is likely its most important advantage. Conventional PDE3 inhibitors target the enzyme regardless of its intracellular location; this can raise cAMP content globally within the cell, resulting in a combination of pro-apoptotic, pro-hypertrophic, and inotropic [66–68]. Blocking the protein–protein interactions that integrate PDE3A into SERCA2 complexes could lead to a selective increase in cAMP content in the vicinity of phospholamban and SERCA2 so as to amplify intracellular Ca^{2+} cycling and increase contractility without the deleterious pro-arrhythmic, pro-apoptotic, and pro-hypertrophic consequences (Figure 4).

On the other hand, the protein–protein interactions that localise PDE3B intracellularly may be targets through which the cardioprotective effects of PDE3B ablation can be elicited without the adverse pro-hypertrophic and pro-arrhythmic consequences of PDE3A inhibition. The feasibility of this approach has been demonstrated in experiments using peptides that block the protein–protein interactions of cyclic nucleotide phosphodiesterases. In one example, peptide-array scanning identified a cell-permeant peptide based on a sequence in the N-terminus of PDE3B through which it is incorporated into an Epac1/PI3Kγ complex in vascular endothelial cells. This peptide has been shown to block the integration of PDE3B into this complex, increasing the activation of Epac1 by cAMP and promoting intracellular tubule formation, cell adhesion, and cell spreading [94].

J. Cardiovasc. Dev. Dis. **2018**, *5*, 10

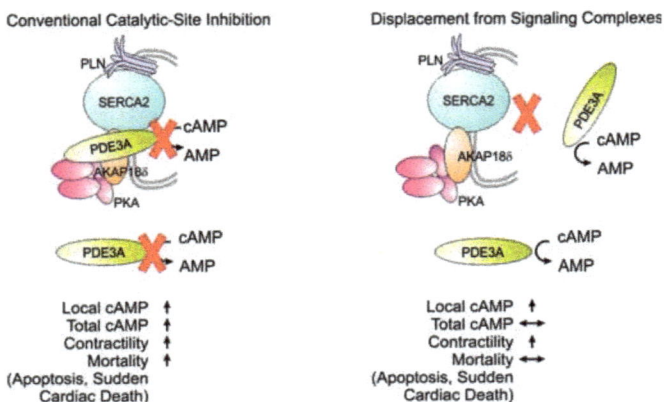

Figure 4. Targeting PDE3A through protein–protein interactions. Conventional PDE3 inhibition activates cAMP-mediated signalling in multiple intracellular compartments, leading possibly to a combination of beneficial and adverse effects. Blocking the protein–protein interactions through which PDE3A is integrated into the SERCA2 complex may stimulate intracellular Ca^{2+} cycling without the adverse effects.

9. Conclusions

Several isoforms in the PDE3 family are expressed in cardiac myocytes, where they have important roles regulating signalling pathways involved in inotropic, pro-apoptotic, and pro-hypertrophic responses. Inhibition of myocardial PDE3 activity is an established therapeutic strategy for increasing contractility in patients with heart failure, but an increase in sudden cardiac death in patients treated chronically with existing PDE3 inhibitors has limited the benefits. Targeting individual PDE3A isoforms in specific intracellular targets could potentially yield inotropic responses without this adverse effect, while targeting PDE3B could have beneficial actions in ischaemia/reperfusion injury. Recent discoveries open the possibility of selectively inhibiting PDE3A or PDE3B at their catalytic sites or, probably more interestingly, of targeting their unique protein–protein interactions to yield compartment-specific effects on intracellular signalling. Time will tell.

Acknowledgments: Matthew Movsesian was supported by Medical Research Funds from the United States Department of Veterans Affairs and a Univa grant from the Eunice Kennedy Shriver National Institute of Child Health and Human Development (R37HD014939; Laurinda Jaffe, Principal Investigator). Faiyaz Ahmad was supported by the NHLBI Intramural Research Program, National Institutes of Health, United States of America. Emilio Hirsch was supported by the grant Telethon GGP14106.

Author Contributions: All three authors wrote the paper. The comments expressed here are those of the authors, and do not reflect official positions of the National Heart, Lung and Blood Institute or National Institutes of Health.

Conflicts of Interest: Matthew Movsesian is the author of patents EP1430140, USPTO 8722866, USPTO 9513288 and USPTO 9513289 issued to the United States Department of Veterans Affairs relating to the targeting of PDE3 isoforms.

J. Cardiovasc. Dev. Dis. **2018**, *5*, 10

Abbreviations

aa	amino acid
AKAP	A-kinase-anchoring protein
β_2-AR	β_2-adrenergic receptor
cAMP	Cyclic adenosine monophosphate
IRS	Insulin-receptor substrate
NHR	N-terminal hydrophobic region
PLN	Phospholamban
PKA	cAMP-dependent protein kinase
PKA-RII	cAMP-dependent protein kinase regulatory subunit II
PKB (AKT)	Protein kinase B
PKC	Protein kinase C
PI3Kγ	Phosphoinositide 3-kinase γ
PIP3	Phosphatidylinositol (3,4,5)-triphosphate
p110γ	Phosphoinositide 3-kinase γ (PI3Kγ) catalytic subunit
p87	PI3Kγ regulatory subunit (also known as p87PIKAP p87-PI3K adapter protein)
SERCA2	Sarcoplasmic/endoplasmic reticulum calcium ATPase-2

References

1. Grant, P.G.; Colman, R.W. Purification and characterization of a human platelet cyclic nucleotide phosphodiesterase. *Biochemistry* **1984**, *23*, 1801–1807. [CrossRef] [PubMed]
2. Boyes, S.; Loten, E.G. Purification of an insulin-sensitive cyclic AMP phosphodiesterase from rat liver. *Eur. J. Biochem.* **1988**, *174*, 303–309. [CrossRef] [PubMed]
3. Degerman, E.; Belfrage, P.; Manganiello, V.C. Structure, localization, and regulation of cGMP-inhibited phosphodiesterase (PDE3). *J. Biol. Chem.* **1997**, *272*, 6823–6826. [CrossRef] [PubMed]
4. DiBianco, R.; Shabetai, R.; Kostuk, W.; Moran, J.; Schlant, R.C.; Wright, R. A comparison of oral milrinone, digoxin, and their combination in the treatment of patients with chronic heart failure. *N. Engl. J. Med.* **1989**, *320*, 677–683. [CrossRef] [PubMed]
5. Uretsky, B.F.; Jessup, M.; Konstam, M.A.; Dec, G.W.; Leier, C.V.; Benotti, J.; Murali, S.; Herrmann, H.C.; Sandberg, J.A. Multicenter trial of oral enoximone in patients with moderate to moderately severe congestive heart failure. Lack of benefit compared with placebo. Enoximone Multicenter Trial Group. *Circulation* **1990**, *82*, 774–780. [CrossRef] [PubMed]
6. Narahara, K.A. Oral enoximone therapy in chronic heart failure: A placebo-controlled randomized trial. The Western Enoximone Study Group. *Am. Heart J.* **1991**, *121*, 1471–1479. [CrossRef]
7. Packer, M.; Carver, J.R.; Rodeheffer, R.J.; Ivanhoe, R.J.; DiBianco, R.; Zeldis, S.M.; Hendrix, G.H.; Bommer, W.J.; Elkayam, U.; Kukin, M.L.; et al. Effect of oral milrinone on mortality in severe chronic heart failure. The PROMISE Study Research Group. *N. Engl. J. Med.* **1991**, *325*, 1468–1475. [CrossRef] [PubMed]
8. Packer, M.; Narahara, K.A.; Elkayam, U.; Sullivan, J.M.; Pearle, D.L.; Massie, B.M.; Creager, M.A. Double-blind, placebo-controlled study of the efficacy of flosequinan in patients with chronic heart failure. Principal Investigators of the REFLECT Study. *J. Am. Coll. Cardiol.* **1993**, *22*, 65–72. [CrossRef]
9. Cohn, J.N.; Goldstein, S.O.; Greenberg, B.H.; Lorell, B.H.; Bourge, R.C.; Jaski, B.E.; Gottlieb, S.O.; McGrew, F., 3rd; DeMets, D.L.; White, B.G. A dose-dependent increase in mortality with vesnarinone among patients with severe heart failure. Vesnarinone Trial Investigators. *N. Engl. J. Med.* **1998**, *339*, 1810–1816. [CrossRef] [PubMed]
10. Amsallem, E.; Kasparian, C.; Haddour, G.; Boissel, J.P.; Nony, P. Phosphodiesterase III inhibitors for heart failure. *Cochrane Database Syst. Rev.* **2005**. [CrossRef] [PubMed]
11. Maurice, D.H.; Ke, H.; Ahmad, F.; Wang, Y.; Chung, J.; Manganiello, V.C. Advances in targeting cyclic nucleotide phosphodiesterases. *Nat. Rev. Drug Discov.* **2014**, *13*, 290–314. [CrossRef] [PubMed]
12. Keravis, T.; Lugnier, C. Cyclic nucleotide phosphodiesterases (PDE) and peptide motifs. *Curr. Pharm. Des.* **2010**, *16*, 1114–1125. [CrossRef] [PubMed]
13. Francis, S.H.; Blount, M.A.; Corbin, J.D. Mammalian cyclic nucleotide phosphodiesterases: Molecular mechanisms and physiological functions. *Physiol. Rev.* **2011**, *91*, 651–690. [CrossRef] [PubMed]

14. Meacci, E.; Taira, M.; Moos, M., Jr.; Smith, C.J.; Movsesian, M.A.; Degerman, E.; Belfrage, P.; Manganiello, V. Molecular cloning and expression of human myocardial cGMP-inhibited cAMP phosphodiesterase. *Proc. Natl. Acad. Sci. USA* **1992**, *89*, 3721–3725. [CrossRef] [PubMed]
15. Miki, T.; Taira, M.; Hockman, S.; Shimada, F.; Lieman, J.; Napolitano, M.; Ward, D.; Taira, M.; Makino, H.; Manganiello, V.C. Characterization of the cDNA and gene encoding human PDE3B, the cGIP1 isoform of the human cyclic GMP-inhibited cyclic nucleotide phosphodiesterase family. *Genomics* **1996**, *36*, 476–485. [CrossRef] [PubMed]
16. Wechsler, J.; Choi, Y.H.; Krall, J.; Ahmad, F.; Manganiello, V.C.; Movsesian, M.A. Isoforms of cyclic nucleotide phosphodiesterase PDE3A in cardiac myocytes. *J. Biol. Chem.* **2002**, *277*, 38072–38078. [CrossRef] [PubMed]
17. Kenan, Y.; Murata, T.; Shakur, Y.; Degerman, E.; Manganiello, V.C. Functions of the N-terminal region of cyclic nucleotide phosphodiesterase 3 (PDE 3) isoforms. *J. Biol. Chem.* **2000**, *275*, 12331–12338. [CrossRef] [PubMed]
18. Shakur, Y.; Takeda, K.; Kenan, Y.; Yu, Z.X.; Rena, G.; Brandt, D.; Houslay, M.D.; Degerman, E.; Ferrans, V.J.; Manganiello, V.C. Membrane localization of cyclic nucleotide phosphodiesterase 3 (PDE3). Two N-terminal domains are required for the efficient targeting to, and association of, PDE3 with endoplasmic reticulum. *J. Biol. Chem.* **2000**, *275*, 38749–38761. [CrossRef] [PubMed]
19. Han, S.J.; Vaccari, S.; Nedachi, T.; Andersen, C.B.; Kovacina, K.S.; Roth, R.A.; Conti, M. Protein kinase B/Akt phosphorylation of PDE3A and its role in mammalian oocyte maturation. *EMBO J.* **2006**, *25*, 5716–5725. [CrossRef] [PubMed]
20. Pozuelo Rubio, M.; Campbell, D.G.; Morrice, N.A.; Mackintosh, C. Phosphodiesterase 3A binds to 14-3-3 proteins in response to PMA-induced phosphorylation of Ser428. *Biochem. J.* **2005**, *392*, 163–172. [CrossRef] [PubMed]
21. Hunter, R.W.; Mackintosh, C.; Hers, I. Protein kinase C-mediated phosphorylation and activation of PDE3A regulate cAMP levels in human platelets. *J. Biol. Chem.* **2009**, *284*, 12339–12348. [CrossRef] [PubMed]
22. Hambleton, R.; Krall, J.; Tikishvili, E.; Honeggar, M.; Ahmad, F.; Manganiello, V.C.; Movsesian, M.A. Isoforms of cyclic nucleotide phosphodiesterase PDE3 and their contribution to cAMP hydrolytic activity in subcellular fractions of human myocardium. *J. Biol. Chem.* **2005**, *280*, 39168–39174. [CrossRef] [PubMed]
23. Leroy, M.J.; Degerman, E.; Taira, M.; Murata, T.; Wang, L.H.; Movsesian, M.A.; Meacci, E.; Manganiello, V.C. Characterization of two recombinant PDE3 (cGMP-inhibited cyclic nucleotide phosphodiesterase) isoforms, RcGIP1 and HcGIP2, expressed in NIH 3006 murine fibroblasts and Sf9 insect cells. *Biochemistry* **1996**, *35*, 10194–10202. [CrossRef] [PubMed]
24. Taira, M.; Hockman, S.C.; Calvo, J.C.; Taira, M.; Belfrage, P.; Manganiello, V.C. Molecular cloning of the rat adipocyte hormone-sensitive cyclic GMP-inhibited cyclic nucleotide phosphodiesterase. *J. Biol. Chem.* **1993**, *268*, 18573–18579. [PubMed]
25. Reinhardt, R.R.; Chin, E.; Zhou, J.; Taira, M.; Murata, T.; Manganiello, V.C.; Bondy, C.A. Distinctive anatomical patterns of gene expression for cGMP-inhibited cyclic nucleotide phosphodiesterases. *J. Clin. Investig.* **1995**, *95*, 1528–1538. [CrossRef] [PubMed]
26. Chung, Y.W.; Lagranha, C.; Chen, Y.; Sun, J.; Tong, G.; Hockman, S.C.; Ahmad, F.; Esfahani, S.G.; Bae, D.H.; Polidovitch, N.; et al. Targeted disruption of PDE3B, but not PDE3A, protects murine heart from ischemia/reperfusion injury. *Proc. Natl. Acad. Sci. USA* **2015**, *112*, E2253–E2262. [CrossRef] [PubMed]
27. Lugnier, C.; Keravis, T.; Le Bec, A.; Pauvert, O.; Proteau, S.; Rousseau, E. Characterization of cyclic nucleotide phosphodiesterase isoforms associated to isolated cardiac nuclei. *Biochim. Biophys. Acta* **1999**, *1472*, 431–446. [CrossRef]
28. Zaccolo, M. cAMP signal transduction in the heart: Understanding spatial control for the development of novel therapeutic strategies. *Br. J. Pharmacol.* **2009**, *158*, 50–60. [CrossRef] [PubMed]
29. Houslay, M.D. Underpinning compartmentalised cAMP signalling through targeted cAMP breakdown. *Trends Biochem. Sci.* **2010**, *35*, 91–100. [CrossRef] [PubMed]
30. Raymond, D.R.; Wilson, L.S.; Carter, R.L.; Maurice, D.H. Numerous distinct PKA-, or EPAC-based, signalling complexes allow selective phosphodiesterase 3 and phosphodiesterase 4 coordination of cell adhesion. *Cell Signal.* **2007**, *19*, 2507–2518. [CrossRef] [PubMed]
31. Scott, J.D.; Santana, L.F. A-kinase anchoring proteins: Getting to the heart of the matter. *Circulation* **2010**, *121*, 1264–1271. [CrossRef] [PubMed]

32. Stangherlin, A.; Zaccolo, M. Local termination of 3′-5′-cyclic adenosine monophosphate signals: The role of A kinase anchoring protein-tethered phosphodiesterases. *J. Cardiovasc. Pharmacol.* **2011**, *58*, 345–353. [CrossRef] [PubMed]

33. Kritzer, M.D.; Li, J.; Dodge-Kafka, K.; Kapiloff, M.S. AKAPs: The architectural underpinnings of local cAMP signaling. *J. Mol. Cell. Cardiol.* **2012**, *52*, 351–358. [CrossRef] [PubMed]

34. Perino, A.; Ghigo, A.; Scott, J.D.; Hirsch, E. Anchoring proteins as regulators of signaling pathways. *Circ. Res.* **2012**, *111*, 482–492. [CrossRef] [PubMed]

35. Movsesian, M.A.; Smith, C.J.; Krall, J.; Bristow, M.R.; Manganiello, V.C. Sarcoplasmic reticulum-associated cyclic adenosine 5′-monophosphate phosphodiesterase activity in normal and failing human hearts. *J. Clin. Investig.* **1991**, *88*, 15–19. [CrossRef] [PubMed]

36. Lugnier, C.; Muller, B.; Le Bec, A.; Beaudry, C.; Rousseau, E. Characterization of indolidan- and rolipram-sensitive cyclic nucleotide phosphodiesterases in canine and human cardiac microsomal fractions. *J. Pharmacol. Exp. Ther.* **1993**, *265*, 1142–1151. [PubMed]

37. Beca, S.; Ahmad, F.; Shen, W.; Liu, J.; Makary, S.; Polidovitch, N.; Sun, J.; Hockman, S.; Chung, Y.W.; Movsesian, M.; et al. Phosphodiesterase type 3A regulates basal myocardial contractility through interacting with sarcoplasmic reticulum calcium ATPase type 2a signaling complexes in mouse heart. *Circ. Res.* **2013**, *112*, 289–297. [CrossRef] [PubMed]

38. Ahmad, F.; Shen, W.; Vandeput, F.; Szabo-Fresnais, N.; Krall, J.; Degerman, E.; Goetz, F.; Klussmann, E.; Movsesian, M.; Manganiello, V. Regulation of sarcoplasmic reticulum Ca^{2+} ATPase 2 (SERCA2) activity by phosphodiesterase 3A (PDE3A) in human myocardium: Phosphorylation-dependent interaction of PDE3A1 with SERCA2. *J. Biol. Chem.* **2015**, *290*, 6763–6776. [CrossRef] [PubMed]

39. Ghigo, A.; Laffargue, M.; Li, M.; Hirsch, E. PI3K and Calcium Signaling in Cardiovascular Disease. *Circ. Res.* **2017**, *121*, 282–292. [CrossRef] [PubMed]

40. Richter, W.; Xie, M.; Scheitrum, C.; Krall, J.; Movsesian, M.A.; Conti, M. Conserved expression and functions of PDE4 in rodent and human heart. *Basic Res. Cardiol.* **2011**, *106*, 249–262. [CrossRef] [PubMed]

41. Lehnart, S.E.; Wehrens, X.H.; Reiken, S.; Warrier, S.; Belevych, A.E.; Harvey, R.D.; Richter, W.; Jin, S.L.; Conti, M.; Marks, A.R. Phosphodiesterase 4D deficiency in the ryanodine-receptor complex promotes heart failure and arrhythmias. *Cell* **2005**, *123*, 25–35. [CrossRef] [PubMed]

42. Kerfant, B.G.; Zhao, D.; Lorenzen-Schmidt, I.; Wilson, L.S.; Cai, S.; Chen, S.R.; Maurice, D.H.; Backx, P.H. PI3Kgamma is required for PDE4, not PDE3, activity in subcellular microdomains containing the sarcoplasmic reticular calcium ATPase in cardiomyocytes. *Circ. Res.* **2007**, *101*, 400–408. [CrossRef] [PubMed]

43. Leroy, J.; Richter, W.; Mika, D.; Castro, L.R.; Abi-Gerges, A.; Xie, M.; Scheitrum, C.; Lefebvre, F.; Schittl, J.; Mateo, P.; et al. Phosphodiesterase 4B in the cardiac L-type Ca(2)(+) channel complex regulates Ca(2)(+) current and protects against ventricular arrhythmias in mice. *J. Clin. Investig.* **2011**, *121*, 2651–2661. [CrossRef] [PubMed]

44. Macphee, C.H.; Reifsnyder, D.H.; Moore, T.A.; Lerea, K.M.; Beavo, J.A. Phosphorylation results in activation of a cAMP phosphodiesterase in human platelets. *J. Biol. Chem.* **1988**, *263*, 10353–10358. [PubMed]

45. Grant, P.G.; Mannarino, A.F.; Colman, R.W. cAMP-mediated phosphorylation of the low-Km cAMP phosphodiesterase markedly stimulates its catalytic activity. *Proc. Natl. Acad. Sci. USA* **1988**, *85*, 9071–9075. [CrossRef] [PubMed]

46. Ahmad, F.; Lindh, R.; Tang, Y.; Ruishalme, I.; Ost, A.; Sahachartsiri, B.; Stralfors, P.; Degerman, E.; Manganiello, V.C. Differential regulation of adipocyte PDE3B in distinct membrane compartments by insulin and the beta3-adrenergic receptor agonist CL316243: Effects of caveolin-1 knockdown on formation/maintenance of macromolecular signalling complexes. *Biochem. J.* **2009**, *424*, 399–410. [CrossRef] [PubMed]

47. Ahmad, F.; Lindh, R.; Tang, Y.; Weston, M.; Degerman, E.; Manganiello, V.C. Insulin-induced formation of macromolecular complexes involved in activation of cyclic nucleotide phosphodiesterase 3B (PDE3B) and its interaction with PKB. *Biochem. J.* **2007**, *404*, 257–268. [CrossRef] [PubMed]

48. Onuma, H.; Osawa, H.; Yamada, K.; Ogura, T.; Tanabe, F.; Granner, D.K.; Makino, H. Identification of the insulin-regulated interaction of phosphodiesterase 3B with 14-3-3 beta protein. *Diabetes* **2002**, *51*, 3362–3367. [CrossRef] [PubMed]

49. Palmer, D.; Jimmo, S.L.; Raymond, D.R.; Wilson, L.S.; Carter, R.L.; Maurice, D.H. Protein kinase A phosphorylation of human phosphodiesterase 3B promotes 14-3-3 protein binding and inhibits phosphatase-catalyzed inactivation. *J. Biol. Chem.* **2007**, *282*, 9411–9419. [CrossRef] [PubMed]

50. Vandeput, F.; Szabo-Fresnais, N.; Ahmad, F.; Kho, C.; Lee, A.; Krall, J.; Dunlop, A.; Hazel, M.W.; Wohlschlegel, J.A.; Hajjar, R.J.; et al. Selective regulation of cyclic nucleotide phosphodiesterase PDE3A isoforms. *Proc. Natl. Acad. Sci. USA* **2013**, *110*, 19778–19783. [CrossRef] [PubMed]

51. Weninger, S.; Van Craenenbroeck, K.; Cameron, R.T.; Vandeput, F.; Movsesian, M.A.; Baillie, G.S.; Lefebvre, R.A. Phosphodiesterase 4 interacts with the 5-HT4(b) receptor to regulate cAMP signaling. *Cell Signal.* **2014**, *26*, 2573–2582. [CrossRef] [PubMed]

52. Ghigo, A.; Perino, A.; Mehel, H.; Zahradnikova, A., Jr.; Morello, F.; Leroy, J.; Nikolaev, V.O.; Damilano, F.; Cimino, J.; De Luca, E.; et al. Phosphoinositide 3-kinase gamma protects against catecholamine-induced ventricular arrhythmia through protein kinase A-mediated regulation of distinct phosphodiesterases. *Circulation* **2012**, *126*, 2073–2083. [CrossRef] [PubMed]

53. Perino, A.; Ghigo, A.; Ferrero, E.; Morello, F.; Santulli, G.; Baillie, G.S.; Damilano, F.; Dunlop, A.J.; Pawson, C.; Walser, R.; et al. Integrating cardiac PIP3 and cAMP signaling through a PKA anchoring function of p110gamma. *Mol. Cell* **2011**, *42*, 84–95. [CrossRef] [PubMed]

54. Marcantoni, A.; Levi, R.C.; Gallo, M.P.; Hirsch, E.; Alloatti, G. Phosphoinositide 3-kinasegamma (PI3Kgamma) controls L-type calcium current (ICa,L) through its positive modulation of type-3 phosphodiesterase (PDE3). *J. Cell. Physiol.* **2006**, *206*, 329–336. [CrossRef] [PubMed]

55. Nikolaev, V.O.; Moshkov, A.; Lyon, A.R.; Miragoli, M.; Novak, P.; Paur, H.; Lohse, M.J.; Korchev, Y.E.; Harding, S.E.; Gorelik, J. Beta2-adrenergic receptor redistribution in heart failure changes cAMP compartmentation. *Science* **2010**, *327*, 1653–1657. [CrossRef] [PubMed]

56. Rondinone, C.M.; Carvalho, E.; Rahn, T.; Manganiello, V.C.; Degerman, E.; Smith, U.P. Phosphorylation of PDE3B by phosphatidylinositol 3-kinase associated with the insulin receptor. *J. Biol. Chem.* **2000**, *275*, 10093–10098. [CrossRef] [PubMed]

57. DiPilato, L.M.; Ahmad, F.; Harms, M.; Seale, P.; Manganiello, V.; Birnbaum, M.J. The Role of PDE3B Phosphorylation in the Inhibition of Lipolysis by Insulin. *Mol. Cell. Biol.* **2015**, *35*, 2752–2760. [CrossRef] [PubMed]

58. Odagiri, K.; Katoh, H.; Kawashima, H.; Tanaka, T.; Ohtani, H.; Saotome, M.; Urushida, T.; Satoh, H.; Hayashi, H. Local control of mitochondrial membrane potential, permeability transition pore and reactive oxygen species by calcium and calmodulin in rat ventricular myocytes. *J. Mol. Cell. Cardiol.* **2009**, *46*, 989–997. [CrossRef] [PubMed]

59. Kitamura, T.; Kitamura, Y.; Kuroda, S.; Hino, Y.; Ando, M.; Kotani, K.; Konishi, H.; Matsuzaki, H.; Kikkawa, U.; Ogawa, W.; et al. Insulin-induced phosphorylation and activation of cyclic nucleotide phosphodiesterase 3B by the serine-threonine kinase Akt. *Mol. Cell. Biol.* **1999**, *19*, 6286–6296. [CrossRef] [PubMed]

60. Onuma, H.; Osawa, H.; Ogura, T.; Tanabe, F.; Nishida, W.; Makino, H. A newly identified 50 kDa protein, which is associated with phosphodiesterase 3B, is phosphorylated by insulin in rat adipocytes. *Biochem. Biophys. Res. Commun.* **2005**, *337*, 976–982. [CrossRef] [PubMed]

61. Nilsson, R.; Ahmad, F.; Sward, K.; Andersson, U.; Weston, M.; Manganiello, V.; Degerman, E. Plasma membrane cyclic nucleotide phosphodiesterase 3B (PDE3B) is associated with caveolae in primary adipocytes. *Cell Signal.* **2006**, *18*, 1713–1721. [CrossRef] [PubMed]

62. Patrucco, E.; Notte, A.; Barberis, L.; Selvetella, G.; Maffei, A.; Brancaccio, M.; Marengo, S.; Russo, G.; Azzolino, O.; Rybalkin, S.D.; et al. PI3Kgamma modulates the cardiac response to chronic pressure overload by distinct kinase-dependent and -independent effects. *Cell* **2004**, *118*, 375–387. [CrossRef] [PubMed]

63. Perino, A.; Beretta, M.; Kilic, A.; Ghigo, A.; Carnevale, D.; Repetto, I.E.; Braccini, L.; Longo, D.; Liebig-Gonglach, M.; Zaglia, T.; et al. Combined inhibition of PI3Kbeta and PI3Kgamma reduces fat mass by enhancing alpha-MSH-dependent sympathetic drive. *Sci. Signal.* **2014**, *7*, ra110. [CrossRef] [PubMed]

64. Damilano, F.; Perino, A.; Hirsch, E. PI3K kinase and scaffold functions in heart. *Ann. N. Y. Acad. Sci.* **2010**, *1188*, 39–45. [CrossRef] [PubMed]

65. Oikawa, M.; Wu, M.; Lim, S.; Knight, W.E.; Miller, C.L.; Cai, Y.; Lu, Y.; Blaxall, B.C.; Takeishi, Y.; Abe, J.; et al. Cyclic nucleotide phosphodiesterase 3A1 protects the heart against ischemia-reperfusion injury. *J. Mol. Cell. Cardiol.* **2013**, *64*, 11–19. [CrossRef] [PubMed]

66. Ding, B.; Abe, J.; Wei, H.; Xu, H.; Che, W.; Aizawa, T.; Liu, W.; Molina, C.A.; Sadoshima, J.; Blaxall, B.C.; et al. A positive feedback loop of phosphodiesterase 3 (PDE3) and inducible cAMP early repressor (ICER) leads to cardiomyocyte apoptosis. *Proc. Natl. Acad. Sci. USA* **2005**, *102*, 14771–14776. [CrossRef] [PubMed]

67. Ding, B.; Abe, J.; Wei, H.; Huang, Q.; Walsh, R.A.; Molina, C.A.; Zhao, A.; Sadoshima, J.; Blaxall, B.C.; Berk, B.C.; et al. Functional role of phosphodiesterase 3 in cardiomyocyte apoptosis: Implication in heart failure. *Circulation* **2005**, *111*, 2469–2476. [CrossRef] [PubMed]

68. Zoccarato, A.; Surdo, N.C.; Aronsen, J.M.; Fields, L.A.; Mancuso, L.; Dodoni, G.; Stangherlin, A.; Livie, C.; Jiang, H.; Sin, Y.Y.; et al. Cardiac Hypertrophy Is Inhibited by a Local Pool of cAMP Regulated by Phosphodiesterase 2. *Circ. Res.* **2015**, *117*, 707–719. [CrossRef] [PubMed]

69. Maass, P.G.; Aydin, A.; Luft, F.C.; Schachterle, C.; Weise, A.; Stricker, S.; Lindschau, C.; Vaegler, M.; Qadri, F.; Toka, H.R.; et al. PDE3A mutations cause autosomal dominant hypertension with brachydactyly. *Nat. Genet.* **2015**, *47*, 647–653. [CrossRef] [PubMed]

70. Boda, H.; Uchida, H.; Takaiso, N.; Ouchi, Y.; Fujita, N.; Kuno, A.; Hata, T.; Nagatani, A.; Funamoto, Y.; Miyata, M.; et al. A PDE3A mutation in familial hypertension and brachydactyly syndrome. *J. Hum. Genet.* **2016**, *61*, 701–703. [CrossRef] [PubMed]

71. Toka, O.; Tank, J.; Schachterle, C.; Aydin, A.; Maass, P.G.; Elitok, S.; Bartels-Klein, E.; Hollfinger, I.; Lindschau, C.; Mai, K.; et al. Clinical Effects of Phosphodiesterase 3A Mutations in Inherited Hypertension With Brachydactyly. *Hypertension* **2015**, *66*, 800–808. [CrossRef] [PubMed]

72. Bristow, M.R.; Ginsburg, R.; Minobe, W.; Cubicciotti, R.S.; Sageman, W.S.; Lurie, K.; Billingham, M.E.; Harrison, D.C.; Stinson, E.B. Decreased catecholamine sensitivity and beta-adrenergic-receptor density in failing human hearts. *N. Engl. J. Med.* **1982**, *307*, 205–211. [CrossRef] [PubMed]

73. Bristow, M.R.; Ginsburg, R.; Umans, V.; Fowler, M.; Minobe, W.; Rasmussen, R.; Zera, P.; Menlove, R.; Shah, P.; Jamieson, S.; et al. Beta 1- and beta 2-adrenergic-receptor subpopulations in nonfailing and failing human ventricular myocardium: Coupling of both receptor subtypes to muscle contraction and selective beta 1-receptor down-regulation in heart failure. *Circ. Res.* **1986**, *59*, 297–309. [CrossRef] [PubMed]

74. Ungerer, M.; Parruti, G.; Bohm, M.; Puzicha, M.; DeBlasi, A.; Erdmann, E.; Lohse, M.J. Expression of beta-arrestins and beta-adrenergic receptor kinases in the failing human heart. *Circ. Res.* **1994**, *74*, 206–213. [CrossRef] [PubMed]

75. Ungerer, M.; Bohm, M.; Elce, J.S.; Erdmann, E.; Lohse, M.J. Altered expression of beta-adrenergic receptor kinase and beta 1-adrenergic receptors in the failing human heart. *Circulation* **1993**, *87*, 454–463. [CrossRef] [PubMed]

76. Neumann, J.; Schmitz, W.; Scholz, H.; von Meyerinck, L.; Doring, V.; Kalmar, P. Increase in myocardial Gi-proteins in heart failure. *Lancet* **1988**, *2*, 936–937. [CrossRef]

77. Feldman, A.M.; Cates, A.E.; Veazey, W.B.; Hershberger, R.E.; Bristow, M.R.; Baughman, K.L.; Baumgartner, W.A.; Van Dop, C. Increase of the 40,000-mol wt pertussis toxin substrate (G protein) in the failing human heart. *J. Clin. Investig.* **1988**, *82*, 189–197. [CrossRef] [PubMed]

78. Feldman, M.D.; Copelas, L.; Gwathmey, J.K.; Phillips, P.; Warren, S.E.; Schoen, F.; Grossman, W.; Morgan, J.P. Deficient production of cyclic AMP: Pharmacologic evidence of an important cause of contractile dysfunction in patients with end-stage heart failure. *Circulation* **1987**, *75*, 331–339. [CrossRef] [PubMed]

79. Danielsen, W.; v der Leyen, H.; Meyer, W.; Neumann, J.; Schmitz, W.; Scholz, H.; Starbatty, J.; Stein, B.; Doring, V.; Kalmar, P. Basal and isoprenaline-stimulated cAMP content in failing versus nonfailing human cardiac preparations. *J. Cardiovasc. Pharmacol.* **1989**, *14*, 171–173. [CrossRef] [PubMed]

80. Bohm, M.; Reiger, B.; Schwinger, R.H.; Erdmann, E. cAMP concentrations, cAMP dependent protein kinase activity, and phospholamban in non-failing and failing myocardium. *Cardiovasc. Res.* **1994**, *28*, 1713–1719. [CrossRef] [PubMed]

81. Beuckelmann, D.J.; Nabauer, M.; Erdmann, E. Intracellular calcium handling in isolated ventricular myocytes from patients with terminal heart failure. *Circulation* **1992**, *85*, 1046–1055. [CrossRef] [PubMed]

82. Baim, D.S.; McDowell, A.V.; Cherniles, J.; Monrad, E.S.; Parker, J.A.; Edelson, J.; Braunwald, E.; Grossman, W. Evaluation of a new bipyridine inotropic agent—Milrinone—In patients with severe congestive heart failure. *N. Engl. J. Med.* **1983**, *309*, 748–756. [CrossRef] [PubMed]

83. Benotti, J.R.; Grossman, W.; Braunwald, E.; Davolos, D.D.; Alousi, A.A. Hemodynamic assessment of amrinone. A new inotropic agent. *N. Engl. J. Med.* **1978**, *299*, 1373–1377. [CrossRef] [PubMed]

84. Jaski, B.E.; Fifer, M.A.; Wright, R.F.; Braunwald, E.; Colucci, W.S. Positive inotropic and vasodilator actions of milrinone in patients with severe congestive heart failure. Dose-response relationships and comparison to nitroprusside. *J. Clin. Investig.* **1985**, *75*, 643–649. [CrossRef] [PubMed]

85. Sinoway, L.S.; Maskin, C.S.; Chadwick, B.; Forman, R.; Sonnenblick, E.H.; Le Jemtel, T.H. Long-term therapy with a new cardiotonic agent, WIN 47203: Drug-dependent improvement in cardiac performance and progression of the underlying disease. *J. Am. Coll. Cardiol.* **1983**, *2*, 327–331. [CrossRef]

86. Maskin, C.S.; Sinoway, L.; Chadwick, B.; Sonnenblick, E.H.; Le Jemtel, T.H. Sustained hemodynamic and clinical effects of a new cardiotonic agent, WIN 47203, in patients with severe congestive heart failure. *Circulation* **1983**, *67*, 1065–1070. [CrossRef] [PubMed]

87. Anderson, J.L. Hemodynamic and clinical benefits with intravenous milrinone in severe chronic heart failure: Results of a multicenter study in the United States. *Am. Heart J.* **1991**, *121*, 1956–1964. [CrossRef]

88. Monrad, E.S.; McKay, R.G.; Baim, D.S.; Colucci, W.S.; Fifer, M.A.; Heller, G.V.; Royal, H.D.; Grossman, W. Improvement in indexes of diastolic performance in patients with congestive heart failure treated with milrinone. *Circulation* **1984**, *70*, 1030–1037. [CrossRef] [PubMed]

89. Pande, R.L.; Hiatt, W.R.; Zhang, P.; Hittel, N.; Creager, M.A. A pooled analysis of the durability and predictors of treatment response of cilostazol in patients with intermittent claudication. *Vasc. Med.* **2010**, *15*, 181–188. [CrossRef] [PubMed]

90. Del Monte, F.; Lebeche, D.; Guerrero, J.L.; Tsuji, T.; Doye, A.A.; Gwathmey, J.K.; Hajjar, R.J. Abrogation of ventricular arrhythmias in a model of ischemia and reperfusion by targeting myocardial calcium cycling. *Proc. Natl. Acad. Sci. USA* **2004**, *101*, 5622–5627. [CrossRef] [PubMed]

91. Lyon, A.R.; Bannister, M.L.; Collins, T.; Pearce, E.; Sepehripour, A.H.; Dubb, S.S.; Garcia, E.; O'Gara, P.; Liang, L.; Kohlbrenner, E.; et al. SERCA2a gene transfer decreases sarcoplasmic reticulum calcium leak and reduces ventricular arrhythmias in a model of chronic heart failure. *Circ. Arrhythm. Electrophysiol.* **2011**, *4*, 362–372. [CrossRef] [PubMed]

92. Duan, L.M.; Yu, H.Y.; Li, Y.L.; Jia, C.J. Design and discovery of 2-(4-(1*H*-tetrazol-5-yl)-1*H*-pyrazol-1-yl)-4-(4-phenyl)thiazole derivatives as cardiotonic agents via inhibition of PDE3. *Bioorg. Med. Chem.* **2015**, *23*, 6111–6117. [CrossRef] [PubMed]

93. Lygren, B.; Carlson, C.R.; Santamaria, K.; Lissandron, V.; McSorley, T.; Litzenberg, J.; Lorenz, D.; Wiesner, B.; Rosenthal, W.; Zaccolo, M.; et al. AKAP complex regulates Ca^{2+} re-uptake into heart sarcoplasmic reticulum. *EMBO Rep.* **2007**, *8*, 1061–1067. [CrossRef] [PubMed]

94. Wilson, L.S.; Baillie, G.S.; Pritchard, L.M.; Umana, B.; Terrin, A.; Zaccolo, M.; Houslay, M.D.; Maurice, D.H. A phosphodiesterase 3B-based signaling complex integrates exchange protein activated by cAMP 1 and phosphatidylinositol 3-kinase signals in human arterial endothelial cells. *J. Biol. Chem.* **2011**, *286*, 16285–16296. [CrossRef] [PubMed]

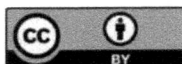

Journal of
Cardiovascular
Development and Disease

MDPI

Review

PDE4-Mediated cAMP Signalling

Bracy A. Fertig and George S. Baillie *

University of Glasgow, Glasgow G12 8QQ, UK; b.fertig.1@research.gla.ac.uk
* Correspondence: george.baillie@glasgow.ac.uk; Tel.: +44-141-330-6388

Received: 19 December 2017; Accepted: 23 January 2018; Published: 31 January 2018

Abstract: cAMP is the archetypal and ubiquitous second messenger utilised for the fine control of many cardiovascular cell signalling systems. The ability of cAMP to elicit cell surface receptor-specific responses relies on its compartmentalisation by cAMP hydrolysing enzymes known as phosphodiesterases. One family of these enzymes, PDE4, is particularly important in the cardiovascular system, where it has been extensively studied and shown to orchestrate complex, localised signalling that underpins many crucial functions of the heart In the cardiac myocyte, cAMP activates PKA, which phosphorylates a small subset of mostly sarcoplasmic substrate proteins that drive β-adrenergic enhancement of cardiac function. The phosphorylation of these substrates, many of which are involved in cardiac excitation-contraction coupling, has been shown to be tightly regulated by highly localised pools of individual PDE4 isoforms. The spatial and temporal regulation of cardiac signalling is made possible by the formation of macromolecular "signalosomes", which often include a cAMP effector, such as PKA, its substrate, PDE4 and an anchoring protein such as an AKAP. Studies described in the present review highlight the importance of this relationship for individual cardiac PKA substrates and we provide an overview of how this signalling paradigm is coordinated to promote efficient adrenergic enhancement of cardiac function. The role of PDE4 also extends to the vascular endothelium, where it regulates vascular permeability and barrier function. In this distinct location, PDE4 interacts with adherens junctions to regulate their stability. These highly specific, non-redundant roles for PDE4 isoforms have far reaching therapeutic potential. PDE inhibitors in the clinic have been plagued with problems due to the active site-directed nature of the compounds which concomitantly attenuate PDE activity in all highly localised "signalosomes".

Keywords: phosphodiesterase 4; cardiac myocyte; vascular endothelium

1. Introduction

Cyclic 3′,5′-adenosine monophosphate (cAMP) was the first second messenger molecule to be discovered, and has been researched tirelessly in the context of numerous physiological systems. Much of the current understanding of cAMP signalling, however, has come from studying its function in the cardiovascular system, where it has major roles in the heart and vessels [1]. In the heart, cAMP influences a multitude of processes from contractility and hypertrophy of myocytes to apoptosis and cell survival [2]. In the vasculature, effects on smooth muscle cell contraction and relaxation, as well as endothelial cell permeability has been attributed to cAMP signalling processes [3]. Additionally, cAMP can modify cell proliferation, migration, differentiation, and response to stress [4–7]. cAMP produces these vast cellular effects by activating four types of effector proteins: protein kinase A (PKA), exchange protein directly activated by cAMP (EPAC), cyclic nucleotide activated ion channels (CNGC), and popeye domain containing proteins (POPDC). The present review will focus on the effects of PKA and EPAC. PKA functions to phosphorylate substrate proteins, while EPAC activates the RAS superfamily of enzymes [8]. The present review will focus on the ways in which phosphodiesterase 4 (PDE4) enzymes modify cAMP's ability to produce these varied physiological effects within the cardiovascular system.

2. cAMP Signalling and Compartmentalisation

The small, highly diffusible molecule, cAMP can be produced by both membrane-bound adenylyl cyclase (mAC) and soluble adenylyl cyclase (sAC) in response to various stimuli, such as the activation of various G_s-coupled receptors, which activates mAC [9]. Its properties suggest that it would quickly diffuse throughout the cell, simultaneously activating all effector proteins almost instantly. In striking contrast, it was shown by Larry Brunton and colleagues in the early 1980s that cAMP can cause multiple discrete receptor specific responses in the same cells [10,11]. To explain this phenomenon, it was quickly postulated, and eventually proven, that compartmentalisation of cAMP signalling underpins receptor specific responses by restricting the number and identity of PKA substrates that get phosphorylated in response to each specific receptor ligation [12,13]. Such fine control of one ubiquitous second messenger that acts to activate only discrete pools of PKA is made possible by the subcellular localisation of proteins that degrade cAMP. This function is attributed to a super-family of enzymes called phosphodiesterases (PDEs). PDEs are the only known route to the hydrolysis of cAMP and this function empowers these enzymes to act as "sinks", reducing cAMP concentration in localised areas preventing the inappropriate phosphorylation of PKA substrates under basal conditions. Following receptor activation, however, this situation can be altered to allow cAMP concentrations to exceed the activation threshold of PKA enzymes tethered to discretely positioned "signalosomes". This situation occurs only when the cAMP concentration in the vicinity of the relevant "signalosomes" is high enough to swamp the PDE component, promoting downstream physiological effects [14]. The integration of PDE4 isoforms into specific "signalosomes" within the heart and the function of these protein complexes will be the subject of this review.

3. PDEs and PDE4-Ology

PDEs are a large super-family of enzymes, which are the products of 11 different gene families, grouped according to their structure, function, and affinity for cAMP and cGMP. Structurally, all PDEs have conserved carboxy-terminal catalytic cores while their amino-terminal regions differ among families, subfamilies, and specific isoforms. The N-terminal regions have a number of functional roles. These include the targeting to specific subcellular locations and to signalosomes, and the modulation of responses to signals from regulatory molecules or post-translational modifications [1,15]. cAMP-specific PDE4s make up the largest family with over 20 isoforms encoded by four genes (A, B, C, and D). Each isoform has a unique N-terminal region, made up of an N-terminal targeting domain (TD). Additionally, the N-terminal region contains upstream conserved regions 1 and 2 (UCR1 and UCR2), which are linked to each other and to the catalytic domain by linker region 1 and 2 (LR1 and LR2) respectively [16]. Based on the presence and size of UCR1 and UCR2, PDE4 isoforms can be categorised into long, short, super-short, and dead-short isoforms (Figure 1); long isoforms have both UCR1 and 2, short isoforms have only UCR2, super-short have a truncated UCR2, and dead-short isoforms lack both UCR domains and have a truncated catalytic domain [17].

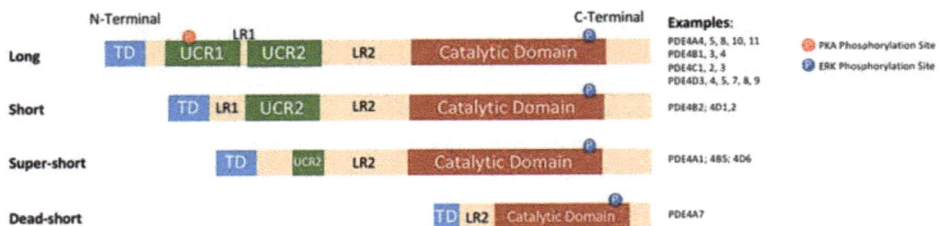

Figure 1. Diversity of domain organisation of PDE4 isoforms TD, transduction domain; LR1/2, linker region 1/2; UCR1/2, upstream conserved region 1/2.

UCR1 and 2 have a number of roles, including the regulation of functional outcomes following PDE4 phosphorylation by protein kinase A (PKA) or extracellular signal-regulated kinase (ERK). The presence or absence of these domains means that phosphorylation can have different, and even opposite, functional effects in different isoforms [18–20].

The catalytic domain of PDE4 has been extensively studied, and X-ray crystal structures have demonstrated the deep hydrophobic pocket made of numerous helices which makes up the active site for the hydrolysis of cAMP [15,21]. The structure of this domain has been integral for the design of family-specific inhibitors, which have been widely used both clinically and experimentally [22,23].

As previously mentioned, the subcellular localisation of PDEs is integral to their function in shaping cAMP gradients and responses. This localisation is often directed by the N-terminal targeting domains, which are highly varied among PDE4 isoforms [24,25], though targeting can also be driven by other regions including the newly identified multi-functional docking domain positioned at the C-terminal end of the catalytic unit [26]. Unique subsets of PDE4 specific interactions allow single isoforms to have multiple non-redundant roles in different tissues, cells and even different micro-domains within the same cell [27]. The disruption of this location dependent function of small pools of highly active PDE4s has been considered as a novel way to circumvent side-effects observed following the systemic inhibition of global PDE4 activity using site-directed PDE4 inhibitors [28].

4. Technological Approaches to Defining Roles for PDE4 Isoforms

Isoform specific roles of PDEs have been identified within the realm of the cardiovascular system and historically, as new technologies have been invented, these have been used to identify specific interactions and functions of PDE4. Often, the first and easiest approach utilised is pharmacological, and employs family-specific inhibitors. However, this strategy gives little information on individual isoforms and can often engender "bulk" cAMP effects due to simultaneous inhibition of all PDE4 enzymes in all locations. Other more targeted approaches include siRNA knockdown and overexpression of dominant-negative PDEs. Both of these allow diminution of the influence of one isoform by either genetic silencing or displacement of endogenous, functional PDEs [29–31]. Often these approaches are sufficient to pinpoint specific cellular functions for single isoforms; however, if one isoform has multiple roles in the same cell, an incomplete understanding of the complexity of PDE4 action can be lost.

The identification of specific protein-protein interactions within PDE signalosomes has been integral to understanding PDE4 function. Peptide array technology has proved to be an accurate way to screen for such interactions and to predict the regions and specific amino acids which are essential for holding signalling complexes together [32–34]. Another advantage of this technique is that it allows the informed design of cell-permeable disruptor peptides, which can interrupt these signalosome interactions. Disruptor peptides provide by far the most specific form of inhibition as only a specific localised pool of the PDE4 isoform of choice is displaced, leaving any other cellular effects of that isoform untouched [28,35].

The development of fluorescent probes which can monitor cAMP dynamics in real time have led to vast advancements in the field. Briefly, these probes contain two fluorescent moieties, a donor and an acceptor, and a cAMP binding domain. When cAMP binds, a conformational change is induced, altering the fluorescent energy transfer between the donor and acceptor, known as fluorescence resonance energy transfer (FRET). The detection of the two emissions allows real time changes in cAMP concentration to be measured [36].

Many of the studies described in the present report employ a combination of these techniques to create robust evidence for the specific roles of PDE4 isoforms in the cardiovascular system.

5. PDE4 in the Heart

Much of the understanding of cAMP compartmentalisation and the role of PDEs comes from extensive studies of the signalling pathway in cardiac myocytes. Generally speaking, four PDE families have been identified as having notable roles in cAMP signalling in the heart: PDE1, PDE2, PDE3, and PDE4 [37]. Despite the identification of localised expression of PDE4 in cardiac myocytes, inhibition of this family was shown to have very limited effects on cardiovascular parameters, such as basal blood pressure, heart rate, and contractility. This can be explained by the fact that PDE4 is a major player not at basal cAMP levels, but during β-adrenergic stimulation, when intracellular [cAMP] is raised. Additionally, it has been shown that redundancy of the PDE network can lead to compensatory effects, in which other families with the same hydrolytic activity attenuate the effects of PDE4 loss of function [38].

In the cardiac myocyte, sympathetic activation leads to β-adrenergic signalling, a major part of the fight or flight response. Briefly, when the receptor is activated, its associated G_s-protein causes the activation of AC, which catalyses the production of cAMP from ATP. cAMP in turn activates various effector proteins; of major importance for this signalling paradigm is PKA, which phosphorylates a number of substrates important for cardiac excitation-contraction coupling, and EPAC, which is of particular importance in the vasculature. These phosphorylation effects lead to positive inotropic and lusitropic effects, increasing the function of the heart for increased circulatory demands [39].

Interestingly, the phosphorylation of these substrate proteins by PKA is tightly regulated by PDE4 enzymes, which associate directly within signalosomes, modifying the signalling in tight compartments. In this way, it is not global signalling which is affected by PDE4, but local, compartmentalised signalling. This concept, developed in the 1980s by Hayes et al. using biochemical means was proven unequivocally using advanced imaging techniques [12]. Optical probes that acted as cAMP FRET reporters, allowed visualisation of the formation of cAMP gradients following submaximal β-adrenergic stimulation. When used in combination with PDE inhibitors, it became apparent that the loss of cAMP hydrolysis within cellular microdomains abrogated the spatial and temporal control of cAMP dynamics that is required to channel receptor-specific physiological outcomes [13,40].

PDE4 and cardiac disease have a complicated relationship [41]. On one hand, PDE inhibition has been shown to enhance cAMP signalling, resulting in increased cardiomyocyte function. In contrast, chronic inhibition of PDEs results in increased mortality, often due to cardiac side effects [41,42]. Finally, PDE4 activity is decreased in heart failure, potentially contributing to disease progression due to faulty regulation of the sympathetic induction of phosphorylation of cardiac excitation-contraction coupling proteins [43,44].

The role of PDE4 in the cardiac myocyte cannot be described in full without delving into the discrete roles of specific isoforms within their discrete subcellular compartments. The next sections of this review will focus on these unique functions. A schematic summary of cardiac PDE signalosomes is shown in Figure 2.

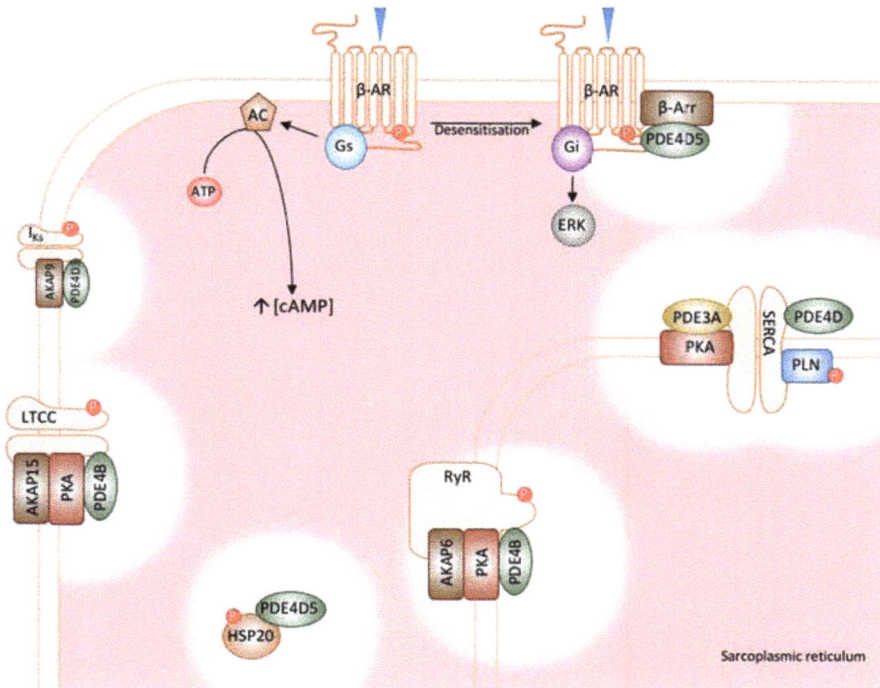

Figure 2. Cardiac PDE signalosomes. PDE4 family members have been shown to integrate into macromolecular complexes with numerous cardiac proteins, many of which are involved in excitation-contraction coupling and calcium handling. PDE4D5 interacts with β-arrestin, regulating receptor desensitisation. PDE4B regulates both the LTCC and RyR, which controls the process of calcium induced calcium release. PDE4D interacts with SERCA, regulating the reuptake of calcium into the SR. PDE4D3 interacts with IKs, modulating basal channel function. Finally, PKE4D5 regulates the cardioprotective effects of HSP20. AC, adenylyl cyclase; AKAP, A-kinase anchoring protein; ATP, adenosine triphosphate; β-AR, β-adrenoceptor; β-Arr, β-arrestin; ERK, extracellular signal regulated kinases; G_i; inhibitory G-protein; G_s, stimulatory G-protein; HSP20, heat shock protein 20; I_{KS}, cardiac I_{KS} potassium channel; LTCC, L-type calcium channel; P, phosphorylation; PKA, protein kinase A PLN, phosphopamban, RyR, ryanodine receptor SERCA, sarcoplasmic reticulum calcium ATPase [35,43,45–49].

5.1. PDE4D5's Role in β-Adrenoceptor Desensitisation

One of the best understood functions of PDE4 in the cardiovascular system is the role of PDE4D5 in the regulation of β_2-adrenergic signalling in the cardiac myocyte. When the β_2-adrenoceptor is stimulated, its coupled G_s protein stimulates AC, which produces cAMP to activate localised PKA. Desensitisation of adrenergic signalling occurs when a negative-feedback loop is created when the receptor itself is phosphorylated by PKA. This phosphorylation switches the receptor's signalling to an inhibitory G protein, G_i, which inhibits AC as well as activating other pathways, such as ERK1/2 [50]. Additionally, the phosphorylation of the receptor by G-protein coupled receptor kinases (GRKs) causes the recruitment of β-arrestin, which further desensitises the receptor by sterically hindering access to the G-protein [51]. However, when it was observed that the recruitment of β-arrestin also increased local cAMP degradation, it became clear that PDE translocation was a crucial function of β-arrestin [52]. In 2003, Baillie and colleagues used pharmacological inhibition and overexpression of dominant negative mutants to show that PDE4D5 is recruited to the β_2-adrenoceptor by β-arrestin. In neonatal rat ventricular myocytes (NRVM), both rolipram (a PDE4 inhibitor) and dominant negative PDE4D5 increased the PKA phosphorylation of the receptor, and the activation of ERK1/2, which is consistent with phenotypic switching of the receptor [53]. In a similar study, siRNA was used to knockdown pan-PDE4D, which caused similar effects, namely, increased PKA phosphorylation of the receptor and ERK activation. The same effects were achieved by the specific knockdown of PDE4D5 and this was the first time a function had been ascribed to an individual PDE4 isoform [29].

Interestingly, PDE4D5 is not the only isoform which has been shown to interact with β-arrestin. In fact, all PDE4 isoforms have this ability due to the presence of the binding site in the conserved catalytic region [52]. The presence of an additional β-arrestin binding site on PDE4D5's unique N-terminal binding domain could confer the specificity of its functioning as it is the "chosen-one" for β-arrestin translocation [46]. Additionally, other pools of PDE4 which are expressed in the cell could be preferentially sequestered in a different cellular location with different binding partners.

The direct interaction of the PDE with β-arrestin, however, is not sufficient to explain these observations. The localisation of a pool of PKA to the β_2-adrenergic receptor has been shown to depend on the scaffolding protein, AKAP79 [29]. This allows the tethered PDE to regulate the activity of this discrete pool of PKA. This determines the phosphorylation status and, thereby, the phenotypic switching of the receptor.

5.2. PDE4D5 Regulates Cardioprotection by HSP20

Another example in which PDE4 has been shown to regulate the phosphorylation of a crucial cardiac signalling protein is in the case of the small heat shock protein 20 (HSP20, HSPB6). HSP20 is part of a diverse, ubiquitously expressed family of small chaperone proteins, whose expression patterns are regulated by cellular stressors [54]. HSP20 has been shown to have a protective role in cardiac myocytes, but only in its phosphorylated state [55–57]. In fact, when HSP20 is phosphorylated by PKA at Ser16, it protects the cell by switching off harmful signalling (NF-kB) and switching on protective signalling (Akt/PKB), inhibiting necrosis and apoptosis, and stabilising the cell's cytoskeleton [58–61]. These protective mechanisms have been studied in the context of a variety of cardiac indications, including ischaemia/reperfusion, chronic β-adrenergic stimulation, and heart failure [61–63]. The importance of phosphorylation has been shown in a variety of mutant studies, in which a non-phosphorylated mutant (S16A) lost its protective effects in I/R injury, and constitutively phosphorylated mutant (S16D) effectively protected cells from apoptosis [55,56].

The importance of PKA phosphorylation for HSP20's cardioprotective abilities led researchers to investigate the role of PDEs in this signalling pathway [35]. Initial experiments showed that pharmacological inhibition of PDE4 augmented the isoprenaline-induced increase in phosphorylated HSP20, confirming the functional role of PDE4. Real time monitoring of cAMP levels using FRET technology gave more insight into PDE4's role in this pathway. Comparing the response of a cAMP FRET probe tethered to HSP20 with an untethered, cytosolic probe showed that PDE4 inhibition caused a greater increase in cAMP in the vicinity of HSP20. This result highlights once again that the location of small active pools of PDE4 is key to the enzyme's control of specific events in cardiac myocytes.

The next step was to determine whether there was a direct interaction. Co-immunoprecipitation studies were used in conjunction with peptide array experiments to show that HSP20 directly interacts with the conserved catalytic region of PDE4D isoforms. The identification of the amino acids important for the docking of HSP20 to PDE4D allowed the design and manufacturing of a cell permeable peptide (peptide 906) which dismantles the interaction. Treatment of NRVM with this peptide not only resulted in an increased phosphorylation of HSP20, but also an attenuation of hypertrophic response to sustained β-adrenergic stimulation [64]. The peptide was also subsequently used in a rodent model of heart disease with great effect [65].

5.3. PDE4D3's Regulation of RyR Phosphorylation

In the clinic, the use of PDE inhibitors has been plagued with cardiac problems, including increased susceptibility to arrhythmia and heart failure. The underlying mechanisms were unknown until Lehnart and colleagues performed an elegant study using PDE4D deficient mice [43]. It was observed that these animals developed a dilated cardiomyopathy which had many characteristics consistent with human chronic heart failure as well as exercise induced ventricular arrhythmias (VT). Upon observation at the cellular level, it was shown that despite normal global cAMP signalling in the PDE4D$^{-/-}$ mice, there was a marked increase in localised cAMP at the cardiomyocyte Z line. This observation coupled with the evidence of previous studies showing that the ryanodine receptor (RyR) is hyperphosphorylated by PKA at Ser2808 in heart failure led the researchers to study the role of PDE4's regulation of RyR phosphorylation in their model [66–69]. Indeed, the PDE4D$^{-/-}$ mice showed both hyperphosphorylation of the RyR as well as diminished levels of calstabin-2 (FKBP12.6), which functions to stabilise RyR and reduce calcium leak from the sarcoplasmic reticulum [70,71]. These changes led to multiple phenotypic observations. In terms of RyR function, the channels had a "leaky" phenotype, similar to that which has been shown in heart failure and exercise induced sudden cardiac death [66,70].

The individual isoform of PDE which associates with RyR to regulate these effects was identified as PDE4D3. This is consistent with PDE4D3 being one of the three PDE4D isoforms expressed in the heart; however, studies completed in rat hearts should be extrapolated with caution due to potential differences in expression patterns of human hearts [72]. The elimination of PDE4D3 in complex with RyR was shown to be highly relevant physiologically as PDE4D3 levels in the complex are also reduced in human heart failure samples. This provided an interesting explanation for the hyperphosphorylation of RyR by PKA despite globally decreased cAMP signalling in failing human cardiac myocytes, as had been previously observed [73].

As the final piece of the puzzle, the group sought to confirm the role of hyperphosphorylated RyR as a causative factor for the observed phenotypes. The PDE4D$^{-/-}$ mice were crossed with mice harbouring a mutation which did not allow PKA phosphorylation of the RyR (S2808A). These mice were protected against both exercise induced sudden cardiac death and myocardial infarction (MI) induced sudden cardiac death, confirming the role of the PDE4D3, PKA, RyR signalosome in the observed phenotypes.

The similarities of the phenotypes observed in PDE4D$^{-/-}$ mice with human cardiac disease provide a compelling argument for the role of aberrant signalling relating to maladjustment of the PDE complement within cardiac "signalosomes" in cardiomyopathy. Additionally, the identification of PDE4D3 in complex with the RyR pinpointed another unique function for an individual PDE4 isoform.

5.4. PDE4D3 Regulates Basal I_{Ks} Activity

The electrical activity of cardiac myocytes is another function where PDE4 has an active input. The slowly activating potassium channel (IKs) is a major repolarising current in the cardiac action potential. IKs exists as a macromolecular complex which comprises KCNQ1 α-subunits and KCNE1 β-subunits which interact with a variety of proteins that regulate the channel's function [74,75]. These include AC9, AKAP-9, PKA, and protein phosphatase-1 [76,77]. As with many other cAMP signalling models in the cardiac myocyte, it was clear that a PDE may be involved in this signalosome, thereby regulating PKA phosphorylation of the α-subunits. In a primarily biochemical study, immunoprecipitation techniques identified that PDE4D3 is spatially confined within this macromolecular complex via a direct interaction with AKAP-9 [49]. Functional experiments in ventricular myocytes using pharmacological inhibitors showed that the PDE4 was able to fine tune the functioning of the channel at basal conditions, probably due to a basally active AC in the vicinity.

5.5. PDE4B Has a Dominant Role in LTCC Regulation

The L-type calcium channel (LTCC) is yet another cardiac excitation-contraction coupling protein whose function is modified by a PDE4 isoform. This protein functions to allow calcium influx through the cardiac myocyte membrane, which triggers the release of calcium from intracellular stores by the RyR, in a process known as calcium-induced calcium release (CICR) [39]. Under conditions of β-adrenergic stimulation, PKA phosphorylates the pore forming subunits of the LTCC, which increases channel activity [78,79]. In combination with RyR phosphorylation, CICR is increased, leading to a positive inotropic effect [39].

Although both PDE4B and PDE4D were both shown to tether to the LTCC signalosome, a study using subfamily specific knockout mice showed that PDE4B exhibits the dominant functional role in the regulation of LTCC phosphorylation and the protection against arrhythmia [47]. Firstly, experiments in wild type mice showed that PDE4 inhibition had no effect on basal calcium current through the LTCC ($I_{Ca,L}$) but markedly increased $I_{Ca,L}$ under conditions of β-adrenergic stimulation. Consistently, in both PDE4B$^{-/-}$ and PDE4D$^{-/-}$ mice, $I_{Ca,L}$ was increased, leading to increased calcium transients and increased contractility. The disease relevance of this research was shown using in vivo pacing in the knockout animals, which resulted in ventricular tachycardia (VT) in PDE4B$^{-/-}$ mice but not in PDE4D$^{-/-}$ mice. This study displayed the dominant functional role of PDE4B in the regulation of phosphorylation of LTCC, which consequently regulates the entry of calcium into the cell and the initiation of CICR.

The role of PDE4B in the protection against arrhythmia is consistent with the observation of decreased PDE4B activity in cardiac hypertrophy [44]. The combination of these two findings could represent at least a partial explanation of the incidence of arrhythmia and sudden cardiac death associated with heart failure.

5.6. PDE4D and PDE3A Regulate PLN Phosphorylation and SERCA Function

The regulation of sarcoplasmic reticular calcium ATPase (SERCA) function relies on both PDE3 and PDE4 isoforms, unlike in other cardiac PDE signalosomes.

SERCA is a calcium channel on the sarcoplasmic reticular membrane which functions to sequester calcium in its intracellular store. Phospholamban (PLN) inhibits its activity, tightly regulating channel function. PLN can be phosphorylated by PKA, which reduces its inhibitory influence, leading to increased SERCA activity and enhanced sarcoplasmic reticulum (SR) calcium load and contractility [80].

Both PDE4D and PDE3A have been shown to integrate into a signalosome containing SERCA, PLN, PKA and other structural and regulatory proteins, thereby regulating PLN phosphorylation and exhibiting a regulation of basal contractile function [48,81]. In separate studies, members of both PDE subfamilies were detected in SERCA immunoprecipitates, showing that these PDEs integrate into the SERCA/PLN signalosome. Knockout of PDE3A in rodents resulted in increased phosphorylation of PLN associated with increased SERCA activity, SR calcium load, and increased contractility, suggesting a major role for this isoform in the SERCA microdomain. However, similar studies in PDE4D knockout rodents produced strikingly similar results, from increased PLN phosphorylation to increased contractility. Taken together, it is apparent that both PDE3A and PDE4D are important modulators of cAMP signalling at the SERCA microdomain as both seem to have comparable effects. Further studies will be necessary to dissect any unique, non-compensated roles of these PDE isoforms on SERCA function.

As evidenced by the examples above, highly localised pools of PDEs and in particular PDE4 have influence on many steps of the cardiac excitation-contraction coupling process. Although the identity of the PDE4 isoforms differ in the distinct locations, the underlying concept of dormant signalosomes being activated following the inhibition, displacement, silencing or overwhelming of a spatially restricted PDE4 cohort prevails. Clearly, the initial concept pioneered by Hayes et al. and subsequently validated using optical cAMP probes has also been upheld in diseases that occur as a result of the malformation of highly tuned cAMP gradients underpinned by loss of localised PDE4 machinery [12].

6. Vascular cAMP Signalling and PDEs

Although cardiac myocytes have taken centre stage in terms of PDE4 research, this group of enzymes also has major roles in the wider cardiovascular system, regulating many characteristics of the vasculature. cAMP signalling is particularly important in the signalling systems of vascular endothelial cells (VECs) where increases in cAMP concentration results in reduced vascular permeability. The literature is clear that PDEs are integral to the fine control of such processes [82]. In conditions of low cGMP, PDE4 is the major regulator of PKA and EPAC activation, both of which influence permeability. In addition to PDE4, PDE2 and PDE3 activity also impinge on VEC permeability, but their influence is changed by increases in cGMP, which activates PDE2 and inhibits PDE3, allowing fine tuning of regulation [82,83]. As in cardiac myocytes, localised signalosomes have been identified as crucial in the maintenance of signalling specificity. The components of compartmentalised signalling complexes in this location include various AC subtypes, PDE2, PDE3, and PDE4 isoforms, and AKAPs. An important study by Maurice and colleagues identified the unique, non-compensated role of PDE4D in the regulation of vascular permeability, confirming the notion of compartmentalised signalling in VECs [3,83].

PDE4D's Role in the Regulation of Vascular Permeability

VEC permeability is largely mediated through adherens junctions (AJ), structures comprised of vascular endothelial cell cadherins (VECAD) which interact with those of neighbouring cells and assemble a complex containing catenins and actinins to the cytoskeleton [84,85]. When VECs are stimulated by agents that increase cAMP, the activation of PKA and EPAC results in the stabilisation of AJs, decreasing cell permeability [83]. Pharmacological inhibition and siRNA-mediated knockdown identified PDE4D and EPAC1 as the mediators of cAMP-dependent changes in permeability [3]. Interestingly, the use of pharmacological inhibition of PDE4 and knockdown of PDE4D yielded conflicting results. As expected, PDE4 inhibition decreased cell permeability; however, in stark contrast, knockdown of PDE4D increased cell permeability. This was explained by a dual role of PDE4D in this cellular compartment. Not only does the PDE regulate EPAC1 activation by hydrolysing cAMP, but it also acts as the tether, localising EPAC1 to the VECAD structures. The identification of PDE4D's function as a scaffold identified a novel role for the family of enzymes. Maurice et al. also employed a disruptor peptide to determine the function of the interaction between EPAC1 and PDE4D. Treatment with this peptide reduced VEC permeability to a similar degree as global PDE4 inhibition (Figure 3). The specific disruption of the PDE4D-EPAC1 interaction proved to be a novel method to alter VEC permeability and barrier function.

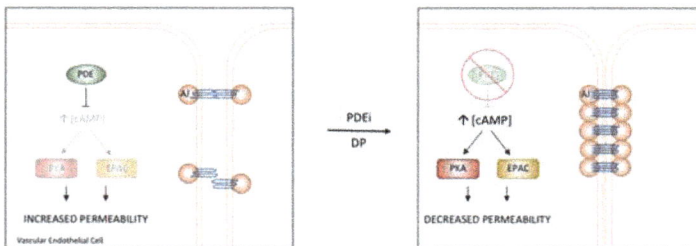

Figure 3. PDE regulation of Vascular Endothelial Permeability. PDE4D has been shown to regulate the permeability of the vascular endothelium through interactions with components of AJs. Treatment with PDE inhibitors or a specific disruptor of the PDE4D/EPAC1 interaction results in increased cAMP and stabilization of AJs, ultimately causing reduced permeability and increased barrier function [3].

7. Future Directions and Outlook

As described in the present review, the study of PDE4 in the cardiovascular system is centered on the discovery of isoform specific roles within signalosomes. Compartmentalisation of distinct PDE4 isoforms underpin their function and allow low cellular concentrations of the enzyme to have a pivotal role in many areas of cardiac signaling. Future development of new technologies, such as the expansion of novel, highly targeted FRET probes, will allow the effects of PDEs on cAMP signalling to be observed in novel ways that were not previously possible [86]. In conjunction with PDE4 gene therapy, PDE4 activators and novel animal models where inducible dominant negative PD4 constructs are expressed, our understanding of the currently accepted roles of PDEs will be increased, and novel roles at additional microdomains will inevitably be uncovered. This information will undoubtedly drive novel therapeutic endeavors to target this versatile enzyme family for the good of humankind.

Conflicts of Interest: The authors declare no conflict of interest.

References

1. Houslay, M.D.; Baillie, G.S.; Maurice, D.H. cAMP-Specific phosphodiesterase-4 enzymes in the cardiovascular system: A molecular toolbox for generating compartmentalized cAMP signaling. *Circ. Res.* **2007**, *100*, 950–966. [CrossRef] [PubMed]
2. Tomita, H.; Nazmy, M.; Kajimoto, K.; Yehia, G.; Molina, C.A.; Sadoshima, J. Inducible cAMP early repressor (ICER) is a negative-feedback regulator of cardiac hypertrophy and an important mediator of cardiac myocyte apoptosis in response to beta-adrenergic receptor stimulation. *Circ. Res.* **2003**, *93*, 12–22. [CrossRef] [PubMed]
3. Rampersad, S.N.; Ovens, J.D.; Huston, E.; Umana, M.B.; Wilson, L.S.; Netherton, S.J.; Lynch, M.J.; Baillie, G.S.; Houslay, M.D.; Maurice, D.H. Cyclic AMP phosphodiesterase 4D (PDE4D) Tethers EPAC1 in a vascular endothelial cadherin (VE-Cad)-based signaling complex and controls cAMP-mediated vascular permeability. *J. Biol. Chem.* **2010**, *285*, 33614–33622. [CrossRef] [PubMed]
4. Fetalvero, K.M.; Shyu, M.; Nomikos, A.P.; Chiu, Y.F.; Wagner, R.J.; Powell, R.J.; Hwa, J.; Martin, K.A. The prostacyclin receptor induces human vascular smooth muscle cell differentiation via the protein kinase A pathway. *Am. J. Physiol. Heart Circ. Physiol.* **2006**, *290*, H1337–H1346. [CrossRef] [PubMed]
5. Johnson, R.; Webb, J.G.; Newman, W.H.; Wang, Z. Regulation of human vascular smooth muscle cell migration by beta-adrenergic receptors. *Am. Surg.* **2006**, *72*, 51–54. [PubMed]
6. Li, R.C.; Cindrova-Davies, T.; Skepper, J.N.; Sellers, L.A. Prostacyclin induces apoptosis of vascular smooth muscle cells by a cAMP-mediated inhibition of extracellular signal-regulated kinase activity and can counteract the mitogenic activity of endothelin-1 or basic fibroblast growth factor. *Circ. Res.* **2004**, *94*, 759–767. [CrossRef] [PubMed]
7. Wu, Y.J.; Bond, M.; Sala-Newby, G.B.; Newby, A.C. Altered S-phase kinase-associated protein-2 levels are a major mediator of cyclic nucleotide-induced inhibition of vascular smooth muscle cell proliferation. *Circ. Res.* **2006**, *98*, 1141–1150. [CrossRef] [PubMed]
8. Cheng, X.; Ji, Z.; Tsalkova, T.; Mei, F. Epac and PKA: A tale of two intracellular cAMP receptors. *Acta Biochim. Biophys. Sin. (Shanghai)* **2008**, *40*, 651–662. [CrossRef] [PubMed]
9. Chen, J.; Levin, L.R.; Buck, J. Role of soluble adenylyl cyclase in the heart. *Am. J. Physiol. Heart Circ. Physiol.* **2012**, *302*, H538–H543. [CrossRef] [PubMed]
10. Hayes, J.S.; Brunton, L.L.; Mayer, S.E. Selective activation of particulate cAMP-dependent protein kinase by isoproterenol and prostaglandin E1. *J. Biol. Chem.* **1980**, *255*, 5113–5119. [PubMed]
11. Beavo, J.A.; Brunton, L.L. Cyclic nucleotide research–still expanding after half a century. *Nat. Rev. Mol. Cell Biol.* **2002**, *3*, 710–718. [CrossRef] [PubMed]
12. Hayes, J.S.; Brunton, L.L. Functional compartments in cyclic nucleotide action. *J. Cycl. Nucleotide Res.* **1982**, *8*, 1–16.
13. Zaccolo, M.; Pozzan, T. Discrete microdomains with high concentration of cAMP in stimulated rat neonatal cardiac myocytes. *Science* **2002**, *295*, 1711–1715. [CrossRef] [PubMed]

14. Baillie, G.S. Compartmentalized signalling: Spatial regulation of cAMP by the action of compartmentalized phosphodiesterases. *FEBS J.* **2009**, *276*, 1790–1799. [CrossRef] [PubMed]

15. Ke, H.; Wang, H. Crystal structures of phosphodiesterases and implications on substrate specificity and inhibitor selectivity. *Curr. Top. Med. Chem.* **2007**, *7*, 391–403. [CrossRef] [PubMed]

16. Bolger, G.B. Molecular biology of the cyclic AMP-specific cyclic nucleotide phosphodiesterases: A diverse family of regulatory enzymes. *Cell. Signal.* **1994**, *6*, 851–859. [CrossRef]

17. Houslay, M.D. PDE4 cAMP-specific phosphodiesterases. *Prog. Nucleic Acid Res. Mol. Biol.* **2001**, *69*, 249–315. [PubMed]

18. Hoffmann, R.; Baillie, G.S.; MacKenzie, S.J.; Yarwood, S.J.; Houslay, M.D. The MAP kinase ERK2 inhibits the cyclic AMP-specific phosphodiesterase HSPDE4D3 by phosphorylating it at Ser579. *EMBO J.* **1999**, *18*, 893–903. [CrossRef] [PubMed]

19. MacKenzie, S.J.; Baillie, G.S.; McPhee, I.; MacKenzie, C.; Seamons, R.; McSorley, T.; Millen, J.; Beard, M.B.; van Heeke, G.; Houslay, M.D. Long PDE4 cAMP specific phosphodiesterases are activated by protein kinase A-mediated phosphorylation of a single serine residue in Upstream Conserved Region 1 (UCR1). *Br. J. Pharmacol.* **2002**, *136*, 421–433. [CrossRef] [PubMed]

20. Sette, C.; Conti, M. Phosphorylation and activation of a cAMP-specific phosphodiesterase by the cAMP-dependent protein kinase. Involvement of serine 54 in the enzyme activation. *J. Biol. Chem.* **1996**, *271*, 16526–16534. [CrossRef] [PubMed]

21. Burgin, A.B.; Magnusson, O.T.; Singh, J.; Witte, P.; Staker, B.L.; Bjornsson, J.M.; Thorsteinsdottir, M.; Hrafnsdottir, S.; Hagen, T.; Kiselyov, A.S.; et al. Design of phosphodiesterase 4D (PDE4D) allosteric modulators for enhancing cognition with improved safety. *Nat. Biotechnol.* **2010**, *28*, 63–70. [CrossRef] [PubMed]

22. Ahmad, F.; Murata, T.; Shimizu, K.; Degerman, E.; Maurice, D.; Manganiello, V. Cyclic nucleotide phosphodiesterases: Important signaling modulators and therapeutic targets. *Oral Dis.* **2015**, *21*, e25–e50. [CrossRef] [PubMed]

23. McCahill, A.C.; Huston, E.; Li, X.; Houslay, M.D. PDE4 associates with different scaffolding proteins: Modulating interactions as treatment for certain diseases. *Handb. Exp. Pharmacol.* **2008**, *186*, 125–166.

24. Houslay, M.D.; Adams, D.R. PDE4 cAMP phosphodiesterases: Modular enzymes that orchestrate signalling cross-talk, desensitization and compartmentalization. *Biochem. J.* **2003**, *370*, 1–18. [CrossRef] [PubMed]

25. Huston, E.; Gall, I.; Houslay, T.M.; Houslay, M.D. Helix-1 of the cAMP-specific phosphodiesterase PDE4A1 regulates its phospholipase-D-dependent redistribution in response to release of Ca^{2+}. *J. Cell Sci.* **2006**, *119*, 3799–3810. [CrossRef] [PubMed]

26. Houslay, K.F.; Christian, F.; MacLeod, R.; Adams, D.R.; Houslay, M.D.; Baillie, G.S. Identification of a multifunctional docking site on the catalytic unit of phosphodiesterase-4 (PDE4) that is utilised by multiple interaction partners. *Biochem. J.* **2017**, *474*, 597–609. [CrossRef] [PubMed]

27. Wills, L.; Ehsan, M.; Whiteley, E.L.; Baillie, G.S. Location, location, location: PDE4D5 function is directed by its unique N-terminal region. *Cell. Signal.* **2016**, *28*, 701–705. [CrossRef] [PubMed]

28. Lee, L.C.; Maurice, D.H.; Baillie, G.S. Targeting protein-protein interactions within the cyclic AMP signaling system as a therapeutic strategy for cardiovascular disease. *Future Med. Chem.* **2013**, *5*, 451–464. [CrossRef] [PubMed]

29. Lynch, M.J.; Baillie, G.S.; Mohamed, A.; Li, X.; Maisonneuve, C.; Klussmann, E.; van Heeke, G.; Houslay, M.D. RNA silencing identifies PDE4D5 as the functionally relevant cAMP phosphodiesterase interacting with beta arrestin to control the protein kinase A/AKAP79-mediated switching of the beta2-adrenergic receptor to activation of ERK in HEK293B2 cells. *J. Biol. Chem.* **2005**, *280*, 33178–33189. [CrossRef] [PubMed]

30. Banan, M.; Puri, N. The ins and outs of RNAi in mammalian cells. *Curr. Pharm. Biotechnol.* **2004**, *5*, 441–450. [CrossRef] [PubMed]

31. McCahill, A.; McSorley, T.; Huston, E.; Hill, E.V.; Lynch, M.J.; Gall, I.; Keryer, G.; Lygren, B.; Tasken, K.; van Heeke, G.; et al. In resting COS1 cells a dominant negative approach shows that specific, anchored PDE4 cAMP phosphodiesterase isoforms gate the activation, by basal cyclic AMP production, of AKAP-tethered protein kinase A type II located in the centrosomal region. *Cell. Signal.* **2005**, *17*, 1158–1173. [CrossRef] [PubMed]

32. Frank, R. The SPOT-synthesis technique. Synthetic peptide arrays on membrane supports–principles and applications. *J. Immunol. Methods* **2002**, *267*, 13–26. [CrossRef]

33. Bolger, G.B.; Baillie, G.S.; Li, X.; Lynch, M.J.; Herzyk, P.; Mohamed, A.; Mitchell, L.H.; McCahill, A.; Hundsrucker, C.; Klussmann, E.; et al. Scanning peptide array analyses identify overlapping binding sites for the signalling scaffold proteins, beta-arrestin and RACK1, in cAMP-specific phosphodiesterase PDE4D5. *Biochem. J.* **2006**, *398*, 23–36. [CrossRef] [PubMed]

34. Baillie, G.S. George Baillie on peptide array, a technique that transformed research on phosphodiesterases. *Future Sci. OA* **2015**, *1*. [CrossRef] [PubMed]

35. Sin, Y.Y.; Edwards, H.V.; Li, X.; Day, J.P.; Christian, F.; Dunlop, A.J.; Adams, D.R.; Zaccolo, M.; Houslay, M.D.; Baillie, G.S. Disruption of the cyclic AMP phosphodiesterase-4 (PDE4)-HSP20 complex attenuates the beta-agonist induced hypertrophic response in cardiac myocytes. *J. Mol. Cell. Cardiol.* **2011**, *50*, 872–883. [CrossRef] [PubMed]

36. Berrera, M.; Dodoni, G.; Monterisi, S.; Pertegato, V.; Zamparo, I.; Zaccolo, M. A toolkit for real-time detection of cAMP: Insights into compartmentalized signaling. *Handb. Exp. Pharmacol.* **2008**, *186*, 285–298.

37. Fischmeister, R.; Castro, L.R.; Abi-Gerges, A.; Rochais, F.; Jurevicius, J.; Leroy, J.; Vandecasteele, G. Compartmentation of cyclic nucleotide signaling in the heart: The role of cyclic nucleotide phosphodiesterases. *Circ. Res.* **2006**, *99*, 816–828. [CrossRef] [PubMed]

38. Zhao, C.Y.; Greenstein, J.L.; Winslow, R.L. Interaction between phosphodiesterases in the regulation of the cardiac beta-adrenergic pathway. *J. Mol. Cell. Cardiol.* **2015**, *88*, 29–38. [CrossRef] [PubMed]

39. Bers, D.M. Cardiac excitation-contraction coupling. *Nature* **2002**, *415*, 198–205. [CrossRef] [PubMed]

40. Mongillo, M.; McSorley, T.; Evellin, S.; Sood, A.; Lissandron, V.; Terrin, A.; Huston, E.; Hannawacker, A.; Lohse, M.J.; Pozzan, T.; et al. Fluorescence resonance energy transfer-based analysis of cAMP dynamics in live neonatal rat cardiac myocytes reveals distinct functions of compartmentalized phosphodiesterases. *Circ. Res.* **2004**, *95*, 67–75. [CrossRef] [PubMed]

41. Lehnart, S.E.; Marks, A.R. Phosphodiesterase 4D and heart failure: A cautionary tale. *Expert Opin. Ther. Targets* **2006**, *10*, 677–688. [CrossRef] [PubMed]

42. Packer, M.; Carver, J.R.; Rodeheffer, R.J.; Ivanhoe, R.J.; DiBianco, R.; Zeldis, S.M.; Hendrix, G.H.; Bommer, W.J.; Elkayam, U.; Kukin, M.L.; et al. Effect of oral milrinone on mortality in severe chronic heart failure. The PROMISE Study Research Group. *N. Engl. J. Med.* **1991**, *325*, 1468–1475. [CrossRef] [PubMed]

43. Lehnart, S.E.; Wehrens, X.H.; Reiken, S.; Warrier, S.; Belevych, A.E.; Harvey, R.D.; Richter, W.; Jin, S.L.; Conti, M.; Marks, A.R. Phosphodiesterase 4D deficiency in the ryanodine-receptor complex promotes heart failure and arrhythmias. *Cell* **2005**, *123*, 25–35. [CrossRef] [PubMed]

44. Abi-Gerges, A.; Richter, W.; Lefebvre, F.; Mateo, P.; Varin, A.; Heymes, C.; Samuel, J.L.; Lugnier, C.; Conti, M.; Fischmeister, R.; et al. Decreased expression and activity of cAMP phosphodiesterases in cardiac hypertrophy and its impact on beta-adrenergic cAMP signals. *Circ. Res.* **2009**, *105*, 784–792. [CrossRef] [PubMed]

45. Maurice, D.H.; Ke, H.; Ahmad, F.; Wang, Y.; Chung, J.; Manganiello, V.C. Advances in targeting cyclic nucleotide phosphodiesterases. *Nat. Rev. Drug Discov.* **2014**, *13*, 290–314. [CrossRef] [PubMed]

46. Bolger, G.B.; McCahill, A.; Huston, E.; Cheung, Y.F.; McSorley, T.; Baillie, G.S.; Houslay, M.D. The unique amino-terminal region of the PDE4D5 cAMP phosphodiesterase isoform confers preferential interaction with beta-arrestins. *J. Biol. Chem.* **2003**, *278*, 49230–49238. [CrossRef] [PubMed]

47. Leroy, J.; Richter, W.; Mika, D.; Castro, L.R.; Abi-Gerges, A.; Xie, M.; Scheitrum, C.; Lefebvre, F.; Schittl, J.; Mateo, P.; et al. Phosphodiesterase 4B in the cardiac L-type Ca^{2+} channel complex regulates Ca^{2+} current and protects against ventricular arrhythmias in mice. *J. Clin. Invest.* **2011**, *121*, 2651–2661. [CrossRef] [PubMed]

48. Beca, S.; Helli, P.B.; Simpson, J.A.; Zhao, D.; Farman, G.P.; Jones, P.; Tian, X.; Wilson, L.S.; Ahmad, F.; Chen, S.R.W.; et al. Phosphodiesterase 4D regulates baseline sarcoplasmic reticulum Ca^{2+} release and cardiac contractility, independently of L-type Ca^{2+} current. *Circ. Res.* **2011**, *109*, 1024–1030. [CrossRef] [PubMed]

49. Terrenoire, C.; Houslay, M.D.; Baillie, G.S.; Kass, R.S. The cardiac IKs potassium channel macromolecular complex includes the phosphodiesterase PDE4D3. *J. Biol. Chem.* **2009**, *284*, 9140–9146. [CrossRef] [PubMed]

50. Daaka, Y.; Luttrell, L.M.; Lefkowitz, R.J. Switching of the coupling of the beta2-adrenergic receptor to different G proteins by protein kinase A. *Nature* **1997**, *390*, 88–91. [PubMed]

51. Krupnick, J.G.; Benovic, J.L. The role of receptor kinases and arrestins in G protein-coupled receptor regulation. *Annu. Rev. Pharmacol. Toxicol.* **1998**, *38*, 289–319. [CrossRef] [PubMed]

52. Perry, S.J.; Baillie, G.S.; Kohout, T.A.; McPhee, I.; Magiera, M.M.; Ang, K.L.; Miller, W.E.; McLean, A.J.; Conti, M.; Houslay, M.D.; et al. Targeting of cyclic AMP degradation to β2-adrenergic receptors by β-arrestins. *Science* **2002**, *298*, 834–836. [CrossRef] [PubMed]

53. Baillie, G.S.; Sood, A.; McPhee, I.; Gall, I.; Perry, S.J.; Lefkowitz, R.J.; Houslay, M.D. β-Arrestin-mediated PDE4 cAMP phosphodiesterase recruitment regulates β-adrenoceptor switching from G_s to G_i. *Proc. Natl. Acad. Sci. USA* **2003**, *100*, 940–945. [CrossRef] [PubMed]

54. Sun, Y.; MacRae, T.H. The small heat shock proteins and their role in human disease. *FEBS J.* **2005**, *272*, 2613–2627. [CrossRef] [PubMed]

55. Fan, G.C.; Chu, G.; Mitton, B.; Song, Q.; Yuan, Q.; Kranias, E.G. Small heat-shock protein Hsp20 phosphorylation inhibits β-agonist-induced cardiac apoptosis. *Circ. Res.* **2004**, *94*, 1474–1482. [CrossRef] [PubMed]

56. Nicolaou, P.; Knoll, R.; Haghighi, K.; Fan, G.C.; Dorn, G.W., 2nd; Hasenfub, G.; Kranias, E.G. Human mutation in the anti-apoptotic heat shock protein 20 abrogates its cardioprotective effects. *J. Biol. Chem.* **2008**, *283*, 33465–33471. [CrossRef] [PubMed]

57. Qian, J.; Ren, X.; Wang, X.; Zhang, P.; Jones, W.K.; Molkentin, J.D.; Fan, G.C.; Kranias, E.G. Blockade of Hsp20 phosphorylation exacerbates cardiac ischemia/reperfusion injury by suppressed autophagy and increased cell death. *Circ. Res.* **2009**, *105*, 1223–1231. [CrossRef] [PubMed]

58. Wang, X.; Zingarelli, B.; O'Connor, M.; Zhang, P.; Adeyemo, A.; Kranias, E.G.; Wang, Y.; Fan, G.C. Overexpression of Hsp20 prevents endotoxin-induced myocardial dysfunction and apoptosis via inhibition of NF-κB activation. *J. Mol. Cell. Cardiol.* **2009**, *47*, 382–390. [CrossRef] [PubMed]

59. Fan, G.C.; Zhou, X.; Wang, X.; Song, G.; Qian, J.; Nicolaou, P.; Chen, G.; Ren, X.; Kranias, E.G. Heat shock protein 20 interacting with phosphorylated Akt reduces doxorubicin-triggered oxidative stress and cardiotoxicity. *Circ. Res.* **2008**, *103*, 1270–1279. [CrossRef] [PubMed]

60. Tessier, D.J.; Komalavilas, P.; Panitch, A.; Joshi, L.; Brophy, C.M. The small heat shock protein (HSP) 20 is dynamically associated with the actin cross-linking protein actinin. *J. Surg. Res.* **2003**, *111*, 152–157. [CrossRef]

61. Zhu, Y.H.; Ma, T.M.; Wang, X. Gene transfer of heat-shock protein 20 protects against ischemia/reperfusion injury in rat hearts. *Acta Pharmacol. Sin.* **2005**, *26*, 1193–1200. [CrossRef] [PubMed]

62. Dohke, T.; Wada, A.; Isono, T.; Fujii, M.; Yamamoto, T.; Tsutamoto, T.; Horie, M. Proteomic analysis reveals significant alternations of cardiac small heat shock protein expression in congestive heart failure. *J. Card. Fail.* **2006**, *12*, 77–84. [CrossRef] [PubMed]

63. Fan, G.C.; Yuan, Q.; Song, G.; Wang, Y.; Chen, G.; Qian, J.; Zhou, X.; Lee, Y.J.; Ashraf, M.; Kranias, E.G. Small heat-shock protein Hsp20 attenuates β-agonist-mediated cardiac remodeling through apoptosis signal-regulating kinase 1. *Circ. Res.* **2006**, *99*, 1233–1242. [CrossRef] [PubMed]

64. Edwards, H.V.; Scott, J.D.; Baillie, G.S. PKA phosphorylation of the small heat-shock protein Hsp20 enhances its cardioprotective effects. *Biochem. Soc. Trans.* **2012**, *40*, 210–214. [CrossRef] [PubMed]

65. Martin, T.P.; Hortigon-Vinagre, M.P.; Findlay, J.E.; Elliott, C.; Currie, S.; Baillie, G.S. Targeted disruption of the heat shock protein 20-phosphodiesterase 4D (PDE4D) interaction protects against pathological cardiac remodelling in a mouse model of hypertrophy. *FEBS Open Bio* **2014**, *4*, 923–927. [CrossRef] [PubMed]

66. Marx, S.O.; Reiken, S.; Hisamatsu, Y.; Jayaraman, T.; Burkhoff, D.; Rosemblit, N.; Marks, A.R. PKA phosphorylation dissociates FKBP12.6 from the calcium release channel (ryanodine receptor): Defective regulation in failing hearts. *Cell* **2000**, *101*, 365–376. [CrossRef]

67. Antos, C.L.; Frey, N.; Marx, S.O.; Reiken, S.; Gaburjakova, M.; Richardson, J.A.; Marks, A.R.; Olson, E.N. Dilated cardiomyopathy and sudden death resulting from constitutive activation of protein kinase A. *Circ. Res.* **2001**, *89*, 997–1004. [CrossRef] [PubMed]

68. Reiken, S.; Gaburjakova, M.; Guatimosim, S.; Gomez, A.M.; D'Armiento, J.; Burkhoff, D.; Wang, J.; Vassort, G.; Lederer, W.J.; Marks, A.R. Protein kinase A phosphorylation of the cardiac calcium release channel (ryanodine receptor) in normal and failing hearts. Role of phosphatases and response to isoproterenol. *J. Biol. Chem.* **2003**, *278*, 444–453. [CrossRef] [PubMed]

69. Reiken, S.; Wehrens, X.H.; Vest, J.A.; Barbone, A.; Klotz, S.; Mancini, D.; Burkhof, D.; Marks, A.R. β-Blockers restore calcium release channel function and improve cardiac muscle performance in human heart failure. *Circulation* **2003**, *107*, 2459–2466. [CrossRef] [PubMed]

70. Wehrens, X.H.; Lehnart, S.E.; Huang, F.; Vest, J.A.; Reiken, S.R.; Mohler, P.J.; Sun, J.; Guatimosim, S.; Song, L.S.; Rosemblit, N.; et al. FKBP12.6 deficiency and defective calcium release channel (ryanodine receptor) function linked to exercise-induced sudden cardiac death. *Cell* **2003**, *113*, 829–840. [CrossRef]

71. Wehrens, X.H.; Lehnart, S.E.; Reiken, S.R.; Deng, S.X.; Vest, J.A.; Cervantes, D.; Coromilas, J.; Landry, D.W.; Marks, A.R. Protection from cardiac arrhythmia through ryanodine receptor-stabilizing protein calstabin2. *Science* **2004**, *304*, 292–296. [CrossRef] [PubMed]

72. Richter, W.; Jin, S.L.C.; Conti, M. Splice variants of the cyclic nucleotide phosphodiesterase PDE4D are differentially expressed and regulated in rat tissue. *Biochem. J.* **2005**, *388*, 803–811. [CrossRef] [PubMed]

73. Regitz-Zagrosek, V.; Hertrampf, R.; Steffen, C.; Hildebrandt, A.; Fleck, E. Myocardial cyclic AMP and norepinephrine content in human heart failure. *Eur. Heart J.* **1994**, *15* (Suppl. D), 7–13. [CrossRef] [PubMed]

74. Sanguinetti, M.C.; Curran, M.E.; Zou, A.; Shen, J.; Spector, P.S.; Atkinson, D.L.; Keating, M.T. Coassembly of K_VLQT1 and minK (IsK) proteins to form cardiac I_{KS} potassium channel. *Nature* **1996**, *384*, 80–83. [CrossRef] [PubMed]

75. Barhanin, J.; Lesage, F.; Guillemare, E.; Fink, M.; Lazdunski, M.; Romey, G. K_VLQT1 and lsK (minK) proteins associate to form the I_{KS} cardiac potassium current. *Nature* **1996**, *384*, 78–80. [CrossRef] [PubMed]

76. Li, Y.; Chen, L.; Kass, R.S.; Dessauer, C.W. The A-kinase anchoring protein Yotiao facilitates complex formation between adenylyl cyclase type 9 and the I_{KS} potassium channel in heart. *J. Biol. Chem.* **2012**, *287*, 29815–29824. [CrossRef] [PubMed]

77. Marx, S.O.; Kurokawa, J.; Reiken, S.; Motoike, H.; D'Armiento, J.; Marks, A.R.; Kass, R.S. Requirement of a macromolecular signaling complex for β adrenergic receptor modulation of the KCNQ1-KCNE1 potassium channel. *Science* **2002**, *295*, 496–499. [CrossRef] [PubMed]

78. Fuller, M.D.; Emrick, M.A.; Sadilek, M.; Scheuer, T.; Catterall, W.A. Molecular mechanism of calcium channel regulation in the fight-or-flight response. *Sci. Signal.* **2010**, *3*, ra70. [CrossRef] [PubMed]

79. Bunemann, M.; Gerhardstein, B.L.; Gao, T.; Hosey, M.M. Functional regulation of L-type calcium channels via protein kinase A-mediated phosphorylation of the beta(2) subunit. *J. Biol. Chem.* **1999**, *274*, 33851–33854. [CrossRef] [PubMed]

80. MacLennan, D.H.; Kranias, E.G. Phospholamban: A crucial regulator of cardiac contractility. *Nat. Rev. Mol. Cell Biol.* **2003**, *4*, 566–577. [CrossRef] [PubMed]

81. Beca, S.; Ahmad, F.; Shen, W.; Liu, J.; Makary, S.; Polidovitch, N.; Sun, J.; Hockman, S.; Chung, Y.W.; Movsesian, M.; et al. Phosphodiesterase type 3A regulates basal myocardial contractility through interacting with sarcoplasmic reticulum calcium ATPase type 2a signaling complexes in mouse heart. *Circ. Res.* **2013**, *112*, 289–297. [CrossRef] [PubMed]

82. Maurice, D.H. Subcellular signaling in the endothelium: Cyclic nucleotides take their place. *Curr. Opin. Pharmacol.* **2011**, *11*, 656–664. [CrossRef] [PubMed]

83. Sayner, S.L.; Alexeyev, M.; Dessauer, C.W.; Stevens, T. Soluble adenylyl cyclase reveals the significance of cAMP compartmentation on pulmonary microvascular endothelial cell barrier. *Circ. Res.* **2006**, *98*, 675–681. [CrossRef] [PubMed]

84. Dejana, E.; Tournier-Lasserve, E.; Weinstein, B.M. The control of vascular integrity by endothelial cell junctions: Molecular basis and pathological implications. *Dev. Cell* **2009**, *16*, 209–221. [CrossRef] [PubMed]

85. Cavallaro, U.; Dejana, E. Adhesion molecule signalling: Not always a sticky business. *Nat. Rev. Mol. Cell Biol.* **2011**, *12*, 189–197. [CrossRef] [PubMed]

86. Surdo, N.C.; Berrera, M.; Koschinski, A.; Brescia, M.; Machado, M.R.; Carr, C.; Wright, P.; Gorelik, J.; Morotti, S.; Grandi, E.; et al. FRET biosensor uncovers cAMP nano-domains at beta-adrenergic targets that dictate precise tuning of cardiac contractility. *Nat. Commun.* **2017**, *8*, 15031. [CrossRef] [PubMed]

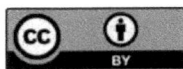

Journal of
*Cardiovascular
Development and Disease*

MDPI

Review

Roles of PDE1 in Pathological Cardiac Remodeling and Dysfunction

Si Chen [1,2], Walter E. Knight [3] and Chen Yan [1,*]

[1] Aab Cardiovascular Research Institute, Department of Medicine, University of Rochester School of Medicine and Dentistry, Rochester, NY 14641, USA; si_chen@urmc.rochester.edu

[2] Department of Pharmacology and Physiology, University of Rochester School of Medicine and Dentistry, Rochester, NY 14641, USA

[3] Division of Cardiology, Department of Medicine, University of Colorado School of Medicine, 12700 E. 19th Avenue, B139, Aurora, CO 80045, USA; wek4@cornell.edu

* Correspondence: chen_yan@urmc.rochester.edu; Tel.: +585-276-7704

Received: 12 March 2018; Accepted: 20 April 2018; Published: 23 April 2018

Abstract: Pathological cardiac hypertrophy and dysfunction is a response to various stress stimuli and can result in reduced cardiac output and heart failure. Cyclic nucleotide signaling regulates several cardiac functions including contractility, remodeling, and fibrosis. Cyclic nucleotide phosphodiesterases (PDEs), by catalyzing the hydrolysis of cyclic nucleotides, are critical in the homeostasis of intracellular cyclic nucleotide signaling and hold great therapeutic potential as drug targets. Recent studies have revealed that the inhibition of the PDE family member PDE1 plays a protective role in pathological cardiac remodeling and dysfunction by the modulation of distinct cyclic nucleotide signaling pathways. This review summarizes recent key findings regarding the roles of PDE1 in the cardiac system that can lead to a better understanding of its therapeutic potential.

Keywords: phosphodiesterases (PDEs); PDE1; cyclic nucleotide; cardiac hypertrophy; cardiac dysfunction

1. Introduction

Heart failure, the inability of the heart to provide sufficient blood to the body, is a leading cause of death in the United States. Heart failure is associated with significant myocardial deterioration, including pathological hypertrophy, fibrosis, and cell death, as well as contractile dysfunction and ventricular arrhythmia [1]. Therefore, identifying novel molecular targets involved in pathological cardiac remodeling and dysfunction is crucial. Cyclic nucleotide signaling is important in numerous biological functions and pathological processes in the cardiovascular system, ranging from short-term muscle contraction/relaxation to long-term cell growth/survival and structural remodeling [2]. Phosphodiesterases (PDEs), by catalyzing the hydrolysis of cyclic nucleotides, play important roles in the regulation of intracellular cyclic nucleotide amplitude, duration, and compartmentalization [3]. Alterations in PDE expression and activity are responsible for disruptions in cyclic nucleotide homeostasis, contributing to disease progression [3]. In this review, we give an overview of the role and therapeutic potential of PDE1 regulation in pathological cardiac remodeling and dysfunction.

2. Pathological Cardiac Remodeling and Heart Failure

The heart is comprised of both cardiac myocytes and non-myocytes, including fibroblasts, endothelial cells, mast cells, and smooth muscle cells, as well as extracellular matrix [4]. In response to pathological conditions such as hypertension, neurohumoral activation, obesity, valvular heart disease, myocardial injury, and genetic mutations, the heart can undergo pathological remodeling, which features an increase in myocyte size, increased levels of myocyte death, and extracellular matrix protein deposition [5]. Cardiac hypertrophy is an adaptive response to increased workload and initially helps to maintain an almost normal function [1]. However, with prolonged stress, the heart can undergo irreversible decompensation, which is associated with a complex array of unfavorable events [1]. These pathological events include myocyte elongation and myocyte loss, which leads to chamber dilation and the thinning of the ventricular walls [1,6]. In addition, chronic stress stimulates cardiac fibroblast activation, characterized by a phenotypic changes to alpha-smooth muscle actin (α-SMA)-positive myofibroblasts [7]. Activated fibroblasts gain functions in cell proliferation, migration, and extracellular matrix (ECM) production, which leads to cardiac fibrosis, a hallmark of pathological cardiac remodeling [7,8]. Moreover, cardiac myocyte death is associated with various types of cardiac disease [9]. Apoptosis, necrosis, and autophagy are the three major types of cell death found in the heart, which induce cardiac arrhythmia, trigger cardiac remodeling, and ultimately lead to cardiac dysfunction [10]. Therefore, limiting cardiac myocyte loss by attenuating cell death has critical implications for the treatment of heart failure.

Numerous signaling pathways and molecular mechanisms have been implicated in cardiac hypertrophy [11]. For example, calcium (Ca^{2+})-dependent signaling molecules such as Ca^{2+}/calmodulin-dependent serine/threonine phosphatase, calcineurin, and the Ca^{2+}/calmodulin- dependent kinase II (CaMKII) play well-known roles in pathological cardiac remodeling [12]. Calcineurin has been implicated in mediating pathological hypertrophy in conjunction with the transcription factor nuclear factor of activated T cells (NFAT) [1,12]. Upon dephosphorylation by calcineurin in the cytosol, NFAT is imported into the nucleus and thus serves to induce a hypertrophic response [1]. The inhibition of calcineurin alleviates cardiac myocyte hypertrophy induced by Ang II or α-adrenergic agonist stimulation in vitro, and by pressure overload and isoproterenol (ISO) treatment in vivo [13]. The expression and phosphorylation of CaMKII can also be induced by an upregulation of intracellular Ca^{2+} levels in the cardiac myocyte [14]. In cardiac hypertrophy, CaMKII exerts its molecular effects by binding to and phosphorylating target proteins such as class II histone deacetylases (HDACs). Upon phosphorylation by CaMKII, several class II HDACs regulate the derepression of myocyte enhancer factor 2 (MEF2)-dependent genes through the nuclear export of HDACs, which contributes critically to hypertrophic signaling in the heart [15].

3. Cyclic Nucleotide Signaling and PDEs in the Heart

3.1. Cyclic 3′,5′ Adenosine Monophosphate (cAMP) Signaling

Cyclic AMP was first isolated and characterized by Sutherland and Rall over a half-century ago [16,17]. A large family of enzymes known as the adenylyl cyclases (ACs) catalyze the synthesis of cAMP from adenosine triphosphate (ATP) in response to a variety of extracellular signals such as hormones, growth factors, and neurotransmitters [18,19]. To date, 10 ACs, including nine membrane ACs and one soluble AC, have been identified [20,21]. Membrane ACs are regulated by G-protein coupled receptors (GPCRs), whereas soluble ACs are regulated by bicarbonate and Ca^{2+} [20–22]. This increase in cAMP leads to the activation of several downstream effector molecules including protein kinase A (PKA), an exchange factor directly activated by cAMP (EPAC), and cyclic nucleotide gated channels (CNGs) [18]. The development of Förster resonance energy transfer (FRET)-based techniques that enable the measurement of cAMP concentrations at the single cell level have demonstrated that cAMP levels are not uniform throughout the entire cell, which may indicate that it regulates different biological functions [23,24].

In the cardiac myocyte, catecholamines stimulate the β-adrenergic receptors (β-ARs), leading to cAMP-mediated activation of PKA signaling, which then is able to phosphorylate L-type Ca^{2+} channels (LTCC) and ryanodine receptors (RYRs) to induce intracellular Ca^{2+} increases, thus stimulating myocyte contractility [25–28]. Furthermore, the PKA-mediated phosphorylation of phospholamban (PLB) leads to enhanced Ca^{2+} re-uptake through the sarcoplasmic/endoplasmic reticulum calcium

ATPase 2 (SERCA2) in the sarcoplasmic reticulum (SR) adjacent to the T-tubule, leading to faster myofilament relaxation [29]. β-AR mediated cAMP signaling can be either detrimental or beneficial to the heart. Acute stimulation of β1-AR/cAMP has beneficial effects on cardiac contractile function, whereas chronic stimulation results in myocyte hypertrophy, apoptosis, and cardiac fibrosis, finally leading to heart failure [30]. Interestingly, it has been found that the activation of cAMP/PKA signaling by stimulating the adenosine A_2 receptor (A_2R) is cardiac-protective: for example, A_2R activation alleviated transverse aortic constriction (TAC)-induced cardiac dysfunction [31]. These studies indicate that different cAMP signaling modules regulate distinct and even opposing effects in cardiac myocytes.

3.2. Cyclic 3′,5′ Guanosine Monophosphate (cGMP) Signaling

Cyclic GMP is generated from GTP by two families of guanylyl cyclases (GCs), with seven particulate GCs (pGCs) activated by natriuretic peptides (NPs) and three soluble GCs (sGCs) activated by nitric oxide (NO) or carbon monoxide (CO) [32,33]. cGMP regulates three major types of effector molecules: cGMP dependent protein kinases (PKG), cGMP-regulated PDEs, and cGMP-gated cation channels [34]. Similar to cAMP, cGMP is highly compartmentalized in the cell, and elicits distinct downstream biological effects [35,36]. There appear to be multiple protective cGMP signaling modules in the heart [37–40]. For example, a study by Frantz and colleagues found that mice with a cardiac myocyte-specific PKGI knockout (KO) developed significant cardiac dysfunction and cardiomyopathy in both Ang II- and TAC-induced cardiac hypertrophic models, with decreased expression of SERCA2 and PLB and altered Ca^{2+} homeostasis [37]. PDE5 inhibition has been shown to attenuate cardiac hypertrophy by targeting NO-sGC-derived cGMP [38,40–43]. PDE9 inhibition also protects against cardiac hypertrophy by targeting NP-pGC-derived cGMP [44]. Similarly, we have also found that PDE1A inhibition attenuates cardiac myocyte hypertrophy in a cGMP-dependent manner [45].

3.3. Different PDE Isozymes in the Heart

The degradation of cyclic nucleotides is catalyzed by PDEs. The PDE superfamily is comprised of 11 structurally related but functionally distinct gene families, PDE1–PDE11, with differences in their cellular functions, structures, catalytic properties, and mechanisms of regulation [3]. All PDEs share a conserved carboxyl-terminal catalytic core of approximately 270 amino acids, with a shared sequence identity of 25–50% between family members [46]. However, the regulatory characteristics of PDEs are determined by their unique amino-terminal regions, which contain elements known to be involved in enzyme phosphorylation, dimerization, auto-inhibition, ligand binding, and protein-protein interaction. These regions thus allow distinct localization and heterogeneity in cyclic nucleotide signaling and enable diverse functions of various PDEs [3,46,47].

Research has clearly established that the degradation of cyclic nucleotides by PDEs is regulated differently under physiological and pathological conditions. In particular, the expression and activity of several PDEs are altered in various types of cardiovascular disease [40,44,45,48,49]. Up to now, at least seven PDE family members have been found in the heart, including PDE1–PDE9 [44,48,50–54]. Among these, PDE4 and PDE8 specifically hydrolyze cAMP, PDE5 and PDE9 specifically hydrolyze cGMP, while PDE1, 2, and 3 can hydrolyze both cAMP and cGMP [3]. Thus, a thorough understanding of the roles of specific PDE isoforms in cardiac pathology and physiology is critical. This review mainly focuses on the roles of two isoforms of PDE1 in the heart (PDE1A and PDE1C).

4. PDE1 and Pathological Cardiac Remodeling and Dysfunction

4.1. PDE1

The PDE1 family was one of the first classes of PDEs to be identified [55]. All PDE1 family members are regulated by the binding of Ca^{2+}/CaM, which is the reason that PDE1 is also referred to as Ca^{2+}/CaM-stimulated PDE [56]. Thus, the Ca^{2+}-dependent activation of PDE1 isozymes plays a critical role in the crosstalk between Ca^{2+} and cyclic nucleotide signaling [57]. The PDE1 family members are encoded by three distinct genes, *PDE1A, 1B,* and *1C,* and alternative splicing of these genes gives rise to a number of functionally distinct isozymes, which allows for differential cell/subcellular expression and Ca^{2+} sensitivity, leading to the finely tuned regulation of cyclic nucleotide signaling [45]. Like other PDEs, PDE1 variants consist of a conserved C-terminal catalytic domain with diverse N-terminal regulatory domains. The N-terminus of all PDE1s contains two CaM binding domains with an inhibitory sequence in between them. It has been suggested that the binding of Ca^{2+}/CaM therefore relieves the inhibition of PDE1 activity [58]. As a consequence, the catalytic activity of PDE1 can be stimulated more than 10-fold upon the binding of Ca^{2+}/CaM [56,59]. Each PDE1 isoform is able to catalyze the hydrolysis of both cAMP and cGMP, but with different substrate affinities. PDE1As hydrolyze cGMP ($Km \approx 5$ µM) with greater affinity than cAMP ($Km \approx 112$ µM) in vitro [59]. PDE1B enzymes also prefer cGMP ($Km \approx 2.4$ µM) to cAMP ($Km \approx 24$ µM) [49]. However, PDE1Cs hydrolyze cAMP and cGMP with a similarly high affinity ($Km \approx 1$ µM) [49,56].

Given the well-established role of Ca^{2+} signaling in pathological cardiac remodeling and the potential role of PDE1 as a mediator for Ca^{2+} to antagonize cyclic nucleotide signaling, understanding the role of PDE1 in cardiac diseases is of great interest. PDE1 expression is highly regulated with differential isozyme localization to specific tissues and cell types [50,58,60,61]. PDE1A expression is relatively low in the normal heart but is upregulated in the diseased heart, which is consistent among humans, rats, and mice [62]. PDE1C expression varies with species: it is high in human, modest in mouse, and low in rat normal heart [45,62,63]. PDE1B expression is barely detectable in the heart [62,63]. In human myocardium, PDE1C has been shown to be localized along the M- and Z-lines of cardiac myocytes in a striated pattern [62]. Taken together, these observations indicate that there are substantial species-specific differences in PDE1 expression in the heart. With the development of PDE1-selective inhibitors and the genetically engineered PDE1 KO mice, the roles of PDE1 in cardiac cells and cardiac disease models have been recently explored in vitro and in vivo. Here we review the expression and regulation of different PDE1 isoforms in pathological cardiac remodeling and dysfunction.

4.2. Role of PDE1A in Cardiac Myocyte Hypertrophy and Fibroblast Activation

PDE1A expression has been found to be significantly upregulated in diseased hearts of various etiologies, such as in mouse hearts with dysfunction induced by chronic ISO infusion, myocardial infarction (MI), and TAC, in rat heart treated with chronic Ang II infusion, as well as in human failing hearts with both dilated and ischemic cardiomyopathy [36,45]. PDE1A induction in diseased hearts appears to occur in both cardiac myocytes as well as in activated cardiac fibroblasts in fibrotic areas [36]. PDE1A upregulation has been also observed in cultured neonatal rat ventricular myocytes (NRVMs) and adult rat ventricular myocytes (ARVMs) given hypertrophic stimuli such as ISO or Ang II [45]. To determine the specific contribution of PDE1A to the regulation of cardiac hypertrophy, Miller et al. utilized the pan PDE1-selective inhibitor IC86340 and PDE1A-specific shRNA to block PDE1A function in rat cardiac myocytes where PDE1C expression is limited [45]. They found that PDE1 inhibition by IC86340 and PDE1A downregulation by shRNA prevent the hypertrophic response induced by phenylephrine (PE) treatment in both NRVMs and ARVMs. PE causes a reduction in cGMP levels in cardiac myocytes, which can be abolished by the PDE1 inhibitor IC86340 or PDE1A shRNA [45]. This suggests that PDE1A plays a critical role in the PE-induced suppression of cGMP signaling in cardiac myocytes, likely through the Ca^{2+}-dependent activation of PDE1A. Consistently, PDE1A suppression of cardiac hypertrophy also occurs in a PKG-dependent manner [45]. These studies indicate that the inhibition of PDE1A alleviates cardiac myocyte hypertrophy by blocking a PE-induced decrease in intracellular cGMP and PKG activity [45]. However, the detailed underlying molecular mechanism by which PDE1A-mediated cGMP/PKG signaling regulates cardiac myocyte hypertrophy remains unknown. PDE5A inhibition also suppressed cardiac myocyte hypertrophy in a cGMP/PKG-dependent manner [38]. However, the mechanisms by which PDE1A and PDE5A mediate the regulation of cardiac myocyte hypertrophy appear to be different. This is supported by the fact that treatment with the PDE5 inhibitor sildenafil together with the PDE1 inhibitor IC86340 or PDE1A shRNA elicited additive effects on antagonizing myocyte hypertrophy, suggesting that two different pathways are involved [45].

In addition to cardiac myocytes, PDE1A is also significantly induced in activated cardiac fibroblasts (α-SMA positive myofibroblasts) within fibrotic areas of rodent and human failing hearts [36]. In vitro, PDE1A can be upregulated in rat cardiac fibroblasts by treatment with pro-fibrotic stimuli such as Ang II and transforming growth factor β (TGF-β) [36]. In addition, the PDE1 family contributes 70% of total cGMP-hydrolyzing PDE activity under Ang II stimulation, suggesting a major role for PDE1 in Ang II-activated fibroblasts [36]. The role of PDE1A in cardiac fibroblast activation (phenotype changing to myofibroblasts) was investigated in primary cultured rat cardiac fibroblasts [36]. Both IC86340 and PDE1A shRNA treatment reduced Ang II- or TGF-β-induced myofibroblast activation and ECM synthesis [36]. PDE1A-mediated myofibroblast transformation and ECM synthesis are dependent on the suppression of both cAMP/Epac1/Rap1 signaling as well as cGMP/PKG signaling [36], which is in line with the dual substrate specificity of PDE1A. FRET-based approaches further showed that IC86340 induces a rapid but transient elevation of cGMP, and preferentially stimulated nuclear and perinuclear cAMP production in activated fibroblasts [36]. The roles of PDE1A-mediated regulation of cAMP/Epac1 and cGMP/PKG in cardiac fibroblasts are consistent with previous findings that the activation of Epac1 [64–66] or cGMP/PKG signaling [38,67,68] exerts anti-fibrotic effect in cardiac fibroblasts.

Recently, Wang et al. generated two different lines of global PDE1A null mice by using the transcription activator-like effector nucleases (TALEN) approach, one containing a frame deletion of 15bp within the catalytic active site of mPDE1A and the other exhibiting a frame shift insertion, for the purpose of studying polycystic kidney disease (ADPKD) [69]. It has been shown that both null lines of mice developed a mild renal cystic disease phenotype on a wild-type background and accelerated the development of phenotype in an ADPKD mouse model (a *pkd2* gene mutant background) at ages $\leq$16 weeks [69]. Additionally, these PDE1A null mice had lower aortic blood pressure and increased left ventricular ejection fraction [69]. However, whether PDE1A deficiency affects stress-induced pathological cardiac remodeling and dysfunction is still not clear.

4.3. Role of PDE1C in Pathological Cardiac Remodeling and Dysfunction

PDE1C represents one of the major PDE activities in the normal human heart [62]. Its role in cardiac remodeling and dysfunction was recently evaluated by Knight et al. using a global PDE1C knockout (PDE1C-KO) mouse strain. In their study, it was found that PDE1C expression is upregulated in both mouse and human failing hearts [49], which is consistent with a recent RNA-sequencing study of human failing heart samples reporting an increase of PDE1C expression in both ischemic heart disease and dilated cardiomyopathy [49,70]. Unlike PDE1A, PDE1C is only expressed in cardiac myocytes and is undetectable in cardiac fibroblasts or myofibroblasts [49]. Interestingly, TAC-induced cardiac remodeling and dysfunction observed in PDE1C wild-type (PDE1C-WT) mice was significantly alleviated in PDE1C-KO mice, as indicated by reduced chamber dilation, myocardial hypertrophy, cardiac myocyte apoptosis, and interstitial fibrosis, as well as attenuated loss of fractional shortening and ejection fraction [49]. This indicates a detrimental role for PDE1C in the development of heart failure induced by chronic pressure overload.

In isolated cardiac cells, PDE1C deficiency abolished Ang II-, PE-, or ISO-induced cardiac myocyte hypertrophy [49]. Ang II- and ISO-induced cell death were also blocked in PDE1C-KO myocytes. In addition, IC86340 attenuated cell death and apoptosis in WT myocytes but had no further effect in PDE1C-KO myocytes, indicating that the protective effect of IC86340 on myocyte death is primarily through PDE1C [49]. The anti-hypertrophic and anti-apoptotic effects of PDE1C deficiency and/or inhibition were mediated in a cAMP/PKA-dependent manner, and the PI3K/AKT signaling pathway appears to be important for this protective effect [49]. However, the detailed molecular mechanisms by which PDE1C regulates cAMP-mediated cardiac-protective signaling pathways deserve to be further investigated. PDE1C expression was barely detectable in WT cardiac fibroblasts or WT myofibroblasts (stimulated with TGF-β) [49]. However, TAC-induced cardiac interstitial fibrosis was attenuated in PDE1C-KO hearts [49]. This raises the hypothesis that myocyte PDE1C regulates fibroblast function through a paracrine-dependent mechanism. Indeed, conditioned medium collected from PDE1C-KO but not PDE1C-WT cardiomyocytes was found to attenuate TGF-β-induced fibroblast activation, suggesting that PDE1C inhibition or deficiency inhibits fibroblast activation through secreted factor(s) from myocytes [49]. However, the secreted factor(s) that mediate this crosstalk between cardiac myocytes and fibroblasts remain unknown.

4.4. PDE1 and Other PDEs: Similarities, Differences, and Potential Interactions

Although PDE1A is able to regulate cGMP levels and cGMP-dependent signaling in cardiac myocytes [45], the specific source(s) of cGMP modulated by PDE1A in cardiac myocytes remains unknown. In vascular SMCs, PDE1A appears to be able to regulate cGMP derived from atrial natriuretic peptide (ANP) stimulation [71]. Several other PDEs have previously been shown to regulate cGMP signaling in cardiomyocytes. For example, PDE5A likely regulates NO-derived cGMP [38] and plays a critical role in mediating various types of cardiac diseases including ischemia/reperfusion (I/R) injury [72,73], doxorubicin cardiotoxicity [74], ischemic and diabetic cardiomyopathy [75], and cardiac hypertrophy [38,76]. PDE5 is expressed at low levels and localized to sarcomeric Z-bands within cardiac myocytes [53]. A recent study found that PDE9, another cGMP-specific PDE, upregulated expression in both mouse and human hypertrophic hearts [44]. The inhibition and genetic deletion of PDE9 was shown to protect the heart against TAC-induced cardiac remodeling and pre-established heart disease [44]. PDE9 couples to NP-derived cGMP [44]. Moreover, PDE2, which preferentially localizes in the membrane fraction of cardiac myocytes, is also critical for cGMP catabolism in cardiac myocytes in response to particulate GC activation [35]. Evidence to date suggests that PDE1C primarily regulates cAMP signaling in cardiac myocytes [49]. PDE1C inhibition/deficiency protects cardiac myocyte from death in a PKA-dependent manner [49]. Also, PDE1C is responsible for the Ang II-mediated suppression of myocyte cAMP levels [49]. These observations suggest that PDE1C antagonizes a protective cAMP signaling pathway in cardiac myocytes. Indeed, our unpublished observations suggest that PDE1C negatively regulates cardiac protective A_2R-cAMP signaling. In contrast, previous studies have shown that PDE3A inhibition potentiates a detrimental cAMP signaling pathway that promotes cardiac myocyte death [48,77–79]. However, PDE4 inhibition has a limited effect on cardiac myocyte death/survival despite the drastic elevation of cAMP upon PDE4 inhibition [48].

Taken together, these findings suggest that in cardiac myocytes there are multiple different, even functionally opposing cyclic nucleotide signaling pathways that are modulated by distinct PDE isozymes. The functional diversity of individual PDEs could be achieved through multiple mechanisms: the association of PDEs with discrete "pools" of cyclic nucleotides, targeted to spatially separated compartments, and complexed with distinct sets of signaling molecules. In addition, the variable enzymatic and regulatory properties make individual PDEs function in different biological conditions, such as basal vs. stimulated, physiological vs. pathological cellular environments, etc. PDE1-mediated functions are associated with intracellular Ca^{2+} levels because PDE1 needs Ca^{2+} to be activated. For example, previous studies have shown that PDE1A is responsible for PE-induced cGMP reduction, while PDE1C is important for Ang II-induced cAMP reduction in cardiac myocytes [45,49]. Moreover, a recent study using FRET approaches further supported the role of Ca^{2+} in the PDE1-mediated regulated cAMP response in cardiac myocytes [80]. Specifically, it has been shown that PDE1 inhibition is able to elicit significant cAMP elevation under stimulation by forskolin but not ISO, under a paced but not basal state, or mimicked by pretreating resting cells with Ca^{2+} elevating agents [80]. It will be of great interest to understand the integratory roles of these different cyclic nucleotide signaling pathways modulated by distinct PDEs in regulating cardiac myocyte functions. Targeting multiple PDEs in combination may represent a compelling strategy. Indeed, a number of recent studies have shown synergistic effects on cyclic nucleotide level and subsequent biological functions resulting from the inhibition of combinations of PDEs [81,82].

5. Therapeutic Potential of PDE1 Inhibition in Pathological Cardiac Remodeling

To evaluate the pharmacological effects of PDE1 inhibition in pathological cardiac remodeling in vivo, the systemic application of IC86340 was evaluated in an ISO-induced mouse hypertrophy and fibrosis model [36,45]. It was found that mice receiving daily IC86340 treatment at the doses of 3 and 6 mg/kg per day elicited a small (10 to 20 mmHg) reduction of blood pressure (BP) with no significant changes in heart rate. The effect on BP reduction is consistent with that of other PDE1 inhibitors such as Lu AF41228/Lu AF58027 and vinpocetine, which have been shown to cause vasodilation and/or lower BP in rodents [71,83]. The effects of PDE1 inhibitors on blood pressure regulation are likely mediated exclusively by PDE1A, but not PDE1C, as PDE1A is expressed in the medial vascular smooth muscle cells (SMCs) responsible for vascular contractile function [84–86]. The role of PDE1A in the regulation of blood pressure has been more directly supported by the recent findings from two lines of PDE1A null mice that showed reduced aortic blood pressure [69]. Additionally, the association of PDE1A single nucleotide polymorphisms (SNPs) with diastolic blood pressure has been revealed by human genetic studies [87,88]. In addition to the effect of IC86340 on BP, there is no correlation between BP and ISO-induced remodeling [89]. In the mouse heart, IC86340 treatment (3 mg/kg per day) attenuated ISO infusion-mediated increases in cardiac hypertrophy, as assessed by increased heart size, heart weight/body weight ratio, and heart weight/tibia length ratio [45]. In addition, enlarged cardiac myocyte cross-sectional area and elevated ANP gene expression were also significantly reduced by IC86340 treatment [45]. Moreover, cardiac fibrosis, as indicated by α-SMC-positive myofibroblasts and collagen deposition, were significantly reduced by IC86340 [36]. These results support a critical role for PDE1 activation in ISO-induced cardiac hypertrophy in vivo. The effects of IC86340 or other PDE1-selective inhibitors deserve to be evaluated in different models of cardiovascular disease in the future.

Vinpocetine is also widely used as a PDE1 inhibitor. It is a derivative of the alkaloid vincamine and has, for several decades now, been used clinically in many countries for the treatment of cerebrovascular disorders such as stroke and dementia [90–92]. In addition to being a PDE1 inhibitor, vinpocetine can act as a blocker for voltage-dependent Na^+ channels as well as act as an inhibitor for IkB kinase (IKK), serving as a critical mediator of inflammatory signaling [93]. The excellent safety profile of vinpocetine has attracted significant interest for exploring the potential therapeutic effects of vinpocetine treatment in various other disease models. Indeed, emerging experimental evidence has shown the beneficial effects of vinpocetine in various inflammatory and cardiovascular disease models. For example, vinpocetine treatment partially restored the sensitivity of the vasculature to nitroglycerin (NTG) in a rat model of NTG tolerance [71]. In addition, vinpocetine significantly attenuated mouse carotid artery wall thickening and neointimal formation induced by ligation injury, and markedly suppressed the spontaneous remodeling of human saphenous vein explants in an ex vivo culture model [94]. High-fat diet-induced atherosclerosis in ApoE-deficient mice was also significantly suppressed by vinpocetine [95,96]. Moreover, the inhibition of PDE1 by vinpocetine has been suggested to play a protective role in cardiac hypertrophy and fibrosis [97]. It has been found that vinpocetine significantly alleviates chronic Ang II-induced cardiac hypertrophy and fibrosis in vivo [97]. Consistently, in isolated cardiac myocytes, vinpocetine attenuates Ang II-induced myocyte hypertrophy in a dose-dependent manner [97]. In addition, vinpocetine blocks TGF-β-induced fibroblast activation [97]. Interestingly, when PDE1 activity is blocked by IC86340, vinpocetine exerts no additional effects on cardiac myocyte hypertrophy and fibroblast activation, likely demonstrating that its protective effects are effective largely through PDE1 inhibition [97]. Taken together, these data indicate that vinpocetine is a drug with multiple pharmacological targets and multiple therapeutic effects [93]. In addition to its direct protective effects on cardiac cells, other biological effects of

J. Cardiovasc. Dev. Dis. **2018**, *5*, 22

vinpocetine may also act together in an indirect beneficial manner for preventing cardiac diseases, including vasodilation, anti-inflammation, and anti-vascular occlusive remodeling [93,94,98–100].

6. Conclusions and Perspective

Experimental evidence has suggested that both PDE1A and PDE1C are important in regulating cardiac structural remodeling and function (Figure 1). However, their regulation, function, and mechanistic actions in the heart appear to be distinct. PDE1A is expressed and functions in both cardiac myocytes and fibroblasts, particularly in response to stimulation with hypertrophic and fibrotic stimuli [36,45]. However, PDE1C is expressed in cardiac myocytes but not fibroblasts [49]. PDE1A and PDE1C both regulate cardiac myocyte hypertrophy induced by pathological stimuli such as Ang II, but via distinct signaling pathways: PDE1A acts through cGMP/PKG while PDE1C acts through cAMP/PKA [45,49]. The differential functions and mechanisms of PDE1A and PDE1C in cardiac hypertrophy stimulated with other growth factors or particularly in response to physiological hypertrophy also deserve to be further investigated. Interestingly, the protective effect of pan PDE1 inhibition on cardiac myocyte death is primarily dependent on PDE1C inhibition [49]. PDE1C deficiency but not PDE1A deficiency blocked myocyte death induced by different death stimuli (our unpublished observations). These results suggest that PDE1C but not PDE1A plays a major role in regulating cardiac myocyte death, at least in isolated cardiac myocytes in vitro. In cardiac fibroblasts, PDE1A directly regulates fibroblast activation and ECM production [36]. However, PDE1C appears to regulate fibroblast function through the myocyte-PDE1C-mediated regulation of unknown secreted factor(s) via a paracrine mechanism [49]. Most knowledge of PDE1A in cardiac myocytes and fibroblasts is derived from experimental observations in cultured primary cells [36,45,49]. Future validation in animal models in vivo is necessary. Taken together, PDE1A and PDE1C regulate distinct cyclic nucleotide signaling pathways and play different roles in the heart. Future development of cardiac cell-specific PDE1A or 1C knockout mice, or genetically modified mice with selectively altered PDE1A or PDE1C, should be helpful in elucidating a more detailed characterization of the role of PDE1 isoforms in cardiac remodeling and dysfunction.

Although both PDE1A and PDE1C exhibit direct biological effects in cardiac myocytes and/or fibroblasts, the two major cell types in the heart, the expression of PDE1 isozymes in other cardiac cell types or in other organs may also indirectly influence cardiac structural remodeling and function [36,45,49]. These tissues/organs include but are not limited to the vasculature, brain, kidney, and lung. PDE1A and 1C have very different expression profiles in many tissues of the human body [63]. PDE1A null mice have been shown to have a mild renal cystic disease and a urine concentrating defect [69]. Moreover, a recent study defined a significant level of expression of PDE1A in sinoatrial nodal tissue, which may be important in regulating sinoatrial nodal pacemaker function [101]. Therefore, when studying cardiac function using global PDE1A knockout mice or systemically applying pan PDE1 inhibitors, the potential effects on heart rate, contractility, BP reduction, and kidney function should be taken into consideration.

To date, all PDE1 inhibitors are pan inhibitors, lacking the ability to distinguish between different PDE1 isozymes. The future development of PDE1 isozyme-selective inhibitors is important for achieving specific pharmacological effects. Taken together, basic research studies in isolated cardiac cells and in experimental cardiac disease models provide strong evidence for roles of PDE1A and PDE1C in pathological cardiac remodeling and dysfunction, suggesting that PDE1A and PDE1C might represent potential novel and promising therapeutic targets.

J. Cardiovasc. Dev. Dis. **2018**, *5*, 22

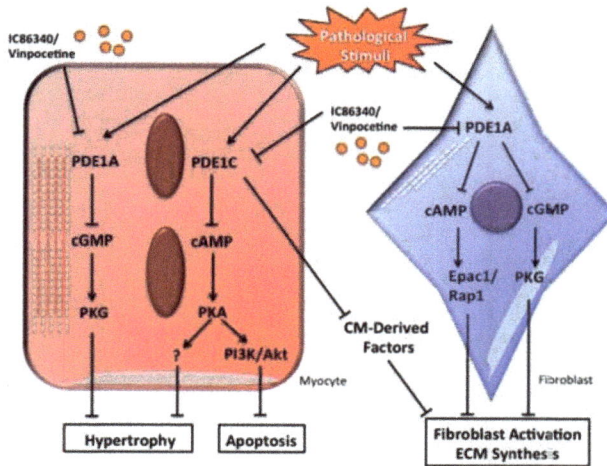

Figure 1. Schematic diagram showing the potential role of PDE1A and PDE1C in regulating pathological cardiac remodeling including cardiac hypertrophy and fibrosis. In cardiac myocytes, PDE1A-dependent regulation of cGMP/PKG signaling alleviates myocyte hypertrophy, PDE1C-dependent regulation of cAMP/PKA signaling suppresses both myocyte hypertrophy and apoptosis. In cardiac fibroblasts, PDE1A-dependent dual regulation of cAMP-Epac1-Rap1 and cGMP-PKG signaling decreases fibroblast activation and ECM synthesis, whereas PDE1C may regulate cardiac fibrosis through paracrine signaling between cardiac myocytes and fibroblasts.

Author Contributions: S.C. conceived the manuscript and prepared the figures. All authors wrote the review.

Acknowledgments: C.Y. was supported by USA NIH HL134910 and HL088400. S.C. was supported by AHA predoctoral fellowship 17PRE33660835.

Conflicts of Interest: The authors declare no conflict of interest.

References

1. Frey, N.; Olson, E.N. Cardiac hypertrophy: The good, the bad, and the ugly. *Annu. Rev. Physiol.* **2003**, *65*, 45–79. [CrossRef] [PubMed]
2. Beavo, J.A.; Brunton, L.L. Cyclic nucleotide research—Still expanding after half a century. *Nat. Rev. Mol. Cell Biol.* **2002**, *3*, 710–718. [CrossRef] [PubMed]
3. Maurice, D.H.; Ke, H.; Ahmad, F.; Wang, Y.; Chung, J.; Manganiello, V.C. Advances in targeting cyclic nucleotide phosphodiesterases. *Nat. Rev. Drug Discov.* **2014**, *13*, 290–314. [CrossRef] [PubMed]
4. Banerjee, I.; Fuseler, J.W.; Price, R.L.; Borg, T.K.; Baudino, T.A. Determination of cell types and numbers during cardiac development in the neonatal and adult rat and mouse. *Am. J. Physiol. Heart Circ. Physiol.* **2007**, *293*, H1883–H1891. [CrossRef] [PubMed]
5. Hill, J.A.; Olson, E.N. Cardiac plasticity. *N. Engl. J. Med.* **2008**, *358*, 1370–1380. [CrossRef] [PubMed]
6. McMullen, J.R.; Jennings, G.L. Differences between pathological and physiological cardiac hypertrophy: Novel therapeutic strategies to treat heart failure. *Clin. Exp. Pharmacol. Physiol.* **2007**, *34*, 255–262. [CrossRef] [PubMed]
7. Porter, K.E.; Turner, N.A. Cardiac fibroblasts: At the heart of myocardial remodeling. *Pharmacol. Ther.* **2009**, *123*, 255–278. [CrossRef] [PubMed]
8. Deb, A.; Ubil, E. Cardiac fibroblast in development and wound healing. *J. Mol. Cell. Cardiol.* **2014**, *70*, 47–55. [CrossRef] [PubMed]
9. Chiong, M.; Wang, Z.V.; Pedrozo, Z.; Cao, D.J.; Troncoso, R.; Ibacache, M.; Criollo, A.; Nemchenko, A.; Hill, J.A.; Lavandero, S. Cardiomyocyte death: Mechanisms and translational implications. *Cell Death Dis.* **2011**, *2*, e244. [CrossRef] [PubMed]

10. Nadal-Ginard, B.; Kajstura, J.; Leri, A.; Anversa, P. Myocyte death, growth, and regeneration in cardiac hypertrophy and failure. *Circ. Res.* **2003**, *92*, 139–150. [CrossRef] [PubMed]

11. Balakumar, P.; Jagadeesh, G. Multifarious molecular signaling cascades of cardiac hypertrophy: Can the muddy waters be cleared? *Pharmacol. Res.* **2010**, *62*, 365–383. [CrossRef] [PubMed]

12. Dewenter, M.; von der Lieth, A.; Katus, H.A.; Backs, J. Calcium Signaling and Transcriptional Regulation in Cardiomyocytes. *Circ. Res.* **2017**, *121*, 1000–1020. [CrossRef] [PubMed]

13. De Windt, L.J.; Lim, H.W.; Bueno, O.F.; Liang, Q.; Delling, U.; Braz, J.C.; Glascock, B.J.; Kimball, T.F.; del Monte, F.; Hajjar, R.J.; et al. Targeted inhibition of calcineurin attenuates cardiac hypertrophy in vivo. *Proc. Natl. Acad. Sci. USA* **2001**, *98*, 3322–3327. [CrossRef] [PubMed]

14. Anderson, M.E.; Brown, J.H.; Bers, D.M. CaMKII in myocardial hypertrophy and heart failure. *J. Mol. Cell. Cardiol.* **2011**, *51*, 468–473. [CrossRef] [PubMed]

15. Zhang, T.; Kohlhaas, M.; Backs, J.; Mishra, S.; Phillips, W.; Dybkova, N.; Chang, S.; Ling, H.; Bers, D.M.; Maier, L.S.; et al. CaMKIIdelta isoforms differentially affect calcium handling but similarly regulate HDAC/MEF2 transcriptional responses. *J. Biol. Chem.* **2007**, *282*, 35078–35087. [CrossRef] [PubMed]

16. Berthet, J.; Rall, T.W.; Sutherland, E.W. The relationship of epinephrine and glucagon to liver phosphorylase. IV. Effect of epinephrine and glucagon on the reactivation of phosphorylase in liver homogenates. *J. Biol. Chem.* **1957**, *224*, 463–475. [PubMed]

17. Rall, T.W.; Sutherland, E.W. Formation of a cyclic adenine ribonucleotide by tissue particles. *J. Biol. Chem.* **1958**, *232*, 1065–1076. [PubMed]

18. Kopperud, R.; Krakstad, C.; Selheim, F.; Doskeland, S.O. cAMP effector mechanisms. Novel twists for an 'old' signaling system. *FEBS Lett.* **2003**, *546*, 121–126. [CrossRef]

19. Gancedo, J.M. Biological roles of cAMP: Variations on a theme in the different kingdoms of life. *Biol. Rev. Camb. Philos. Soc.* **2013**, *88*, 645–668. [CrossRef] [PubMed]

20. Hanoune, J.; Defer, N. Regulation and role of adenylyl cyclase isoforms. *Annu. Rev. Pharmacol. Toxicol.* **2001**, *41*, 145–174. [CrossRef] [PubMed]

21. Steegborn, C. Structure, mechanism, and regulation of soluble adenylyl cyclases—Similarities and differences to transmembrane adenylyl cyclases. *Biochim. Biophys. Acta* **2014**, *1842*, 2535–2547. [CrossRef] [PubMed]

22. Tresguerres, M.; Levin, L.R.; Buck, J. Intracellular cAMP signaling by soluble adenylyl cyclase. *Kidney Int.* **2011**, *79*, 1277–1288. [CrossRef] [PubMed]

23. Willoughby, D.; Cooper, D.M. Live-cell imaging of cAMP dynamics. *Nat. Methods* **2008**, *5*, 29–36. [CrossRef] [PubMed]

24. Leroy, J.; Abi-Gerges, A.; Nikolaev, V.O.; Richter, W.; Lechene, P.; Mazet, J.L.; Conti, M.; Fischmeister, R.; Vandecasteele, G. Spatiotemporal dynamics of beta-adrenergic cAMP signals and L-type Ca^{2+} channel regulation in adult rat ventricular myocytes: Role of phosphodiesterases. *Circ. Res.* **2008**, *102*, 1091–1100. [CrossRef] [PubMed]

25. Scriven, D.R.; Dan, P.; Moore, E.D. Distribution of proteins implicated in excitation-contraction coupling in rat ventricular myocytes. *Biophys. J.* **2000**, *79*, 2682–2691. [CrossRef]

26. Trafford, A.W.; Diaz, M.E.; Negretti, N.; Eisner, D.A. Enhanced Ca^{2+} current and decreased Ca^{2+} efflux restore sarcoplasmic reticulum Ca^{2+} content after depletion. *Circ. Res.* **1997**, *81*, 477–484. [CrossRef] [PubMed]

27. Chen, X.; Piacentino, V., 3rd; Furukawa, S.; Goldman, B.; Margulies, K.B.; Houser, S.R. L-type Ca^{2+} channel density and regulation are altered in failing human ventricular myocytes and recover after support with mechanical assist devices. *Circ. Res.* **2002**, *91*, 517–524. [CrossRef] [PubMed]

28. Marx, S.O.; Reiken, S.; Hisamatsu, Y.; Gaburjakova, M.; Gaburjakova, J.; Yang, Y.M.; Rosemblit, N.; Marks, A.R. Phosphorylation-dependent regulation of ryanodine receptors: A novel role for leucine/isoleucine zippers. *J. Cell Biol.* **2001**, *153*, 699–708. [CrossRef] [PubMed]

29. Brittsan, A.G.; Kranias, E.G. Phospholamban and cardiac contractile function. *J. Mol. Cell. Cardiol.* **2000**, *32*, 2131–2139. [CrossRef] [PubMed]

30. Guellich, A.; Mehel, H.; Fischmeister, R. Cyclic AMP synthesis and hydrolysis in the normal and failing heart. *Pflugers Arch.* **2014**, *466*, 1163–1175. [CrossRef] [PubMed]

31. Hamad, E.A.; Zhu, W.; Chan, T.O.; Myers, V.; Gao, E.; Li, X.; Zhang, J.; Song, J.; Zhang, X.Q.; Cheung, J.Y.; et al. Cardioprotection of controlled and cardiac-specific over-expression of A(2A)-adenosine receptor in the pressure overload. *PLoS ONE* **2012**, *7*, e39919. [CrossRef] [PubMed]

32. Lukowski, R.; Krieg, T.; Rybalkin, S.D.; Beavo, J.; Hofmann, F. Turning on cGMP-dependent pathways to treat cardiac dysfunctions: Boom, bust, and beyond. *Trends Pharmacol. Sci.* **2014**, *35*, 404–413. [CrossRef] [PubMed]

33. Potter, L.R. Guanylyl cyclase structure, function and regulation. *Cell Signal.* **2011**, *23*, 1921–1926. [CrossRef] [PubMed]

34. Tsai, E.J.; Kass, D.A. Cyclic GMP signaling in cardiovascular pathophysiology and therapeutics. *Pharmacol. Ther.* **2009**, *122*, 216–238. [CrossRef] [PubMed]

35. Castro, L.R.; Verde, I.; Cooper, D.M.; Fischmeister, R. Cyclic guanosine monophosphate compartmentation in rat cardiac myocytes. *Circulation* **2006**, *113*, 2221–2228. [CrossRef] [PubMed]

36. Miller, C.L.; Cai, Y.; Oikawa, M.; Thomas, T.; Dostmann, W.R.; Zaccolo, M.; Fujiwara, K.; Yan, C. Cyclic nucleotide phosphodiesterase 1A: A key regulator of cardiac fibroblast activation and extracellular matrix remodeling in the heart. *Basic Res. Cardiol.* **2011**, *106*, 1023–1039. [CrossRef] [PubMed]

37. Frantz, S.; Klaiber, M.; Baba, H.A.; Oberwinkler, H.; Volker, K.; Gabetaner, B.; Bayer, B.; Abebetaer, M.; Schuh, K.; Feil, R.; et al. Stress-dependent dilated cardiomyopathy in mice with cardiomyocyte-restricted inactivation of cyclic GMP-dependent protein kinase I. *Eur Heart J.* **2013**, *34*, 1233–1244. [CrossRef] [PubMed]

38. Takimoto, E.; Champion, H.C.; Li, M.; Belardi, D.; Ren, S.; Rodriguez, E.R.; Bedja, D.; Gabrielson, K.L.; Wang, Y.; Kass, D.A. Chronic inhibition of cyclic GMP phosphodiesterase 5A prevents and reverses cardiac hypertrophy. *Nat. Med.* **2005**, *11*, 214–222. [CrossRef] [PubMed]

39. Wegener, J.W.; Nawrath, H.; Wolfsgruber, W.; Kuhbandner, S.; Werner, C.; Hofmann, F.; Feil, R. cGMP-dependent protein kinase I mediates the negative inotropic effect of cGMP in the murine myocardium. *Circ. Res.* **2002**, *90*, 18–20. [CrossRef] [PubMed]

40. Patrucco, E.; Domes, K.; Sbroggio, M.; Blaich, A.; Schlossmann, J.; Desch, M.; Rybalkin, S.D.; Beavo, J.A.; Lukowski, R.; Hofmann, F. Roles of cGMP-dependent protein kinase I (cGKI) and PDE5 in the regulation of Ang II-induced cardiac hypertrophy and fibrosis. *Proc. Natl. Acad. Sci. USA* **2014**, *111*, 12925–12929. [CrossRef] [PubMed]

41. Lu, Z.; Xu, X.; Hu, X.; Lee, S.; Traverse, J.H.; Zhu, G.; Fassett, J.; Tao, Y.; Zhang, P.; dos Remedios, C.; et al. Oxidative stress regulates left ventricular PDE5 expression in the failing heart. *Circulation* **2010**, *121*, 1474–1483. [CrossRef] [PubMed]

42. Nagayama, T.; Hsu, S.; Zhang, M.; Koitabashi, N.; Bedja, D.; Gabrielson, K.L.; Takimoto, E.; Kass, D.A. Sildenafil stops progressive chamber, cellular, and molecular remodeling and improves calcium handling and function in hearts with pre-existing advanced hypertrophy caused by pressure overload. *J. Am. Coll. Cardiol.* **2009**, *53*, 207–215. [CrossRef] [PubMed]

43. Takimoto, E.; Belardi, D.; Tocchetti, C.G.; Vahebi, S.; Cormaci, G.; Ketner, E.A.; Moens, A.L.; Champion, H.C.; Kass, D.A. Compartmentalization of cardiac β-adrenergic inotropy modulation by phosphodiesterase type 5. *Circulation* **2007**, *115*, 2159–2167. [CrossRef] [PubMed]

44. Lee, D.I.; Zhu, G.; Sasaki, T.; Cho, G.S.; Hamdani, N.; Holewinski, R.; Jo, S.H.; Danner, T.; Zhang, M.; Rainer, P.P.; et al. Phosphodiesterase 9A controls nitric-oxide-independent cGMP and hypertrophic heart disease. *Nature* **2015**, *519*, 472–476. [CrossRef] [PubMed]

45. Miller, C.L.; Oikawa, M.; Cai, Y.; Wojtovich, A.P.; Nagel, D.J.; Xu, X.; Xu, H.; Florio, V.; Rybalkin, S.D.; Beavo, J.A.; et al. Role of Ca^{2+}/calmodulin-stimulated cyclic nucleotide phosphodiesterase 1 in mediating cardiomyocyte hypertrophy. *Circ. Res.* **2009**, *105*, 956–964. [CrossRef] [PubMed]

46. Bobin, P.; Belacel-Ouari, M.; Bedioune, I.; Zhang, L.; Leroy, J.; Leblais, V.; Fischmeister, R.; Vandecasteele, G. Cyclic nucleotide phosphodiesterases in heart and vessels: A therapeutic perspective. *Arch. Cardiovasc. Dis.* **2016**, *109*, 431–443. [CrossRef] [PubMed]

47. Omori, K.; Kotera, J. Overview of PDEs and their regulation. *Circ. Res.* **2007**, *100*, 309–327. [CrossRef] [PubMed]

48. Ding, B.; Abe, J.I.; Wei, H.; Huang, Q.; Walsh, R.A.; Molina, C.A.; Zhao, A.; Sadoshima, J.; Blaxall, B.C.; Berk, B.C.; et al. Functional role of phosphodiesterase 3 in cardiomyocyte apoptosis: Implication in heart failure. *Circulation* **2005**, *111*, 2469–2476. [CrossRef] [PubMed]

49. Knight, W.E.; Chen, S.; Zhang, Y.; Oikawa, M.; Wu, M.; Zhou, Q.; Miller, C.L.; Cai, Y.; Mickelsen, D.M.; Moravec, C.; et al. PDE1C deficiency antagonizes pathological cardiac remodeling and dysfunction. *Proc. Natl. Acad. Sci. USA* **2016**, *113*, E7116–E7125. [CrossRef] [PubMed]

50. Sonnenburg, W.K.; Rybalkin, S.D.; Bornfeldt, K.E.; Kwak, K.S.; Rybalkina, I.G.; Beavo, J.A. Identification, quantitation, and cellular localization of PDE1 calmodulin-stimulated cyclic nucleotide phosphodiesterases. *Methods* **1998**, *14*, 3–19. [CrossRef] [PubMed]

51. Stephenson, D.T.; Coskran, T.M.; Wilhelms, M.B.; Adamowicz, W.O.; O'Donnell, M.M.; Muravnick, K.B.; Menniti, F.S.; Kleiman, R.J.; Morton, D. Immunohistochemical localization of phosphodiesterase 2A in multiple mammalian species. *J. Histochem. Cytochem.* **2009**, *57*, 933–949. [CrossRef] [PubMed]

52. Richter, W.; Xie, M.; Scheitrum, C.; Krall, J.; Movsesian, M.A.; Conti, M. Conserved expression and functions of PDE4 in rodent and human heart. *Basic Res. Cardiol.* **2011**, *106*, 249–262. [CrossRef] [PubMed]

53. Takimoto, E.; Champion, H.C.; Belardi, D.; Moslehi, J.; Mongillo, M.; Mergia, E.; Montrose, D.C.; Isoda, T.; Aufiero, K.; Zaccolo, M.; et al. cGMP catabolism by phosphodiesterase 5A regulates cardiac adrenergic stimulation by NOS3-dependent mechanism. *Circ. Res.* **2005**, *96*, 100–109. [CrossRef] [PubMed]

54. Patrucco, E.; Albergine, M.S.; Santana, L.F.; Beavo, J.A. Phosphodiesterase 8A (PDE8A) regulates excitation-contraction coupling in ventricular myocytes. *J. Mol. Cell. Cardiol.* **2010**, *49*, 330–333. [CrossRef] [PubMed]

55. Cheung, W.Y. Cyclic 3′,5′-nucleotide phosphodiesterase. Demonstration of an activator. *Biochem. Biophys. Res. Commun.* **1970**, *38*, 533–538. [CrossRef]

56. Bender, A.T.; Beavo, J.A. Cyclic nucleotide phosphodiesterases: Molecular regulation to clinical use. *Pharmacol. Rev.* **2006**, *58*, 488–520. [CrossRef] [PubMed]

57. Yan, C.; Kim, D.; Aizawa, T.; Berk, B.C. Functional interplay between angiotensin II and nitric oxide: Cyclic GMP as a key mediator. *Arterioscler. Thromb. Vasc. Biol.* **2003**, *23*, 26–36. [CrossRef] [PubMed]

58. Sonnenburg, W.K.; Seger, D.; Kwak, K.S.; Huang, J.; Charbonneau, H.; Beavo, J.A. Identification of inhibitory and calmodulin-binding domains of the PDE1A1 and PDE1A2 calmodulin-stimulated cyclic nucleotide phosphodiesterases. *J. Biol. Chem.* **1995**, *270*, 30989–31000. [CrossRef] [PubMed]

59. Chan, S.; Yan, C. PDE1 isozymes, key regulators of pathological vascular remodeling. *Curr. Opin. Pharmacol.* **2011**, *11*, 720–724. [CrossRef] [PubMed]

60. Yan, C.; Zhao, A.Z.; Bentley, J.K.; Beavo, J.A. The calmodulin-dependent phosphodiesterase gene PDE1C encodes several functionally different splice variants in a tissue-specific manner. *J. Biol. Chem.* **1996**, *271*, 25699–25706. [CrossRef] [PubMed]

61. Yu, J.; Wolda, S.L.; Frazier, A.L.; Florio, V.A.; Martins, T.J.; Snyder, P.B.; Harris, E.A.; McCaw, K.N.; Farrell, C.A.; Steiner, B.; et al. Identification and characterisation of a human calmodulin-stimulated phosphodiesterase PDE1B1. *Cell. Signal.* **1997**, *9*, 519–529. [CrossRef]

62. Vandeput, F.; Wolda, S.L.; Krall, J.; Hambleton, R.; Uher, L.; McCaw, K.N.; Radwanski, P.B.; Florio, V.; Movsesian, M.A. Cyclic Nucleotide Phosphodiesterase PDE1C1 in Human Cardiac Myocytes. *J. Biol. Chem.* **2007**, *282*, 32749–32757. [CrossRef] [PubMed]

63. Lakics, V.; Karran, E.H.; Boess, F.G. Quantitative comparison of phosphodiesterase mRNA distribution in human brain and peripheral tissues. *Neuropharmacology* **2010**, *59*, 367–374. [CrossRef] [PubMed]

64. Yokoyama, U.; Patel, H.H.; Lai, N.C.; Aroonsakool, N.; Roth, D.M.; Insel, P.A. The cyclic AMP effector Epac integrates pro- and anti-fibrotic signals. *Proc. Natl. Acad. Sci. USA* **2008**, *105*, 6386–6391. [CrossRef] [PubMed]

65. Olmedo, I.; Munoz, C.; Guzman, N.; Catalan, M.; Vivar, R.; Ayala, P.; Humeres, C.; Aranguiz, P.; Garcia, L.; Velarde, V.; et al. EPAC expression and function in cardiac fibroblasts and myofibroblasts. *Toxicol. Appl. Pharmacol.* **2013**, *272*, 414–422. [CrossRef] [PubMed]

66. Insel, P.A.; Murray, F.; Yokoyama, U.; Romano, S.; Yun, H.; Brown, L.; Snead, A.; Lu, D.; Aroonsakool, N. cAMP and Epac in the regulation of tissue fibrosis. *Br. J. Pharmacol.* **2012**, *166*, 447–456. [CrossRef] [PubMed]

67. Buxton, I.L.; Duan, D. Cyclic GMP/protein kinase G phosphorylation of Smad3 blocks transforming growth factor-beta-induced nuclear Smad translocation: A key antifibrogenic mechanism of atrial natriuretic peptide. *Circ. Res.* **2008**, *102*, 151–153. [CrossRef] [PubMed]

68. Li, P.; Wang, D.; Lucas, J.; Oparil, S.; Xing, D.; Cao, X.; Novak, L.; Renfrow, M.B.; Chen, Y.F. Atrial natriuretic peptide inhibits transforming growth factor beta-induced Smad signaling and myofibroblast transformation in mouse cardiac fibroblasts. *Circ. Res.* **2008**, *102*, 185–192. [CrossRef] [PubMed]

69. Wang, X.; Yamada, S.; LaRiviere, W.B.; Ye, H.; Bakeberg, J.L.; Irazabal, M.V.; Chebib, F.T.; van Deursen, J.; Harris, P.C.; Sussman, C.R.; et al. Generation and phenotypic characterization of Pde1a mutant mice. *PLoS ONE* **2017**, *12*, e0181087. [CrossRef] [PubMed]

70. Liu, Y.; Morley, M.; Brandimarto, J.; Hannenhalli, S.; Hu, Y.; Ashley, E.A.; Tang, W.H.; Moravec, C.S.; Margulies, K.B.; Cappola, T.P.; et al. RNA-Seq identifies novel myocardial gene expression signatures of heart failure. *Genomics* **2015**, *105*, 83–89. [CrossRef] [PubMed]

71. Kim, D.; Rybalkin, S.D.; Pi, X.; Wang, Y.; Zhang, C.; Munzel, T.; Beavo, J.A.; Berk, B.C.; Yan, C. Upregulation of phosphodiesterase 1A1 expression is associated with the development of nitrate tolerance. *Circulation* **2001**, *104*, 2338–2343. [CrossRef] [PubMed]

72. Ockaili, R.; Salloum, F.; Hawkins, J.; Kukreja, R.C. Sildenafil (Viagra) induces powerful cardioprotective effect via opening of mitochondrial K(ATP) channels in rabbits. *Am. J. Physiol. Heart Circ. Physiol.* **2002**, *283*, H1263–H1269. [CrossRef] [PubMed]

73. Das, A.; Xi, L.; Kukreja, R.C. Phosphodiesterase-5 inhibitor sildenafil preconditions adult cardiac myocytes against necrosis and apoptosis. Essential role of nitric oxide signaling. *J. Biol. Chem.* **2005**, *280*, 12944–12955. [CrossRef] [PubMed]

74. Fisher, P.W.; Salloum, F.; Das, A.; Hyder, H.; Kukreja, R.C. Phosphodiesterase-5 inhibition with sildenafil attenuates cardiomyocyte apoptosis and left ventricular dysfunction in a chronic model of doxorubicin cardiotoxicity. *Circulation* **2005**, *111*, 1601–1610. [CrossRef] [PubMed]

75. Giannetta, E.; Isidori, A.M.; Galea, N.; Carbone, I.; Mandosi, E.; Vizza, C.D.; Naro, F.; Morano, S.; Fedele, F.; Lenzi, A. Chronic Inhibition of cGMP phosphodiesterase 5A improves diabetic cardiomyopathy: A randomized, controlled clinical trial using magnetic resonance imaging with myocardial tagging. *Circulation* **2012**, *125*, 2323–2333. [CrossRef] [PubMed]

76. Das, A.; Durrant, D.; Salloum, F.N.; Xi, L.; Kukreja, R.C. PDE5 inhibitors as therapeutics for heart disease, diabetes and cancer. *Pharmacol. Ther.* **2015**, *147*, 12–21. [CrossRef] [PubMed]

77. Ding, B.; Abe, J.; Wei, H.; Xu, H.; Che, W.; Aizawa, T.; Liu, W.; Molina, C.A.; Sadoshima, J.; Blaxall, B.C.; et al. A positive feedback loop of phosphodiesterase 3 (PDE3) and inducible cAMP early repressor (ICER) leads to cardiomyocyte apoptosis. *Proc. Natl. Acad. Sci. USA* **2005**, *102*, 14771–14776. [CrossRef] [PubMed]

78. Yan, C.; Miller, C.L.; Abe, J. Regulation of phosphodiesterase 3 and inducible cAMP early repressor in the heart. *Circ. Res.* **2007**, *100*, 489–501. [CrossRef] [PubMed]

79. Oikawa, M.; Wu, M.; Lim, S.; Knight, W.E.; Miller, C.L.; Cai, Y.; Lu, Y.; Blaxall, B.C.; Takeishi, Y.; Abe, J.; et al. Cyclic nucleotide phosphodiesterase 3A1 protects the heart against ischemia-reperfusion injury. *J. Mol. Cell. Cardiol.* **2013**, *64*, 11–19. [CrossRef] [PubMed]

80. Sprenger, J.U.; Bork, N.I.; Herting, J.; Fischer, T.H.; Nikolaev, V.O. Interactions of Calcium Fluctuations during Cardiomyocyte Contraction with Real-Time cAMP Dynamics Detected by FRET. *PLoS ONE* **2016**, *11*, e0167974. [CrossRef] [PubMed]

81. Kraynik, S.M.; Miyaoka, R.S.; Beavo, J.A. PDE3 and PDE4 isozyme-selective inhibitors are both required for synergistic activation of brown adipose tissue. *Mol. Pharmacol.* **2013**, *83*, 1155–1165. [CrossRef] [PubMed]

82. Beltejar, M.G.; Lau, H.T.; Golkowski, M.G.; Ong, S.E.; Beavo, J.A. Analyses of PDE-regulated phosphoproteomes reveal unique and specific cAMP-signaling modules in T cells. *Proc. Natl. Acad. Sci. USA* **2017**, *114*, E6240–E6249. [CrossRef] [PubMed]

83. Laursen, M.; Beck, L.; Kehler, J.; Christoffersen, C.T.; Bundgaard, C.; Mogensen, S.; Mow, T.J.; Pinilla, E.; Knudsen, J.S.; Hedegaard, E.R.; et al. Novel selective PDE type 1 inhibitors cause vasodilatation and lower blood pressure in rats. *Br. J. Pharmacol.* **2017**, *174*, 2563–2575. [CrossRef] [PubMed]

84. Nagel, D.J.; Aizawa, T.; Jeon, K.-I.; Liu, W.; Mohan, A.; Wei, H.; Miano, J.M.; Florio, V.A.; Gao, P.; Korshunov, V.A.; et al. Role of nuclear Ca^{2+}/calmodulin-stimulated phosphodiesterase 1A in vascular smooth muscle cell growth and survival. *Circ. Res.* **2006**, *98*, 777–784. [CrossRef] [PubMed]

85. Rybalkin, S.D.; Bornfeldt, K.E.; Sonnenburg, W.K.; Rybalkina, I.G.; Kwak, K.S.; Hanson, K.; Krebs, E.G.; Beavo, J.A. Calmodulin-stimulated cyclic nucleotide phosphodiesterase (PDE1C) is induced in human arterial smooth muscle cells of the synthetic, proliferative phenotype. *J. Clin. Investig.* **1997**, *100*, 2611–2621. [CrossRef] [PubMed]

86. Cai, Y.; Nagel, D.J.; Zhou, Q.; Cygnar, K.D.; Zhao, H.; Li, F.; Pi, X.; Knight, P.A.; Yan, C. Role of cAMP-phosphodiesterase 1C signaling in regulating growth factor receptor stability, vascular smooth muscle cell growth, migration, and neointimal hyperplasia. *Circ. Res.* **2015**, *116*, 1120–1132. [CrossRef] [PubMed]

87. Bautista Nino, P.K.; Durik, M.; Danser, A.H.; de Vries, R.; Musterd-Bhaggoe, U.M.; Meima, M.E.; Kavousi, M.; Ghanbari, M.; Hoeijmakers, J.H.; O'Donnell, C.J.; et al. Phosphodiesterase 1 regulation is a key mechanism in vascular aging. *Clin. Sci.* **2015**, *129*, 1061–1075. [CrossRef] [PubMed]

88. Yan, C. Cyclic nucleotide phosphodiesterase 1 and vascular aging. *Clin. Sci.* **2015**, *129*, 1077–1081. [CrossRef] [PubMed]

89. Saadane, N.; Alpert, L.; Chalifour, L.E. Expression of immediate early genes, GATA-4, and Nkx-2.5 in adrenergic-induced cardiac hypertrophy and during regression in adult mice. *Br. J. Pharmacol.* **1999**, *127*, 1165–1176. [CrossRef] [PubMed]

90. Jincai, W.; Tingfang, D.; Yongheng, Z.; Zhongmin, L.; Kaihua, Z.; Xiaohong, L. Effects of vinpocetine and ozagrel on behavioral recovery of rats after global brain ischemia. *J. Clin. Neurosci.* **2014**, *21*, 661–663. [CrossRef] [PubMed]

91. Bonoczk, P.; Panczel, G.; Nagy, Z. Vinpocetine increases cerebral blood flow and oxygenation in stroke patients: A near infrared spectroscopy and transcranial Doppler study. *Eur. J. Ultrasound* **2002**, *15*, 85–91. [CrossRef]

92. Vas, A.; Gulyas, B.; Szabo, Z.; Bonoczk, P.; Csiba, L.; Kiss, B.; Karpati, E.; Panczel, G.; Nagy, Z. Clinical and non-clinical investigations using positron emission tomography, near infrared spectroscopy and transcranial Doppler methods on the neuroprotective drug vinpocetine: A summary of evidences. *J. Neurol. Sci.* **2002**, *203–204*, 259–262. [CrossRef]

93. Zhang, Y.S.; Li, J.D.; Yan, C. An update on vinpocetine: New discoveries and clinical implications. *Eur. J. Pharmacol.* **2018**, *819*, 30–34. [CrossRef] [PubMed]

94. Cai, Y.; Knight, W.E.; Guo, S.; Li, J.D.; Knight, P.A.; Yan, C. Vinpocetine suppresses pathological vascular remodeling by inhibiting vascular smooth muscle cell proliferation and migration. *J. Pharmacol. Exp. Ther.* **2012**, *343*, 479–488. [CrossRef] [PubMed]

95. Cai, Y.; Li, J.-D.; Yan, C. Vinpocetine Attenuates Lipid Accumulation and Atherosclerosis Formation. *Biochem. Biophys. Res. Commun.* **2013**, in press. [CrossRef] [PubMed]

96. Zhuang, J.; Peng, W.; Li, H.; Lu, Y.; Wang, K.; Fan, F.; Li, S.; Xu, Y. Inhibitory effects of vinpocetine on the progression of atherosclerosis are mediated by Akt/NF-κB dependent mechanisms in apoE$^{-/-}$ mice. *PLoS ONE* **2013**, *8*, e82509. [CrossRef] [PubMed]

97. Wu, M.P.; Zhang, Y.S.; Xu, X.; Zhou, Q.; Li, J.D.; Yan, C. Vinpocetine Attenuates Pathological Cardiac Remodeling by Inhibiting Cardiac Hypertrophy and Fibrosis. *Cardiovasc. Drugs Ther.* **2017**, *31*, 157–166. [CrossRef] [PubMed]

98. Jeon, K.I.; Xu, X.; Aizawa, T.; Lim, J.H.; Jono, H.; Kwon, D.S.; Abe, J.; Berk, B.C.; Li, J.D.; Yan, C. Vinpocetine inhibits NF-kappaB-dependent inflammation via an IKK-dependent but PDE-independent mechanism. *Proc. Natl. Acad. Sci. USA* **2010**, *107*, 9795–9800. [CrossRef] [PubMed]

99. Ruiz-Miyazawa, K.W.; Pinho-Ribeiro, F.A.; Zarpelon, A.C.; Staurengo-Ferrari, L.; Silva, R.L.; Alves-Filho, J.C.; Cunha, T.M.; Cunha, F.Q.; Casagrande, R.; Verri, W.A., Jr. Vinpocetine reduces lipopolysaccharide-induced inflammatory pain and neutrophil recruitment in mice by targeting oxidative stress, cytokines and NF-κB. *Chem. Biol. Interact.* **2015**, *237*, 9–17. [CrossRef] [PubMed]

100. Evgenov, O.V.; Busch, C.J.; Evgenov, N.V.; Liu, R.; Petersen, B.; Falkowski, G.E.; Petho, B.; Vas, A.M.; Bloch, K.D.; Zapol, W.M.; et al. Inhibition of phosphodiesterase 1 augments the pulmonary vasodilator response to inhaled nitric oxide in awake lambs with acute pulmonary hypertension. *Am. J. Physiol. Lung Cell. Mol. Physiol.* **2006**, *290*, L723–L729. [CrossRef] [PubMed]

101. Lukyanenko, Y.O.; Younes, A.; Lyashkov, A.E.; Tarasov, K.V.; Riordon, D.R.; Lee, J.; Sirenko, S.G.; Kobrinsky, E.; Ziman, B.; Tarasova, Y.S.; et al. Ca^{2+}/calmodulin-activated phosphodiesterase 1A is highly expressed in rabbit cardiac sinoatrial nodal cells and regulates pacemaker function. *J. Mol. Cell. Cardiol.* **2016**, *98*, 73–82. [CrossRef] [PubMed]

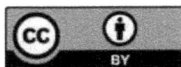

Journal of
Cardiovascular
Development and Disease

MDPI

Communication

Phosphodiesterases 3 and 4 Differentially Regulate the Funny Current, I_f, in Mouse Sinoatrial Node Myocytes

Joshua R. St. Clair [1], Eric D. Larson [1], Emily J. Sharpe [1], Zhandi Liao [1] and Catherine Proenza [1,2,*]

[1] Department of Physiology and Biophysics, University of Colorado School of Medicine, Aurora, CO 80045, USA; joshua.stclair@ucdenver.edu (J.R.S.); eric.larson@ucdenver.edu (E.D.L.); emily.sharpe@ucdenver.edu (E.J.S.); zdliao@ucdavis.edu (Z.L.)
[2] Department of Medicine, Division of Cardiology, University of Colorado School of Medicine, Aurora, CO 80045, USA
* Correspondence: catherine.proenza@ucdenver.edu; Tel.: +1-303-724-2522

Received: 30 June 2017; Accepted: 19 July 2017; Published: 1 August 2017

Abstract: Cardiac pacemaking, at rest and during the sympathetic fight-or-flight response, depends on cAMP ($3',5'$-cyclic adenosine monophosphate) signaling in sinoatrial node myocytes (SAMs). The cardiac "funny current" (I_f) is among the cAMP-sensitive effectors that drive pacemaking in SAMs. I_f is produced by hyperpolarization-activated, cyclic nucleotide-sensitive (HCN) channels. Voltage-dependent gating of HCN channels is potentiated by cAMP, which acts either by binding directly to the channels or by activating the cAMP-dependent protein kinase (PKA), which phosphorylates them. PKA activity is required for signaling between β adrenergic receptors (βARs) and HCN channels in SAMs but the mechanism that constrains cAMP signaling to a PKA-dependent pathway is unknown. Phosphodiesterases (PDEs) hydrolyze cAMP and form cAMP signaling domains in other types of cardiomyocytes. Here we examine the role of PDEs in regulation of I_f in SAMs. I_f was recorded in whole-cell voltage-clamp experiments from acutely-isolated mouse SAMs in the absence or presence of PDE and PKA inhibitors, and before and after βAR stimulation. General PDE inhibition caused a PKA-independent depolarizing shift in the midpoint activation voltage ($V_{1/2}$) of I_f at rest and removed the requirement for PKA in βAR-to-HCN signaling. PDE4 inhibition produced a similar PKA-independent depolarizing shift in the $V_{1/2}$ of I_f at rest, but did not remove the requirement for PKA in βAR-to-HCN signaling. PDE3 inhibition produced PKA-dependent changes in I_f both at rest and in response to βAR stimulation. Our results suggest that PDE3 and PDE4 isoforms create distinct cAMP signaling domains that differentially constrain access of cAMP to HCN channels and establish the requirement for PKA in signaling between βARs and HCN channels in SAMs.

Keywords: sinoatrial node; HCN channel; funny current (I_f); cardiac pacemaking; cardiomyocyte; cell compartmentalization; phosphodiesterases; cyclic AMP (cAMP); ion channel; patch clamp

1. Introduction

Cardiac pacemaking, at rest and during the sympathetic fight-or-flight response, depends on cAMP signaling in sinoatrial node myocytes (SAMs). SAMs are highly-specialized cells that drive pacemaking by firing spontaneous action potentials (APs). Spontaneous APs in SAMs result from a spontaneous depolarization during diastole that drives the membrane potential to its threshold to initiate the subsequent AP. The diastolic depolarization in SAMs arises as a function of the coordinated activity of a unique complement of ion channels that work in concert with intracellular Ca^{2+}

signaling [1–4]. $3',5'$-cyclic adenosine monophosphate (cAMP) is a critical regulator of pacemaking in SAMs. The resting cytoplasmic concentration of cAMP is thought to be higher in SAMs than in other cardiac myocytes [5] and sympathetic nervous system stimulation increases heart rate by activating β adrenergic receptors (βARs) and further increasing cAMP in SAMs.

The "funny current" (I_f) is a hallmark of SAMs and is among the many cAMP-sensitive effectors that contribute to spontaneous pacemaker activity in SAMs. I_f is produced by hyperpolarization-activated, cyclic nucleotide-sensitive (HCN) ion channels. HCN4 is the predominant HCN channel isoform in the sinoatrial node of all mammals; it is expressed at high levels in SAMs and is used as a marker of the sinoatrial node [6–9]. I_f is activated by membrane hyperpolarization and is a mixed cationic conductance with a reversal potential of approximately -30 mV in physiological solutions [10,11]. Thus, I_f is inward at diastolic potentials, and it is thought to contribute to the diastolic depolarization phase of the sinoatrial AP. In accordance with a critical role for I_f in pacemaking, mutations in HCN4 channels cause sinoatrial node dysfunction in human patients and animal models [12–14] and HCN channel blockers decrease the heart rate [15,16].

cAMP potentiates voltage-dependent gating of HCN4 channels either by binding directly to a conserved cyclic nucleotide binding domain in the proximal C-terminus [17,18] or by protein kinase A (PKA)-mediated phosphorylation of the distal C-terminus [11]. In either case, cAMP causes a depolarizing shift in the midpoint activation voltage ($V_{1/2}$). We previously showed that PKA activity is necessary for cAMP-dependent signaling between βARs and HCN channels in SAMs; inhibition of PKA with an inhibitory peptide, PKI, significantly reduced the shift in $V_{1/2}$ produced by βAR stimulation [11]. However, we have also shown that HCN channels in SAMs can be activated by cAMP even in the absence of PKA activity [19], presumably by binding directly to the channels. Thus, the requirement for PKA in βAR-to-HCN4 channel signaling in SAMs could arise as a function of compartmentalization or restricted diffusion of cAMP [19].

Although cAMP is a small, soluble molecule, it does not behave as a freely-diffusing molecule in many types of cells [20–27]. cAMP concentration in cells is determined by a balance between production by adenylyl cyclases and degradation by cyclic nucleotide phosphodiesterases (PDEs) PDEs have been shown to form functional diffusion barriers in other types of cardiac myocytes [28–32]. PDEs are organized into 11 families, of which the PDE3 and PDE4 families are the most abundant in the mouse sinoatrial node [33]. Functional studies using subtype-specific inhibitors have shown that the PDE3 and PDE4 families regulate the beating rate of mouse right atrial preparations [34], as well as the AP firing rate and Ca^{2+} currents in isolated mouse SAMs [33]. PDE4 is specific for cAMP, although it has a relatively low affinity (2–8 µM). In contrast, PDE3 can hydrolyze both cAMP and cGMP, but has a high affinity for cAMP (10–100 nM). Hydrolysis of cAMP by PDE3 is inhibited by cGMP due to a ~10-fold slower maximum reaction rate for cGMP [35,36].

In this study we tested the hypothesis that PDEs contribute to regulation of I_f in SAMs by creating functional cAMP signaling domains. Indeed, we found that the PDE3 and PDE4 isoforms play distinct roles in regulation of I_f, such that PDE4s control access of cAMP to HCN channels at rest, while PDE3s interact functionally with PKA to constrain signaling between βARs and HCN channels in SAMs.

2. Materials and Methods

2.1. Ethical Approval

This study was carried out in accordance with the US Animal Welfare Act and the National Research Council's *Guide for the Care and Use of Laboratory Animals* and was conducted according to a protocol that was approved by the University of Colorado-Anschutz Medical Campus Institutional Animal Care and Use Committee (protocol number 84814(06)1E). Six- to eight-week old male C57BL/6J mice were obtained from Jackson Laboratories (Bar Harbor, ME, USA; Cat. #000664). Animals were anesthetized by isofluorane inhalation and euthanized under anesthesia by cervical dislocation.

2.2. Sinoatrial Myocyte Isolation

Sinoatrial myocytes were isolated as we have previously described [11,19,37–42]. Briefly, hearts were removed into heparinized (10 U/mL) Tyrodes solution at 35 °C (in mM: 140 NaCl, 5.4 KCl, 1.2 KH_2PO_4, 1.8 $MgCl_2$, 1 $CaCl_2$, 5 HEPES, and 5.55 glucose, with pH adjusted to 7.4 with NaOH). The sinoatrial node, as defined by the borders of the crista terminalis, the interatrial septum, and the inferior and superior vena cavae, was excised and digested in an enzyme cocktail consisting of collagenase type II (Worthington Biochemical, NJ, USA), protease type XIV (Sigma Aldrich, St. Louis, MO, USA), and elastase (Worthington Biochemical, Lakewood, NJ, USA) for 25–30 min at 35 °C in a modified Tyrodes solution (in mM: 140 NaCl, 5.4 KCl, 1.2 KH_2PO_4, 5 HEPES, 18.5 glucose, 0.066 $CaCl_2$, 50 taurine, and 1 mg/mL BSA; pH adjusted to 6.9 with NaOH). Tissue was transferred to a modified KB solution (in mM: 100 potassium glutamate, 10 potassium aspartate, 25 KCl, 10 KH_2PO_4, 2 $MgSO_4$, 20 taurine, 5 creatine, 0.5 EGTA, 20 glucose, 5 HEPES, and 0.1% BSA; pH adjusted to 7.2 with KOH) at 35 °C, and cells were dissociated by trituration with a fire-polished glass pipet for ~10 min. Ca^{2+} was gradually reintroduced, and dissociated cells were maintained at room temperature for up to 8 h prior to electrophysiological recordings.

2.3. Sinoatrial Myocyte Electrophysiology

For electrophysiology, an aliquot of the sinoatrial node myocyte suspension was transferred to a glass-bottomed recording chamber on the stage of an inverted microscope. Individual SAMs were identified by spontaneous contractions, characteristic morphology [11,19,37–42], capacitance <45 pS, and the presence of I_f. Borosilicate glass pipettes had resistances of 1–3 MΩ when filled with an intracellular solution containing (in mM): 135 potassium aspartate, 6.6 sodium phosphocreatine, 1 $MgCl_2$, 1 $CaCl_2$, 10 HEPES, 10 EGTA, 4 Mg-ATP; pH adjusted to 7.2 with KOH. SAMs were constantly perfused (1–2 mL/min) with Tyrodes solution containing 1 mM $BaCl_2$ to block K^+ currents. A 1 mM stock solution of isoproterenol hydrochloride (ISO; Calbiochem/EMD Millipore, Billerica, MA, USA) in 1 mM ascorbic acid was stored as frozen aliquots, which were thawed on the day of experimentation and added to the perfusing Tyrodes solution to a final concentration of 1 μM as indicated.

Whole cell voltage clamp recordings were performed >2 min after achieving the whole cell recording configuration, to allow for intracellular perfusion with the pipette solution. To determine the voltage dependence of I_f, families of currents were elicited by 3 s hyperpolarizing voltage steps ranging from −60 mV up to −170 mV in 10 mV increments from a holding potential of −35 mV, as previously described [11,19,37–42]. Although steady state activation of I_f is not attained within 3 s for more depolarized potentials owing to the very slow kinetics of activation of I_f, the protocol is an experimentally-feasible means to approximate and compare the voltage-dependence of activation of I_f in the presence of different inhibitors (see [11]). Conductance (G) was calculated from the inward currents as:

$$G = I/(V_m − V_r) \tag{1}$$

where I is the time-dependent component of I_f, V_m is the applied membrane voltage (corrected for a +14 mV junction potential error, calculated using JPCalc [43]), and V_r is the reversal potential for I_f under these experimental conditions (−30 mV; [10,11]). Conductances were plotted as a function of voltage, and isochronal midpoint activation voltages ($V_{1/2}$) were determined for each cell by fitting with a Boltzmann function:

$$f(V) = V_{min} + \frac{V_{max} − V_{min}}{1 + e^{\frac{z_d F}{RT}(V−V_{1/2})}} \tag{2}$$

where V_{min} and V_{max} are the voltages corresponding to the minimum and maximum currents, Z_d is the charge valence, R is the gas constant, T is temperature, and F is the Faraday constant. The conductance-voltage relationship was determined for each individual cell included in the study and all individual GVs reached saturation. Averaged GV relationships are extrapolated to −170 for all conditions to facilitate comparisons. All experiments were conducted at room temperature in order to access the full range of activation midpoints for I_f (approximately -110 to -130 mV). Three cells were considered outliers and were excluded from the datasets because their midpoint activation voltages were greater than two standard deviations from the mean.

The isoproterenol- (ISO-) dependent shift in voltage dependence ($\Delta V_{1/2}$-ISO) was determined from paired recordings in individual cells before and after wash-on of 1 μM ISO in the absence or presence of PDE inhibitors. Current elicited by 1 s test pulses to -120 mV every 5–10 s was monitored during the ISO wash-on. The second GV protocol was begun when the increased current due to the ISO-dependent shift in $V_{1/2}$ reached steady state (within 1–2 min). PDE inhibitors were present in the extracellular solution as follows: total PDE inhibition with 100 μM 3-isobutyl-1-methylxanthine (IBMX; Tocris Bioscience, Bristol, UK), PDE4 inhibition with 10 μM rolipram (roli; Tocris Bioscience) or PDE3 inhibition with 10 or 50 μM milrinone (milr; Tocris Bioscience). The PKA inhibitory peptide 6-22 amide (PKI; Tocris Bioscience) was added to the intracellular (patch pipette) solution as noted at a final concentration of 10 μM. The adenylyl cyclase inhibitor MDL-12,330A (MDL) was applied at a final concentration of 10 μM in the bath solution.

2.4. Statistical Analysis

Data are presented as mean $\pm$ SEM. Statistical significance was evaluated by paired or unpaired two-tailed *t* tests or one-way ANOVAs with post-hoc tests as indicated. A *p* value of <0.05 was considered to be statistically significant.

3. Results

3.1. Phosphodiesterases Restrict Access of cAMP to HCN Channels at Rest

To evaluate the overall effects of PDEs on I_f in mouse SAMs, we applied the general, non-subtype-selective PDE inhibitor, 3-isobutyl-1-methylxanthine (IBMX; 100 μM in the extracellular solution) to acutely isolated SAMs in whole-cell voltage-clamp experiments. We found that IBMX shifted the midpoint activation voltage ($V_{1/2}$) of I_f by ~15 mV to more depolarized potentials (Figure 1A,C; Table 1), consistent with an increase in cAMP concentration in the vicinity of the HCN channels. Thus PDEs limit access of basal cAMP to HCN channels at rest.

Since we previously found that PKA activity is required for the cAMP-dependent activation of I_f by βARs in SAMs [11], we next asked whether PKA is also required for the cAMP liberated by IBMX to activate I_f. To this end, we evaluated the effects of IBMX on I_f in SAMs in which PKA was inhibited by the pseudosubstrate inhibitory peptide, PKI 6-22 amide (PKI; 10 μM in the patch pipette). We found that IBMX had essentially identical effects in the presence or absence of PKI; the $V_{1/2}$ of I_f did not differ in IBMX versus IBMX plus PKI (Figure 1C). Thus, in contrast to the cAMP generated upon βAR stimulation, the basal cAMP released upon PDE inhibition can activate HCN channels in SAMs independent of PKA activity.

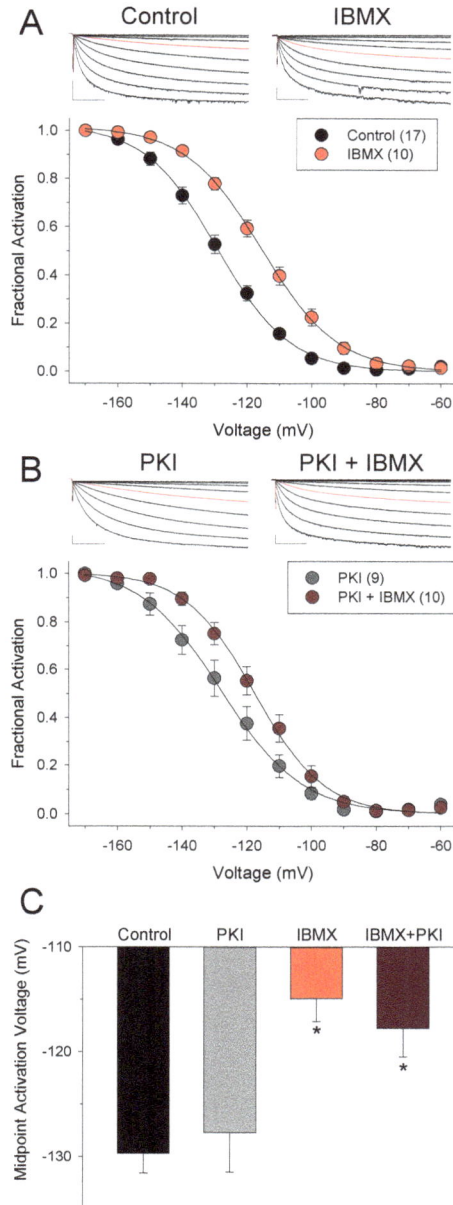

Figure 1. General PDE inhibition activates I_f in SAMs at rest via a PKA-independent mechanism. (**A,B**) Average ($\pm$SEM) normalized conductance-voltage plots for I_f in control (*black*), IBMX (100 μM in extracellular solution; *red*), PKI (10 μM in patch pipette; *grey*), or IBMX plus PKI (*dark red*). Numbers in parentheses in the legends indicate the number of cells in each dataset. Insets show representative I_f current families. Red traces show currents elicited by voltage steps to -120 mV to illustrate shifts in voltage dependence. Scale bars, 200 pA, 500 ms; and (**C**) average ($\pm$SEM) $V_{1/2}$ for I_f for the indicated conditions. Asterisks indicate $p < 0.05$ versus control; one-way ANOVA with Holm-Sidak post-test.

Table 1. Midpoint activation voltages for I_f in mouse sinoatrial myocytes. $V_{1/2}$ values for I_f were determined in the absence or presence of PDE inhibitors (IBMX 100 μM, rolipram 10 μM, milrinone 10 μM, or 50 μM as indicated) in the extracellular solution with and without the PKA inhibitory peptide, PKI (10 μM) in the pipette solution. For each cell, $V_{1/2}$ values were determined before or after wash-on of 1 μM isoproterenol in the extracellular solution; $\Delta V_{1/2(ISO)}$ is the average ISO-induced shift in $V_{1/2}$. Data for cAMP (1 mM in the patch pipette) and MDL-12,330A (10 μM in the extracellular solution) are provided for comparison from [13].

Treatment	$V_{1/2}$ before ISO (mV)	$V_{1/2}$ after ISO (mV)	$\Delta V_{1/2}$-ISO (mV)	n	*p* Value Control vs. ISO (Paired *t*-Test)
CONTROL	−129.7 ± 1.9	−119.6 ± 1.5	10.1 ± 1.2	17	0.000000237
+PKI	−127.7 ± 3.8	−123.6 ± 3.5	4.1 ± 0.7	9	0.00188
IBMX	−114.9 ± 2.2	−110.1 ± 2.8	4.8 ± 1.9	10	0.0328
+PKI	−117.7 ± 2.7	−110.6 ± 2.7	7.1 ± 1.1	10	0.000128
ROLIPRAM	−117.4 ± 1.6	−113.4 ± 2.2	4.0 ± 1.1	9	0.00712
+PKI	−118.9 ± 3.0	−118.8 ± 2.8	0.1 ± 1.9	7	0.967
MILRINONE (10 μM)	−124.0 ± 4.3	−121.1 ± 4.7	2.9 ± 1.7	8	0.123
+PKI	−119.3 ± 4.7	−112.5 ± 4.8	6.8 ± 2.4	10	0.0206
MILRINONE (50 μM)	−124.1 ± 1.9	−122.2 ± 2.0	1.8 ± 1.0	10	0.104
+PKI	−116.8 ± 1.3	−110.9 ± 1.8	5.9 ± 1.2	11	0.000648
MDL-12,330A	−131.1 ± 1.9	−132.0 ± 2.2	−0.9 ± 1.1	7	0.469
1 mM cAMP	−112.0 ± 1.6	-	-	10	-
3 mM cAMP	−114.1 ± 1.9	-	-	7	-

3.2. Different Effects of PDE4 and PDE3 on I_f under Basal Conditions

PDE4 activity is thought to regulate sinoatrial node pacemaker activity in a number of species, based on experiments using rolipram, a PDE4 family inhibitor [33,34,44,45]. To determine the role of PDE4 in basal regulation of I_f in mouse SAMs, we evaluated the effects of rolipram (10 μM in the bath solution) on the $V_{1/2}$ of I_f. We found that rolipram caused a significant depolarizing shift in $V_{1/2}$ which was indistinguishable from the shift produced by IBMX (Figure 2A,C; Table 1). As in the case of IBMX, the rolipram-liberated cAMP did not require PKA activity in order to activate HCN channels, since the $V_{1/2}$ values did not differ in rolipram alone compared to rolipram plus PKI (Figure 2C; Table 1).

The PDE3 family is also thought to affect sinoatrial node function; inhibition of PDE3 increases basal pacemaker activity in isolated SAMs and atrial preparations from mice [33,34]. In contrast to IBMX or rolipram, we found that the PDE3 family inhibitor, milrinone (10 or 50 μM) produced only a modest, statistically insignificant, depolarizing shift in the $V_{1/2}$ of I_f in SAMs when applied by itself (Figure 3A,C; Table 1). However, when milrinone was applied in the presence of PKI, it produced a significant depolarizing shift in $V_{1/2}$ of I_f, which was similar in magnitude to the shifts produced by IBMX or rolipram (Figure 3; Table 1).

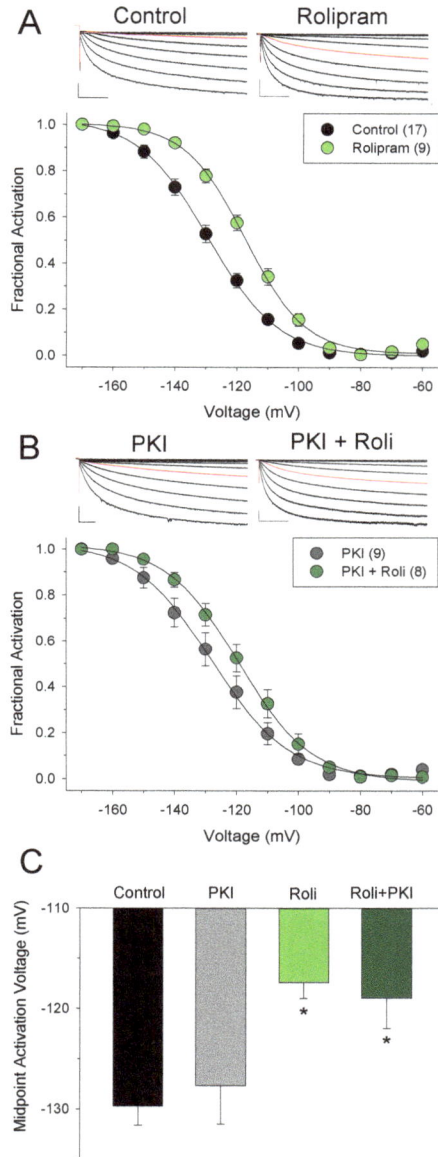

Figure 2. PDE4 inhibition activates I_f in SAMs at rest via a PKA-independent mechanism. (**A,B**) Average (±SEM) normalized conductance-voltage plots for I_f in control (*black*), rolipram (10 μM in the extracellular solution; *green*), PKI (10 μM in the patch pipette; *grey*), or PKI plus rolipram (*dark green*). Numbers in parentheses in the legends indicate the number of cells in each dataset. *Insets* show representative I_f current families. Red traces elicited by voltage steps to −120 mV illustrate shifts in the voltage dependence. Scale bars, 100 pA, 500 ms. for control, 500 pA, 500 ms for PKI; and (**C**) shows the average (±SEM) $V_{1/2}$ for I_f for indicated conditions. *Asterisks* indicate $p < 0.05$ versus control; one-way ANOVA with Holm-Sidak post-test.

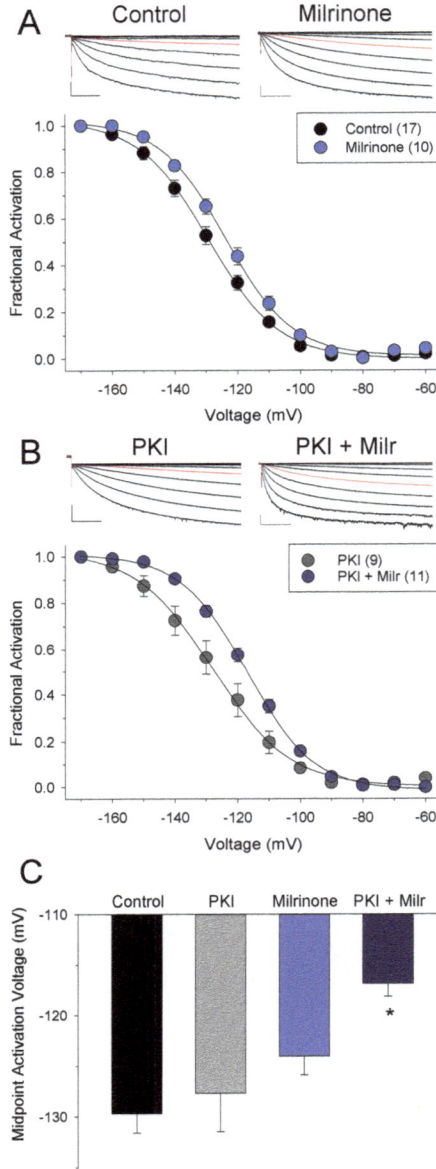

Figure 3. Effects of PDE3 inhibition on I_f at rest. (**A,B**) Average ($\pm$SEM) normalized conductance-voltage plots for I_f in control (black), milrinone (50 µM in the extracellular solution; *blue*), PKI (10 µM in the patch pipette; *grey*), or milrinone plus PKI (*dark blue*). Numbers in parentheses in the legends indicate the number of cells in each dataset. Insets show representative I_f current families. Red traces elicited by voltage steps to -120 mV illustrate shifts in the voltage dependence. Scale bars, 100 pA, 500 ms for control, 500 pA, 500 ms for PKI; and (**C**) shows the average ($\pm$SEM) $V_{1/2}$ for I_f for indicated conditions. Asterisk indicates $p < 0.05$ versus control; one-way ANOVA with Holm-Sidak post-test.

3.3. PDEs Establish the Requirement for PKA Activity in Signaling between βARs and HCN Channels in SAMs

To evaluate the role of PDEs in establishing the requirement for PKA in βAR-to-HCN channel signaling in SAMs, we assayed the shift in $V_{1/2}$ in individual cells in response to the wash-on of the βAR agonist, isoproterenol ($\Delta V_{1/2}$-ISO). $\Delta V_{1/2}$-ISO shifts were determined in the absence or presence of PDE inhibitors and PKI. In control Tyrode's solution, the wash-on of ISO produced a ~10 mV depolarizing shift in the $V_{1/2}$ of I_f (Figure 4A). In the presence of PKI in the patch pipette (but the absence of any PDE inhibitors), ISO still produced a significant shift in $V_{1/2}$ in paired recordings from individual cells, but the magnitude of this shift was significantly reduced compared to control (Figure 4A; Table 1). In cells treated with IBMX, ISO produced a significant ~5 mV depolarizing shift in $V_{1/2}$, in addition to the ~15 mV shift already caused by IBMX (Figure 4B; Table 1). We attribute the reduced $\Delta V_{1/2}$-ISO in IBMX versus control (Figure 4B versus Figure 4A) to a ceiling effect, because the absolute value of the $V_{1/2}$ in IBMX plus ISO (approximately −110 mV) did not differ from that produced by a saturating concentration of cAMP introduced via the patch pipette (approximately −112 mV; Table 1). Whereas PKI significantly decreased the $\Delta V_{1/2}$-ISO under control conditions (Figure 4A), it did not reduce $\Delta V_{1/2}$-ISO when PDEs were inhibited by IBMX (Figure 4B). Thus, PDEs contribute to the formation of the PKA-dependent signaling pathway between βARs and HCN channels in SAMs, apparently by restricting the ability of βAR-stimulated cAMP to access the channels.

The contributions of the PDE4 and PDE3 families to the PKA-dependent βAR-to-HCN channel signaling pathway were evaluated using rolipram or milrinone. In cells treated with rolipram, ISO produced a significant depolarizing shift in the $V_{1/2}$ of I_f (Figure 4C; Table 1). As in the case of IBMX, this ISO-dependent shift was reduced in magnitude compared to the shift in control conditions, and again, the reduction is attributed to a ceiling effect because the $V_{1/2}$ for rolipram plus ISO did not differ from that of saturating cAMP (Table 1). However, in contrast to the situation of general PDE block with IBMX, block of PDE4s with rolipram did not relieve the requirement for PKA in βAR-to-HCN channel signaling in SAMs. In fact, PKI completely abolished the ability of ISO to shift the $V_{1/2}$ in the presence of rolipram ($p = 0.967$ versus a hypothetical mean shift of 0; Figure 4C; Table 1). Thus, PDE4 does not appear to contribute to the PKA dependent βAR-to-HCN signaling pathway.

While the ability of ISO to shift the $V_{1/2}$ was nearly eliminated by the PDE3 inhibitor milrinone when it was applied alone ($p = 0.104$ versus a hypothetical mean shift of 0; Figure 4D; Table 1), simultaneous inhibition of both PDE3 and PKA, with milrinone plus PKI, restored the ability of ISO to shift in $V_{1/2}$ of I_f (Figure 4D; Table 1) consistent with a role for PDE3 in the formation of the PKA dependent βAR-to-HCN signaling pathway and, again, indicative of an interaction between PKA and PDE3 in the regulation of I_f in SAMs.

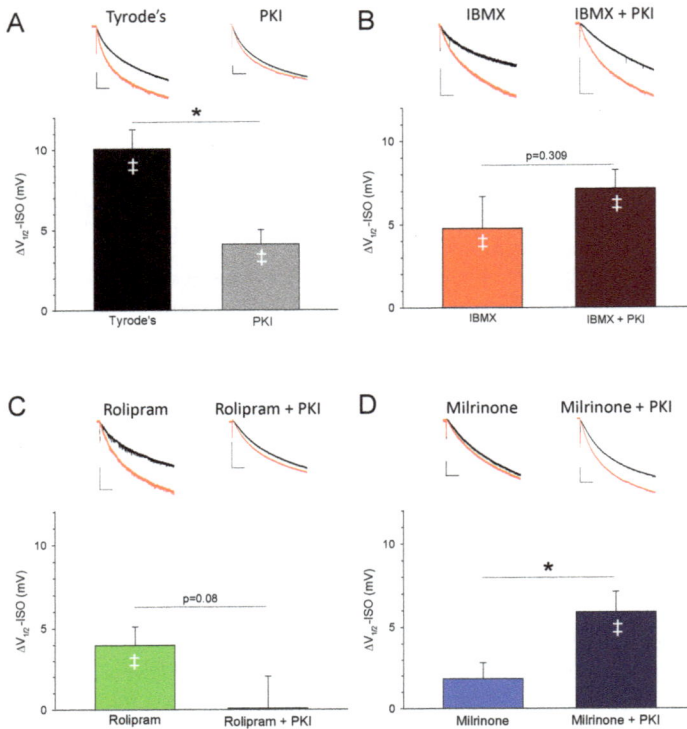

Figure 4. Effects of PDE inhibition on the ability of ISO to shift the voltage-dependence of I_f. The shift in $V_{1/2}$ of I_f in response to ISO ($\Delta V_{1/2}$-ISO) was determined for individual cells by measuring $V_{1/2}$ values before and after wash-on of ISO in (**A**) control Tyrode's extracellular solution (*black*) or Tyrode's solution with PKI (10 µM) in the patch pipette (*grey*); (**B**) IBMX (100 µM in the extracellular solution; *red*) or IBMX with PKI in the pipette (*dark red*); (**C**) rolipram (10 µM in the extracellular solution; *light green*) or rolipram with PKI in the pipette (*dark green*); and (**D**) milrinone (50 µM; *blue*) or milrinone with PKI in the pipette (*dark blue*). Dashed lines indicate the $\Delta V_{1/2}$-ISO shift in control conditions for comparison. Asterisks indicate $p < 0.05$ compared to the corresponding condition without PKI; *t*-tests. Double daggers indicate a significant shift in response to ISO ($p < 0.05$ versus a hypothetical shift of 0 mV; one-sample *t*-tests). Insets represent the hyperpolarization-activated currents elicited by single voltage steps to near the midpoint activation voltage for each condition from individual cells before (black) and after (red) wash-on of ISO in the absence (left) or presence (right) of PKI. Scale bars: Tyrode's, 200 pA; PKI, 200 pA; IBMX, 50 pA; IMBX + PKI, 100 pA; rolipram, 100 pA; rolipram + PKI, 200 pA; milrinone, 100 pA; milrinone + PKI, 200 pA. All time scale bars, 500 ms.

4. Discussion

In this study we examined the role of phosphodiesterases in cAMP-dependent regulation of I_f in acutely-isolated sinoatrial node myocytes from mice. We found that the PDE3 and PDE4 isoforms contribute to formation of at least two functional cAMP signaling domains that control I_f in SAMs. The PDE4 family restricts access of cAMP to HCN channels under basal conditions, but does not appear to play a role in the formation of the PKA-dependent βAR-to-HCN channel signaling pathway. Meanwhile, the PDE3 family interacts functionally with PKA to regulate I_f at rest and contributes to the formation of the PKA-dependent pathway between βARs and HCN channels in SAMs.

Our interpretation of the results assumes that the pharmacological agents we used are relatively selective and that the degree of block achieved is fairly complete. While we cannot exclude the possibility of some off-target block, our results using PKI, IBMX, rolipram and milrinone cannot be explained by isoform cross-reactivity amongst the blockers. For example, although high concentrations of the PDE3 blocker milrinone (>10 µM) can also inhibit PDE4, lower concentrations are thought to be specific for PDE3 [33,35,46]. We tested the effects of 10 µM milrinone on I_f and observed a minimal response (Table 1). To ensure that we had reached a maximal effective concentration in mouse SAMs, and to compare our results to other studies [45], we also evaluated the effects of 50 µM milrinone. We found no difference in the response of I_f to 10 or 50 µM milrinone (Table 1 [11]). Moreover, the effects of milrinone were qualitatively different from the effects of either the general PDE inhibitor, IBMX, or the PDE4 inhibitor, rolipram. Thus, we conclude that (1) PDE3, alone, has minimal effects on I_f (although it interacts functionally with PKA, see below), and (2) the effects of milrinone on I_f in our experiments did not reflect appreciable block of PDE4.

A key finding of our study is that the shifts in the basal $V_{1/2}$ of I_f produced by IBMX or rolipram were similar in the presence and absence of the PKA inhibitory peptide, PKI. The shifts produced by PDE inhibition alone (without PKA inhibition) could reflect combined effects of direct cAMP binding and PKA phosphorylation, whereas those in the presence of PKI presumably result from a direct effect of cAMP alone. We interpret the similar effects in the presence and absence of PKI as an indication that the cAMP liberated upon total PDE inhibition or PDE4 inhibition activates I_f without a requirement for PKA activity. However, this interpretation assumes that PKI blocks a substantial fraction of the PKA activity near HCN channels in SAMs. We feel that this assumption is justified based on our finding that PKI significantly reduced the shift in $V_{1/2}$ in response to ISO under the same conditions (Figure 4A; Table 1; [11]). A more direct assessment of PKA activity (e.g., PKA assays in sinoatrial node homogenates) would be difficult to interpret because data from tissue extracts is a poor proxy for PKA activity within temporally- and spatially-restricted cAMP signaling domains in SAMs.

The results of the present study extend our previous observations that, although PKA activity is required for βAR signaling to HCN channels in SAMs [11], it is still possible for cAMP to activate I_f in SAMs even in the absence of PKA activity [19]. Taken together, the previous and new data suggest a working model in which members of the PDE4 family form a functional "barrier" that isolates HCN channels from the high basal cAMP in SAMs. Disruption of this barrier with either rolipram or IBMX permits cAMP to access HCN channels, where it activates them via a PKA-independent mechanism (presumably via direct binding to the cyclic nucleotide binding domain of the channels). In our model, PDE3 family members are proposed to form a distinct functional barrier that prevents the cAMP generated upon βAR stimulation from reaching HCN channels directly, thereby constraining βAR signaling to HCN channels to a PKA-dependent pathway. Additional work will be required to determine whether these barriers represent distinct cAMP compartments in SAMs and whether the PKA-dependent activation of I_f by βAR stimulation results from phosphorylation of HCN channels by PKA, or if it occurs as a result of an indirect mechanism, such as control of cAMP production—e.g., by Ca^{2+}-activated adenylyl cyclases [47]—with the resulting cAMP then potentiating I_f by binding directly to HCN channels.

Our observations of differing effects when PDE3 and PKA were inhibited together, instead of individually, indicates a complex functional interaction between PDE3 and PKA in the regulation of I_f in SAMs. The data preclude a simple model in which PDE3 simply acts to restrict the cAMP source that controls PKA regulation of I_f. Instead, there must be co-regulation between PDE3 and PKA. Possible nodes of cross-talk between PDE3 and PKA include the activation of PDE3 by PKA and the inhibition of PDE3 hydrolysis of cAMP by cGMP [35,36]. In the first scenario, inhibition of PKA with PKI would also inhibit PDE3, thereby increasing cAMP, and allowing it to act by binding directly to HCN channels. Consistent with this notion, we found that milrinone, alone, had no significant effect on the $V_{1/2}$ of I_f, but produced a significant depolarizing shift when it was applied in the presence of PKI (Figure 3, Table 1). Meanwhile, a role for cGMP is suggested by the observation of high levels of

J. Cardiovasc. Dev. Dis. **2017**, *4*, 10

soluble guanylyl cyclase and cGMP in the sinoatrial node [48]. Indeed, cGMP-mediated inhibition of PDE3 has been suggested to increase cAMP concentration and accelerate AP firing rate in mouse sinoatrial nodes [49]. cGMP-mediated inhibition of PDE3 has also been shown to modulate cAMP levels in subcellular compartments involved in βAR signaling in ventricular myocytes [50].

Our data complement results of previous studies in which PDEs have been shown to regulate pacemaker activity of the sinoatrial node. Our observations of depolarizing shifts in the voltage dependence of I_f in response to PDE inhibition are in agreement with the notions that the resting cAMP concentration is relatively high in SAMs and that it is limited by constitutive PDE activity [5,33,45,47]. The role of PDE4 in limiting the basal cAMP concentration in the vicinity of HCN channels in our study is in agreement with the observations of Hua et al. [33], who found that inhibition of PDE4 with rolipram (10 μM) increased AP firing rate and $I_{Ca,L}$ in isolated mouse SAMs to a greater extent than did PDE3 inhibition with milrinone (10 μM). Our data suggest that I_f works along with $I_{Ca,L}$ to mediate the increase in AP firing rate in response to PDE4 inhibition. Galindo-Tovar and Kaumann [34] used rolipram (1 μM) along with the PDE3 inhibitor cilostamide (300 nM) to show that both PDE3 and PDE4 contribute to control of basal firing rate in isolated mouse right atria via actions on a cAMP compartment that is distinct from that mediated by βARs. These data are in good agreement with our observations of multiple functional cAMP signaling domains formed by PDEs in SAMs and of PDE4-dependent regulation of I_f under basal conditions. However, they also suggest that additional PDE3-dependent mechanisms may also contribute to pacemaker activity in the mouse sinoatrial node. Interestingly, βAR-induced tachycardia across many species is resistant to PDE inhibition, suggesting that cAMP signaling between βARs and relevant effectors for the fight-or-flight increase in heart rate is not controlled by PDEs [51,52]. Hence, βAR regulation of I_f appears to serve primarily as a frequency adaptation mechanism rather than a primary driver of the sympathetic heart rate response. Vinogradova et al. [45] used milrinone (50 μM) to suggest that PDE3 may be the dominant isoform controlling basal firing rate in rabbit SAMs. However, we did not observe a difference between 10 μM and 50 μM milrinone in mouse SAMs, and saw effects of milrinone only in combination with PKA inhibition. Taken together, these data suggest that there may be species-dependent differences in the roles of different PDE isoforms in regulation of sinoatrial node activity.

5. Conclusions

In summary, our results indicate that the PDE3 and PDE4 isoforms create functionally-distinct cAMP signaling domains in mouse SAMs that regulate I_f at rest and in response to βAR stimulation. Specifically, the PDE4 family restricts access of cAMP to HCN4 channels under basal conditions, and the PDE3 family contributes to the formation of a preferred PKA-dependent pathway between βARs and HCN channels. Given that I_f is a critical factor in sinoatrial node pacemaker activity, it is likely that these mechanisms contribute to the regulation of heart rate.

Acknowledgments: We thank Hicham Bichraoui and Christian Rickert for helpful discussions and critical reading of the manuscript. This work was supported by a grant from the National Heart Lung and Blood Institute (R01-HL088427) to CP. EJS was supported by 5T32-AG000279 from the National Institute on Aging and F31-HL132408 from the National Heart Lung and Blood Institute. The content is solely the responsibility of the authors and does not necessarily represent the official views of the National Institutes of Health.

Author Contributions: J.R.S. and C.P. designed the experiments. J.R.S., Z.L., E.D.L., E.J.S., and C.P. performed and analyzed the experiments and wrote the manuscript. All authors approved the final version of the manuscript and are accountable for all aspects of the work. All persons designated as authors, and all those who qualify for authorship, are listed.

Conflicts of Interest: The founding sponsors had no role in the design of the study; in the collection, analyses, or interpretation of data; in the writing of the manuscript, and in the decision to publish the results.

Abbreviations

AP	action potential
βAR	adrenergic receptor
cAMP	3′,5′-cyclic adenosine monophosphate
HCN channel	hyperpolarization-activated, cyclic nucleotide-sensitive ion channel
IBMX	3-isobutyl-1-methylxanthine
I_f	funny current
ISO	isoproterenol
milr	milrinone
PDE	phosphodiesterase
PKA	cAMP-dependent protein kinase
PKI	PKA inhibitory peptide
roli	rolipram
SAM	sinoatrial node myocyte
$V_{1/2}$	midpoint activation voltage

References

1. Mangoni, M.; Nargeot, J. Genesis and regulation of the heart automaticity. *Physiol. Rev.* **2008**, *88*, 919–982. [CrossRef] [PubMed]
2. Lakatta, E.G.; DiFrancesco, D. What keeps us ticking: A funny current, a calcium clock, or both? *J. Mol. Cell. Cardiol.* **2009**, *47*, 157–170. [CrossRef] [PubMed]
3. DiFrancesco, D. The role of the funny current in pacemaker activity. *Circ. Res.* **2010**, *106*, 434–446. [CrossRef] [PubMed]
4. Lakatta, E.G.; Maltsev, V.A.; Vinogradova, T.M. A coupled SYSTEM of intracellular Ca^{2+} clocks and surface membrane voltage clocks controls the timekeeping mechanism of the heart's pacemaker. *Circ. Res* **2010**, *106*, 659–673. [CrossRef] [PubMed]
5. Vinogradova, T.; Lyashkov, A.; Zhu, W.; Ruknudin, A.; Sirenko, S.; Yang, D.; Deo, S.; Barlow, M.; Johnson, S.; Caffrey, J.; et al. High basal protein kinase A-dependent phosphorylation drives rhythmic internal Ca^{2+} store oscillations and spontaneous beating of cardiac pacemaker cells. *Circ. Res.* **2006**, *98*, 505–514. [CrossRef] [PubMed]
6. Liu, J.; Dobrzynski, H.; Yanni, J.; Boyett, M.R.; Lei, M. Organisation of the mouse sinoatrial node: Structure and expression of HCN channels. *Cardiovasc. Res.* **2007**, *73*, 729–738. [CrossRef] [PubMed]
7. Marionneau, C.; Couette, B.; Liu, J.; Li, H.; Mangoni, M.E.; Nargeot, J.; Lei, M.; Escande, D.; Demolombe, S. Specific pattern of ionic channel gene expression associated with pacemaker activity in the mouse heart. *J. Physiol.* **2005**, *562*, 223–234. [CrossRef] [PubMed]
8. Moosmang, S.; Stieber, J.; Zong, X.; Biel, M.; Hofmann, F.; Ludwig, A. Cellular expression and functional characterization of four hyperpolarization-activated pacemaker channels in cardiac and neuronal tissues. *Eur. J. Biochem.* **2001**, *268*, 1646–1652. [CrossRef] [PubMed]
9. Shi, W.; Wymore, R.; Yu, H.; Wu, J.; Wymore, R.T.; Pan, Z.; Robinson, R.B.; Dixon, J.E.; McKinnon, D.; Cohen, I.S. Distribution and Prevalence of Hyperpolarization-Activated Cation Channel (HCN) mRNA Expression in Cardiac Tissues. *Circ. Res.* **1999**, *85*, e1–e6. [CrossRef] [PubMed]
10. Mangoni, M.E.; Nargeot, J. Properties of the hyperpolarization-activated current (I(f)) in isolated mouse sino-atrial cells. *Cardiovasc. Res.* **2001**, *52*, 51–64. [CrossRef]
11. Liao, Z.; Lockhead, D.; Larson, E.; Proenza, C. Phosphorylation and modulation of hyperpolarization-activated HCN4 channels by protein kinase A in the mouse sinoatrial node. *J. Gen. Physiol.* **2010**, *136*, 247–258. [CrossRef] [PubMed]
12. Verkerk, A.O.; Wilders, R. Pacemaker activity of the human sinoatrial node An update on the effects of mutations in HCN4 on the hyperpolarization-activated current. *Int. J. Mol. Sci.* **2015**, *16*, 3071–3094. [CrossRef] [PubMed]
13. Baruscotti, M.; Bucchi, A.; Milanesi, R.; Paina, M.; Barbuti, A.; Gnecchi-Ruscone, T.; Bianco, E.; Vitali-Serdoz, L.; Cappato, R.; DiFrancesco, D. A gain-of-function mutation in the cardiac pacemaker HCN4 channel increasing cAMP sensitivity is associated with familial Inappropriate Sinus Tachycardia. *Eur. Heart J.* **2017**, *38*, 280–288. [CrossRef] [PubMed]

14. Herrmann, S.; Hofmann, F.; Stieber, J.; Ludwig, A. HCN channels in the heart: Lessons from mouse mutants. *Br. J. Pharmacol.* **2012**, *166*, 501–509. [CrossRef] [PubMed]

15. Borer, J.S. Drug insight: If inhibitors as specific heart-rate-reducing agents. *Nat. Clin. Pract. Cardiovasc. Med.* **2004**, *1*, 103–109. [CrossRef] [PubMed]

16. Roubille, F.; Tardif, J.-C. New Therapeutic Targets in Cardiology Heart Failure and Arrhythmia: HCN Channels. *Circulation* **2013**, *127*, 1986–1996. [CrossRef] [PubMed]

17. DiFrancesco, D.; Tortora, P. Direct activation of cardiac pacemaker channels by intracellular cyclic AMP. *Nature* **1991**, *351*, 145–147. [CrossRef] [PubMed]

18. Zagotta, W.N.; Olivier, N.B.; Black, K.D.; Young, E.C.; Olson, R.; Gouaux, E. Structural basis for modulation and agonist specificity of HCN pacemaker channels. *Nature* **2003**, *425*, 200–205. [CrossRef] [PubMed]

19. St. Clair, J.R.; Liao, Z.; Larson, E.D.; Proenza, C. PKA-independent activation of I(f) by cAMP in mouse sinoatrial myocytes. *Channels* **2013**, *7*, 318–321.

20. Conti, M.; Mika, D.; Richter, W. Cyclic AMP compartments and signaling specificity: Role of cyclic nucleotide phosphodiesterases. *J. Gen. Physiol.* **2014**, *143*, 29–38. [CrossRef] [PubMed]

21. Dodge-Kafka, K.L.; Langeberg, L.; Scott, J.D. Compartmentation of Cyclic Nucleotide Signaling in the Heart the Role of A-Kinase Anchoring Proteins. *Circ. Res.* **2006**, *98*, 993–1001. [CrossRef] [PubMed]

22. Karpen, J.W. Perspectives on: Cyclic nucleotide microdomains and signaling specificity. *J. Gen. Physiol.* **2014**, *143*, 5–7. [CrossRef] [PubMed]

23. Perera, R.K.; Nikolaev, V.O. Compartmentation of cAMP signalling in cardiomyocytes in health and disease. *Acta Physiol.* **2013**, *207*, 650–662. [CrossRef] [PubMed]

24. Richards, M.; Lomas, O.; Jalink, K.; Ford, K.L.; Vaughan-Jones, R.D.; Lefkimmiatis, K.; Swietach, P. Intracellular tortuosity underlies slow cAMP diffusion in adult ventricular myocytes. *Cardiovasc. Res.* **2016**, *110*, 395–407. [CrossRef] [PubMed]

25. Warrier, S.; Ramamurthy, G.; Eckert, R.L.; Nikolaev, V.O.; Lohse, M.J.; Harvey, R.D. cAMP microdomains and L-type Ca^{2+} channel regulation in guinea-pig ventricular myocytes. *J. Physiol.* **2007**, *580*, 765–776. [CrossRef] [PubMed]

26. Xiang, Y. Compartmentalization of beta-adrenergic signals in cardiomyocytes. *Circ. Res.* **2011**, *109*, 231–244. [CrossRef] [PubMed]

27. Zaccolo, M. cAMP signal transduction in the heart: Understanding spatial control for the development of novel therapeutic strategies. *Br. J. Pharmacol.* **2009**, *158*, 50–60. [CrossRef] [PubMed]

28. Jurevicius, J.; Fischmeister, R. cAMP compartmentation is responsible for a local activation of cardiac Ca^{2+} channels by beta-adrenergic agonists. *Proc. Natl. Acad. Sci. USA* **1996**, *93*, 295–299. [CrossRef] [PubMed]

29. Steinberg, S.F.; Brunton, L.L. Compartmentation of G Protein-Coupled Signaling Pathways in Cardiac Myocytes. *Annu. Rev. Pharmacol. Toxicol.* **2001**, *41*, 751–773. [CrossRef] [PubMed]

30. Zaccolo, M.; Pozzan, T. Discrete microdomains with high concentration of cAMP in stimulated rat neonatal cardiac myocytes. *Science* **2002**, *295*, 1711–1715. [CrossRef] [PubMed]

31. Jurevicius, J.; Skeberdis, V.A.; Fischmeister, R. Role of cyclic nucleotide phosphodiesterase isoforms in cAMP compartmentation following beta2-adrenergic stimulation of $I_{Ca,L}$ in frog ventricular myocytes. *J. Physiol.* **2003**, *551*, 239–252. [CrossRef] [PubMed]

32. Mongillo, M.; McSorley, T.; Evellin, S.; Sood, A.; Lissandron, V.; Terrin, A.; Huston, E.; Hannawacker, A.; Lohse, M.J.; Pozzan, T.; et al. Fluorescence Resonance Energy Transfer-Based Analysis of cAMP Dynamics in Live Neonatal Rat Cardiac Myocytes Reveals Distinct Functions of Compartmentalized Phosphodiesterases. *Circ. Res.* **2004**, *95*, 67–75. [CrossRef] [PubMed]

33. Hua, R.; Adamczyk, A.; Robbins, C.; Ray, G.; Rose, R. Distinct patterns of constitutive phosphodiesterase activity in mouse sinoatrial node and atrial myocardium. *PLoS ONE* **2012**, *7*, e47652. [CrossRef] [PubMed]

34. Galindo-Tovar, A.; Kaumann, A.J. Phosphodiesterase-4 blunts inotropism and arrhythmias but not sinoatrial tachycardia of (−)-adrenaline mediated through mouse cardiac β1-adrenoceptors. *Br. J. Pharmacol.* **2008**, *153*, 710–720. [CrossRef] [PubMed]

35. Shakur, Y.; Fong, M.; Hensley, J.; Cone, J.; Movsesian, M.; Kambayashi, J.; Yoshitake, M.; Liu, Y. Comparison of the effects of cilostazol and milrinone on cAMP-PDE activity, intracellular cAMP and calcium in the heart. *Cardiovasc. Drugs Ther. Spons. Int. Soc. Cardiovasc. Pharmacother.* **2002**, *16*, 417–427. [CrossRef]

36. Zaccolo, M.; Movsesian, M. cAMP and cGMP signaling cross-talk: Role of phosphodiesterases and implications for cardiac pathophysiology. *Circ. Res.* **2007**, *100*, 1569–1578. [CrossRef] [PubMed]

37. Liao, Z.; St. Clair, J.R.; Larson, E.D.; Proenza, C. Myristoylated peptides potentiate the funny current (I(f)) in sinoatrial myocytes. *Channels* **2011**, *5*, 115–119. [CrossRef] [PubMed]
38. Groenke, S.; Larson, E.D.; Alber, S.; Zhang, R.; Lamp, S.T.; Ren, X.; Nakano, H.; Jordan, M.C.; Karagueuzian, H.S.; Roos, K.P.; et al. Complete atrial-specific knockout of sodium-calcium exchange eliminates sinoatrial node pacemaker activity. *PLoS ONE* **2013**, *8*, e81633. [CrossRef] [PubMed]
39. St. Clair, J.R.; Sharpe, E.J.; Proenza, C. Culture and adenoviral infection of sinoatrial node myocytes from adult mice. *Am. J. Physiol. Heart Circ. Physiol.* **2015**, *309*, H490–H498. [CrossRef] [PubMed]
40. Larson, E.D.; St. Clair, J.R.; Sumner, W.A.; Bannister, R.A.; Proenza, C. Depressed pacemaker activity of sinoatrial node myocytes contributes to the age-dependent decline in maximum heart rate. *Proc. Natl. Acad. Sci. USA* **2013**, *110*, 18011–18016. [CrossRef] [PubMed]
41. Sharpe, E.J.; St. Clair, J.R.; Proenza, C. Methods for the Isolation, Culture, and Functional Characterization of Sinoatrial Node Myocytes from Adult Mice. *J. Vis. Exp.* **2016**. [CrossRef] [PubMed]
42. Sharpe, E.J.; Larson, E.D.; Proenza, C. Cyclic AMP reverses the effects of aging on pacemaker activity and I_f in sinoatrial node myocytes. *J. Gen. Physiol.* **2017**, *149*, 237–247. [CrossRef] [PubMed]
43. Barry, P.H. JPCalc, a software package for calculating liquid junction potential corrections in patch-clamp, intracellular, epithelial and bilayer measurements and for correcting junction potential measurements. *J. Neurosci. Methods* **1994**, *51*, 107–116. [CrossRef]
44. Kaumann, A.J.; Galindo-Tovar, A.; Escudero, E.; Vargas, M.L. Phosphodiesterases do not limit beta1-adrenoceptor-mediated sinoatrial tachycardia: Evidence with PDE3 and PDE4 in rabbits and PDE1–5 in rats. *Naunyn. Schmiedebergs Arch. Pharmacol.* **2009**, *380*, 421–430. [CrossRef] [PubMed]
45. Vinogradova, T.; Sirenko, S.; Lyashkov, A.; Younes, A.; Li, Y.; Zhu, W.; Yang, D.; Ruknudin, A.; Spurgeon, H.; Lakatta, E. Constitutive phosphodiesterase activity restricts spontaneous beating rate of cardiac pacemaker cells by suppressing local Ca^{2+} releases. *Circ. Res.* **2008**, *102*, 761–769. [CrossRef] [PubMed]
46. Kerfant, B.-G.; Zhao, D.; Lorenzen-Schmidt, I.; Wilson, L.S.; Cai, S.; Chen, S.R.W.; Maurice, D.H.; Backx, P.H. PI3Kγ Is Required for PDE4, not PDE3, Activity in Subcellular Microdomains Containing the Sarcoplasmic Reticular Calcium ATPase in Cardiomyocytes. *Circ. Res.* **2007**, *101*, 400–408. [CrossRef] [PubMed]
47. Mattick, P.; Parrington, J.; Odia, E.; Simpson, A.; Collins, T.; Terrar, D. Ca^{2+}-stimulated adenylyl cyclase isoform AC1 is preferentially expressed in guinea-pig sino-atrial node cells and modulates the I(f) pacemaker current. *J. Physiol.* **2007**, *582*, 1195–1203. [CrossRef] [PubMed]
48. Brahmajothi, M.V.; Campbell, D.L. Heterogeneous expression of NO-activated soluble guanylyl cyclase in mammalian heart: Implications for NO- and redox-mediated indirect versus direct regulation of cardiac ion channel function. *Channels* **2007**, *1*, 353–365. [CrossRef] [PubMed]
49. Abramochkin, D.V.; Konovalova, O.P.; Kamkin, A.; Sitdikova, G.F. Carbon monoxide modulates electrical activity of murine myocardium via cGMP-dependent mechanisms. *J. Physiol. Biochem.* **2015**, *71*, 107–119. [CrossRef] [PubMed]
50. Stangherlin, A.; Gesellchen, F.; Zoccarato, A.; Terrin, A.; Fields, L.A.; Berrera, M.; Surdo, N.C.; Craig, M.A.; Smith, G.; Hamilton, G.; et al. cGMP Signals Modulate cAMP Levels in a Compartment-Specific Manner to Regulate Catecholamine-Dependent Signaling in Cardiac Myocytes. *Circ. Res.* **2011**, *108*, 929–939. [CrossRef] [PubMed]
51. Galindo-Tovar, A.; Vargas, M.L.; Kaumann, A.J. Inhibitors of phosphodiesterases PDE2, PDE3, and PDE4 do not increase the sinoatrial tachycardia of noradrenaline and prostaglandin PGE1 in mice. *Naunyn. Schmiedebergs Arch. Pharmacol.* **2016**, *389*, 177–186. [CrossRef] [PubMed]
52. Kaumann, A.J. Phosphodiesterases reduce spontaneous sinoatrial beating but not the "fight or flight" tachycardia elicited by agonists through Gs-protein-coupled receptors. *Trends Pharmacol. Sci.* **2011**, *32*, 377–383. [CrossRef] [PubMed]

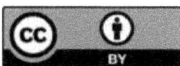

Journal of
*Cardiovascular
Development and Disease*

MDPI

Review

Roles of A-Kinase Anchoring Proteins and Phosphodiesterases in the Cardiovascular System

Maria Ercu [1] and Enno Klussmann [1,2,*]

1   Max Delbrück Center for Molecular Medicine Berlin (MDC), Berlin 13125, Germany;
    maria.ercu@mdc-berlin.de
2   DZHK (German Centre for Cardiovascular Research), partner site Berlin 13347, Germany
*   Correspondence: enno.klussmann@mdc-berlin.de; Tel.: +49-(0)30-9406-2596; Fax: +49-(0)30-9406-2593

Received: 31 January 2018; Accepted: 18 February 2018; Published: 20 February 2018

Abstract: A-kinase anchoring proteins (AKAPs) and cyclic nucleotide phosphodiesterases (PDEs) are essential enzymes in the cyclic adenosine $3'$-$5'$ monophosphate (cAMP) signaling cascade. They establish local cAMP pools by controlling the intensity, duration and compartmentalization of cyclic nucleotide-dependent signaling. Various members of the AKAP and PDE families are expressed in the cardiovascular system and direct important processes maintaining homeostatic functioning of the heart and vasculature, e.g., the endothelial barrier function and excitation-contraction coupling. Dysregulation of AKAP and PDE function is associated with pathophysiological conditions in the cardiovascular system including heart failure, hypertension and atherosclerosis. A number of diseases, including autosomal dominant hypertension with brachydactyly (HTNB) and type I long-QT syndrome (LQT1), result from mutations in genes encoding for distinct members of the two classes of enzymes. This review provides an overview over the AKAPs and PDEs relevant for cAMP compartmentalization in the heart and vasculature and discusses their pathophysiological role as well as highlights the potential benefits of targeting these proteins and their protein-protein interactions for the treatment of cardiovascular diseases.

Keywords: cAMP; compartmentalization; A-kinase anchoring proteins (AKAP); cyclic nucleotide phosphodiesterases (PDE); PDE inhibitors

1. Introduction

Cardiovascular diseases (CVD) represent the leading cause of death worldwide and hypertension is the main risk factor for such conditions [1]. Treatments targeting the causes of cardiovascular diseases such as hypertension or heart failure are rare [2].

The second messenger cyclic adenosine $3'$-$5'$ monophosphate (cAMP) is ubiquitous and functions as a signal transducer of many extracellular cues [3]. It regulates a variety of biological processes that are essential for, among others, proper cardiac function and it is involved in disease [4,5]. cAMP exerts its effects via activation of downstream effector proteins, i.e., cAMP-dependent protein kinase A (PKA), exchange proteins activated by cAMP (Epac) and cyclic nucleotide-gated ion channels (CNG), hyperpolarization-activated cyclic nucleotide-gated channels (HCN) and the recently identified Popeye domain containing (POPDC) proteins [6–8].

The plethora of extracellular signals, the limited number of intracellular cAMP effectors and the requirement of a specific biological response to each of the external signals imply a tight control of the intracellular signaling. This is achieved through signaling in defined cellular compartments. Local cAMP pools are established by the interplay of essentially four processes within the cell, namely cAMP synthesis, its diffusion, formation of multi-protein signaling complexes and cAMP degradation. In the heart, stimulation of β-adrenoceptors (β-ARs) triggers the activation the α-subunits of the stimulatory G proteins (G_s), which in turn stimulate adenylyl cyclases (ACs) to convert ATP to cAMP [9]. The formation of multi-protein signaling complexes in the cAMP signaling pathway is orchestrated by the family of A-kinase anchoring proteins (AKAPs), which act as scaffolds and engage in direct protein-protein interactions, including with PKA, and target them to defined subcellular compartments [10–15]. AKAPs play essential roles both in the heart and vascular physiology by coordinating complexes involved in the regulation of various processes including endothelial-barrier function [16,17] cardiac contraction and relaxation [18–21] and action potential duration [22,23]. AKAPs apparently play a role in several pathophysiological conditions in the cardiovascular system, e.g., in the heart their dysregulation is associated with heart failure [24,25].

Termination of cAMP signaling is predominantly achieved by hydrolysis of the phosphodiester bond within the second messenger, a reaction catalyzed by cyclic nucleotide phosphodiesterases (PDEs) [26]. Various PDE families regulate different aspects of cardiac and vascular muscle functions [27], such as the endothelial barrier function [28,29], the Ca^{2+} handling and thus contractility [30] and the basal pacemaking activity [31]. PDEs are also involved in the pathological cardiac remodeling and dysfunction [4,32–35].

The aim of this review is to provide an overview over the AKAPs and PDEs that are relevant in the compartmentalization of cAMP signaling in the cardiovascular system, to discuss their role in physiology and pathophysiology and the potential of these proteins and their protein-protein interactions as pharmacological targets in cardiovascular diseases.

2. A-kinase Anchoring Proteins (AKAPs)

AKAPs are a family of over 40 different scaffolding proteins and are key players in the spatio-temporal control of cAMP-dependent signaling by targeting PKA and additional signaling proteins including ACs, PDEs, further protein kinases and phosphatases to specific subcellular compartments [11,36–38]. PKA is the major downstream effector of cAMP. It is a serine/threonine kinase with broad specificity that controls many cellular processes, e.g., metabolism, cell growth, cell division and cardiac myocyte contraction [39]. It is a heterotetramer that consists of two catalytic subunits (Cα, Cβ or Cγ) kept in an inactive state by two regulatory RI (RIα or RIβ) or RII (RIIα or RIIβ) subunits that are organized as homodimers in the holoenzyme [40]. Upon cAMP binding to the R subunits, the C subunits are released and thus activated and subsequently phosphorylate local substrates [39]. This view was recently confirmed by quantitative mass spectrometric analyses [41]. However, PKA holoenzyme can also be active, as indicated by early biochemical experiments [42,43]. This notion was supported by recent fluorescence resonance energy transfer (FRET) imaging-based experiments, which suggested that physiological cAMP levels promote only minimal dissociation of the C subunits from the holoenzyme, thereby limiting the range of PKA action to the substrates in the immediate proximity [44]. Thus, it appears that both PKA holoenzyme and/or the dissociated C subunits can be active.

The structural feature that all AKAPs share is their ability to bind PKA via their A-kinase binding domains (AKBs), a structurally conserved amphipathic helix of 14–18 amino acids that docks into the hydrophobic groove formed by the N-terminal dimerization/docking (D/D) domains upon R subunits' dimerization (Figure 1) [45–48]. Despite the fact that most AKAPs bind to PKA-RII subunits [37,49], there are the so-called dual specific AKAPs [50] that can bind both RI and RII subunits as well as AKAPs that specifically bind RI subunits (e.g., sphingosine kinase interacting protein (SKIP) and small membrane (sm) AKAP) [51–53]. Recently, hydrophilic anchor points have been identified within and outside the amphipathic helix forming the AKB that are involved in determining the affinity of the binding between an AKAP and the D/D domain. These observations suggest that targeting the amino acids that act as anchor points could lower the binding affinity or even prevent the interaction, making them candidates for pharmacological targeting. Moreover, targeting the anchor points makes the development of selective inhibitors of specific AKAP-PKA interactions feasible [48]. Selective inhibitory agents would be valuable tools for the investigation of cellular functions of individual AKAP-PKA interactions and could be starting points for drug development efforts.

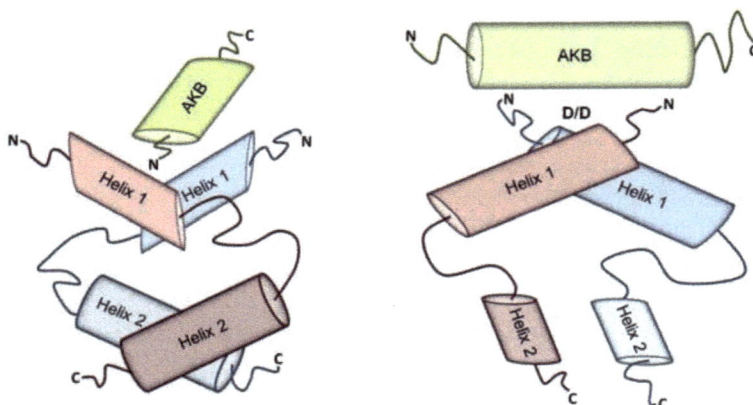

Figure 1. Schematic representation of A-kinase anchoring proteins (AKAP)-protein kinase A (PKA) interactions displayed at two different angles. The amphipathic AKB helix of AKAPs docks into the hydrophobic groove formed by the dimers of the N-terminal D/D domains of regulatory subunits of PKA. *AKB* A-kinase-binding domain; *D/D* dimerization and docking domain.

2.1. AKAP Subcellular Localization

Targeting of AKAPs to specific subcellular compartments is essential for a coordinated cAMP-dependent signaling response, including accurate PKA-catalyzed substrate phosphorylation [54]. AKAPs can be directed to various cellular compartments, including the plasma membrane (PM, e.g., AKAP18α, AKAP18β, AKAP79 [55–57]), the sarcoplasmic reticulum (SR, e.g., AKAP18δ [20]), the cytosol (e.g., SKIP, GSKIP [51,58–61]), the cytoskeleton (e.g., gravin, ezrin [62]), the mitochondria (e.g., D-AKAP1 [63]) and the nucleus (e.g., pericentrin and AKAP350 [64,65]).

2.2. AKAPs in the Cardiovascular System

Several AKAPs are expressed in the cardiovascular system (Table 1). They regulate a variety of processes and are key proteins in maintaining the homeostatic functioning of the heart and vasculature [66]. For instance, gravin and AKAP220 are involved in maintaining the vascular integrity [16,17]. Homeostasis of the vascular tone is achieved through tight control of the balance between contraction and relaxation of vascular smooth muscle cells (VSMC), processes in which AKAP79 is involved [67,68]. Ca^{2+} handling and thus cardiac myocyte contractility is regulated by several macromolecular protein complexes whose platforms are AKAPs, e.g., AKAP18α, γ and δ, mAKAPβ [19–21,69]. The AKAP Yotiao is the key player in cardiac myocyte repolarization that follows contraction [22]. Several AKAPs are involved in stress response-induced cardiac myocyte hypertrophy, including AKAP-Lbc and mAKAPβ [70,71]. AKAP79 and gravin are important for the recycling of $β_1$-ARs and $β_2$-ARs, respectively [72,73].

Table 1. Overview of AKAPs expressed in the heart and vasculature and of the cardiovascular processes that they regulate.

Common Name	Gene Name	Alternative Name	Regulated Cardiovascular Process
D-AKAP1	*AKAP1*	AKAP121/ AKAP149/AKAP84	Cardiac stress response
D-AKAP2	*AKAP10*	-	Cardiac repolarization
AKAP9 (long isoform)	*AKAP9*	-	Endothelial barrier function
AKAP18α AKAP18γ AKAP18δ	*AKAP7*	-	Excitation-contraction coupling

Table 1. *Cont.*

Common Name	Gene Name	Alternative Name	Regulated Cardiovascular Process
AKAP79	*AKAP5*	AKAP75/AKAP150	Vascular tone; Excitation-contraction coupling; β-AR desensitization/resensitization cycle
AKAP220	*AKAP11*	-	Endothelial barrier function
AKAP-Lbc	*AKAP13*	Brx-1/Proto-Lbc/ Ht31	Cardiac stress response
mAKAPβ	*AKAP6*	AKAP100	Excitation-contraction coupling; Cardiac stress response
AKAP Yotiao	*AKAP9*	GC-NAP	Cardiac repolarization
Gravin	*AKAP12*	AKAP250	Endothelial barrier function; β-AR desensitization/resensitization cycle
SKIP	*SPHKAP*	-	Cardiac stress response

2.2.1. AKAPs Regulating the Endothelial Barrier Function

The vascular endothelium lining the intima of blood vessels consists of a layer of endothelial cells tightly adherent to each other through cell-cell junctions. A healthy endothelium plays an essential role in the proper functioning of the vascular system. It regulates macromolecular permeability and anti-inflammatory, anti-thrombotic and anti-hypertrophic responses. Inflammatory conditions trigger pathological changes in the vascular system that lead to endothelial dysfunction, a state in which pathologically activated endothelial cells lose their barrier properties and initiate expression of pro-inflammatory adhesion molecules on their surface [74]. This results in increased vascular permeability allowing the infiltration of various molecules such as lipoproteins into the sub-endothelial space, and of circulating immune cells (e.g., monocytes). Ultimately, this leads to severe pathological conditions including atherosclerosis, allergy and sepsis [75,76].

AKAP-mediated PKA compartmentalization is essential for the maintenance of proper endothelial barrier function [16,17,77]. The vascular endothelium integrity is mainly dependent on tight junctions (TJs), important in sealing space between adjacent cells, and on adherens junctions, which assure direct contacts with the actin cytoskeleton of neighboring cells, thus providing mechanical strength. AKAP220 associates with PKA, β-catenin and the endothelial adherens junctions protein VE-cadherin, tethering PKA in close proximity to the cell-cell junctions [16]. Gravin (also known as AKAP12 or AKAP250) promotes vascular integrity by regulating the actin cytoskeleton via p21-activated kinase family proteins 2 (PAK2), an actin cytoskeletal regulator and afadin (AF6), a linker of the actin cytoskeleton with intercellular adhesion molecules [17]. Rac1 is a member of the Rho family of small GTPases, which upon activation strengthens the adherens junctions and the cortical actin skeleton, thereby preserving the endothelial barrier [78]. Simultaneous depletion of gravin and AKAP220 inhibited cAMP-mediated Rac1 activation, underlining the importance of these AKAPs in preventing endothelial dysfunction [16].

One other member of the AKAP family is involved in maintaining vascular integrity, the long isoform of AKAP9. Following Epac1 activation, AKAP9 contributes to microtubule growth regulation and is essential for preserving the endothelial barrier [79].

2.2.2. AKAPs Regulating the Vascular Tone

Homeostasis of the vascular tone is maintained by a tight balance between dilation and constriction of blood vessel endothelium; the main regulator is the renin-angiotensin-aldosterone system (RAAS). The main effector molecule of this system is angiotensin II (AngII), which exerts most of its effects via angiotensin type I receptors (AT_1R). For instance, arterial smooth muscle contraction is induced by AngII-dependent stimulation of AT_1R, localized at the sarcolemma, and subsequent activation of phospholipase C (PLC), which catalyzes the hydrolysis of phosphatidylinositol 4,5-bisphosphate (PIP2) to diacylglycerol (DAG) and inositol 1,4,5-trisphosphate (IP3). DAG activates protein kinase C (PKC), which in turn phosphorylates L-type Ca^{2+} ($Ca_V1.2$) channels, thereby increasing their open probability and increasing Ca^{2+} entry into the cytosol [75].

In arterial smooth muscle cells, the activity of a specific subpopulation of $Ca_V1.2$ channels is regulated by AKAP79 (AKAP5/AKAP75/AKAP150)-dependent targeting of PKCα to the sarcolemma, which facilitates phosphorylation of the channels and increases their open probablility [80]. By affecting the opening probability of specific $Ca_V1.2$ channels, the AKAP79 complex regulates the so-called "$Ca_V1.2$ sparklets", which refers to local elevations of intracellular Ca^{2+} pools that directly induce contraction of the VSMCs. The sparklets increase the vascular tone [67]. In addition, AKAP79 facilitates and most probably stabilizes the coupling of small clusters of adjacent $Ca_V1.2$ channels, which can then open synchronously and generate large $Ca_V1.2$ sparklets, thus increasing the contractile force [81,82]. Prolonged $Ca_V1.2$ channel activity and thus persistent $Ca_V1.2$ sparklets could lead to vascular dysfunction and eventually contribute to AngII-induced hypertension [80].

Transient receptor potential vanilloid 4 (TRPV4) channels are Ca^{2+} permeant channels that unlike the $Ca_V1.2$ channels, promote relaxation upon activation. Both $Ca_V1.2$- and TRPV4-mediated Ca^{2+} influxes activate adjacent ryanodine receptors (RyR), leading to release of Ca^{2+} from the SR into the cytosol in the form of Ca^{2+} sparks. While the $Ca_V1.2$-mediated Ca^{2+} influx increases contraction, the local TRPV4-generated Ca^{2+} sparks activate the large-conductance, Ca^{2+}-activated K^+ (BK) channels, which promote membrane hyperpolarization and closure of the $Ca_V1.2$ channels, ultimately resulting in relaxation [83,84]. In the arterial smooth muscle cells, AngII increased TRPV4 activity via PKC, which is tethered to the sarcolemma in close proximity of the channel by AKAP79, thus opposing the $Ca_V1.2$ channel-induced vasoconstriction [68].

In conclusion, AKAP79 plays an essential role in the control of arterial vascular tone by regulating two opposing processes, contraction and relaxation of arterial myocytes.

2.2.3. AKAPs Controlling Excitation-Contraction Coupling

The cycling of Ca^{2+} between the cytosol and the SR is at the basis of cardiac contraction and relaxation. Key players in these processes are L-type Ca^{2+} $Ca_V1.2$ channels, RyR_2, SR Ca^{2+} ATPase 2 (SERCA2) and the Na^+/Ca^{2+} exchanger. More specifically, upon sarcolemma depolarization, $Ca_V1.2$ channels located at the T tubules open allowing Ca^{2+} influx into the cardiac myocyte. This causes Ca^{2+}-induced Ca^{2+} release from the SR into the cytosol through RyR_2 located at the SR. The Ca^{2+}, upon interaction with troponin T located on the thin myofibers, promotes contraction. Relaxation occurs via SERCA2-mediated Ca^{2+} re-uptake into the SR and through Ca^{2+} transport out of the cell by Na^+/Ca^{2+} exchangers [85]. SERCA2 is activated upon the phosphorylation and subsequent dissociation of phospholamban (PLN), a SR phosphoprotein [20,86,87].

β-ARs introduce a further layer into the regulation of cardiac myocyte contractility. Their stimulation induces PKA-dependent phosphorylation of several proteins involved in Ca^{2+} handling, e.g., the $Ca_V1.2$ channels, RyR_2 and PLN. These phosphorylations are facilitated by distinct AKAPs.

AKAP18α is a membrane-associated scaffolding protein and is the smallest AKAP7 gene transcript, comprising 81 amino acids. AKAP18α promotes cardiac contractility by mediating the PKA-dependent phosphorylation of $Ca_V1.2$ channels at Serine 1928 (Ser1928) on its α subunit and at multiple sites on its β subunit, which enhances the open probability of the channel and increases the Ca^{2+} current [69,88]. The activity of a subset of $Ca_V1.2$ channels associated with caveolin-3 (Cav3) is regulated by PKA phosphorylation of the specific channel subpopulation mediated by an AKAP79 (AKAP5/AKAP75/AKAP150)-based macromolecular complex consisting of β-AR, PKA, AC5/6 and protein phosphatase calcineurin (PP2B) [89]. The muscle selective AKAP, mAKAPβ (a short version of mAKAP) associates with RyR_2 at the SR and thereby facilitates the PKA phosphorylation of the channel, leading to enhanced opening of the channel and subsequent enhanced Ca^{2+} release from the SR into the cytosol [19]. In addition, mAKAPβ interacts with the Na^+/Ca^{2+} exchanger 1 at the sarcolemma and promotes the PKA-dependent activation of the exchanger, resulting in increased Ca^{2+}

efflux [90,91]. AKAP18δ (rat heart) and AKAP18γ (human heart) facilitate the PKA phosphorylation of PLN and promote its dissociation from SERCA2 and hence activation of the ATPase, thus enhancing the re-uptake of Ca^{2+} into the SR [20,21,92].

2.2.4. AKAPs Regulating Cardiac Repolarization

The cardiac repolarization phase is initiated by the slow heart potassium current (I_{Ks}) moving outwards through the I_{Ks} potassium channel, a macromolecular complex consisting of a pore-forming α subunit (KCNQ1) and a regulatory β subunit (KCNE1) along other intracellular proteins [93]. The AKAP Yotiao, the smallest transcript of the *AKAP9* gene, is essential for cardiac repolarization since it mediates the PKA-dependent phosphorylation of KCNQ1 and therefore regulates the activity of the I_{Ks} potassium channel [22]. Mutations in the KCNQ1 subunit or Yotiao increase the duration of the action potential and lead to type I long-QT syndrome (LQT1), a channelopathy that can elicit fatal arrhythmia [94]. Another AKAP that contributes to the regulation of cardiac action potentials is the dual specific D-AKAP2 (AKAP10). A single-nucleotide polymorphism (SNP) in its PKA binding domain causes a decrease in the PR interval in the electrocardiogram, which in turn can cause arrhythmias and sudden cardiac death [54,95–97].

2.2.5. AKAPs Involved in Cardiac Stress Response

Cardiac hypertrophy is a stress-induced adaptation to maintain normal heart function [23,25]. At the cellular level, it is characterized by the upregulation of specific genes that promote the non-mitotic growth of cardiac myocytes [98]. AKAP-Lbc encodes in addition to its AKAP function for a guanine nucleotide exchange factor (GEF) that directly binds and activates the GTP-binding protein RhoA [99–102]. The interaction is involved in both cardiac development [103] and pathological cardiac myocyte hypertrophy [70]. $α_1$-AR stimulation enhances the RhoGEF activity of AKAP-Lbc, which in turn activates RhoA, contributing to a pathological increase in the hypertrophic response [70]. PKA-mediated phosphorylation at Ser1565 of AKAP-Lbc leads to the recruitment of 14-3-3 proteins, which inhibit the Rho-GEF activity of the anchoring protein [104]. Also, an AKAP-Lbc-dependent signalosome mediates the activation and cytosolic release of activated protein kinase D (PKD), which has been shown to promote cardiac hypertrophy by facilitating the nuclear export of histone deacetylase 5 (HDAC5) [105,106].

Another AKAP that plays a central role in modulating stress signal-induced hypertrophic pathways is mAKAPβ. It coordinates a variety of cAMP-responsive enzymes. This anchoring protein is targeted to the nuclear envelope of cardiac myocytes via an interaction with nesprin-1α [107]. At the SR it can integrate and transduce a variety of hypertrophic signals [71]. For instance, mAKAPβ-mediated PKA phosphorylation and subsequent activation of RyR_2 located at the nuclear envelope promotes the activation and nuclear translocation of the pro-hypertrophic transcription factor nuclear factor of activated T cells (NFAT) [108]. In addition, a mAKAPβ-based signalosome consisting of PKA, PDE4D3, Epac1, ERK5 and PP2A promotes ERK5-induced cardiomyocyte hypertrophy [71,109]. Cardiac remodeling can also be regulated by hypoxia, a process in which a mAKAP-based protein complex consisting of hypoxia-inducible factor 1α (HIF-1α), prolyl hydroxylase domain protein (PHD), the von Hippel-Lindau protein (pVHL) and the E3 ligase designated seven in absentia homolog 2 (Siah2) plays a role. More specifically, when oxygen levels are reduced, mAKAP promotes the degradation of PHD and thereby facilitates an increase in HIF-1α levels, which regulates transcription of genes that promote cell survival [110].

Other AKAPs that are thought to be involved in the cardiac stress response are D-AKAP1 and SKIP [111,112]. D-AKAP1 is a scaffolding protein of the outer mitochondrial membrane, which is protective against cardiac hypertrophy since its overexpression leads to cardiac myocyte cell size reduction and inhibition of the β-AR agonist isoproterenol-induced hypertrophy [111]. Moreover, D-AKAP1 expression maintains the mitochondrial structure and function in the heart and reduces the infarct size, cardiac remodeling and mortality under conditions of ischemia, i.e., after myocardial infarction [113].

SKIP plays an important role in the generation of the cardioprotective and anti-apoptotic lysophospholipid sphingosine-1-phosphate (S1P) produced upon myocardial ischemia-reperfusion injury [112]. It is involved in the regulation of sphingosine kinase type 1 (SPHK1), which upon activation phosphorylates sphingosine to form S1P [114].

2.2.6. AKAPs Involved in the β-ARs Desensitization/Resensitization Cycle

Upon activation, β-ARs are phosphorylated and subsequently bind β-arrestin, which prevents further ligand binding leading to receptor desensitization. The phosphorylated β-ARs are internalized and reach the early endosomes where they undergo resensitization after PP2A-mediated dephosphorylation. Upon resensitization, the non-phosphorylated receptors are recycled to the plasma membrane where they can bind further ligands. Therefore, β-AR desensitization and resensitization are essential processes in maintaining the proper functioning of the receptor [115].

Gravin and AKAP79 are important in the desensitization/resensitization cycle [72,73]. A gravin-based complex consisting of PKA, PKC, PP2B, β-arrestin and G protein-linked receptor kinase 2 (GRK2) is essential for the desensitization and resensitization of the β_2-ARs, with which it interacts at their C-terminal tail [72]. AKAP79 mediates the PKA-dependent phosphorylation of the β_1-ARs by also binding to the C terminus of the receptor, leading to their recycling and resensitization [73].

2.3. Aberrant cAMP Compartmentalization Can be Visualized

Dysregulation of local cAMP signaling is associated with cardiovascular diseases, e.g., maladaptive cardiac remodeling and heart failure [116,117]. FRET-based imaging using genetically encoded sensors (cAMP-binding and PKA activity reporters) is utilized to visualize local cAMP signaling components and real-time changes in cAMP levels with high spatio-temporal resolution [118–121]. Such sensors can be targeted to various subcellular locations including in cardiac myocytes in close proximity of sarcolemmal ion channels and SR proteins involved in Ca^{2+} handling, e.g., RyR_2 and SERCA2a [122–125]. In addition, the FRET-based reporters can be used for cAMP imaging in intact cardiac tissue as well as in ex vivo and in vivo hearts [126]. For monitoring activities of signaling molecules in their cognate microdomains, FRET approaches have also been combined with other techniques such as scanning ion-conductance microscopy (SICM), a non-optical method that allows the imaging of both cell membrane morphology and functional parameters at resolutions in the nanometer range [127–130].

3. Cyclic Nucleotide Phosphodiesterases (PDEs)

Hydrolysis by PDEs is the main route for lowering of intracellular levels of cAMP and cGMP and is essential for the spatio-temporal regulation of cyclic nucleotide-dependent signaling [26]. The PDE superfamily consists of 21 genes that give rise to more than 100 proteins due to differential transcription initiation sites and alternative splicing. PDEs are classified into 11 families (PDE1–PDE11). They differ in their primary structures, substrate specificities, mechanisms of regulation and kinetic properties [131]. Some PDE families selectively hydrolyze cAMP or cGMP, while others, the so-called dual specific PDEs, catalyze the hydrolysis of both second messengers (Figure 2) [132].

PDEs display a common general structure consisting of three components: a family-specific N-terminal regulatory domain, a conserved catalytic domain (25–52 % homology) and a C-terminal domain that can be either phosphorylated by the mitogen-activated protein kinase (MAPK) or prenylated [131,133–135]. The regulatory domains contain various structural features involved in the regulation (i.e., sites for covalent modifications, e.g., phosphorylation), binding of regulatory molecules (e.g., Ca^{2+}-binding protein calmodulin), localization (targeting domains and protein-protein interaction motifs, e.g., AKAP-binding motifs) and dimerization (e.g., GAF domains) of the enzymes [131,136,137].

The catalytic domains feature in the active site a Zn^{2+} binding motif and an additional divalent metal binding site that is most probably occupied by Mg^{2+}, but could also correspond to Mn^{2+} and Co^{2+} [138].

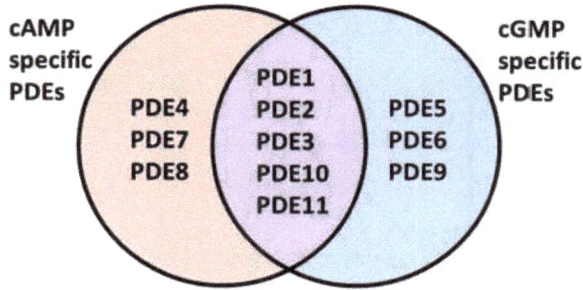

Figure 2. Substrate specificity of individual phosphodiesterase (PDE) families.

3.1. PDE Subcellular Localization

The subcellular localization of PDEs is key in achieving compartmentalized cyclic nucleotide signaling and, therefore, in the generation of specific physiological responses [136]. PDEs are located at various intracellular locations, e.g., the cytosol (e.g., PDE3A3 and PDE5 [139,140]), plasma membrane (e.g., PDE2A, PDE3A1, PDE6α, PDE6β [139,141,142]), the Golgi–centrosome (e.g., PDE7A1 [143]) and nuclear regions (e.g., PDE9A1, PDE9A16, PDE9A17 [144]).

3.2. PDEs in the Cardiovascular System

Members from most PDE families are expressed in the cardiovascular system and regulate a variety of processes essential for the proper functioning of the heart and vasculature (Table 2). The PDE families 2, 3, 4 and 5, for example, regulate the endothelial barrier function and are, therefore, of utmost importance in maintaining vascular integrity [28,145,146]. Several members of the PDE families 2, 3, 4, 5 and 8 are involved in the control of cardiac contractility [30,120,147–150]. In addition, the basal pace-making activity of the sinoatrial (SA) node of the heart is regulated by two PDE families, namely PDE3 and PDE4 [151]. In addition, various PDE family members, PDE1A, PDE3A, PDE4B, PDE4D, PDE5 and PDE9A, are implicated in the cardiac stress response, which triggers pathological cardiac remodeling and ultimately cardiac dysfunction (e.g., heart failure and arrhythmias) [34,152–156].

Table 2. Overview of the PDE families expressed in the cardiovascular system and the corresponding cardiovascular processes that they regulate.

PDE Family	PDE Gene	Substrate Specificity	Regulated Cardiovascular Process
PDE1	PDE1A PDE1B PDE1C	cAMP, cGMP	Cardiac stress response
PDE2	PDE2A	cAMP, cGMP	Endothelial barrier function; Excitation-contraction coupling
PDE3	PDE3A PDE3B	cAMP, cGMP	Endothelial barrier function; Excitation-contraction coupling; Basal pacemaking activity of the SA node; Cardiac stress response
PDE4	PDE4A PDE4B PDE4C PDE4D	cAMP	Endothelial barrier function; Excitation-contraction coupling; Basal pacemaking activity of the SA node; Cardiac stress response

Table 2. *Cont.*

PDE Family	PDE Gene	Substrate Specificity	Regulated Cardiovascular Process
PDE5	PDE5A	cGMP	Endothelial barrier function; Excitation-contraction coupling; Cardiac stress response
PDE8	PDE8A PDE8B	cAMP	Excitation-contraction coupling
PDE9	PDE9A	cGMP	Cardiac stress response

3.2.1. PDE3A and Autosomal Dominant Hypertension with Brachydactyly (HTNB)

PDE3A along with PDE3B belongs to the PDE3 family, also known as the cGMP-inhibited cAMP PDE family, which is able to hydrolyze both cAMP and cGMP in a competitive manner. PDE3A is highly expressed and plays important roles in VSMCs, cardiac myocytes, platelets and oocytes, whereas PDE3B is mainly expressed in adipose and soft tissue. Upon alternative splicing, three PDE3A isoforms are generated, namely PDE3A1 (136 kDa), PDE3A2 (118 kDa) and PDE3A3 (94 kDa) (Figure 3A). They are located in different cellular compartments. PDE3A1 is the main isoform found in human cardiac myocytes and is predominantly located at membranes. It contains two N-terminal hydrophobic regions (NHR), of which the first one consists of four transmembrane domains. PDE3A2, which lacks the first but contains the second NHR can be both membrane-associated and cytosolic and is the main variant found in VSMCs. PDE3A3 is found only in the cytosol, since it lacks both previously mentioned hydrophobic regions. All three isoforms possess the same catalytic region and present high similarities regarding their catalytic activity and inhibitor sensitivity (Figure 3A) [157,158].

Mutations in genes encoding for distinct PDE family members can have detrimental effects and cause specific human diseases. One such example is represented by the Mendelian syndrome Autosomal-dominant hypertension with brachydactyly type E (HTNB), caused by missense mutations in the gene encoding for PDE3A [159]. The syndrome is characterized by an age-dependent progressive hypertension, brachydactyly type E and blood vessel hyperplasia [159]. If untreated, blood pressure increases by 50 mm Hg and patients die from stroke before age 50 years. Surprisingly, hypertension-associated end organ damage such as cardiac hypertrophy, kidney damage or hypertensive retinopathy is low [160,161].

Eight mutations in *PDE3A* were discovered in eight unrelated families from Turkey, France, the United States, South Africa, Canada, Netherlands and Japan. All these mutations were missense, gain of function mutations and found in close proximity to each other. The identified mutations cause amino acid substitutions in a region between amino acids 445 and 449 and increases of PKA-mediated phosphorylation of serine residues 428 and 438 of PDE3A1 and PDE3A2. The region is not present in PDE3A3 (Figure 3A) [159]. The substitutions lead to increased cAMP affinity and hydrolytic activity of the enzymes (Figure 3B). In addition, the hyperactive enzyme is erroneously localized in microsomal fractions from HeLa cells, suggesting that aberrant compartmentalization is detrimental in the cardiovascular system [159,161]. VSMCs from patients expressing the hyperactive version of the enzyme with the T445N substitution display higher proliferation rates, explaining the vascular phenotype.

In the human heart, PKA-mediated phosphorylation of PDE3A1 induces its recruitment to an AKAP18-based signalosome in the heart that controls the Ca^{2+} reuptake into the SR and thereby participates in the control of cardiac relaxation [21]. An extended overview over functions of PDE3 in the heart was provided in recent reviews (e.g., [162,163]).

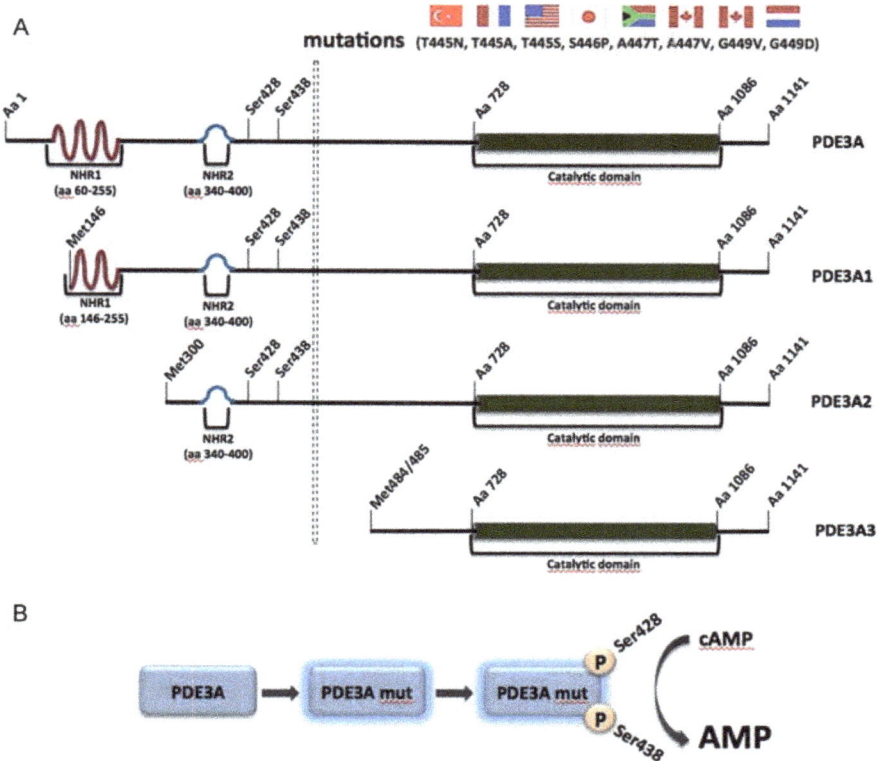

Figure 3. Schematic representation of the PDE3A gene, PDE3A protein isoforms and the hyperphosphorylation caused by the identified mutations. (**A**) Eight mutations have been identified in families from the countries indicated by the flags. The mutations cluster within a region of the gene encoding amino acids 445 and 449. The mutations cause hyperphosphorylations of Ser428 and Ser438. The N-terminal hydrophobic region (NHR) 1 of PDE3A1 comprises four transmembrane domains, while NHR2 contains no typical transmembrane region but a cluster of hydrophobic amino acids. PDE3A2 contains only NHR2 and PDE3A3 lacks all N-terminal hydrophobic regions (for details see text). (**B**) The hyperphosphorylation increases cyclic adenosine 3′-5′ monophosphate (cAMP) hydrolysis, causing low cAMP levels.

3.3. PDE Inhibitors

Due to their essential physiological and pathological roles in cyclic nucleotide signaling, PDEs are considered pharmacological targets for a variety of cardiovascular diseases, including atherosclerosis, hypertension, heart failure and intermittent claudication [26,164–166]. Several inhibitors of PDE3, 4 and 5 are approved as drugs, some of which are used for the treatment of cardiovascular diseases.

3.3.1. PDE3

The PDE3 inhibitor cilostazol is an antiplatelet agent with vasodilatory and antiproliferative properties. It has been widely studied in a number of cardiovascular diseases including coronary and peripheral artery diseases and cerebrovascular disease [167]. Cilostazol is administered for the treatment of peripheral arterial circulatory disorders and also used as an antiplatelet agent in patients that underwent carotid artery stenting [168,169]. In addition, it is also approved for the treatment of intermittent claudication-induced symptoms [170–172]. Cilostazol appears to be a promising therapeutic agent for secondary prevention of stroke and was shown to improve right ventricular systolic function as well as to decrease pulmonary artery pressure [167,173]. PDE3 inhibitors inhibit neointima formation in a rat balloon double-injury model displaying neither cytotoxicity nor effects on VSMC migration, and thus are considered targets in preventing acute re-occlusion after angioplasties, e.g., percutaneous transluminal coronary angioplasty (PTCA) [174].

Milrinone is another PDE3 inhibitor. It has inotropic and vasodilatory properties, and is widely used in patients with end-stage heart failure in order to temporarily improve cardiac contractility (positive inotropic effect) and decrease vascular resistance. Taking into account that long-term administration of milrinone can induce apoptosis of cardiac myocytes, cardiac arrhythmias, hypotension and increases cardiovascular mortality, it is only used in a selected group of patients [170,175–177]. A potential explanation for the long-term PDE3 inhibitor therapy-induced mortality could be the fact that PDE3A inhibition induces cardiac myocyte apoptosis via a PDE3A-inducible cAMP early repressor (ICER) feedback loop. More specifically, PDE3A inhibition leads to PKA activation and ICER protein stabilization, which, in turn, promotes cardiac myocyte apoptosis. Therefore, therapeutic strategies that would diminish PDE3A activity without affecting the PDE3A-ICER feedback loop could promote the beneficial effects while by-passing the side effects [152,162]. Current research aims at determining the effects of milrinone on pulmonary hypertension and right ventricular failure, where it is believed to be particularly helpful [176].

3.3.2. PDE4

The PDE4 family is encoded by four genes, *PDE4A, PDE4B, PDE4C* and *PDE4D* [178] and was shown to be involved in the excitation-contraction coupling regulation, especially in rodents. It has been recently suggested that PDE4 inhibitors could be beneficial in treating sepsis in infants with cardio-renal syndrome (CRS) since they are effective in improving cardiac function in a rat model suffering from sepsis-induced acute cardiac dysfunction and kidney injury [179]. In addition, PDE4 depletion stabilized the endothelial barrier by reducing the atrial natriuretic peptide (ANP)-induced vascular permeability and, therefore, was efficient in maintaining the plasma volume [180]. Despite the fact that PDE4A, PDE4B and PDE4D are expressed in the human and rodent heart, with PDE4D being the predominant isoform found in the human heart [181], there is no approval for a PDE4 inhibitor for the treatment of cardiovascular diseases. A highly selective PDE4 inhibitor, roflumilast, has been approved in various countries for the treatment of chronic obstructive pulmonary disease (COPD), a chronic inflammatory lung disease characterized by heavily breathing due to obstructive airflow from the lungs as well as a decline of lung function over time [182–184]. Another inhibitor, apremilast is employed for the treatment of psoriasis [185].

3.3.3. PDE5

PDE5A is the sole gene coding for the PDE5 family, which plays an essential role in the cardiovascular system. PDE5 expression is low in the healthy cardiac tissue, whereas it is upregulated in the diseased heart [155,186]. PDE5 inhibition counteracts cardiac remodeling and fibrosis of isolated cardiac fibroblasts via repression of transforming growth factor (TGF)-β1-induced Smad signaling [187]. PDE5 depletion inhibits left ventricular remodeling induced by hypertrophic and pro-fibrotic stimuli [188]. Reduction in PDE5 expression was beneficial for chronic heart failure patients by enhancing the endothelium-dependent, flow-mediated vasodilation [189]. In addition, high PDE5 expression was identified in the hypertrophic human right ventricle and its inhibition enhanced contractility, particularly important for pulmonary hypertension [186]. PDE5 inhibitors such as sildenafil, vardenafil and tadalafil are approved for the treatment of erectile dysfunction and pulmonary hypertension but are not yet approved for the treatment of other cardiovascular diseases [26]. Nevertheless, recent studies suggest potential therapeutic benefits for PDE5 inhibitors, i.e., sildenafil and tadalafil in the treatment of myocardial infarction, ischemia/reperfusion injury, endothelial dysfunction, cardiac hypertrophy and heart failure [190,191].

3.3.4. Potential for PDE1, PDE2, PDE8 and PDE9 Inhibitors

PDE1, PDE2, PDE8 and PDE9 inhibition is considered a therapeutic opportunity for the treatment of cardiovascular diseases but inhibitors are not approved.

The PDE1 family is encoded by three distinct genes, *PDE1A, PDE1B* and *PDE1C*, and is the only PDE family activated by calcium/calmodulin (Ca^{2+}/CaM) binding [192,193]. Due to their potential to dilate coronary arteries, inhibition of PDE1 enzymes may be beneficial for the treatment of coronary artery disease (CAD) and angina pectoris [194]. Nuclear PDE1A is important for the proliferation of VSMCs and, therefore, could contribute to neointima formation in diseases, e.g., atherosclerosis and restenosis [195]. Thus, diminishing its expression could decrease pathological neointima development. In addition, inhibition of the PDE1 family might improve cardiopathy and pulmonary arterial hypertension since it decreases the structural remodeling process underlying these two conditions [196].

PDE2A is the only gene coding for the PDE2 family and plays a central role in the cardiac $Ca_V1.2$ current regulation. The expression is up-regulated in human failing hearts [197,198]. Inhibition of PDE2 had a positive inotropic effect in dogs and mice, whereas its overexpression decreased the heart rate in mice. Interestingly, in a heart-specific PDE2-transgenic mouse model, increased PDE2 abundance prevents ventricular arrhythmias by inhibiting Ca^{2+} leak from the SR and helps in maintaining the contractile function of the heart after myocardial infarction [199]. On the contrary, a recent study in patients that had experienced an acute myocardial infarction (AMI) suggests that inhibition of endothelial PDE2A could have a beneficial effect and improve the clinical outcome. Hypoxia and pro-inflammatory cytokines such as tumor necrosis factor-α (TNF-α) promote PDE2A activation, which results in diminished submembrane cAMP levels and endothelial barrier disruption. This facilitates the extravasation of activated neutrophils and leads to inflammation in the early post-myocardial infarction phase [29].

The PDE8 family comprises two members, PDE8A and PDE8B and regulates excitation-contraction coupling in ventricular myocytes. More specifically, it has been suggested that PDE8A controls at least one cAMP pool involved in the cardiac myocyte-dependent Ca^{2+} cycling regulation. It was also observed that PDE8A deletion caused both increased RyR_2 leak as well as enhanced Ca^{2+} refilling of the SR [150].

The PDE9 family is encoded by a single gene, *PDE9A*, and consists of more than 20 different splice variants. PDE9A expression was identified in human and rodent hearts, where its expression increased upon hypertrophy and heart failure development [156,200]. PDE9A depletion had a protective effect for the heart against pathological remodeling caused by pressure overload and it reversed a previously established heart disease without requiring the activity of NO synthase [156].

4. Concluding Remarks

Compartmentalized cyclic nucleotide signaling is found at the basis of precision of cellular signaling and its dysregulation is associated with various pathological conditions including several cardiovascular diseases. Local pools of cAMP are established by the interplay of cAMP synthesis, diffusion, degradation as well as positioning of the relevant signaling proteins. AKAPs and PDEs are essential players in these processes since they orchestrate the formation of multi-protein signaling complexes and terminate local cAMP signaling, respectively. This interplay ensures the spatio-temporal regulation of cyclic nucleotide-dependent signaling. Despite the fact that both molecules are key elements in the cAMP signaling pathway, very little is known with respect to their direct interaction or their interplay in the cardiovascular system. However, a few PDE-containing AKAP complexes have been identified; examples are the SERCA2/AKAP18 signalosome, which incorporates PDE3A1 upon its phosphorylation and is important for cardiac contractility, and the

PDE4D3 containing mAKAPβ-based signalosome involved in cardiomyocyte hypertrophy regulation ([21,71,109]). Alterations in AKAP expression and their protein-protein interactions are associated with various cardiovascular diseases [12,24]. Hence the development of pharmacological agents targeting such dysregulated signaling components for evaluating their relevance as pharmacological targets is needed. First examples show that targeting AKAPs and their protein-protein interactions with small molecules is possible. For instance, an AKAP-PKA interaction inhibitor, FMP-API-1 [201] was identified. Recently, a novel small molecule, Scaff10-8, was developed, which inhibits the interaction of AKAP-Lbc and RhoA and prevents the AKAP-Lbc-mediated RhoA activation, an event pathologically activated in models of cardiac hypertrophy [102]. Further molecules directed against the AKAP-Lbc-RhoA interface have recently been identified and may serve to guide to further preclinical drug development efforts [202,203].

Approved inhibitors of PDEs target the catalytic activities of PDEs. However, the catalytic domains of the various members of individual families are identical and inhibition of one inhibits all. This lack of selectivity presumably explains PDE inhibitor therapy-associated side effects, which are frequent and dramatic over long-term administration [158]. PDE isoform-selective inhibition may be achieved through disruption of specific protein-protein interactions. and therefore the displacement of particular PDE isoforms from their subcellular compartments [204].

In conclusion, targeting proteins directing compartmentalized cAMP signaling, in particular AKAPs and PDEs, not only serves to understanding their role in heart and vascular physiology and pathophysiology but also has therapeutic potential for the treatment of a wide range of cardiovascular diseases.

Acknowledgments: This work was supported by grants from the Else Kröner-Fresenius-Stiftung (2013_A145), the German-Israeli Foundation (G.I.F. I-1210-286.13/2012), the German Centre for Cardiovascular Research (DZHK 81X210012 and B18-005 SE), the Deutsche Forschungsgemeinschaft (DFG KL1415/7-1) and the Bundesministerium für Bildung und Forschung (BMBF; 16GW0179K) to EK.

Conflicts of Interest: The authors declare no conflict of interest.

References

1. Lawes, C.M.; Vander Hoorn, S.; Rodgers, A.; Hypertension, I.S.o. Global burden of blood-pressure-related disease, 2001. *Lancet* **2008**, *371*, 1513–1518. [CrossRef]
2. Bolívar, J.J. Essential hypertension: An approach to its etiology and neurogenic pathophysiology. *Int. J. Hypertens.* **2013**, *2013*, 547809. [CrossRef] [PubMed]
3. Beavo, J.A.; Brunton, L.L. Cyclic nucleotide research—Still expanding after half a century. *Nat. Rev. Mol. Cell Biol.* **2002**, *3*, 710–718. [CrossRef] [PubMed]
4. Fischmeister, R.; Castro, L.R.; Abi-Gerges, A.; Rochais, F.; Jurevicius, J.; Leroy, J.; Vandecasteele, G. Compartmentation of cyclic nucleotide signaling in the heart: The role of cyclic nucleotide phosphodiesterases. *Circ. Res.* **2006**, *99*, 816–828. [CrossRef] [PubMed]
5. Perera, R.K.; Nikolaev, V.O. Compartmentation of cAMP signalling in cardiomyocytes in health and disease. *Acta Physiol (Oxf)* **2013**, *207*, 650–662. [CrossRef] [PubMed]
6. Lorenz, R.; Bertinetti, D.; Herberg, F.W. cAMP-dependent protein kinase and cGMP-dependent protein kinase as cyclic nucleotide effectors. *Handb. Exp. Pharmacol.* **2017**, *238*, 105–122. [PubMed]
7. Lezoualc'h, F.; Fazal, L.; Laudette, M.; Conte, C. Cyclic AMP sensor epac proteins and their role in cardiovascular function and disease. *Circ. Res.* **2016**, *118*, 881–897. [CrossRef] [PubMed]
8. Brand, T.; Schindler, R. New kids on the block: The popeye domain containing (popdc) protein family acting as a novel class of cAMP effector proteins in striated muscle. *Cell Signal.* **2017**, *40*, 156–165. [CrossRef] [PubMed]
9. Pierce, K.L.; Premont, R.T.; Lefkowitz, R.J. Seven-transmembrane receptors. *Nat. Rev. Mol. Cell Biol.* **2002**, *3*, 639–650. [CrossRef] [PubMed]
10. Szaszák, M.; Christian, F.; Rosenthal, W.; Klussmann, E. Compartmentalized cAMP signalling in regulated exocytic processes in non-neuronal cells. *Cell Signal.* **2008**, *20*, 590–601. [CrossRef] [PubMed]

11. Skroblin, P.; Grossmann, S.; Schafer, G.; Rosenthal, W.; Klussmann, E. Mechanisms of protein kinase A anchoring. *Int Rev. Cell Mol. Biol* **2010**, *283*, 235–330. [PubMed]
12. Dema, A.; Perets, E.; Schulz, M.S.; Deák, V.A.; Klussmann, E. Pharmacological targeting of AKAP-directed compartmentalized cAMP signalling. *Cell Signal.* **2015**, *27*, 2474–2487. [CrossRef] [PubMed]
13. Pidoux, G.; Taskén, K. Specificity and spatial dynamics of protein kinase A signaling organized by A-kinase-anchoring proteins. *J. Mol. Endocrinol.* **2010**, *44*, 271–284. [CrossRef] [PubMed]
14. Scott, J.D.; Dessauer, C.W.; Taskén, K. Creating order from chaos: Cellular regulation by kinase anchoring. *Annu Rev. Pharmacol Toxicol* **2013**, *53*, 187–210. [CrossRef] [PubMed]
15. Nikolaev, V.O.; Zaccolo, M. *Microdomains in the Cardiovascular System*; Springer International Publishing: Cham, Switzerland, 2017.
16. Radeva, M.Y.; Kugelmann, D.; Spindler, V.; Waschke, J. PKA compartmentalization via AKAP220 and AKAP12 contributes to endothelial barrier regulation. *PLoS One* **2014**, *9*, e106733. [CrossRef] [PubMed]
17. Kwon, H.B.; Choi, Y.K.; Lim, J.J.; Kwon, S.H.; Her, S.; Kim, H.J.; Lim, K.J.; Ahn, J.C.; Kim, Y.M.; Bae, M.K.; et al. AKAP12 regulates vascular integrity in zebrafish. *Exp. Mol. Med.* **2012**, *44*, 225–235. [CrossRef] [PubMed]
18. Gray, P.C.; Johnson, B.D.; Westenbroek, R.E.; Hays, L.G.; Yates, J.R.; Scheuer, T.; Catterall, W.A.; Murphy, B.J. Primary structure and function of an A kinase anchoring protein associated with calcium channels. *Neuron* **1998**, *20*, 1017–1026. [CrossRef]
19. Marx, S.O.; Reiken, S.; Hisamatsu, Y.; Jayaraman, T.; Burkhoff, D.; Rosemblit, N.; Marks, A.R. Pka phosphorylation dissociates fkbp12.6 from the calcium release channel (ryanodine receptor): Defective regulation in failing hearts. *Cell* **2000**, *101*, 365–376. [CrossRef]
20. Lygren, B.; Carlson, C.R.; Santamaria, K.; Lissandron, V.; McSorley, T.; Litzenberg, J.; Lorenz, D.; Wiesner, B.; Rosenthal, W.; Zaccolo, M.; et al. AKAP complex regulates Ca^{2+} re-uptake into heart sarcoplasmic reticulum. *EMBO Rep.* **2007**, *8*, 1061–1067. [CrossRef] [PubMed]
21. Ahmad, F.; Shen, W.; Vandeput, F.; Szabo-Fresnais, N.; Krall, J.; Degerman, E.; Goetz, F.; Klussmann, E.; Movsesian, M.; Manganiello, V. Regulation of sarcoplasmic reticulum Ca^{2+} atpase 2 (serca2) activity by phosphodiesterase 3a (pde3a) in human myocardium: Phosphorylation-dependent interaction of pde3a1 with serca2. *J. Biol. Chem.* **2015**, *290*, 6763–6776. [CrossRef] [PubMed]
22. Marx, S.O.; Kurokawa, J.; Reiken, S.; Motoike, H.; D'Armiento, J.; Marks, A.R; Kass, R.S. Requirement of a macromolecular signaling complex for beta adrenergic receptor modulation of the kcnq1-kcne1 potassium channel. *Science* **2002**, *295*, 496–499. [CrossRef] [PubMed]
23. Frey, N.; Katus, H.A.; Olson, E.N.; Hill, J.A. Hypertrophy of the heart: A new therapeutic target? *Circulation* **2004**, *109*, 1580–1589. [CrossRef] [PubMed]
24. Deák, V.A.; Klussmann, E. Pharmacological interference with protein-protein interactions of akinase anchoring proteins as a strategy for the treatment of disease. *Curr. Drug Targets* **2016**, *17*, 1147–1171. [CrossRef] [PubMed]
25. Diviani, D.; Reggi, E.; Arambasic, M.; Caso, S.; Maric, D. Emerging roles of A-kinase anchoring proteins in cardiovascular pathophysiology. *Biochim. Biophys. Acta* **2016**, *1863*, 1926–1936. [CrossRef] [PubMed]
26. Maurice, D.H.; Ke, H.; Ahmad, F.; Wang, Y.; Chung, J.; Manganiello, V.C. Advances in targeting cyclic nucleotide phosphodiesterases. *Nat. Rev. Drug Discov.* **2014**, *13*, 290–314. [CrossRef] [PubMed]
27. Kim, G.E.; Kass, D.A. Cardiac phosphodiesterases and their modulation for treating heart disease. *Handb. Exp. Pharmacol.* **2017**, *243*, 249–269. [PubMed]
28. Surapisitchat, J.; Jeon, K.I.; Yan, C.; Beavo, J.A. Differential regulation of endothelial cell permeability by cgmp via phosphodiesterases 2 and 3. *Circ. Res.* **2007**, *101*, 811–818. [CrossRef] [PubMed]
29. Chen, W.; Spitzl, A.; Mathes, D.; Nikolaev, V.O.; Werner, F.; Weirather, J.; Špiranec, K.; Röck, K.; Fischer, J.W.; Kämmerer, U.; et al. Endothelial actions of anp enhance myocardial inflammatory infiltration in the early phase after acute infarction. *Circ. Res.* **2016**, *119*, 237–248. [CrossRef] [PubMed]
30. Yan, C.; Miller, C.L.; Abe, J. Regulation of phosphodiesterase 3 and inducible cAMP early repressor in the heart. *Circ. Res.* **2007**, *100*, 489–501. [CrossRef] [PubMed]
31. Galindo-Tovar, A.; Vargas, M.L.; Kaumann, A.J. Phosphodiesterases PDE3 and PDE4 jointly control the inotropic effects but not chronotropic effects of (-)-cgp12177 despite PDE4-evoked sinoatrial bradycardia in rat atrium. *Naunyn-Schmiedeberg's Arch. Pharmacol.* **2009**, *379*, 379–384. [CrossRef] [PubMed]

32. Ding, B.; Abe, J.I.; Wei, H.; Huang, Q.; Walsh, R.A.; Molina, C.A.; Zhao, A.; Sadoshima, J.; Blaxall, B.C.; Berk, B.C.; et al. Functional role of phosphodiesterase 3 in cardiomyocyte apoptosis: Implication in heart failure. *Circulation* **2005**, *111*, 2469–2476. [CrossRef] [PubMed]

33. Abi-Gerges, A.; Richter, W.; Lefebvre, F.; Mateo, P.; Varin, A.; Heymes, C.; Samuel, J.L.; Lugnier, C.; Conti, M.; Fischmeister, R.; et al. Decreased expression and activity of cAMP phosphodiesterases in cardiac hypertrophy and its impact on beta-adrenergic cAMP signals. *Circ. Res.* **2009**, *105*, 784–792. [CrossRef] [PubMed]

34. Miller, C.L.; Oikawa, M.; Cai, Y.; Wojtovich, A.P.; Nagel, D.J.; Xu, X.; Xu, H.; Florio, V.; Rybalkin, S.D.; Beavo, J.A.; et al. Role of Ca^{2+}/calmodulin-stimulated cyclic nucleotide phosphodiesterase 1 in mediating cardiomyocyte hypertrophy. *Circ. Res.* **2009**, *105*, 956–964. [CrossRef] [PubMed]

35. Bobin, P.; Belacel-Ouari, M.; Bedioune, I.; Zhang, L.; Leroy, J.; Leblais, V.; Fischmeister, R.; Vandecasteele, G. Cyclic nucleotide phosphodiesterases in heart and vessels: A therapeutic perspective. *Arch. Cardiovasc. Dis.* **2016**, *109*, 431–443. [CrossRef] [PubMed]

36. Rababa'h, A.; Singh, S.; Suryavanshi, S.V.; Altarabsheh, S.E.; Deo, S.V.; McConnell, B.K. Compartmentalization role of A-kinase anchoring proteins (AKAPs) in mediating protein kinase A (PKA) signaling and cardiomyocyte hypertrophy. *Int. J. Mol. Sci.* **2014**, *16*, 218–229. [CrossRef] [PubMed]

37. Welch, E.J.; Jones, B.W.; Scott, J.D. Networking with AKAPs: Context-dependent regulation of anchored enzymes. *Mol. Interv.* **2010**, *10*, 86–97. [CrossRef] [PubMed]

38. Langeberg, L.K.; Scott, J.D. Signalling scaffolds and local organization of cellular behaviour. *Nat. Rev. Mol. Cell Biol.* **2015**, *16*, 232–244. [CrossRef] [PubMed]

39. Francis, S.H.; Corbin, J.D. Structure and function of cyclic nucleotide-dependent protein kinases. *Annu. Rev. Physiol.* **1994**, *56*, 237–272. [CrossRef] [PubMed]

40. Taylor, S.S.; Ilouz, R.; Zhang, P.; Kornev, A.P. Assembly of allosteric macromolecular switches: Lessons from PKA. *Nat. Rev. Mol. Cell Biol.* **2012**, *13*, 646–658. [CrossRef] [PubMed]

41. Walker-Gray, R.; Stengel, F.; Gold, M.G. Mechanisms for restraining cAMP-dependent protein kinase revealed by subunit quantitation and cross-linking approaches. *Proc. Natl. Acad. Sci. USA* **2017**, *114*, 10414–10419. [CrossRef] [PubMed]

42. Yang, S.; Fletcher, W.H.; Johnson, D.A. Regulation of cAMP-dependent protein kinase: Enzyme activation without dissociation. *Biochemistry* **1995**, *34*, 6267–6271. [CrossRef] [PubMed]

43. Kopperud, R.; Christensen, A.E.; Kjarland, E.; Viste, K.; Kleivdal, H.; Doskeland, S.O. Formation of inactive cAMP-saturated holoenzyme of cAMP-dependent protein kinase under physiological conditions. *J. Biol. Chem.* **2002**, *277*, 13443–13448. [CrossRef] [PubMed]

44. Smith, F.D.; Esseltine, J.L.; Nygren, P.J.; Veesler, D.; Byrne, D.P.; Vonderach, M.; Strashnov, I.; Eyers, C.E.; Eyers, P.A.; Langeberg, L.K.; et al. Local protein kinase A action proceeds through intact holoenzymes. *Science* **2017**, *356*, 1288–1293. [CrossRef] [PubMed]

45. Ruehr, M.L.; Zakhary, D.R.; Damron, D.S.; Bond, M. Cyclic amp-dependent protein kinase binding to A-kinase anchoring proteins in living cells by fluorescence resonance energy transfer of green fluorescent protein fusion proteins. *J. Biol. Chem.* **1999**, *274*, 33092–33096. [CrossRef] [PubMed]

46. Gold, M.G.; Lygren, B.; Dokurno, P.; Hoshi, N.; McConnachie, G.; Tasken, K.; Carlson, C.R.; Scott, J.D.; Barford, D. Molecular basis of akap specificity for PKA regulatory subunits. *Mol. Cell* **2006**, *24*, 383–395. [CrossRef] [PubMed]

47. Kinderman, F.S.; Kim, C.; von Daake, S.; Ma, Y.; Pham, B.Q.; Spraggon, G.; Xuong, N.H.; Jennings, P.A.; Taylor, S.S. A dynamic mechanism for akap binding to rii isoforms of cAMP-dependent protein kinase. *Mol. Cell* **2006**, *24*, 397–408. [CrossRef] [PubMed]

48. Götz, F.; Roske, Y.; Schulz, M.S.; Autenrieth, K.; Bertinetti, D.; Faelber, K.; Zühlke, K.; Kreuchwig, A.; Kennedy, E.J.; Krause, G.; et al. AKAP18:Pka-riiα structure reveals crucial anchor points for recognition of regulatory subunits of PKA. *Biochem. J.* **2016**, *473*, 1881–1894. [CrossRef] [PubMed]

49. McSorley, T.; Stefan, E.; Henn, V.; Wiesner, B.; Baillie, G.S.; Houslay, M.D.; Rosenthal, W.; Klussmann, E. Spatial organisation of AKAP18 and PDE4 isoforms in renal collecting duct principal cells. *Eur. J. Cell. Biol.* **2006**, *85*, 673–678. [CrossRef] [PubMed]

50. Huang, L.J.; Durick, K.; Weiner, J.A.; Chun, J.; Taylor, S.S. Identification of a novel protein kinase A anchoring protein that binds both type i and type ii regulatory subunits. *J. Biol. Chem.* **1997**, *272*, 8057–8064. [CrossRef] [PubMed]

51. Kovanich, D.; van der Heyden, M.A.; Aye, T.T.; van Veen, T.A.; Heck, A.J.; Scholten, A. Sphingosine kinase interacting protein is an A-kinase anchoring protein specific for type i cAMP-dependent protein kinase. *Chembiochem* **2010**, *11*, 963–971. [CrossRef] [PubMed]

52. Means, C.K.; Lygren, B.; Langeberg, L.K.; Jain, A.; Dixon, R.E.; Vega, A.L.; Gold, M.G.; Petrosyan, S.; Taylor, S.S.; Murphy, A.N.; et al. An entirely specific type i a-kinase anchoring protein that can sequester two molecules of protein kinase A at mitochondria. *Proc. Natl. Acad. Sci. USA* **2011**, *108*, E1227–E1235. [CrossRef] [PubMed]

53. Burgers, P.P.; Ma, Y.; Margarucci, L.; Mackey, M.; van der Heyden, M.A.; Ellisman, M.; Scholten, A.; Taylor, S.S.; Heck, A.J. A small novel A-kinase anchoring protein (AKAP) that localizes specifically protein kinase A-regulatory subunit i (PKA-ri) to the plasma membrane. *J. Biol. Chem.* **2012**, *287*, 43789–43797. [CrossRef] [PubMed]

54. Tröger, J.; Moutty, M.C.; Skroblin, P.; Klussmann, E. A-kinase anchoring proteins as potential drug targets. *Br. J. Pharmacol.* **2012**, *166*, 420–433. [CrossRef] [PubMed]

55. Fraser, I.D.; Tavalin, S.J.; Lester, L.B.; Langeberg, L.K.; Westphal, A.M.; Dean, R.A.; Marrion, N.V.; Scott, J.D. A novel lipid-anchored A-kinase anchoring protein facilitates cAMP-responsive membrane events. *EMBO J.* **1998**, *17*, 2261–2272. [CrossRef] [PubMed]

56. Trotter, K.W.; Fraser, I.D.; Scott, G.K.; Stutts, M.J.; Scott, J.D.; Milgram, S.L. Alternative splicing regulates the subcellular localization of A-kinase anchoring protein 18 isoforms. *J. Cell Biol.* **1999**, *147*, 1481–1492. [CrossRef] [PubMed]

57. Dell'Acqua, M.L.; Faux, M.C.; Thorburn, J.; Thorburn, A.; Scott, J.D. Membrane-targeting sequences on AKAP79 bind phosphatidylinositol-4,5-bisphosphate. *EMBO J.* **1998**, *17*, 2246–2260. [CrossRef] [PubMed]

58. Hundsrucker, C.; Skroblin, P.; Christian, F.; Zenn, H.M.; Popara, V.; Joshi, M.; Eichhorst, J.; Wiesner, B.; Herberg, F.W.; Reif, B.; et al. Glycogen synthase kinase 3β interaction protein functions as an A-kinase anchoring protein. *J. Biol. Chem.* **2010**, *285*, 5507–5521. [CrossRef] [PubMed]

59. Deák, V.A.; Skroblin, P.; Dittmayer, C.; Knobeloch, K.P.; Bachmann, S.; Klussmann, E. The A-kinase anchoring protein gskip regulates gsk3β activity and controls palatal shelf fusion in mice. *J. Biol. Chem.* **2016**, *291*, 681–690. [CrossRef] [PubMed]

60. Dema, A.; Schröter, M.F.; Perets, E.; Skroblin, P.; Moutty, M.C.; Deák, V.A.; Birchmeier, W.; Klussmann, E. The A-kinase anchoring protein (AKAP) glycogen synthase kinase 3β interaction protein (gskip) regulates β-catenin through its interactions with both protein kinase a (PKA) and gsk3β. *J. Biol. Chem.* **2016**, *291*, 19618–19630. [CrossRef] [PubMed]

61. Scholten, A.; Poh, M.K.; van Veen, T.A.; van Breukelen, B.; Vos, M.A.; Heck, A.J. Analysis of the cGMP/cAMP interactome using a chemical proteomics approach in mammalian heart tissue validates sphingosine kinase type 1-interacting protein as a genuine and highly abundant AKAP. *J. Proteom. Res.* **2006**, *5*, 1435–1447. [CrossRef] [PubMed]

62. Taskén, K.; Aandahl, E.M. Localized effects of cAMP mediated by distinct routes of protein kinase a. *Physiol. Rev.* **2004**, *84*, 137–167. [CrossRef] [PubMed]

63. Huang, L.J.; Wang, L.; Ma, Y.; Durick, K.; Perkins, G.; Deerinck, T.J.; Ellisman, M.H.; Taylor, S.S. Nh2-terminal targeting motifs direct dual specificity A-kinase-anchoring protein 1 (d-AKAP1) to either mitochondria or endoplasmic reticulum. *J. Cell. Biol* **1999**, *145*, 951–959. [CrossRef] [PubMed]

64. Diviani, D.; Langeberg, L.K.; Doxsey, S.J.; Scott, J.D. Pericentrin anchors protein kinase a at the centrosome through a newly identified rii-binding domain. *Curr. Biol.* **2000**, *10*, 417–420. [CrossRef]

65. Gillingham, A.K.; Munro, S. The pact domain, a conserved centrosomal targeting motif in the coiled-coil proteins AKAP450 and pericentrin. *EMBO Rep.* **2000**, *1*, 524–529. [CrossRef] [PubMed]

66. Scott, J.D.; Santana, L.F. A-kinase anchoring proteins: Getting to the heart of the matter. *Circulation* **2010**, *121*, 1264–1271. [CrossRef] [PubMed]

67. Navedo, M.F.; Santana, L.F. Cav1.2 sparklets in heart and vascular smooth muscle. *J. Mol. Cell. Cardiol.* **2013**, *58*, 67–76. [CrossRef] [PubMed]

68. Mercado, J.; Baylie, R.; Navedo, M.F.; Yuan, C.; Scott, J.D.; Nelson, M.T.; Brayden, J.E.; Santana, L.F. Local control of trpv4 channels by AKAP150-targeted PKC in arterial smooth muscle. *J. Gen. Physiol.* **2014**, *143*, 559–575. [CrossRef] [PubMed]

69. Hulme, J.T.; Westenbroek, R.E.; Scheuer, T.; Catterall, W.A. Phosphorylation of serine 1928 in the distal C-terminal domain of cardiac cav1.2 channels during β1-adrenergic regulation. *Proc. Natl. Acad. Sci. USA* **2006**, *103*, 16574–16579. [CrossRef] [PubMed]

70. Appert-Collin, A.; Cotecchia, S.; Nenniger-Tosato, M.; Pedrazzini, T.; Diviani, D. The A-kinase anchoring protein (AKAP)-lbc-signaling complex mediates alpha1 adrenergic receptor-induced cardiomyocyte hypertrophy. *Proc. Natl Acad Sci USA* **2007**, *104*, 10140–10145. [CrossRef] [PubMed]

71. Dodge-Kafka, K.L.; Soughayer, J.; Pare, G.C.; Carlisle Michel, J.J.; Langeberg, L.K.; Kapiloff, M.S.; Scott, J.D. The protein kinase a anchoring protein mAKAP coordinates two integrated cAMP effector pathways. *Nature* **2005**, *437*, 574–578. [CrossRef] [PubMed]

72. Fan, G.; Shumay, E.; Wang, H.; Malbon, C.C. The scaffold protein gravin (cAMP-dependent protein kinase-anchoring protein 250) binds the β2-adrenergic receptor via the receptor cytoplasmic Arg-329 to Leu-413 domain and provides a mobile scaffold during desensitization. *J. Biol. Chem.* **2001**, *276*, 24005–24014. [CrossRef] [PubMed]

73. Gardner, L.A.; Tavalin, S.J.; Goehring, A.S.; Scott, J.D.; Bahouth, S.W. AKAP79-mediated targeting of the cyclic AMP-dependent protein kinase to the β1-adrenergic receptor promotes recycling and functional resensitization of the receptor. *J. Biol. Chem.* **2006**, *281*, 33537–33553. [CrossRef] [PubMed]

74. Chiu, J.J.; Chien, S. Effects of disturbed flow on vascular endothelium: Pathophysiological basis and clinical perspectives. *Physiol. Rev.* **2011**, *91*, 327–387. [CrossRef] [PubMed]

75. Mehta, D.; Malik, A.B. Signaling mechanisms regulating endothelial permeability. *Physiol. Rev.* **2006**, *86*, 279–367. [CrossRef] [PubMed]

76. Cinel, I.; Dellinger, R.P. Advances in pathogenesis and management of sepsis. *Curr. Opin. Infect. Dis.* **2007**, *20*, 345–352. [CrossRef] [PubMed]

77. Choi, Y.K.; Kim, J.H.; Kim, W.J.; Lee, H.Y.; Park, J.A.; Lee, S.W.; Yoon, D.K.; Kim, H.H.; Chung, H.; Yu, Y.S.; et al. AKAP12 regulates human blood-retinal barrier formation by downregulation of hypoxia-inducible factor-1α. *J. Neurosci.* **2007**, *27*, 4472–4481. [CrossRef] [PubMed]

78. Schlegel, N.; Waschke, J. cAMP with other signaling cues converges on rac1 to stabilize the endothelial barrier—A signaling pathway compromised in inflammation. *Cell Tissue Res.* **2014**, *355*, 587–596. [CrossRef] [PubMed]

79. Sehrawat, S.; Ernandez, T.; Cullere, X.; Takahashi, M.; Ono, Y.; Komarova, Y.; Mayadas, T.N. AKAP9 regulation of microtubule dynamics promotes epac1-induced endothelial barrier properties. *Blood* **2011**, *117*, 708–718. [CrossRef] [PubMed]

80. Navedo, M.F.; Nieves-Cintron, M.; Amberg, G.C.; Yuan, C.; Votaw, V.S.; Lederer, W.J.; McKnight, G.S.; Santana, L.F. AKAP150 is required for stuttering persistent Ca^{2+} sparklets and angiotensin ii-induced hypertension. *Circ. Res.* **2008**, *102*, e1–e11. [CrossRef] [PubMed]

81. Navedo, M.F.; Cheng, E.P.; Yuan, C.; Votaw, S.; Molkentin, J.D.; Scott, J.D.; Santana, L.F. Increased coupled gating of l-type Ca^{2+} channels during hypertension and timothy syndrome. *Circ. Res.* **2010**, *106*, 748–756. [CrossRef] [PubMed]

82. Dixon, R.E.; Cheng, E.P.; Mercado, J.L.; Santana, L.F. L-type Ca^{2+} channel function during timothy syndrome. *Trends Cardiovasc. Med.* **2012**, *22*, 72–76. [CrossRef] [PubMed]

83. Earley, S.; Heppner, T.J.; Nelson, M.T.; Brayden, J.E. Trpv4 forms a novel Ca^{2+} signaling complex with ryanodine receptors and bkca channels. *Circ. Res.* **2005**, *97*, 1270–1279. [CrossRef] [PubMed]

84. Earley, S.; Pauyo, T.; Drapp, R.; Tavares, M.J.; Liedtke, W.; Brayden, J.E. Trpv4-dependent dilation of peripheral resistance arteries influences arterial pressure. *Am. J. Physiol. Heart Circ. Physiol.* **2009**, *297*, H1096–H1102. [CrossRef] [PubMed]

85. Bers, D.M. Cardiac excitation-contraction coupling. *Nature* **2002**, *415*, 198–205. [CrossRef] [PubMed]

86. Szentesi, P.; Pignier, C.; Egger, M.; Kranias, E.G.; Niggli, E. Sarcoplasmic reticulum Ca^{2+} refilling controls recovery from Ca^{2+}-induced Ca^{2+} release refractoriness in heart muscle. *Circ. Res.* **2004**, *95*, 807–813. [CrossRef] [PubMed]

87. Kranias, E.G.; Hajjar, R.J. Modulation of cardiac contractility by the phospholamban/serca2a regulatome. *Circ. Res.* **2012**, *110*, 1646–1660. [CrossRef] [PubMed]

88. Bünemann, M.; Gerhardstein, B.L.; Gao, T.; Hosey, M.M. Functional regulation of l-type calcium channels via protein kinase A-mediated phosphorylation of the β2 subunit. *J. Biol. Chem.* **1999**, *274*, 33851–33854. [CrossRef] [PubMed]

89. Nichols, C.B.; Rossow, C.F.; Navedo, M.F.; Westenbroek, R.E.; Catterall, W.A.; Santana, L.F.; McKnight, G.S. Sympathetic stimulation of adult cardiomyocytes requires association of AKAP5 with a subpopulation of l-type calcium channels. *Circ. Res.* **2010**, *107*, 747–756. [CrossRef] [PubMed]

90. Schulze, D.H.; Muqhal, M.; Lederer, W.J.; Ruknudin, A.M. Sodium/calcium exchanger (ncx1) macromolecular complex. *J. Biol. Chem.* **2003**, *278*, 28849–28855. [CrossRef] [PubMed]

91. Ruknudin, A.; He, S.; Lederer, W.J.; Schulze, D.H. Functional differences between cardiac and renal isoforms of the rat Na$^+$-Ca^{2+} exchanger ncx1 expressed in xenopus oocytes. *J. Physiol.* **2000**, *529*, 599–610. [CrossRef] [PubMed]

92. Johnson, K.R.; Nicodemus-Johnson, J.; Carnegie, G.K.; Danziger, R.S. Molecular evolution of A-kinase anchoring protein (AKAP)-7: Implications in comparative PKA compartmentalization. *BMC Evol. Biol.* **2012**, *12*, 125. [CrossRef] [PubMed]

93. Nerbonne, J.M.; Kass, R.S. Molecular physiology of cardiac repolarization. *Physiol. Rev.* **2005**, *85*, 1205–1253. [CrossRef] [PubMed]

94. Lu, J.T.; Kass, R.S. Recent progress in congenital long qt syndrome. *Curr. Opin. Cardiol.* **2010**, *25*, 216–221. [CrossRef] [PubMed]

95. Kammerer, S.; Burns-Hamuro, L.L.; Ma, Y.; Hamon, S.C.; Canaves, J.M.; Shi, M.M.; Nelson, M.R.; Sing, C.F.; Cantor, C.R.; Taylor, S.S.; et al. Amino acid variant in the kinase binding domain of dual-specific a kinase-anchoring protein 2: A disease susceptibility polymorphism. *Proc. Natl. Acad. Sci. USA* **2003**, *100*, 4066–4071. [CrossRef] [PubMed]

96. Tingley, W.G.; Pawlikowska, L.; Zaroff, J.G.; Kim, T.; Nguyen, T.; Young, S.G.; Vranizan, K.; Kwok, P.Y.; Whooley, M.A.; Conklin, B.R. Gene-trapped mouse embryonic stem cell-derived cardiac myocytes and human genetics implicate AKAP10 in heart rhythm regulation. *Proc. Natl. Acad. Sci. USA* **2007**, *104*, 8461–8466. [CrossRef] [PubMed]

97. Łoniewska, B.; Kaczmarczyk, M.; Clark, J.S.; Gorący, I.; Horodnicka-Józwa, A.; Ciechanowicz, A. Association of functional genetic variants of A-kinase anchoring protein 10 with qt interval length in full-term polish newborns. *Arch. Med. Sci.* **2015**, *11*, 149–154. [CrossRef] [PubMed]

98. Frey, N.; Olson, E.N. Cardiac hypertrophy: The good, the bad, and the ugly. *Annu. Rev. Physiol.* **2003**, *65*, 45–79. [CrossRef] [PubMed]

99. Diviani, D.; Soderling, J.; Scott, J.D. AKAP-lbc anchors protein kinase A and nucleates Gα$_{12}$-selective rho-mediated stress fiber formation. *J. Biol. Chem.* **2001**, *276*, 44247–44257. [CrossRef] [PubMed]

100. Klussmann, E.; Edemir, B.; Pepperle, B.; Tamma, G.; Henn, V.; Klauschenz, E.; Hundsrucker, C.; Maric, K.; Rosenthal, W. Ht31: The first protein kinase A anchoring protein to integrate protein kinase A and rho signaling. *FEBS Lett.* **2001**, *507*, 264–268. [CrossRef]

101. Abdul Azeez, K.R.; Knapp, S.; Fernandes, J.M.; Klussmann, E.; Elkins, J.M. The crystal structure of the rhoa-AKAP-lbc dh-ph domain complex. *Biochem. J.* **2014**, *464*, 231–239. [CrossRef] [PubMed]

102. Schrade, K.; Tröger, J.; Eldahshan, A.; Zühlke, K.; Abdul Azeez, K.R.; Elkins, J.M.; Neuenschwander, M.; Oder, A.; Elkewedi, M.; Jaksch, S.; et al. An AKAP-lbc-rhoa interaction inhibitor promotes the translocation of aquaporin-2 to the plasma membrane of renal collecting duct principal cells. *PLoS One* **2018**, *13*, e0191423. [CrossRef] [PubMed]

103. Mayers, C.M.; Wadell, J.; McLean, K.; Venere, M.; Malik, M.; Shibata, T.; Driggers, P.H.; Kino, T.; Guo, X.C.; Koide, H.; et al. The rho guanine nucleotide exchange factor AKAP13 (brx) is essential for cardiac development in mice. *J. Biol. Chem.* **2010**, *285*, 12344–12354. [CrossRef] [PubMed]

104. Diviani, D.; Abuin, L.; Cotecchia, S.; Pansier, L. Anchoring of both PKA and 14-3-3 inhibits the rho-gef activity of the AKAP-lbc signaling complex. *EMBO J.* **2004**, *23*, 2811–2820. [CrossRef] [PubMed]

105. Carnegie, G.K.; Smith, F.D.; McConnachie, G.; Langeberg, L.K.; Scott, J.D. AKAP-lbc nucleates a protein kinase D activation scaffold. *Mol. Cell* **2004**, *15*, 889–899. [CrossRef] [PubMed]

106. Carnegie, G.K.; Soughayer, J.; Smith, F.D.; Pedroja, B.S.; Zhang, F.; Diviani, D.; Bristow, M.R.; Kunkel, M.T.; Newton, A.C.; Langeberg, L.K.; et al. AKAP-lbc mobilizes a cardiac hypertrophy signaling pathway. *Mol. Cell* **2008**, *32*, 169–179. [CrossRef] [PubMed]

107. Pare, G.C.; Easlick, J.L.; Mislow, J.M.; McNally, E.M.; Kapiloff, M.S. Nesprin-1alpha contributes to the targeting of mAKAP to the cardiac myocyte nuclear envelope. *Exp. Cell Res.* **2005**, *303*, 388–399. [CrossRef] [PubMed]

108. Zhang, L.; Malik, S.; Kelley, G.G.; Kapiloff, M.S.; Smrcka, A.V. Phospholipase c epsilon scaffolds to muscle-specific a kinase anchoring protein (mAKAPβ) and integrates multiple hypertrophic stimuli in cardiac myocytes. *J. Biol. Chem.* **2011**, *286*, 23012–23021. [CrossRef] [PubMed]

109. Dodge-Kafka, K.L.; Bauman, A.; Mayer, N.; Henson, E.; Heredia, L.; Ahn, J.; McAvoy, T.; Nairn, A.C.; Kapiloff, M.S. Camp-stimulated protein phosphatase 2a activity associated with muscle a kinase-anchoring protein (mAKAP) signaling complexes inhibits the phosphorylation and activity of the cAMP-specific phosphodiesterase pde4d3. *J. Biol. Chem.* **2010**, *285*, 11078–11086. [CrossRef] [PubMed]

110. Wong, W.; Goehring, A.S.; Kapiloff, M.S.; Langeberg, L.K.; Scott, J.D. MAKAP compartmentalizes oxygen-dependent control of hif-1α. *Sci. Signal.* **2008**, *1*, ra18. [CrossRef] [PubMed]

111. Abrenica, B.; AlShaaban, M.; Czubryt, M.P. The a-kinase anchor protein AKAP121 is a negative regulator of cardiomyocyte hypertrophy. *J. Mol. Cell. Cardiol* **2009**, *46*, 674–681. [CrossRef] [PubMed]

112. Means, C.K.; Xiao, C.Y.; Li, Z.; Zhang, T.; Omens, J.H.; Ishii, I.; Chun, J.; Brown, J.H. Sphingosine 1-phosphate s1p2 and s1p3 receptor-mediated akt activation protects against in vivo myocardial ischemia-reperfusion injury. *Am. J. Physiol. Heart Circ. Physiol.* **2007**, *292*, H2944–H2951. [CrossRef] [PubMed]

113. Schiattarella, G.G.; Cattaneo, F.; Pironti, G.; Magliulo, F.; Carotenuto, G.; Pirozzi, M.; Polishchuk, R.; Borzacchiello, D.; Paolillo, R.; Oliveti, M.; et al. AKAP1 deficiency promotes mitochondrial aberrations and exacerbates cardiac injury following permanent coronary ligation via enhanced mitophagy and apoptosis. *PLoS One* **2016**, *11*, e0154076. [CrossRef] [PubMed]

114. Lacaná, E.; Maceyka, M.; Milstien, S.; Spiegel, S. Cloning and characterization of a protein kinase a anchoring protein (AKAP)-related protein that interacts with and regulates sphingosine kinase 1 activity. *J. Biol. Chem.* **2002**, *277*, 32947–32953. [CrossRef] [PubMed]

115. Vasudevan, N.T.; Mohan, M.L.; Goswami, S.K.; Naga Prasad, S.V. Regulation of β-adrenergic receptor function: An emphasis on receptor resensitization. *Cell Cycle* **2011**, *10*, 3684–3691. [CrossRef] [PubMed]

116. Lohse, M.J.; Engelhardt, S.; Eschenhagen, T. What is the role of β-adrenergic signaling in heart failure? *Circ. Res.* **2003**, *93*, 896–906. [CrossRef] [PubMed]

117. Gold, M.G.; Gonen, T.; Scott, J.D. Local cAMP signaling in disease at a glance. *J. Cell Sci.* **2013**, *126*, 4537–4543. [CrossRef] [PubMed]

118. Berisha, F.; Nikolaev, V.O. Cyclic nucleotide imaging and cardiovascular disease. *Pharmacol. Ther.* **2017**, *175*, 107–115. [CrossRef] [PubMed]

119. Froese, A.; Nikolaev, V.O. Imaging alterations of cardiomyocyte cAMP microdomains in disease. *Front. Pharmacol.* **2015**, *6*, 172. [CrossRef] [PubMed]

120. Pavlaki, N.; Nikolaev, V.O. Imaging of PDE2- and PDE3-mediated cGMP-to-cAMP cross-talk in cardiomyocytes. *J. Cardiovasc. Dev. Dis.* **2018**, *5*, 4. [CrossRef] [PubMed]

121. Musheshe, N.; Schmidt, M.; Zaccolo, M. cAMP: From long-range second messenger to nanodomain signalling. *Trends Pharmacol. Sci.* **2017**, *39*, 209–222. [CrossRef] [PubMed]

122. Thestrup, T.; Litzlbauer, J.; Bartholomäus, I.; Mues, M.; Russo, L.; Dana, H.; Kovalchuk, Y.; Liang, Y.; Kalamakis, G.; Laukat, Y.; et al. Optimized ratiometric calcium sensors for functional in vivo imaging of neurons and t lymphocytes. *Nat. Methods* **2014**, *11*, 175–182. [CrossRef] [PubMed]

123. Sprenger, J.U.; Nikolaev, V.O. Biophysical techniques for detection of cAMP and cGMP in living cells. *Int J. Mol. Sci.* **2013**, *14*, 8025–8046. [CrossRef] [PubMed]

124. Perera, R.K.; Sprenger, J.U.; Steinbrecher, J.H.; Hübscher, D.; Lehnart, S.E.; Abesser, M.; Schuh, K.; El-Armouche, A.; Nikolaev, V.O. Microdomain switch of cGMP-regulated phosphodiesterases leads to anp-induced augmentation of β-adrenoceptor-stimulated contractility in early cardiac hypertrophy. *Circ. Res.* **2015**, *116*, 1304–1311. [CrossRef] [PubMed]

125. Sprenger, J.U.; Perera, R.K.; Steinbrecher, J.H.; Lehnart, S.E.; Maier, L.S.; Hasenfuss, G.; Nikolaev, V.O. In vivo model with targeted cAMP biosensor reveals changes in receptor-microdomain communication in cardiac disease. *Nat. Commun.* **2015**, *6*, 6965. [CrossRef] [PubMed]

126. Jungen, C.; Scherschel, K.; Eickholt, C.; Kuklik, P.; Klatt, N.; Bork, N.; Salzbrunn, T.; Alken, F.; Angendohr, S.; Klene, C.; et al. Disruption of cardiac cholinergic neurons enhances susceptibility to ventricular arrhythmias. *Nat. Commun.* **2017**, *8*, 14155. [CrossRef] [PubMed]

127. Sanchez-Alonso, J.L.; Bhargava, A.; O'Hara, T.; Glukhov, A.V.; Schobesberger, S.; Bhogal, N.; Sikkel, M.B.; Mansfield, C.; Korchev, Y.E.; Lyon, A.R.; et al. Microdomain-specific modulation of l-type calcium channels leads to triggered ventricular arrhythmia in heart failure. *Circ. Res.* **2016**, *119*, 944–955. [CrossRef] [PubMed]

128. Calebiro, D.; Rieken, F.; Wagner, J.; Sungkaworn, T.; Zabel, U.; Borzi, A.; Cocucci, E.; Zürn, A.; Lohse, M.J. Single-molecule analysis of fluorescently labeled g-protein-coupled receptors reveals complexes with distinct dynamics and organization. *Proc. Natl Acad Sci USA* **2013**, *110*, 743–748. [CrossRef] [PubMed]

129. Miragoli, M.; Moshkov, A.; Novak, P.; Shevchuk, A.; Nikolaev, V.O.; El-Hamarsy, I.; Potter, C.M.; Wright, P.; Kadir, S.H.; Lyon, A.R.; et al. Scanning ion conductance microscopy: A convergent high-resolution technology for multi-parametric analysis of living cardiovascular cells. *J. R Soc. Interface* **2011**, *8*, 913–925. [CrossRef] [PubMed]

130. Nikolaev, V.O.; Moshkov, A.; Lyon, A.R.; Miragoli, M.; Novak, P.; Paur, H.; Lohse, M.J.; Korchev, Y.E.; Harding, S.E.; Gorelik, J. β2-adrenergic receptor redistribution in heart failure changes cAMP compartmentation. *Science* **2010**, *327*, 1653–1657. [CrossRef] [PubMed]

131. Conti, M.; Beavo, J. Biochemistry and physiology of cyclic nucleotide phosphodiesterases: Essential components in cyclic nucleotide signaling. *Annu. Rev. Biochem.* **2007**, *76*, 481–511. [CrossRef] [PubMed]

132. Maurice, D.H.; Palmer, D.; Tilley, D.G.; Dunkerley, H.A.; Netherton, S.J.; Raymond, D.R.; Elbatarny, H.S.; Jimmo, S.L. Cyclic nucleotide phosphodiesterase activity, expression, and targeting in cells of the cardiovascular system. *Mol. Pharmacol.* **2003**, *64*, 533–546. [CrossRef] [PubMed]

133. Keravis, T.; Lugnier, C. Cyclic nucleotide phosphodiesterases (PDE) and peptide motifs. *Curr. Pharm. Des.* **2010**, *16*, 1114–1125. [CrossRef] [PubMed]

134. Anant, J.S.; Ong, O.C.; Xie, H.Y.; Clarke, S.; O'Brien, P.J.; Fung, B.K. In vivo differential prenylation of retinal cyclic gmp phosphodiesterase catalytic subunits. *J. Biol. Chem.* **1992**, *267*, 687–690. [PubMed]

135. Baillie, G.S.; MacKenzie, S.J.; McPhee, I.; Houslay, M.D. Sub-family selective actions in the ability of erk2 map kinase to phosphorylate and regulate the activity of PDE4 cyclic AMP-specific phosphodiesterases. *Br. J. Pharmacol.* **2000**, *131*, 811–819. [CrossRef] [PubMed]

136. Omori, K.; Kotera, J. Overview of pdes and their regulation. *Circ. Res.* **2007**, *100*, 309–327. [CrossRef] [PubMed]

137. Francis, S.H.; Blount, M.A.; Corbin, J.D. Mammalian cyclic nucleotide phosphodiesterases: Molecular mechanisms and physiological functions. *Physiol. Rev.* **2011**, *91*, 651–690. [CrossRef] [PubMed]

138. Ke, H.; Wang, H. Crystal structures of phosphodiesterases and implications on substrate specificity and inhibitor selectivity. *Curr. Top. Med. Chem.* **2007**, *7*, 391–403. [CrossRef] [PubMed]

139. Wechsler, J.; Choi, Y.H.; Krall, J.; Ahmad, F.; Manganiello, V.C.; Movsesian, M.A. Isoforms of cyclic nucleotide phosphodiesterase PDE3a in cardiac myocytes. *J. Biol. Chem.* **2002**, *277*, 38072–38078. [CrossRef] [PubMed]

140. Senzaki, H.; Smith, C.J.; Juang, G.J.; Isoda, T.; Mayer, S.P.; Ohler, A.; Paolocci, N.; Tomaselli, G.F.; Hare, J.M.; Kass, D.A. Cardiac phosphodiesterase 5 (cGMP-specific) modulates β-adrenergic signaling in vivo and is down-regulated in heart failure. *FASEB J.* **2001**, *15*, 1718–1726. [CrossRef] [PubMed]

141. Rosman, G.J.; Martins, T.J.; Sonnenburg, W.K.; Beavo, J.A.; Ferguson, K.; Loughney, K. Isolation and characterization of human cdnas encoding a cGMP-stimulated 3',5'-cyclic nucleotide phosphodiesterase. *Gene* **1997**, *191*, 89–95. [CrossRef]

142. Zhang, H.; Liu, X.H.; Zhang, K.; Chen, C.K.; Frederick, J.M.; Prestwich, G.D.; Baehr, W. Photoreceptor cgmp phosphodiesterase delta subunit (pdedelta) functions as a prenyl-binding protein. *J. Biol. Chem.* **2004**, *279*, 407–413. [CrossRef] [PubMed]

143. Han, P.; Sonati, P.; Rubin, C.; Michaeli, T. Pde7a1, a cAMP-specific phosphodiesterase, inhibits cAMP-dependent protein kinase by a direct interaction with c. *J. Biol. Chem.* **2006**, *281*, 15050–15057. [CrossRef] [PubMed]

144. Wang, P.; Wu, P.; Egan, R.W.; Billah, M.M. Identification and characterization of a new human type 9 cGMP-specific phosphodiesterase splice variant (PDE9a5). Differential tissue distribution and subcellular localization of PDE9a variants. *Gene* **2003**, *314*, 15–27. [CrossRef]

145. Sayner, S.; Stevens, T. Soluble adenylate cyclase reveals the significance of compartmentalized cAMP on endothelial cell barrier function. *Biochem. Soc. Trans.* **2006**, *34*, 492–494. [CrossRef] [PubMed]

146. Creighton, J.; Zhu, B.; Alexeyev, M.; Stevens, T. Spectrin-anchored phosphodiesterase 4d4 restricts cAMP from disrupting microtubules and inducing endothelial cell gap formation. *J. Cell. Sci.* **2008**, *121*, 110–119. [CrossRef] [PubMed]

147. Mongillo, M.; Tocchetti, C.G.; Terrin, A.; Lissandron, V.; Cheung, Y.F.; Dostmann, W.R.; Pozzan, T.; Kass, D.A.; Paolocci, N.; Houslay, M.D.; et al. Compartmentalized phosphodiesterase-2 activity blunts β-adrenergic cardiac inotropy via an no/cGMP-dependent pathway. *Circ. Res.* **2006**, *98*, 226–234. [CrossRef] [PubMed]

148. Beca, S.; Helli, P.B.; Simpson, J.A.; Zhao, D.; Farman, G.P.; Jones, P.; Tian, X.; Wilson, L.S.; Ahmad, F.; Chen, S.R.W.; et al. Phosphodiesterase 4d regulates baseline sarcoplasmic reticulum Ca^{2+} release and cardiac contractility, independently of l-type Ca^{2+} current. *Circ. Res.* **2011**, *109*, 1024–1030. [CrossRef] [PubMed]

149. Borlaug, B.A.; Melenovsky, V.; Marhin, T.; Fitzgerald, P.; Kass, D.A. Sildenafil inhibits β-adrenergic-stimulated cardiac contractility in humans. *Circulation* **2005**, *112*, 2642–2649. [CrossRef] [PubMed]

150. Patrucco, E.; Albergine, M.S.; Santana, L.F.; Beavo, J.A. Phosphodiesterase 8a (PDE8a) regulates excitation-contraction coupling in ventricular myocytes. *J. Mol. Cell. Cardiol.* **2010**, *49*, 330–333. [CrossRef] [PubMed]

151. Galindo-Tovar, A.; Kaumann, A.J. Phosphodiesterase-4 blunts inotropism and arrhythmias but not sinoatrial tachycardia of (−)-adrenaline mediated through mouse cardiac β(1)-adrenoceptors. *Br. J. Pharmacol.* **2008**, *153*, 710–720. [CrossRef] [PubMed]

152. Ding, B.; Abe, J.; Wei, H.; Xu, H.; Che, W.; Aizawa, T.; Liu, W.; Molina, C.A.; Sadoshima, J.; Blaxall, B.C.; et al. A positive feedback loop of phosphodiesterase 3 (PDE3) and inducible cAMP early repressor (icer) leads to cardiomyocyte apoptosis. *Proc. Natl. Acad. Sci. USA* **2005**, *102*, 14771–14776. [CrossRef] [PubMed]

153. Leroy, J.; Richter, W.; Mika, D.; Castro, L.R.; Abi-Gerges, A.; Xie, M.; Scheitrum, C.; Lefebvre, F.; Schittl, J.; Mateo, P.; et al. Phosphodiesterase 4b in the cardiac l-type Ca^{2+} channel complex regulates Ca^{2+} current and protects against ventricular arrhythmias in mice. *J. Clin. Invest.* **2011**, *121*, 2651–2661. [CrossRef] [PubMed]

154. Lehnart, S.E.; Wehrens, X.H.; Reiken, S.; Warrier, S.; Belevych, A.E.; Harvey, R.D.; Richter, W.; Jin, S.L.; Conti, M.; Marks, A.R. Phosphodiesterase 4d deficiency in the ryanodine-receptor complex promotes heart failure and arrhythmias. *Cell* **2005**, *123*, 25–35. [CrossRef] [PubMed]

155. Pokreisz, P.; Vandenwijngaert, S.; Bito, V.; Van den Bergh, A.; Lenaerts, I.; Busch, C.; Marsboom, G.; Gheysens, O.; Vermeersch, P.; Biesmans, L.; et al. Ventricular phosphodiesterase-5 expression is increased in patients with advanced heart failure and contributes to adverse ventricular remodeling after myocardial infarction in mice. *Circulation* **2009**, *119*, 408–416. [CrossRef] [PubMed]

156. Lee, D.I.; Zhu, G.; Sasaki, T.; Cho, G.S.; Hamdani, N.; Holewinski, R.; Jo, S.H.; Danner, T.; Zhang, M.; Rainer, P.P.; et al. Phosphodiesterase 9a controls nitric-oxide-independent cGMP and hypertrophic heart disease. *Nature* **2015**, *519*, 472–476. [CrossRef] [PubMed]

157. Hambleton, R.; Krall, J.; Tikishvili, E.; Honeggar, M.; Ahmad, F.; Manganiello, V.C.; Movsesian, M.A. Isoforms of cyclic nucleotide phosphodiesterase pde3 and their contribution to cAMP hydrolytic activity in subcellular fractions of human myocardium. *J. Biol. Chem.* **2005**, *280*, 39168–39174. [CrossRef] [PubMed]

158. Ahmad, F.; Murata, T.; Shimizu, K.; Degerman, E.; Maurice, D.; Manganiello, V. Cyclic nucleotide phosphodiesterases: Important signaling modulators and therapeutic targets. *Oral Dis.* **2015**, *21*, e25–e50. [CrossRef] [PubMed]

159. Maass, P.G.; Aydin, A.; Luft, F.C.; Schächterle, C.; Weise, A.; Stricker, S.; Lindschau, C.; Vaegler, M.; Qadri, F.; Toka, H.R.; et al. PDE3a mutations cause autosomal dominant hypertension with brachydactyly. *Nat. Genet.* **2015**, *47*, 647–653. [CrossRef] [PubMed]

160. Hattenbach, L.O.; Toka, H.R.; Toka, O.; Schuster, H.; Luft, F.C. Absence of hypertensive retinopathy in a turkish kindred with autosomal dominant hypertension and brachydactyly. *Br. J. Ophthalmol.* **1998**, *82*, 1363–1365. [CrossRef] [PubMed]

161. Toka, O.; Tank, J.; Schächterle, C.; Aydin, A.; Maass, P.G.; Elitok, S.; Bartels-Klein, E.; Hollfinger, I.; Lindschau, C.; Mai, K.; et al. Clinical effects of phosphodiesterase 3a mutations in inherited hypertension with brachydactyly. *Hypertension* **2015**, *66*, 800–808. [CrossRef] [PubMed]

162. Movsesian, M. Novel approaches to targeting PDE3 in cardiovascular disease. *Pharmacol. Ther.* **2016**, *163*, 74–81. [CrossRef] [PubMed]

163. Movsesian, M.; Ahmad, F.; Hirsch, E. Functions of PDE3 isoforms in cardiac muscle. *J. Cardiovasc. Dev. Dis* **2018**, *5*, 10. [CrossRef] [PubMed]

164. Francis, S.H.; Conti, M.; Houslay, M.D. Handbook of Experimental Pharmacology 204. In *Phosphodiesterases as Drug Targets*; Springer International Publishing: Cham, Switzerland, 2011.

165. Knight, W.; Yan, C. Therapeutic potential of pde modulation in treating heart disease. *Future Med. Chem.* **2013**, *5*, 1607–1620. [CrossRef] [PubMed]

166. Liu, Y.; Shakur, Y.; Kambayashi, J. Phosphodiesterases as targets for intermittent claudication. *Handb Exp. Pharmacol.* **2011**, 211–236.

167. Rogers, K.C.; Oliphant, C.S.; Finks, S.W. Clinical efficacy and safety of cilostazol: A critical review of the literature. *Drugs* **2015**, *75*, 377–395. [CrossRef] [PubMed]

168. Hiatt, W.R.; Money, S.R.; Brass, E.P. Long-term safety of cilostazol in patients with peripheral artery disease: The castle study (cilostazol: A study in long-term effects). *J. Vasc. Surg.* **2008**, *47*, 330–336. [CrossRef] [PubMed]

169. Takigawa, T.; Matsumaru, Y.; Hayakawa, M.; Nemoto, S.; Matsumura, A. Cilostazol reduces restenosis after carotid artery stenting. *J. Vasc. Surg.* **2010**, *51*, 51–56. [CrossRef] [PubMed]

170. Cone, J.; Wang, S.; Tandon, N.; Fong, M.; Sun, B.; Sakurai, K.; Yoshitake, M.; Kambayashi, J.; Liu, Y. Comparison of the effects of cilostazol and milrinone on intracellular cAMP levels and cellular function in platelets and cardiac cells. *J. Cardiovasc. Pharmacol.* **1999**, *34*, 497–504. [CrossRef] [PubMed]

171. Faxon, D.P.; Creager, M.A.; Smith, S.C.; Pasternak, R.C.; Olin, J.W.; Bettmann, M.A.; Criqui, M.H.; Milani, R.V.; Loscalzo, J.; Kaufman, J.A.; et al. Atherosclerotic vascular disease conference: Executive summary: Atherosclerotic vascular disease conference proceeding for healthcare professionals from a special writing group of the american heart association. *Circulation* **2004**, *109*, 2595–2604. [CrossRef] [PubMed]

172. Gresele, P.; Momi, S.; Falcinelli, E. Anti-platelet therapy: Phosphodiesterase inhibitors. *Br. J. Clin. Pharmacol.* **2011**, *72*, 634–646. [CrossRef] [PubMed]

173. Sahin, M.; Alizade, E.; Pala, S.; Alici, G.; Ozkan, B.; Akgun, T.; Emiroglu, Y.; Demir, S.; Yazicioglu, M.V.; Turkmen, M.M. The effect of cilostazol on right heart function and pulmonary pressure. *Cardiovasc. Ther.* **2013**, *31*, e88–e93. [CrossRef] [PubMed]

174. Inoue, Y.; Toga, K.; Sudo, T.; Tachibana, K.; Tochizawa, S.; Kimura, Y.; Yoshida, Y.; Hidaka, H. Suppression of arterial intimal hyperplasia by cilostamide, a cyclic nucleotide phosphodiesterase 3 inhibitor, in a rat balloon double-injury model. *Br. J. Pharmacol.* **2000**, *130*, 231–241. [CrossRef] [PubMed]

175. Overgaard, C.B.; Dzavík, V. Inotropes and vasopressors: Review of physiology and clinical use in cardiovascular disease. *Circulation* **2008**, *118*, 1047–1056. [CrossRef] [PubMed]

176. Tariq, S.; Aronow, W.S. Use of inotropic agents in treatment of systolic heart failure. *Int J. Mol. Sci.* **2015**, *16*, 29060–29068. [CrossRef] [PubMed]

177. Movsesian, M. New pharmacologic interventions to increase cardiac contractility: Challenges and opportunities. *Curr. Opin. Cardiol.* **2015**, *30*, 285–291. [CrossRef] [PubMed]

178. Klussmann, E. Protein-protein interactions of PDE4 family members—Functions, interactions and therapeutic value. *Cell Signal.* **2016**, *28*, 713–718. [CrossRef] [PubMed]

179. Sims, C.R.; Singh, S.P.; Mu, S.; Gokden, N.; Zakaria, D.; Nguyen, T.C.; Mayeux, P.R. Rolipram improves outcome in a rat model of infant sepsis-induced cardiorenal syndrome. *Front. Pharmacol.* **2017**, *8*, 237. [CrossRef] [PubMed]

180. Lin, Y.C.; Samardzic, H.; Adamson, R.H.; Renkin, E.M.; Clark, J.F.; Reed, R.K.; Curry, F.R. Phosphodiesterase 4 inhibition attenuates atrial natriuretic peptide-induced vascular hyperpermeability and loss of plasma volume. *J. Physiol.* **2011**, *589*, 341–353. [CrossRef] [PubMed]

181. Richter, W.; Xie, M.; Scheitrum, C.; Krall, J.; Movsesian, M.A.; Conti, M. Conserved expression and functions of PDE4 in rodent and human heart. *Basic Res. Cardiol.* **2011**, *106*, 249–262. [CrossRef] [PubMed]

182. Rabe, K.F. Update on roflumilast, a phosphodiesterase 4 inhibitor for the treatment of chronic obstructive pulmonary disease. *Br. J. Pharmacol.* **2011**, *163*, 53–67. [CrossRef] [PubMed]

183. Tenor, H.; Hatzelmann, A.; Beume, R.; Lahu, G.; Zech, K.; Bethke, T.D. Pharmacology, clinical efficacy, and tolerability of phosphodiesterase-4 inhibitors: Impact of human pharmacokinetics. *Handb Exp. Pharmacol.* **2011**, 85–119.

184. Sakkas, L.I.; Mavropoulos, A.; Bogdanos, D.P. Phosphodiesterase 4 inhibitors in immune-mediated diseases: Mode of action, clinical applications, current and future perspectives. *Curr. Med. Chem.* **2017**, *24*, 3054–3067. [CrossRef] [PubMed]

185. Keating, G.M. Apremilast: A review in psoriasis and psoriatic arthritis. *Drugs* **2017**, *77*, 459–472. [CrossRef] [PubMed]

186. Nagendran, J.; Archer, S.L.; Soliman, D.; Gurtu, V.; Moudgil, R.; Haromy, A; St Aubin, C.; Webster, L.; Rebeyka, I.M.; Ross, D.B.; et al. Phosphodiesterase type 5 is highly expressed in the hypertrophied human right ventricle, and acute inhibition of phosphodiesterase type 5 improves contractility. *Circulation* **2007**, *116*, 238–248. [CrossRef] [PubMed]

187. Gong, W.; Yan, M.; Chen, J.; Chaugai, S.; Chen, C.; Wang, D. Chronic inhibition of cyclic guanosine monophosphate-specific phosphodiesterase 5 prevented cardiac fibrosis through inhibition of transforming growth factor β-induced smad signaling. *Front. Med.* **2014**, *8*, 445–455. [CrossRef] [PubMed]

188. Guazzi, M.; van Heerebeek, L.; Paulus, W.J. Phosphodiesterase-5 inhibition in heart failure with preserved ejection fraction: Trading therapy for prevention. *Eur J. Heart Fail.* **2017**, *19*, 337–339. [CrossRef] [PubMed]

189. Katz, S.D.; Balidemaj, K.; Homma, S.; Wu, H.; Wang, J.; Maybaum, S. Acute type 5 phosphodiesterase inhibition with sildenafil enhances flow-mediated vasodilation in patients with chronic heart failure. *J. Am. Coll. Cardiol.* **2000**, *36*, 845–851. [CrossRef]

190. Kukreja, R.C.; Salloum, F.N.; Das, A.; Koka, S.; Ockaili, R.A.; Xi, L. Emerging new uses of phosphodiesterase-5 inhibitors in cardiovascular diseases. *Exp. Clin. Cardiol.* **2011**, *16*, e30–35. [PubMed]

191. Pofi, R.; Gianfrilli, D.; Badagliacca, R.; Di Dato, C.; Venneri, M.A.; Giannetta, E. Everything you ever wanted to know about phosphodiesterase 5 inhibitors and the heart (but never dared ask): How do they work? *J. Endocrinol. Invest.* **2016**, *39*, 131–142. [CrossRef] [PubMed]

192. Sonnenburg, W.K.; Seger, D.; Beavo, J.A. Molecular cloning of a cdna encoding the "61-kda" Calmodulin-stimulated cyclic nucleotide phosphodiesterase. Tissue-specific expression of structurally related isoforms. *J. Biol. Chem.* **1993**, *268*, 645–652. [PubMed]

193. Goraya, T.A.; Cooper, D.M. Ca^{2+}-calmodulin-dependent phosphodiesterase (pde1): Current perspectives. *Cell Signal.* **2005**, *17*, 789–797. [CrossRef] [PubMed]

194. Saeki, T.; Adachi, H.; Takase, Y.; Yoshitake, S.; Souda, S.; Saito, I. A selective type v phosphodiesterase inhibitor, e4021, dilates porcine large coronary artery. *J. Pharmacol. Exp. Ther.* **1995**, *272*, 825–831. [PubMed]

195. Nagel, D.J.; Aizawa, T.; Jeon, K.I.; Liu, W.; Mohan, A.; Wei, H.; Miano, J.M.; Florio, V.A.; Gao, P.; Korshunov, V.A.; et al. Role of nuclear Ca^{2+}/calmodulin-stimulated phosphodiesterase 1a in vascular smooth muscle cell growth and survival. *Circ. Res.* **2006**, *98*, 777–784. [CrossRef] [PubMed]

196. Schermuly, R.T.; Pullamsetti, S.S.; Kwapiszewska, G.; Dumitrascu, R.; Tian, X.; Weissmann, N.; Ghofrani, H.A.; Kaulen, C.; Dunkern, T.; Schudt, C.; et al. Phosphodiesterase 1 upregulation in pulmonary arterial hypertension: Target for reverse-remodeling therapy. *Circulation* **2007**, *115*, 2331–2339. [CrossRef] [PubMed]

197. Fischmeister, R.; Castro, L.; Abi-Gerges, A.; Rochais, F.; Vandecasteele, G. Species- and tissue-dependent effects of no and cyclic gmp on cardiac ion channels. *Comp. Biochem. Physiol. A Mol. Integr. Physiol.* **2005**, *142*, 136–143. [CrossRef] [PubMed]

198. Mehel, H.; Emons, J.; Vettel, C.; Wittköpper, K.; Seppelt, D.; Dewenter, M.; Lutz, S.; Sossalla, S.; Maier, L.S.; Lechêne, P.; et al. Phosphodiesterase-2 is up-regulated in human failing hearts and blunts β-adrenergic responses in cardiomyocytes. *J. Am. Coll. Cardiol.* **2013**, *62*, 1596–1606. [CrossRef] [PubMed]

199. Vettel, C.; Lindner, M.; Dewenter, M.; Lorenz, K.; Schanbacher, C.; Riedel, M.; Lämmle, S.; Meinecke, S.; Mason, F.E.; Sossalla, S.; et al. Phosphodiesterase 2 protects against catecholamine-induced arrhythmia and preserves contractile function after myocardial infarction. *Circ. Res.* **2017**, *120*, 120–132. [CrossRef] [PubMed]

200. Rentero, C.; Monfort, A.; Puigdomènech, P. Identification and distribution of different mrna variants produced by differential splicing in the human phosphodiesterase 9a gene. *Biochem. Biophys. Res. Commun.* **2003**, *301*, 686–692. [CrossRef]

201. Christian, F.; Szaszák, M.; Friedl, S.; Drewianka, S.; Lorenz, D.; Goncalves, A.; Furkert, J.; Vargas, C.; Schmieder, P.; Götz, F.; et al. Small molecule AKAP-protein kinase a (PKA) interaction disruptors that activate PKA interfere with compartmentalized cAMP signaling in cardiac myocytes. *J. Biol. Chem.* **2011**, *286*, 9079–9096. [CrossRef] [PubMed]

202. Khan, A.; Munir, M.; Aiman, S.; Wadood, A.; Khan, A.U. The in silico identification of small molecules for protein-protein interaction inhibition in AKAP-lbc-rhoa signaling complex. *Comput. Biol. Chem.* **2017**, *67*, 84–91. [CrossRef] [PubMed]

203. Diviani, D.; Raimondi, F.; Del Vescovo, C.D.; Dreyer, E.; Reggi, E.; Osman, H.; Ruggieri, L.; Gonano, C.; Cavin, S.; Box, C.L.; et al. Small-molecule protein-protein interaction inhibitor of oncogenic rho signaling. *Cell Chem. Biol.* **2016**, *23*, 1135–1146. [CrossRef] [PubMed]
204. Serrels, B.; Sandilands, E.; Serrels, A.; Baillie, G.; Houslay, M.D.; Brunton, V.G.; Canel, M.; Machesky, L.M.; Anderson, K.I.; Frame, M.C. A complex between fak, rack1, and PDE4d5 controls spreading initiation and cancer cell polarity. *Curr. Biol.* **2010**, *20*, 1086–1092. [CrossRef] [PubMed]

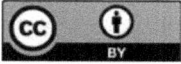

Journal of
*Cardiovascular
Development and Disease*

MDPI

Review

A-Kinase Anchoring Protein-Lbc: A Molecular Scaffold Involved in Cardiac Protection

Dario Diviani *, Halima Osman and Erica Reggi

Département de Pharmacologie et de Toxicologie, Faculté de Biologie et de Médecine, Lausanne 1005, Switzerland; Halima.Osman@unil.ch (H.O.); Erica.Reggi@unil.ch (E.R.)
* Correspondence: Dario.diviani@unil.ch; Tel.: +41-21-692-5404

Received: 12 January 2018; Accepted: 6 February 2018; Published: 8 February 2018

Abstract: Heart failure is a lethal disease that can develop after myocardial infarction, hypertension, or anticancer therapy. In the damaged heart, loss of function is mainly due to cardiomyocyte death and associated cardiac remodeling and fibrosis. In this context, A-kinase anchoring proteins (AKAPs) constitute a family of scaffolding proteins that facilitate the spatiotemporal activation of the cyclic adenosine monophosphate (AMP)-dependent protein kinase (PKA) and other transduction enzymes involved in cardiac remodeling. AKAP-Lbc, a cardiac enriched anchoring protein, has been shown to act as a key coordinator of the activity of signaling pathways involved in cardiac protection and remodeling. This review will summarize and discuss recent advances highlighting the role of the AKAP-Lbc signalosome in orchestrating adaptive responses in the stressed heart.

Keywords: A-kinase anchoring protein (AKAP); protein kinase A; cyclic AMP; cardiomyocyte; cardiac protection; signal transduction

1. Introduction

The heart responds to various stresses and insults such as increased blood pressure, myocardial infarction, and exposure to drugs and toxicants by undergoing a remodeling process that leads to heart failure, a lethal condition in which the cardiac output cannot satisfy the oxygen needs of the body [1–3]. Cardiac remodeling can be associated with an initial adaptive phase where ventricular cardiomyocytes undergo compensatory hypertrophy to maintain cardiac function [4,5]. However, in the long term, hypertrophy predisposes to adverse ventricular events associated with cardiomyocyte death, fibrosis, and progressive cardiac dysfunction [3,6,7]. Heart failure has an annual incidence of 1% in the population over 65 and a five-year survival rate after diagnosis lower than 50% [4]. This underscores the urgent need of identifying new therapies for this syndrome. In this respect, defining key protective signaling pathways favoring survival of cardiomyocyte subjected to stress could provide new opportunities to prevent cardiac remodeling and dysfunction under pathophysiological situations associated with heart injury or insults.

A-kinase anchoring proteins (AKAPs) are molecular scaffolds that act as signal organizers. They ensure coordination of multiple signaling pathways at discrete microdomains of cardiomyocytes and cardiac fibroblasts by locally recruiting the cAMP-dependent protein kinase (PKA) as well as other signaling enzymes [8–11]. Anchoring of PKA is mediated by conserved domains constituted by amphipathic helices of about 20 amino acids [12,13], whereas targeting of AKAP-based signaling complexes to distinct subcellular sites is achieved through specialized protein- or lipid-binding domains located on the anchoring proteins [10]. Among the multitude of signaling molecules recruited by AKAPs one can find kinases, phosphodiesterases (PDEs), adenylyl cyclases (ACs), phosphatases, and GTPases [14–20]. In this respect, the assembly of signaling enzymes displaying opposing action (i.e., kinases and phosphatases) allows bidirectional regulation of transduction events, whereas the clustering of activators and downstream targets (i.e., ACs and PKA substrates) promotes signal potentiation [18].

So far, about 17 AKAPs have been identified in cardiac tissues [21–23] and shown to regulate various homeostatic, adaptive as well as pathophysiological functions including heart rhythm and action potential propagation, calcium cycling and cardiac contraction, cardiac remodeling and heart failure, as well as cardiac protection [5,24–26]. This suggests that modulating the ability of AKAP complexes to locally coordinate the activity of signaling molecules might have major impact on the function of the stressed and/or diseased heart and could be exploited to promote protection and maintain cardiac function. In particular, AKAP-Lbc (AKAP13), a heart-enriched anchoring protein [17], has been shown to organize diverse signaling pathways favoring protection against a cardiac stresses including pressure overload, as well as drugs and toxicants [27–29]. The current minireview article will focus on the role of this multifunctional anchoring protein in favoring adaptive and survival responses in the injured heart. In recent years, additional AKAPs have been show to confer cardiomyocyte protection either in vitro or in vivo including D-AKAP-1 (AKAP1), AKAP79/150 (AKAP5) mAKAP (AKAP6) and AKAP12. For more information about the cardioprotective role of these AKAP-based signaling complexes we refer the reader to other recent publications [30–36].

2. The Role of the cAMP/PKA Pathways in Cardiac Protection

Studies undertaken during the last 20 years indicate that activation of the cAMP/PKA signaling pathway can protect cardiomyocytes against cell death and damage induced by ischemia/reperfusion, anthracycline treatment, hyperglycemic stress, and pressure overload. Early experiments performed using isolated rats hearts demonstrated that cardiac cAMP levels and PKA activity are increased during ischemic preconditioning and that suppression of cAMP signaling attenuates myocardial protection against sustained ischemia [37,38]. Several additional studies later showed that preconditioning of mouse, rat or rabbit hearts with various Gs-coupled receptor agonists including isoproterenol (ISO) [39], glucagon-like peptide 1 (GLP-1) [40], adrenomedullin [41], corticotropin releasing factor [42], and adiponectin [43], confers protection against subsequent ischemia and reduces infarct size in a PKA-dependent manner. Similarly, PKA has also been shown to mediate the protective effects of the GLP-1 receptor agonist exendin-4 against hyperglycemia-induced cardiomyocyte apoptosis [44], of the antidiabetic drug metformin against anthracycline cardiotoxicity [45], and of adrenomedullin 2 against pressure-overload induced cardiac remodeling [46].

These protective effects rely on the ability of PKA to regulate multiple effector proteins and responses in cardiomyocytes. On the one hand, protection against ischemia/reperfusion has been shown to rely on the ability of PKA to (1) inhibit calpain-dependent proteolysis and degradation of structural proteins in cardiomyocytes [38]; (2) increase the opening of the mitochondrial Ca^{2+}-activated K^+ (mitoK(Ca)) channels and improve the efficiency of mitochondrial energy production [41]; (3) promote phosphorylation and enhance the cardioprotective effects of the small heat-shock protein HSP20 [47,48]; (4) reduce inhibitor of Kappa B (IκB) phosphorylation and nuclear factor Kappa B (NF-κB) activation [43]; (5) reduce nicotinamide adenine dinucleotide phosphate (NADPH) oxidase overexpression and superoxide overproduction [43]; and (6) improve calcium handling through phospholamban (PLB) phosphorylation and sarcoplasmic reticulum Ca^{2+} ATPase 2 (SERCA2) activation [49].

On the other hand, protection against pathological cardiac remodeling requires PKA mediated-regulation of histone deacetylases (HDACs) 4 and 5 [50,51]. These two signaling molecules control the activity of transcription factors, such as the myocyte enhancer factor 2 (MEF2), crucially involved in the regulation of gene programs associated with cardiac remodeling [52]. PKA induces HDAC4 proteolysis and the formation of an N-terminal HDAC cleavage product that inhibits the activity of MEF2 [50]. Moreover, the kinase also phosphorylates HDAC5, which, in turn, prevents its nuclear export, leading to the inhibition of MEF2-dependent transcription and fetal gene expression [51]. However, since these later findings where obtained using primary cultures of cardiomyocytes as a model system, investigation should be pursued to determine whether regulation of HDAC function by PKA has anti-remodeling effects in hearts subjected to various forms of stress.

Interestingly, PKA reduces detrimental cardiac remodeling not only by protecting cardiomyocytes from dysfunction and death but also by inhibiting cardiac fibrosis. In this respect, it has been recently shown that activation of PKA signaling by prostaglandin E_2 receptor 4 (EP4) agonists significantly prevented progression of myocardial fibrosis in response to pressure overload [53]. Experiments performed using isolated cardiac fibroblasts subsequently indicated that PKA activation suppresses collagen overproduction induced by the profibrotic agonist transforming growth factor β1 (TGF-β1) [53]. This suggests that PKA might attenuate the formation interstitial cardiac fibrosis, and consequent heart dysfunction through the reduction of excessive extracellular matrix deposition.

The studies described above were carried out using activators or inhibitors that impact cardiac PKA signaling in a global manner and do not allow the precise identification of specific PKA functions in the heart. To circumvent this problem, several studies now adopt more targeted approaches and investigate the function of individual AKAP-PKA signaling complexes in specific cardiac cellular populations.

3. AKAP-Lbc Signaling and Cardiac Protection

AKAP-Lbc (AKAP13) is a cardiac enriched anchoring protein [17], which functions as a scaffold for multiple signaling enzymes as well as a guanine nucleotide exchange factor (GEF) that selectively activates the small molecular weight GTPases RhoA and RhoC [17,23,54]. The exchange of GDP for GTP and the binding to Rho-GTPases is ensured by tandem Dbl-homology (DH) and plekstrin-homology (PH) domains located in the middle of the anchoring protein [17,54,55]. This central catalytic core is surrounded by N-terminal and C-terminal sequences, which provide anchoring sites for signaling molecules [23], and inhibit the basal Rho-GEF activity of AKAP-Lbc in the absence of stimulatory signals [17]. Deletion of these key regulatory regions, which has been shown to occur in chronic myeloid leukemia (CML) patients as the consequence of a chromosomal translocation between chromosomes 15 and 7, significantly increases the basal Rho-GEF activity and promotes oncogenic transformation [55,56].

The Rho-GEF activity of AKAP-Lbc is enhanced by G-protein-coupled receptors (GPCRs) linked to the heterotrimeric G protein G12 such as α1-adrenergic receptors (α1-ARs) [57]. In this respect, it has been shown that the α subunit of G12 (Gα12) can directly activate AKAP-Lbc by binding to a docking site located in its C-terminus. This interaction is proposed to suppress autoinhibitory intramolecular bonds between C-terminal regulatory sequences and the GEF region of the anchoring protein [58].

Initial in vitro studies performed in primary cultures of rat neonatal cardiomyocytes (NVMs) indicated that AKAP-Lbc acts as a mediator of the hypertrophic effects induced by α1-AR and endothelin 1 receptor (ET1-R) agonists [57,59]. These findings served as base for subsequent in vivo investigations showing that the anchoring protein mediates early adaptive growth responses that allow the heart to functionally compensate biomechanical or neurohumoral stresses [27,28]. Finally, in recent years, it became evident that AKAP-Lbc also coordinates and regulates signaling molecules such as the mitogen activated protein kinase (MAPK) p38α [27,60], protein kinase D1 (PKD1) [28,59], and the heat shock protein 20 (HSP20) [61], that promote adaptive and/or cytoprotective responses in cardiomyocytes. The following sections will discuss how coordination of distinct signaling pathways by the AKAP-Lbc signaling complex contributes to cardiomyocyte adaptation and protection against to various stressors and toxicants.

3.1. AKAP-Lbc Mediates Protection against Pressure Overload-Induced Cardiac Dysfunction

Left ventricular pressure overload can be triggered by chronically elevated systemic blood pressure or obstructions of the outflow tract such as aortic valve stenosis. It initially leads to cardiac hypertrophy, which eventually may become maladaptive and predispose to heart failure. It is estimated that chronic hypertension doubles the risk of developing heart failure [4]. Experimentally, pressure overload can be induced in the mouse by transverse aortic constriction (TAC). Cardiac AKAP-Lbc is significantly upregulated in mice subjected to TAC as well as in patients with hypertrophic cardiomyopathy [27,28,59]. It assembles a macromolecular signaling complex coordinating the activity of transduction enzymes such as p38α and PKD1 that have a direct impact on compensatory hypertrophy and maintenance of cardiac function during the early phase of cardiac remodeling.

3.1.1. The Role of AKAP-Lbc-Mediated Regulation of p38α

The role of p38α in cardiac adaptation to stress has been subject of discussion over the last decade. Initial investigations suggested that chronic (constitutive) activation or inhibition of cardiac p38α does not affect hypertrophy [62–66]. However, subsequent studies overturned this view by showing that inducible activation of p38α signaling in adult hearts promotes cardiomyocyte growth [67,68]. In cardiomyocytes, AKAP-Lbc forms a p38-activating transduction unit that includes p38α and its upstream activators protein kinase N α (PKNα), mixed lineage kinase-like mitogen-activated protein triple kinase (MLTK), and mitogen-activated protein kinase kinase 3 (MKK3) (Figure 1) [27]. Cardiomyocyte-specific overexpression of a molecular disruptor of the interaction between AKAP-Lbc and PKNα inhibits pressure overload-induced p38α activation and compensatory cardiac hypertrophy. This leads to the appearance of early signs of heart failure including left ventricular dilation, increased cardiomyocyte apoptosis, and depressed cardiac function [27]. The ability of the AKAP-Lbc/p38α complex to promote compensatory hypertrophy is linked to the induction of mammalian target of rapamycin (mTOR) and the consequent increase in protein synthesis (Figure 1) [27]. These results indicate that AKAP-Lbc facilitates activation of p38α and mTOR in response to abrupt increases in the afterload to promote hypertrophy and reduce cell death, which temporarily preserves the function of the stressed heart. While the pathway linking the AKAP-Lbc/p38α complex and mTOR is currently unknown, recent findings indicate that p38 can enhance cardioprotective mTOR signaling by regulating the activity of the tuberous sclerosis complex (TSC) [69].

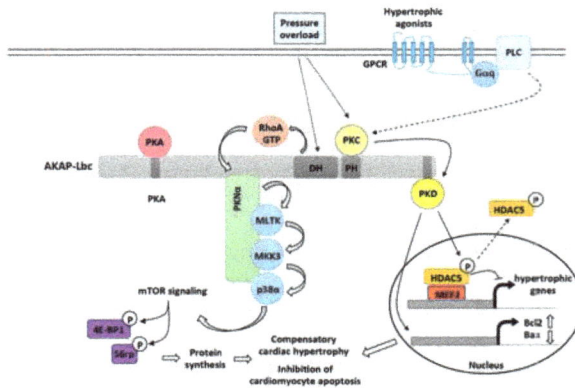

Figure 1. The role of the AKAP-Lbc signaling complex in mediating compensatory cardiac hypertrophy and cardiac protection in response to hemodynamic and neurohumoral stresses. Upon pressure overload, AKAP-Lbc promotes the formation of RhoA-GTP, which, in turn, triggers a signaling cascade involving anchored PKNα, MLTK, MKK3 and p38α. Activated p38α, through an unknown mechanism, enhances mTOR activity resulting in increased phosphorylation of 4E-BP1 and ribosomal protein S6 (S6rp), which leads to enhanced protein synthesis and cardiomyocyte growth Pressure overload as well as activation of Gq-coupled receptors by hypertrophic agonists (ET-1, Angiotensin II) also promote the activation of AKAP-Lbc-anchored PKD1, which, in turn, phosphorylates HDAC5 and favors its nuclear export. As a result, MEF2 becomes activated and promotes transcription of hypertrophic genes. Activated PKD1 plays protective roles during compensatory hypertrophy by inducing the expression of antiapoptotic genes such as Bcl-2 and by inhibiting transcription of pro-apoptotic genes such as Bax.

3.1.2. The Role of AKAP-Lbc-Mediated Regulation of PKD1

Early work by Carnegie et al. showed that AKAP-Lbc can interact with PKD1 and PKCη (Figure 1) [70]. They could demonstrate that stimulation of rat NVMs with agonists binding Gq-coupled receptors, such as α1-ARs and ET1-Rs, enhances PKC activity, which, in turn, phosphorylates anchored PKD1 at serine 944 and 948 to induce its activation. PKD1 is released from the complex when PKA phosphorylates serine 2737 located in the PKD-binding site of AKAP-Lbc. Free PKD1 can then phosphorylate HDAC5 an inhibitor of the prohypertrophic transcription factor MEF2. This facilitates its HDAC5 nuclear export, derepression of MEF2 and activation of hypertrophic gene transcription (Figure 1) [59].

Subsequent in vivo studies showed that gene-trap mice expressing a PKD1 binding deficient mutant of AKAP-Lbc were not able to sustain compensatory cardiac hypertrophy in response TAC or chronic treatment with hypertrophic agonists [28]. The impaired adaptive response to stress was associated with exacerbated cardiomyocyte apoptosis, early-dilated cardiomyopathy and heart failure. Interestingly, increased apoptosis was linked to a marked transcriptional downregulation of antiapoptotic genes such as Bcl2 and the upregulation of the mRNA encoding pro-apoptotic proteins such as Bax, Gzmm, and Dnm1l (Figure 1) [71]. Therefore, AKAP-Lbc-anchored PKD1 facilitates activation of hypertrophic and cytoprotective gene programs to ensure cardiomyocyte survival and adaptation during the early phase of cardiac remodeling.

3.2. AKAP-Lbc Mediates Protection against Doxorubicin-Induced Cardiomyocyte Toxicity

Doxorubicin (Dox) is an anthracycline antibiotic used for the past four decades as an anticancer agent to treat a variety of tumors including leukemia and breast cancer. It exerts its antineoplastic activity by impairing DNA replication, mainly through the inhibition of topoisomerase II, and by promoting the formation of reactive oxygen species (ROS). However, this drug displays severe cardiac side effects, which limit its clinical application and have become a serious concern for cancer survivors [72,73]. Doxorubicin-induced chronic cardiotoxicity is dose-dependent and usually occurs within the first year after treatment. The incidence is about 4% for a doxorubicin dose of 500–550 mg/m^2, 18% for a dose of 551–600 mg/m^2 and 36% for a dose exceeding 600 mg/m^2 [74].

Cardiotoxicity is associated with the ability of Dox to alter Ca^{2+} homeostasis, to affect the expression of sarcomeric proteins, to inhibit the electron transport chain and energy production, and to promote the formation of ROS both in the mitochondria and in the cytoplasm of cardiomyocytes through a series of redox reactions that require iron [75].

ROS production enhances oxidation of DNA [76], proteins and lipids [77], thus causing mitochondrial damage and the activation of cardiomyocyte apoptosis. These effects are reinforced by the profound inhibitory action of Dox on the expression of cytoprotective signaling proteins such the kinase Akt1 and antiapoptotic regulators such as Bcl2 and BclxL [78–80]. In the clinic, the only currently available drug that can partially diminish these cardiotoxic effects is dexrazoxane, an iron chelator that reduces Dox-induced ROS formation [81]. However, the fact that a significant number of patients receiving Dox still develop severe cardiac morbidity underscores the urgency of new therapeutical strategies. In this respect, recent research efforts are now focused on identifying cardioprotective signaling pathways that could efficiently reduce cardiac side effects [82].

Several evidences suggest that the activation of α1-ARs significantly reduces the toxic effects that Dox exerts on cardiomyocytes [83]. Indeed, phenylephrine (PE) and dabuzalgron, two α1-AR agonists, confer significant protection against Dox-induced cardiomyocyte apoptosis, pathological cardiac remodeling, and depressed heart function in mice [80,84]. Interestingly, recent studies performed on rat NVMs indicate that these protective effects could be mediated in part by AKAP-Lbc [29]. In particular, it has been shown that short-hairpin RNA (shRNA)-mediated suppression of AKAP-Lbc expression in ventricular myocytes strongly impairs the ability of the α1-AR agonist phenylephrine (PE) to reduce Dox-induced cardiomyocyte apoptosis. AKAP-Lbc-mediated cardiomyocyte protection requires the recruitment of PKD1 and the activation of two PKD1-dependent prosurvival signaling cascades (Figure 2) [29].

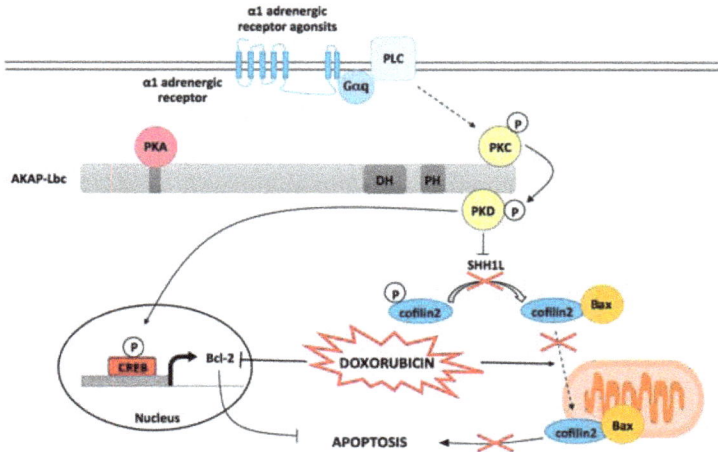

Figure 2. The role of AKAP-Lbc in mediating protection against Dox induced cardiomyocyte toxicity. Scaffolding of PKD by AKAP-Lbc facilitates α1-AR-mediated PKD1 activation resulting in the phosphorylation and inactivation of the phosphatase SSH1L. As a consequence, phosphorylated cofilin2 accumulates and remains sequestrated in the cytoplasm. This inhibits Dox-induced translocation of cofilin2/Bax complexes to mitochondria, and subsequent mitochondrial dysfunction and apoptosis. Activated PKD1 also favors cAMP regulatory element binding protein (CREB)-mediated transcriptional activation of the antiapoptotic gene Bcl-2 otherwise down regulated by Dox treatment.

In the first pathway, the AKAP-Lbc-anchored pool of PKD1 mediates the phosphorylation and activation of the transcription factor cAMP regulatory element binding protein (CREB), which, in turn, promotes upregulation of the antiapoptotic gene Bcl2. This efficiently prevents Dox-induced Bcl2 transcriptional downregulation (Figure 2). In the second pathway, AKAP-Lbc-facilitated activation of PKD1 leads to the phosphorylation and deactivation of the cofilin2-phosphatase slingshot-1L (SSH1L), which increases cofilin2 phosphorylation. This blocks Dox-induced translocation of cofilin2 and Bax complexes to mitochondria, which reduces mitochondrial dysfunction, cytochrome C release, caspase 3 activation and apoptosis (Figure 2) [29,85].

Knowing that PKD1 also favors protection against hypoxia and oxidative stress [85], and adaptation against pressure overload-induced early cardiac remodeling [28], one could suggest that this kinase might confer cardiomyocyte protection against a variety of stresses.

It has been shown that infusion of α1-AR agonists such as PE in mice induce a significant upregulation of cardiac AKAP-Lbc expression [57]. This raises the possibility that AKAP-Lbc-mediated cardioprotective signaling could be enhanced by α1-AR agonists in vivo. Based on this assumption, future studies will need to determine the impact of cardiac AKAP-Lbc suppression and overexpression on Dox-induced chronic cardiac side effects.

3.3. The Cardioprotective Role of the AKAP-Lbc/HSP20 Complex

The small heat shock protein HSP20 has been shown to confer sustained protection against cardiac stresses and insults including chronic β-adrenergic stimulation, ischemia/reperfusion (I/R) and Dox exposure. Indeed, transgenic mice with cardiomyocyte-specific overexpression of HSP20 are protected against apoptosis induced by chronic ISO or Dox infusion and develop significantly smaller infarcts when subjected to I/R [47,48,86,87]. HSP20 mediates its antiapoptotic effects through the inhibition of apoptosis signal-regulating kinase 1 (Ask1) and Bax (Figure 3) and the preservation of the pro-survival activity of Akt1 [48,87]. Interestingly, these cardioprotective effects were shown to require phosphorylation of HSP20 on serine 16 by PKA [88]. This was suggested by studies showing that overexpression of a constitutively phosphorylated mutant (S16D) of HSP20 protects adult cardiomyocytes from apoptosis induced by β-adrenergic agonists [47]. In a screening for polymorphisms associated with human dilated cardiomyopathy, it was later found that a single base change of C to T at nucleotide 59 in the N-terminus of HSP20, resulting in an amino acid substitution from proline 20 to leucine (P20L), strongly impaired PKA-mediated phosphorylation of HSP20 [89].

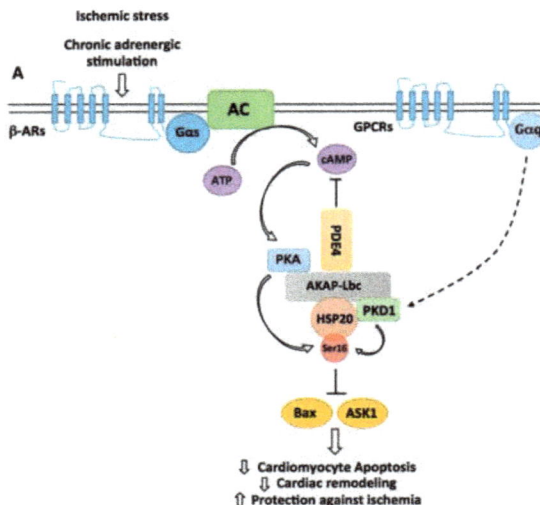

Figure 3. Regulation of HSP20-mediated cardiomyocyte protection by AKAP-Lbc. By recruiting phosphodiesterases 4 (PDE4), AKAP-Lbc maintains a low local concentration of cAMP, which prevents activation of anchored PKA. Chronic β-adrenergic stimulation induces a sustained production of cAMP, which saturates PDE4 and promotes anchored PKA activation. Activated PKA phosphorylates AKAP-Lbc-bound HSP20 on serine 16, an event that has been shown to enhance the cardioprotective function of HSP20. Indeed, phosphorylated HSP20 has been shown to suppress Ask1-dependent signaling and to inhibit Bax leading to reduced cardiomyocyte apoptosis, decreased pathological cardiac remodeling, and increased protection against ischemia. PKD1 can form a complex with HSP20 and promote its phosphorylation on serine 16. The relative contribution of PKA vs. PKD1 to the phosphorylation of HSP20 in vivo remains to be elucidated.

Accordingly, in vitro experiments confirmed that HSP20 P20L was unable to confer protection against I/R-induced cardiomyocyte apoptosis [90]. Recent studies indicate that AKAP-Lbc facilitates PKA-mediated phosphorylation of HSP20 (Figure 3). In particular, it has been shown that AKAP-Lbc stably interacts with HSP20, thus providing a physical link between PKA and the HSP [89]. Importantly, knockdown of AKAP-Lbc and overexpression of a PKA-binding deficient mutant of the anchoring protein in rat NVMs reduce the phosphorylation of HSP20 on serine 16 and increase isoproterenol-induced cardiomyocyte apoptosis [88]. This suggests that phosphorylation of HSP20 by AKAP-Lbc-anchored PKA mediates cardiomyocyte protection. However, it remains to be established whether the anchoring protein favors cardioprotective phosphorylation of HSP20 also in vivo. To this end, future experiments might investigate whether the knockout of AKAP-Lbc in adult hearts affects phospho-HSP20-dependent protective signaling.

The phosphorylation status of HSP20 is also regulated by PDE4 family members, which directly interact with the heat shock protein (Figure 3) [91]. Recruitment of PDE4 maintains the local concentration of cAMP low, which reduces PKA activation and HSP20 phosphorylation under basal conditions. Upon chronic β-adrenergic stimulation, cAMP levels rise in cardiomyocytes and overcome the hydrolyzing capacity of the PDE, what favors HSP20 phosphorylation [91]. Knowing that PDE4 also interacts with AKAP-Lbc [92], one might raise the hypothesis that AKAP-Lbc might serve as a molecular organizer coordinating the activity of PKA and PDE4 to confer spatiotemporal regulation of HSP20 phosphorylation and antiapoptotic function.

It has been shown that serine 16 of HSP20 is also a substrate for PKD1 phosphorylation [93]. This suggests that PKD1 could mediate part of its cardioprotective effects through the regulation of HSP20. The kinase has been shown to directly associate with HSP20 [93] but one could assume that AKAP-Lbc could also target PKD1 in proximity of HSP20 [70]. Based on these new findings, it would be interesting to evaluate the relative importance of PKA versus PKD1 as HSP20 kinases in vivo and to determine their impact on the cardioprotective function of HSP20.

4. Conclusions and Perspectives

The ability of AKAPs to integrate and process multiple signals allows them to regulate several physiological and pathological cardiac functions including contraction, heart rhythm, adaptation to stress and transition to heart failure [10,23,24]. In this context, AKAP-Lbc has the peculiarity of coordinating signaling pathways regulating the heart response to hemodynamic or chemical stresses.

While a number of studies have highlighted the protective role of AKAP-Lbc during the compensated hypertrophic growth of the heart induced by pressure overload and neurohumoral stress, it is currently not known whether this anchoring protein is also involved in later phases of cardiac remodeling. On the one hand, one could speculate that AKAP-Lbc-mediated activation of PKD1, p38α, and mTOR for periods of time that extend beyond the initial phase of compensation might promote deleterious effects through the sustained induction of the fetal gene program and alteration of cardiac contractility [59,94]. On the other hand, however, recent studies indicate that chronic PKD1 and mTOR activation might actually promote cardioprotective effects through the induction of antiapoptotic gene programs [85,95]. To address these contrasting hypotheses future studies using inducible cardiomyocyte-specific AKAP-Lbc knockout mice will need to address the impact of suppressing AKAP-Lbc expression at the end of the compensatory phase on subsequent pathological remodeling.

By facilitating the activation of PKD1 in cardiomyocytes, AKAP-Lbc inhibits cardiomyocyte apoptosis and protects mitochondrial function in response to abrupt increases in the left ventricular afterload and anthracycline (doxorubicin) exposure [28,29]. These antiapoptotic effects are mediated by the upregulation of Bcl2, the inhibition of the translocation of cofilin2 and Bax to mitochondria, and possibly HSP20. Therefore, strategies aimed at stimulating the activity of AKAP-Lbc-anchored PKD1 might represent a possible way to prevent early cardiac dysfunction in the stressed heart. Knowing that α1-ARs are upstream activators of the AKAP-Lbc/PKD1 signaling pathway, one could propose the use of α1-ARs selective agonists as cardioprotective agents. In this context, dabuzalgron, an oral α1A-AR agonist that was originally developed to treat urinary incontinence, could be repurposed to reduce the cardiac side effects of Dox-based anticancer chemotherapy and possibly to limit cardiomyocyte apoptosis in hemodynamically challenged hearts [84].

We recently identified a small molecule able to inhibit AKAP-Lbc-mediated RhoA activation and oncogenic signaling in metastatic prostate cancer cells [96]. While these studies suggest that AKAP-Lbc might represent a potential target in anticancer therapy, one has to consider that compounds inhibiting AKAP-Lbc signaling could potentially interfere with the protective function of the anchoring protein in cardiac cells. Based on this possibility, it will be crucial to carefully evaluate the chronic effect of such molecules on cardiac function.

In conclusion, based on the experimental evidence accumulated over the past decade one could postulate that manipulating the activity of cardioprotective signaling enzymes anchored to AKAP-Lbc might confer early cardiac protection. However, additional investigations will be necessary to decipher the impact of interfering with the AKAP-Lbc signaling properties on late cardiac remodeling and transition to heart failure.

Acknowledgments: This work was supported by grant 31003A_175838 of the Swiss National Science Foundation (to D.D.).

Author Contributions: D.D. conceived the outline of the manuscript; D.D., H.O. and E.R. prepared the manuscript and the Figures.

Conflicts of Interest: The authors declare no conflict of interest.

References

1. Towbin, J.A.; Bowles, N.E. The failing heart. *Nature* **2002**, *415*, 227–233. [CrossRef] [PubMed]
2. Xin, M.; Olson, E.N.; Bassel-Duby, R. Mending broken hearts: Cardiac development as a basis for adult heart regeneration and repair. *Nat. Rev. Mol. Cell Biol.* **2013**, *14*, 529–541. [CrossRef] [PubMed]
3. Weber, K.T.; Sun, Y.; Diez, J. Fibrosis: A living tissue and the infarcted heart. *J. Am. Coll. Cardiol.* **2008**, *52*, 2029–2031. [CrossRef] [PubMed]
4. Burchfield, J.S.; Xie, M.; Hill, J.A. Pathological ventricular remodeling: Mechanisms: Part 1 of 2. *Circulation* **2013**, *128*, 388–400. [CrossRef] [PubMed]
5. Diviani, D.; Maric, D.; Lopez, I.P.; Cavin, S.; del Vescovo, C.D. A-kinase anchoring proteins: Molecular regulators of the cardiac stress response. *Biochim. Biophys. Acta* **2013**, *1833*, 901–908. [CrossRef] [PubMed]
6. Sharma, K.; Kass, D.A. Heart failure with preserved ejection fraction: Mechanisms, clinical features, and therapies. *Circ. Res.* **2014**, *115*, 79–96. [CrossRef] [PubMed]
7. Morissette, M.R.; Rosenzweig, A. Targeting survival signaling in heart failure. *Curr. Opin. Pharmacol.* **2005**, *5*, 165–170. [CrossRef] [PubMed]
8. Esseltine, J.L.; Scott, J.D. AKAP signaling complexes: Pointing towards the next generation of therapeutic targets? *Trends Pharmacol. Sci.* **2013**, *34*, 648–655. [CrossRef] [PubMed]
9. Langeberg, L.K.; Scott, J.D. Signalling scaffolds and local organization of cellular behaviour. *Nat. Rev. Mol. Cell Biol.* **2015**, *16*, 232–244. [CrossRef] [PubMed]
10. Dema, A.; Perets, E.; Schulz, M.S.; Deak, V.A.; Klussmann, E. Pharmacological targeting of AKAP-directed compartmentalized cAMP signalling. *Cell. Signal.* **2015**, *27*, 2474–2487. [CrossRef] [PubMed]
11. Cavin, S.; Maric, D.; Diviani, D. A-kinase anchoring protein-Lbc promotes pro-fibrotic signaling in cardiac fibroblasts. *Biochim. Biophys. Acta* **2014**, *1843*, 335–345. [CrossRef] [PubMed]
12. Gold, M.G.; Lygren, B.; Dokurno, P.; Hoshi, N.; McConnachie, G.; Tasken, K.; Carlson, C.R.; Scott, J.D.; Barford, D. Molecular basis of AKAP specificity for PKA regulatory subunits. *Mol. Cell* **2006**, *24*, 383–395. [CrossRef] [PubMed]
13. Kinderman, F.S.; Kim, C.; von Daake, S.; Ma, Y.; Pham, B.Q.; Spraggon, G.; Xuong, N.H.; Jennings, P.A.; Taylor, S.S. A dynamic mechanism for AKAP binding to RII isoforms of cAMP-dependent protein kinase. *Mol. Cell* **2006**, *24*, 397–408. [CrossRef] [PubMed]
14. Klussmann, E. Protein-protein interactions of PDE4 family members—Functions, interactions and therapeutic value. *Cell. Signal* **2016**, *28*, 713–718. [CrossRef] [PubMed]
15. Dessauer, C.W. Adenylyl cyclase—A-kinase anchoring protein complexes: The next dimension in cAMP signaling. *Mol. Pharmacol.* **2009**, *76*, 935–941. [CrossRef] [PubMed]
16. Kapiloff, M.S.; Piggott, L.A.; Sadana, R.; Li, J.; Heredia, L.A.; Henson, E.; Efendiev, R.; Dessauer, C.W. An adenylyl cyclase-mAKAPβ signaling complex regulates cAMP levels in cardiac myocytes. *J. Biol. Chem.* **2009**, *284*, 23540–23546. [CrossRef] [PubMed]
17. Diviani, D.; Soderling, J.; Scott, J.D. AKAP-Lbc anchors protein kinase A and nucleates Gα 12-selective Rho-mediated stress fiber formation. *J. Biol. Chem.* **2001**, *276*, 44247–44257. [CrossRef] [PubMed]
18. Scott, J.D.; Dessauer, C.W.; Tasken, K. Creating order from chaos: Cellular regulation by kinase anchoring. *Annu. Rev. Pharmacol. Toxicol.* **2013**, *53*, 187–210. [CrossRef] [PubMed]

19. Redden, J.M.; Dodge-Kafka, K.L. AKAP phosphatase complexes in the heart. *J. Cardiovasc. Pharmacol.* **2011**, *58*, 354–362. [CrossRef] [PubMed]
20. Wild, A.R.; Dell'Acqua, M.L. Potential for therapeutic targeting of AKAP signaling complexes in nervous system disorders. *Pharmacol. Ther.* **2017**. [CrossRef] [PubMed]
21. Aye, T.T.; Mohammed, S.; van den Toorn, H.W.; van Veen, T.A.; van der Heyden, M.A.; Scholten, A.; Heck, A.J. Selectivity in enrichment of cAMP-dependent protein kinase regulatory subunits type I and type II and their interactors using modified cAMP affinity resins. *Mol. Cell. Proteom.* **2009**, *8*, 1015–1028. [CrossRef] [PubMed]
22. Aye, T.T.; Soni, S.; van Veen, T.A.; van der Heyden, M.A.; Cappadona, S.; Varro, A.; de Weger, R.A.; de Jonge, N.; Vos, M.A.; Heck, A.J.; et al. Reorganized PKA-AKAP associations in the failing human heart. *J. Mol. Cell. Cardiol.* **2012**, *52*, 511–518. [CrossRef] [PubMed]
23. Diviani, D.; Reggi, E.; Arambasic, M.; Caso, S.; Maric, D. Emerging roles of A-kinase anchoring proteins in cardiovascular pathophysiology. *Biochim. Biophys. Acta* **2016**, *1863*, 1926–1936. [CrossRef] [PubMed]
24. Scott, J.D.; Santana, L.F. A-kinase anchoring proteins: Getting to the heart of the matter. *Circulation* **2010**, *121*, 1264–1271. [CrossRef] [PubMed]
25. Kritzer, M.D.; Li, J.; Dodge-Kafka, K.; Kapiloff, M.S. AKAPs: The architectural underpinnings of local cAMP signaling. *J. Mol. Cell. Cardiol.* **2012**, *52*, 351–358. [CrossRef] [PubMed]
26. Perino, A.; Ghigo, A.; Ferrero, E.; Morello, F.; Santulli, G.; Baillie, G.S.; Damilano, F.; Dunlop, A.J.; Pawson, C.; Walser, R.; et al. Integrating cardiac PIP3 and cAMP signaling through a PKA anchoring function of p110gamma. *Mol. Cell* **2011**, *42*, 84–95. [CrossRef] [PubMed]
27. Lopez, I.P.; Cariolato, L.; Maric, D.; Gillet, L.; Abriel, H.; Diviani, D. A-kinase anchoring protein Lbc coordinates a p38 activating signaling complex controlling compensatory cardiac hypertrophy. *Mol. Cell. Biol.* **2013**, *33*, 2903–2917. [CrossRef] [PubMed]
28. Taglieri, D.M.; Johnson, K.R.; Burmeister, B.T.; Monasky, M.M.; Spindler, M.J.; DeSantiago, J.; Banach, K.; Conklin, B.R.; Carnegie, G.K. The C-terminus of the long AKAP13 isoform (AKAP-Lbc) is critical for development of compensatory cardiac hypertrophy. *J. Mol. Cell. Cardiol.* **2014**, *66*, 27–40. [CrossRef] [PubMed]
29. Caso, S.; Maric, D.; Arambasic, M.; Cotecchia, S.; Diviani, D. AKAP-Lbc mediates protection against doxorubicin-induced cardiomyocyte toxicity. *Biochim. Biophys. Acta* **2017**, *1864*, 2336–2346. [CrossRef] [PubMed]
30. Wong, W.; Goehring, A.S.; Kapiloff, M.S.; Langeberg, L.K.; Scott, J.D. mAKAP compartmentalizes oxygen-dependent control of HIF-1α, Science Signaling. *Sci. Signal.* **2008**, *1*, ra18. [CrossRef] [PubMed]
31. Li, X.; Matta, S.M.; Sullivan, R.D.; Bahouth, S.W. Carvedilol reverses cardiac insufficiency in AKAP5 knockout mice by normalizing the activities of calcineurin and CaMKII. *Cardiovasc. Res.* **2014**, *104*, 270–279. [CrossRef] [PubMed]
32. Perrino, C.; Feliciello, A.; Schiattarella, G.G.; Esposito, G.; Guerriero, R.; Zaccaro, L.; del Gatto, A.; Saviano, M.; Garbi, C.; Carangi, R.; et al. AKAP121 downregulation impairs protective cAMP signals, promotes mitochondrial dysfunction, and increases oxidative stress. *Cardiovasc. Res.* **2010**, *88*, 101–110. [CrossRef] [PubMed]
33. Kim, H.; Scimia, M.C.; Wilkinson, D.; Trelles, R.D.; Wood, M.R.; Bowtell, D.; Dillin, A.; Mercola, M.; Ronai, Z.A. Fine-tuning of Drp1/Fis1 availability by AKAP121/Siah2 regulates mitochondrial adaptation to hypoxia. *Mol. Cell* **2011**, *44*, 532–544. [CrossRef] [PubMed]
34. Selvaraju, V.; Suresh, S.C.; Thirunavukkarasu, M.; Mannu, J.; Foye, J.L.C.; Mathur, P.P.; Palesty, J.A.; Sanchez, J.A.; McFadden, D.W.; Maulik, N. Regulation of A-Kinase-Anchoring Protein 12 by Heat Shock Protein A12B to Prevent Ventricular Dysfunction Following Acute Myocardial Infarction in Diabetic Rats. *J. Cardiovasc. Transl. Res.* **2017**, *10*, 209–220. [CrossRef] [PubMed]
35. Li, L.; Li, J.; Drum, B.M.; Chen, Y.; Yin, H.; Guo, X.; Luckey, S.W.; Gilbert, M.L.; McKnight, G.S.; Scott, J.D.; et al. Loss of AKAP150 promotes pathological remodelling and heart failure propensity by disrupting calcium cycling and contractile reserve. *Cardiovasc. Res.* **2017**, *113*, 147–159. [CrossRef] [PubMed]
36. Schiattarella, G.G.; Cattaneo, F.; Pironti, G.; Magliulo, F.; Carotenuto, G.; Pirozzi, M.; Polishchuk, R.; Borzacchiello, D.; Paolillo, R.; Oliveti, M.; et al. Akap1 Deficiency Promotes Mitochondrial Aberrations and Exacerbates Cardiac Injury Following Permanent Coronary Ligation via Enhanced Mitophagy and Apoptosis. *PLoS ONE* **2016**, *11*, e0154076. [CrossRef] [PubMed]
37. Lochner, A.; Genade, S.; Tromp, E.; Podzuweit, T.; Moolman, J.A. Ischemic preconditioning and the β-adrenergic signal transduction pathway. *Circulation* **1999**, *100*, 958–966. [CrossRef] [PubMed]

38. Inserte, J.; Garcia-Dorado, D.; Ruiz-Meana, M.; Agullo, L.; Pina, P.; Soler-Soler, J. Ischemic preconditioning attenuates calpain-mediated degradation of structural proteins through a protein kinase A-dependent mechanism. *Cardiovasc. Res.* **2004**, *64*, 105–114. [CrossRef] [PubMed]

39. Salie, R.; Moolman, J.A.; Lochner, A. The role of β-adrenergic receptors in the cardioprotective effects of β-preconditioning (βPC). *Cardiovasc. Drugs Ther.* **2011**, *25*, 31–46. [CrossRef] [PubMed]

40. Ye, Y.; Keyes, K.T.; Zhang, C.; Perez-Polo, J.R.; Lin, Y.; Birnbaum, Y. The myocardial infarct size-limiting effect of sitagliptin is PKA-dependent, whereas the protective effect of pioglitazone is partially dependent on PKA. *Am. J. Physiol. Heart Circ. Physiol.* **2010**, *298*, H1454–H1465. [CrossRef] [PubMed]

41. Nishida, H.; Sato, T.; Miyazaki, M.; Nakaya, H. Infarct size limitation by adrenomedullin: Protein kinase A but not PI3-kinase is linked to mitochondrial KCa channels. *Cardiovasc. Res.* **2008**, *77*, 398–405. [CrossRef] [PubMed]

42. Jonassen, A.K.; Wergeland, A.; Helgeland, E.; Mjos, O.D.; Brar, B.K. Activation of corticotropin releasing factor receptor type 2 in the heart by corticotropin releasing factor offers cytoprotection against ischemic injury via PKA and PKC dependent signaling. *Regul. Pept.* **2012**, *174*, 90–97. [CrossRef] [PubMed]

43. Zhang, Y.; Wang, X.L.; Zhao, J.; Wang, Y.J.; Lau, W.B.; Yuan, Y.X.; Gao, E.H.; Koch, W.J.; Ma, X.L. Adiponectin inhibits oxidative/nitrative stress during myocardial ischemia and reperfusion via PKA signaling. *Am. J. Physiol. Endocrinol. Metab.* **2013**, *305*, E1436–E1443. [CrossRef] [PubMed]

44. Younce, C.W.; Burmeister, M.A.; Ayala, J.E. Exendin-4 attenuates high glucose-induced cardiomyocyte apoptosis via inhibition of endoplasmic reticulum stress and activation of SERCA2a. *Am. J. Physiol. Cell Physiol.* **2013**, *304*, C508–C518. [CrossRef] [PubMed]

45. Kobashigawa, L.C.; Xu, Y.C.; Padbury, J.F.; Tseng, Y.T.; Yano, N. Metformin protects cardiomyocyte from doxorubicin induced cytotoxicity through an AMP-activated protein kinase dependent signaling pathway: An in vitro study. *PLoS ONE* **2014**, *9*, e104888. [CrossRef] [PubMed]

46. Chen, H.; Wang, X.; Tong, M.; Wu, D.; Wu, S.; Chen, J.; Wang, X.; Wang, X.; Kang, Y.; Tang, H.; et al. Intermedin suppresses pressure overload cardiac hypertrophy through activation of autophagy. *PLoS ONE* **2013**, *8*, e64757. [CrossRef] [PubMed]

47. Fan, G.C.; Chu, G.; Mitton, B.; Song, Q.; Yuan, Q.; Kranias, E.G. Small heat-shock protein Hsp20 phosphorylation inhibits β-agonist-induced cardiac apoptosis. *Circ. Res.* **2004**, *94*, 1474–1482. [CrossRef] [PubMed]

48. Fan, G.C.; Yuan, Q.; Song, G.; Wang, Y.; Chen, G.; Qian, J.; Zhou, X.; Lee, Y.J.; Ashraf, M.; Kranias, E.G. Small heat-shock protein Hsp20 attenuates β-agonist-mediated cardiac remodeling through apoptosis signal-regulating kinase 1. *Circ. Res.* **2006**, *99*, 1233–1242. [CrossRef] [PubMed]

49. McCarroll, C.S.; He, W.; Foote, K.; Bradley, A.; McGlynn, K.; Vidler, F.; Nixon, C.; Nather, K.; Fattah, C.; Riddell, A.; et al. Runx1 Deficiency Protects Against Adverse Cardiac Remodeling After Myocardial Infarction. *Circulation* **2018**, *137*, 57–70. [CrossRef] [PubMed]

50. Backs, J.; Worst, B.C.; Lehmann, L.H.; Patrick, D.M.; Jebessa, Z.; Kreusser, M.M.; Sun, Q.; Chen, L.; Heft, C.; Katus, H.A.; et al. Selective repression of MEF2 activity by PKA-dependent proteolysis of HDAC4. *J. Cell Biol.* **2011**, *195*, 403–415. [CrossRef] [PubMed]

51. Ha, C.H.; Kim, J.Y.; Zhao, J.; Wang, W.; Jhun, B.S.; Wong, C.; Jin, Z.G. PKA phosphorylates histone deacetylase 5 and prevents its nuclear export, leading to the inhibition of gene transcription and cardiomyocyte hypertrophy. *Proc. Natl. Acad. Sci. USA* **2010**, *107*, 15467–15472. [CrossRef] [PubMed]

52. Zhang, C.L.; McKinsey, T.A.; Chang, S.; Antos, C.L.; Hill, J.A.; Olson, E.N. Class II histone deacetylases act as signal-responsive repressors of cardiac hypertrophy. *Cell* **2002**, *110*, 479–488. [CrossRef]

53. Wang, Q.; Oka, T.; Yamagami, K.; Lee, J.K.; Akazawa, H.; Naito, A.T.; Yasui, T.; Ishizu, T.; Nakaoka, Y.; Sakata, Y.; et al. An EP4 Receptor Agonist Inhibits Cardiac Fibrosis Through Activation of PKA Signaling in Hypertrophied Heart. *Int. Heart J.* **2017**, *58*, 107–114. [CrossRef] [PubMed]

54. Azeez, K.R.A.; Knapp, S.; Fernandes, J.M.; Klussmann, E.; Elkins, J.M. The crystal structure of the RhoA-AKAP-Lbc DH-PH domain complex. *Biochem. J.* **2014**, *464*, 231–239. [CrossRef] [PubMed]

55. Zheng, Y.; Olson, M.F.; Hall, A.; Cerione, R.A.; Toksoz, D. Direct involvement of the small GTP-binding protein Rho in lbc oncogene function. *J. Biol. Chem.* **1995**, *270*, 9031–9034. [CrossRef] [PubMed]

56. Toksoz, D.; Williams, D.A. Novel human oncogene lbc detected by transfection with distinct homology regions to signal transduction products. *Oncogene* **1994**, *9*, 621–628. [PubMed]
57. Appert-Collin, A.; Cotecchia, S.; Nenniger-Tosato, M.; Pedrazzini, T.; Diviani, D. The A-kinase anchoring protein (AKAP)-Lbc-signaling complex mediates α1 adrenergic receptor-induced cardiomyocyte hypertrophy. *Proc. Natl. Acad. Sci. USA* **2007**, *104*, 10140–10145. [CrossRef] [PubMed]
58. Martin, J.W.; Cavagnini, K.S.; Brawley, D.N.; Berkley, C.Y.; Smolski, W.; Garcia, R.G.; Towne, A.L.; Sims, J.R.; Meigs, T.E. A Gα12-specific Binding Domain in AKAP-Lbc and p114RhoGEF. *J. Mol. Signal.* **2016**, *11*. [CrossRef]
59. Carnegie, G.K.; Soughayer, J.; Smith, F.D.; Pedroja, B.S.; Zhang, F.; Diviani, D.; Bristow, M.R.; Kunkel, M.T.; Newton, A.C.; Langeberg, L.K.; et al. AKAP-Lbc mobilizes a cardiac hypertrophy signaling pathway. *Mol. Cell* **2008**, *32*, 169–179. [CrossRef] [PubMed]
60. Cariolato, L.; Cavin, S.; Diviani, D. A-Kinase Anchoring Protein (AKAP)-Lbc Anchors a PKN-based Signaling Complex Involved in α1-Adrenergic Receptor-induced p38 Activation. *J. Biol. Chem.* **2011**, *286*, 7925–7937. [CrossRef] [PubMed]
61. Edwards, H.V.; Scott, J.D.; Baillie, G.S. The A-kinase-anchoring protein AKAP-Lbc facilitates cardioprotective PKA phosphorylation of Hsp20 on Ser(16). *Biochem. J.* **2012**, *446*, 437–443. [CrossRef] [PubMed]
62. Liao, P.; Georgakopoulos, D.; Kovacs, A.; Zheng, M.; Lerner, D.; Pu, H.; Saffitz, J.; Chien, K.; Xiao, R.P.; Kass, D.A.; et al. The in vivo role of p38 MAP kinases in cardiac remodeling and restrictive cardiomyopathy. *Proc. Natl. Acad. Sci. USA* **2001**, *98*, 12283–12288. [CrossRef] [PubMed]
63. Nishida, K.; Yamaguchi, O.; Hirotani, S.; Hikoso, S.; Higuchi, Y.; Watanabe, T.; Takeda, T.; Osuka, S.; Morita, T.; Kondoh, G.; et al. p38α mitogen-activated protein kinase plays a critical role in cardiomyocyte survival but not in cardiac hypertrophic growth in response to pressure overload. *Mol. Cell. Biol.* **2004**, *24*, 10611–10620. [CrossRef] [PubMed]
64. Braz, J.C.; Bueno, O.F.; Liang, Q.; Wilkins, B.J.; Dai, Y.S.; Parsons, S.; Braunwart, J.; Glascock, B.J.; Klevitsky, R.; Kimball, T.F.; et al. Targeted inhibition of p38 MAPK promotes hypertrophic cardiomyopathy through upregulation of calcineurin-NFAT signaling. *J. Clin. Investig.* **2003**, *111*, 1475–1486. [CrossRef] [PubMed]
65. Zhang, S.; Weinheimer, C.; Courtois, M.; Kovacs, A.; Zhang, C.E.; Cheng, A.M.; Wang, Y.; Muslin, A.J. The role of the Grb2-p38 MAPK signaling pathway in cardiac hypertrophy and fibrosis. *J. Clin. Investig.* **2003**, *111*, 833–841. [CrossRef] [PubMed]
66. Martindale, J.J.; Wall, J.A.; Martinez-Longoria, D.M.; Aryal, P.; Rockman, H.A.; Guo, Y.; Bolli, R.; Glembotski, C.C. Overexpression of mitogen-activated protein kinase kinase 6 in the heart improves functional recovery from ischemia in vitro and protects against myocardial infarction in vivo. *J. Biol. Chem.* **2005**, *280*, 669–676. [CrossRef] [PubMed]
67. Streicher, J.M.; Ren, S.; Herschman, H.; Wang, Y. MAPK-Activated Protein Kinase-2 in Cardiac Hypertrophy and Cyclooxygenase-2 Regulation in Heart. *Circ. Res.* **2010**, *106*, 1434–1443. [CrossRef] [PubMed]
68. Marber, M.S.; Rose, B.; Wang, Y. The p38 mitogen-activated protein kinase pathway—A potential target for intervention in infarction, hypertrophy, and heart failure. *J. Mol. Cell. Cardiol.* **2011**, *51*, 485–490. [CrossRef] [PubMed]
69. Hernandez, G.; Lal, H.; Fidalgo, M.; Guerrero, A.; Zalvide, J.; Force, T.; Pombo, C.M. A novel cardioprotective p38-MAPK/mTOR pathway. *Exp. Cell Res.* **2011**, *317*, 2938–2949. [CrossRef] [PubMed]
70. Carnegie, G.K.; Smith, F.D.; McConnachie, G.; Langeberg, L.K.; Scott, J.D. AKAP-Lbc nucleates a protein kinase D activation scaffold. *Mol. Cell* **2004**, *15*, 889–899. [CrossRef] [PubMed]
71. Johnson, K.R.; Nicodemus-Johnson, J.; Spindler, M.J.; Carnegie, G.K. Genome-Wide Gene Expression Analysis Shows AKAP13-Mediated PKD1 Signaling Regulates the Transcriptional Response to Cardiac Hypertrophy. *PLoS ONE* **2015**, *10*, e0132474. [CrossRef] [PubMed]
72. Brown, S.A.; Sandhu, N.; Herrmann, J. Systems biology approaches to adverse drug effects: The example of cardio-oncology. *Nat. Rev. Clin. Oncol.* **2015**, *12*, 718–731. [CrossRef] [PubMed]
73. Cardinale, D.; Colombo, A.; Bacchiani, G.; Tedeschi, I.; Meroni, C.A.; Veglia, F.; Civelli, M.; Lamantia, G.; Colombo, N.; Curigliano, G.; et al. Early detection of anthracycline cardiotoxicity and improvement with heart failure therapy. *Circulation* **2015**, *131*, 1981–1988. [CrossRef] [PubMed]
74. Chatterjee, K.; Zhang, J.; Honbo, N.; Karliner, J.S. Doxorubicin cardiomyopathy. *Cardiology* **2010**, *115*, 155–162. [CrossRef] [PubMed]

75. Octavia, Y.; Tocchetti, C.G.; Gabrielson, K.L.; Janssens, S.; Crijns, H.J.; Moens, A.L. Doxorubicin-induced cardiomyopathy: From molecular mechanisms to therapeutic strategies. *J. Mol. Cell. Cardiol.* **2012**, *52*, 1213–1225. [CrossRef] [PubMed]

76. Palmeira, C.M.; Serrano, J.; Kuehl, D.W.; Wallace, K.B. Preferential oxidation of cardiac mitochondrial DNA following acute intoxication with doxorubicin. *Biochim. Biophys. Acta* **1997**, *1321*, 101–106. [CrossRef]

77. Fajardo, G.; Zhao, M.; Berry, G.; Wong, L.J.; Mochly-Rosen, D.; Bernstein, D. β2-adrenergic receptors mediate cardioprotection through crosstalk with mitochondrial cell death pathways. *J. Mol. Cell. Cardiol.* **2011**, *51*, 781–789. [CrossRef] [PubMed]

78. Kobe, B.; Heierhorst, J.; Feil, S.C.; Parker, M.W.; Benian, G.M.; Weiss, K.R.; Kemp, B.E. Giant protein kinases: Domain interactions and structural basis of autoregulation. *EMBO J.* **1996**, *15*, 6810–6821. [PubMed]

79. De Francesco, E.M.; Rocca, C.; Scavello, F.; Amelio, D.; Pasqua, T.; Rigiracciolo, D.C.; Scarpelli, A.; Avino, S.; Cirillo, F.; Amodio, N.; et al. Protective Role of GPER Agonist G-1 on Cardiotoxicity Induced by Doxorubicin. *J. Cell. Physiol.* **2017**, *232*, 1640–1649. [CrossRef] [PubMed]

80. Aries, A.; Paradis, P.; Lefebvre, C.; Schwartz, R.J.; Nemer, M. Essential role of GATA-4 in cell survival and drug-induced cardiotoxicity. *Proc. Natl. Acad. Sci. USA* **2004**, *101*, 6975–6980. [CrossRef] [PubMed]

81. Lebrecht, D.; Geist, A.; Ketelsen, U.P.; Haberstroh, J.; Setzer, B.; Walker, U.A. Dexrazoxane prevents doxorubicin-induced long-term cardiotoxicity and protects myocardial mitochondria from genetic and functional lesions in rats. *Br. J. Pharmacol.* **2007**, *151*, 771–778. [CrossRef] [PubMed]

82. Ghigo, A.; Li, M.; Hirsch, E. New signal transduction paradigms in anthracycline-induced cardiotoxicity. *Biochim. Biophys. Acta* **2016**, *1863*, 1916–1925. [CrossRef] [PubMed]

83. Huang, Y.; Wright, C.D.; Merkwan, C.L.; Baye, N.L.; Liang, Q.; Simpson, P.C.; O'Connell, T.D. An α1A-adrenergic-extracellular signal-regulated kinase survival signaling pathway in cardiac myocytes. *Circulation* **2007**, *115*, 763–772. [CrossRef] [PubMed]

84. Beak, J.; Huang, W.; Parker, J.S.; Hicks, S.T.; Patterson, C.; Simpson, P.C.; Ma, A.; Jin, J.; Jensen, B.C. An Oral Selective α-1A Adrenergic Receptor Agonist Prevents Doxorubicin Cardiotoxicity. *JACC Basic Transl. Sci.* **2017**, *2*, 39–53. [CrossRef] [PubMed]

85. Xiang, S.Y.; Ouyang, K.; Yung, B.S.; Miyamoto, S.; Smrcka, A.V.; Chen, J.; Brown, J.H. PLCepsilon, PKD1, and SSH1L transduce RhoA signaling to protect mitochondria from oxidative stress in the heart. *Sci. Signal.* **2013**, *6*, ra108. [CrossRef] [PubMed]

86. Fan, G.C.; Ren, X.; Qian, J.; Yuan, Q.; Nicolaou, P.; Wang, Y.; Jones, W.K.; Chu, G.; Kranias, E.G. Novel cardioprotective role of a small heat-shock protein, Hsp20, against ischemia/reperfusion injury. *Circulation* **2005**, *111*, 1792–1799. [CrossRef] [PubMed]

87. Fan, G.C.; Zhou, X.; Wang, X.; Song, G.; Qian, J.; Nicolaou, P.; Chen, G.; Ren, X.; Kranias, E.G. Heat shock protein 20 interacting with phosphorylated Akt reduces doxorubicin-triggered oxidative stress and cardiotoxicity. *Circ. Res.* **2008**, *103*, 1270–1279. [CrossRef] [PubMed]

88. Edwards, H.V.; Scott, J.D.; Baillie, G.S. PKA phosphorylation of the small heat-shock protein Hsp20 enhances its cardioprotective effects. *Biochem. Soc. Trans.* **2012**, *40*, 210–214. [CrossRef] [PubMed]

89. Nicolaou, P.; Knoll, R.; Haghighi, K.; Fan, G.C.; Dorn, G.W., 2nd; Hasenfub, G.; Kranias, E.G. Human mutation in the anti-apoptotic heat shock protein 20 abrogates its cardioprotective effects. *J. Biol. Chem.* **2008**, *283*, 33465–33471. [CrossRef] [PubMed]

90. Niethammer, M.; Kim, E.; Sheng, M. Interaction between the C terminus of NMDA receptor subunits and multiple members of the PSD-95 family of membrane-associated granylate kinases. *J. Neurosci.* **1996**, *16*, 2157–2163. [PubMed]

91. Sin, Y.Y.; Edwards, H.V.; Li, X.; Day, J.P.; Christian, F.; Dunlop, A.J.; Adams, D.R.; Zaccolo, M.; Houslay, M.D.; Baillie, G.S. Disruption of the cyclic AMP phosphodiesterase-4 (PDE4)-HSP20 complex attenuates the β-agonist induced hypertrophic response in cardiac myocytes. *J. Mol. Cell. Cardiol.* **2011**, *50*, 872–883. [CrossRef] [PubMed]

92. Wang, L.; Burmeister, B.T.; Johnson, K.R.; Baillie, G.S.; Karginov, A.V.; Skidgel, R.A.; O'Bryan, J.P.; Carnegie, G.K. UCR1C is a novel activator of phosphodiesterase 4 (PDE4) long isoforms and attenuates cardiomyocyte hypertrophy. *Cell. Signal.* **2015**, *27*, 908–922. [CrossRef] [PubMed]

93. Sin, Y.Y.; Baillie, G.S. Heat shock protein 20 (HSP20) is a novel substrate for protein kinase D1 (PKD1). *Cell Biochem. Funct.* **2015**, *33*, 421–426. [CrossRef] [PubMed]

94. Hill, J.A.; Olson, E.N. Cardiac plasticity. *N. Eng. J. Med.* **2008**, *358*, 1370–1380. [CrossRef] [PubMed]

J. Cardiovasc. Dev. Dis. **2018**, *5*, 12

95. Shende, P.; Plaisance, I.; Morandi, C.; Pellieux, C.; Berthonneche, C.; Zorzato, F.; Krishnan, J.; Lerch, R.; Hall, M.N.; Ruegg, M.A.; et al. Cardiac raptor ablation impairs adaptive hypertrophy, alters metabolic gene expression, and causes heart failure in mice. *Circulation* **2011**, *123*, 1073. [CrossRef] [PubMed]
96. Diviani, D.; Raimondi, F.; Del Vescovo, C.D.; Dreyer, E.; Reggi, E.; Osman, H.; Ruggieri, L.; Gonano, C.; Cavin, S.; Box, C.L.; et al. Small-Molecule Protein-Protein Interaction Inhibitor of Oncogenic Rho Signaling. *Cell Chem. Biol.* **2016**, *23*, 1135–1146.

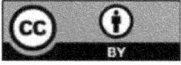

Journal of
Cardiovascular
Development and Disease

MDPI

Review

Epac Function and cAMP Scaffolds in the Heart and Lung

Marion Laudette [1,†]**, Haoxiao Zuo** [2,3,*,†]**, Frank Lezoualc'h** [1] **and Martina Schmidt** [2,3]

1   Inserm UMR-1048, Institut des Maladies Métaboliques et Cardiovasculaires, Université Toulouse III,
    31432 Toulouse, France; marion.laudette@inserm.fr (M.L.); Frank.Lezoualch@inserm.fr (F.L.)
2   Department of Molecular Pharmacology, University of Groningen, 9713AV Groningen, The Netherlands;
    m.schmidt@rug.nl
3   Groningen Research Institute for Asthma and COPD (GRIAC), University Medical Center Groningen,
    University of Groningen, 9713AV Groningen, The Netherlands
*   Correspondence: h.zuo@rug.nl; Tel.: +31-50-363-3321
†   These authors contributed equally to this work.

Received: 12 January 2018; Accepted: 29 January 2018; Published: 3 February 2018

Abstract: Evidence collected over the last ten years indicates that Epac and cAMP scaffold proteins play a critical role in integrating and transducing multiple signaling pathways at the basis of cardiac and lung physiopathology. Some of the deleterious effects of Epac, such as cardiomyocyte hypertrophy and arrhythmia, initially described in vitro, have been confirmed in genetically modified mice for Epac1 and Epac2. Similar recent findings have been collected in the lung. The following sections will describe how Epac and cAMP signalosomes in different subcellular compartments may contribute to cardiac and lung diseases.

Keywords: cAMP; Epac; compartmentalization; A-kinase anchoring proteins; phosphodiesterases

1. Introduction

In the current manuscript, we aim to highlight the most recent insights into signaling by one of the most ancient second messengers cyclic AMP (cAMP). We focus on novel aspects of cAMP scaffolds maintained by a diverse subset of proteins, among them receptors, exchange proteins, phosphodiesterases, and A-kinase anchoring proteins. We will start with the cardiac system and will then proceed with the lung.

2. Epac in Cardiac Disease

Cyclic AMP (cAMP) is one the most important second messengers in the heart because it regulates many physiological processes, such as cardiac contractility and relaxation. The β-adrenergic receptor (β-AR) belongs to the G protein-coupled receptor (GPCR) superfamily, and is essential for the adaptation of cardiac performance to physiological needs. Upon stimulation of β-AR by noradrenaline (released from cardiac sympathetic nervous endings) and circulating adrenaline, cAMP is produced and activates protein kinase A (PKA), which phosphorylates many of the components involved in the excitation-coupling mechanisms, such as L-type the calcium channel (LTCC), phospholamban (PLB), cardiac myosin binding protein C (cMyBPC), and the ryanodine receptor 2 (RyR2), to modulate their activity [1]. Activation of LTCCs produces an inward Ca^{2+} current (ICa) that activates RyR2 through the mechanism known as Ca^{2+}-induced Ca^{2+} release (CICR), which raises cytosolic Ca^{2+} concentration and activates contraction. Whereas PKA-dependent LTCC and RyR2 phosphorylation results in mobilization of Ca^{2+} available for contraction, PKA-mediated phosphorylation of phospholamban, a peptide inhibitor of sarcoplasmic reticulum (SR) Ca^{2+}-ATPase promotes increased Ca^{2+} reuptake in the SR, thereby removing Ca^{2+} from the cytoplasm and accounting for relaxation [1]. In addition, binding of cAMP to hyperpolarization-activated cyclic nucleotide-gated (HCN) channels that carry the pacemaker current, increases heart rate in response to a sympathetic stimulation (chronotropic effect). From the three β-adrenergic subtypes expressed in the mammalian heart, regulation of cardiac function is ascribed to the β_1- and β_2-adrenergic receptor subtypes [2].

Although acute stimulation of the β-AR pathway has beneficial effects on heart function, a sustained activation of β-AR contributes to the development of pathological cardiac remodeling by inducing ventricular hypertrophy, fibrosis, and ultimately, arrhythmia and heart failure (HF), one of the most prevalent causes of mortality globally [3–5]. Toxic effects of sustained β-AR stimulation are consistent with the finding that in HF patients, elevated plasma catecholamine levels correlate with the degree of ventricular dysfunction and mortality [6]. However, β-blocker therapy in HF may appear counterintuitive, as catecholamines represent the main trigger of cardiac contractility and relaxation. Indeed, β-blockers restore the adrenergic signaling system which is desensitized by high and chronic concentrations of catecholamines [3]. Thus, it is not so much to block the whole adrenergic signaling which seems important, but rather to modulate its different aspects. It is in this context that several research groups are interested in understanding the role of exchange proteins directly activated by cAMP (Epac) proteins in the development of cardiac arrhythmia and HF [4].

Evidence collected over the last ten years indicates that Epac proteins play a critical role in integrating and transducing multiple signaling pathways at the basis of cardiac physiopathology. Some of the deleterious effects of Epac, such as cardiomyocyte hypertrophy and arrhythmia, initially described in vitro, have been confirmed in genetically modified mice for Epac1 and Epac2. The following sections will describe how Epac signalosomes in different subcellular compartments of the cardiomyocyte may contribute to cardiac disease.

2.1. Epac Signalosome in Pathological Cardiac Remodeling

Given the importance of the β-AR-cAMP pathway in cardiac pathophysiology, several studies aim to investigate the role of Epac proteins in the development of cardiac remodeling and HF. Remodeling pathological disorder comprises multiple attacks of which the best described are the modification of the geometry of the cardiac cavity associated with cardiomyocyte hypertrophy, fibrosis, and alterations of calcium handling and energy metabolism [7]. In the long term, these changes affect cardiac contractility and favor progression of HF, a process predominantly relying on cardiac signaling in response to the β_1-AR subtype.

Among the two Epac isoforms, Epac1 expression was found to be upregulated in various models of cardiac hypertrophy, such as chronic catecholamine infusion and pressure overload induced by thoracic aortic constriction, as well as in the end stages of human HF [8,9]. On the contrary, the anti-hypertrophic action of some hormones and microRNA, including the growth hormone-releasing hormone and microRNA-133, involves Epac1 inhibition [10,11]. A more direct evidence of Epac1's role in the regulation of cardiac remodeling came from the observation that Epac1 overexpression, or its direct activation with the Epac1 preferential agonist, 8-pCPT-2-O-Me-cAMP (8-CPT), increased various markers of cardiomyocyte hypertrophy, such as protein synthesis and hypertrophic genes in primary ventricular myocytes [8,12,13]. It is hypothesized that in the setting of cardiac remodeling, adaptive autophagy antagonizes Epac1-induced cardiac hypertrophy [14]. In vitro studies revealed that the pharmacological inhibition of Epac1 by a tetrahydroquinoline analogue, CE3F4, prevented the induction of cardiomyocyte hypertrophy markers in response to a prolonged β-AR stimulation in rat ventricular myocytes [14–16]. These findings indicate that Epac1 signaling may provide a novel means for the treatment of pathological cardiac hypertrophy. It is worth mentioning that Epac1 has also been recently identified as a potential mediator of radiation-induced cardiomyocyte hypertrophy, suggesting that this cAMP-sensor is involved in the side effects of anticancer therapy [17].

Compelling evidence indicates that Epac1 signalosome is highly compartmentalized and occurs in several micro subcellular compartments, such as the plasma membrane, sarcoplasm, and the nuclear/perinuclear region of cardiomyocytes [8,18–20]. A macromolecular complex containing the scaffolding protein β-arrestin, Epac1, and Ca^{2+}/calmodulin-dependent protein kinase II (CaMKII), has been reported in the heart [21]. Epac1 constitutively interacts with the β-arrestin in the cytoplasm under basal conditions. Stimulation of $β_1$-AR, but not $β_2$-AR, induces the recruitment of β-arrestin–Epac1 signaling complex at the plasma membrane, whereby it activates a pro-hypertrophic signaling cascade involving the small GTPases Rap2 and Ras, and CaMKII [22]. This acts as a trigger for histone deacetylase type 4 (HDAC4) nuclear export, which initiates a pro-hypertrophic gene program (Figure 1). Interestingly, Epac1 is prevented from undertaking similar signaling at the $β_2$-AR, as the cAMP-hydrolyzing enzyme, phosphodiesterase (PDE)4D5, impedes the interaction of Epac1 with β-arrestin, and therefore its recruitment to activated $β_2$-AR. Of particular importance, disruption of PDE4D5–β-arrestin complex formation with a cell-permeant peptide promotes binding of Epac1–β-arrestin to $β_2$-AR and, consequently $β_2$-AR signaling switches to a $β_1$-AR-like pro-hypertrophic signaling to increase cardiac myocyte remodeling [22]. Taken together, these data provide evidence that Epac compartmentalization contributes to the functional differences between cardiac β-AR subtypes.

Besides its sarcolemma distribution, Epac1 is also concentrated in the nuclear/perinuclear region of cardiomyocytes, positioned well to regulate nuclear signaling [8,20]. Specifically, it was shown that Epac1 is scaffolded at the nuclear envelope with phospholipase C (PLC)ε and muscle-specific A-kinase anchoring proteins (AKAPs) to regulate the hypertrophic gene program in primary cardiomyocytes [19,23,24] (Figure 1). Interestingly, a detailed analysis of Ca^{2+} mobilization in different microdomains demonstrated that Epac (probably Epac1) preferentially elevated Ca^{2+} in the nucleoplasm, correlating with the perinuclear/nuclear localization of Epac1 [25]. Additional in vitro studies showed that Epac1, via its downstream effector, the small G protein Rap2, activated PLC to promote the production of inositol 1,4,5-trisphosphate (IP_3) [26]. Based on this finding, a working hypothesis has been proposed, whereby Epac1 can activate PLC, causing nuclear Ca^{2+} increase via perinuclear IP_3 receptor (IP3-R), which results in the activation of Ca^{2+}-dependent transcription factors involved in cardiac remodeling [25,27] (Figure 1). Consistently, in cultured cardiomyocytes, it has been reported that Epac activates CaMKII to induce the nuclear export of HDAC4 de-repressing the transcription factor myocyte enhancer factor 2 (MEF2) which activates gene transcription, essential for the hypertrophic program [25,26]. Collectively, these findings point to Epac1 role in activating the excitation–transcription coupling, the process by which Ca^{2+} activates gene transcription [27]. Additional Epac hypertrophic signaling have been described and include the GTPase H-Ras, the Ca^{2+} sensitive protein, calcineurin, and its downstream effector, nuclear factor of activated T cells (NFAT), which are key mediators of cardiac remodeling [8,26].

More recently, the study of Epac gene deleted mice has made it possible to better understand the role of these proteins in cardiac pathological remodeling. Global knockout (KO) mice for Epac1 or Epac2, or double full KO for Epac1 and Epac2, do not present any cardiac abnormality, suggesting that these guanine-nucleotide exchange factors activated by cyclic adenosine monophosphate (cAMP-GEFs) do not play a major role during cardiac development [14,28,29]. None of the deletions appreciably affected basal cardiac function. Although Epac has been shown to influence myofilament Ca^{2+} sensitivity in rat cardiomyocytes [18,30], the effects of Epac activation in cell contractility remain controversial, and may depend on the steady-state Ca^{2+} levels at which the myocyte is functioning [18,31–33]. Overall, Epac proteins do not play a major role in the physiological regulation of cardiomyocyte contractility in response to acute β-AR stimulation, compared with PKA, which is the main cAMP effector in this process [29,34]. However, Epac1 genetic inhibition specifically reduces cardiac remodeling induced by chronic activation of β-AR, which confirms the importance of Epac1 in the β-adrenergic signaling during cardiac stress condition [14,28]. Moreover, Epac1 deleted cardiomyocytes prevented 8-CPT-dependent HDAC5 translocation, consistent with its involvement in pathological hypertrophy [20]. Of note, in another model of cardiac hypertrophy induced by aortic stenosis, Epac1 knockdown fails to prevent cardiac hypertrophy, but only fibrosis and cardiomyocyte apoptosis, suggesting that the cardioprotective effects of Epac1 deletion with respect to hypertrophy depend on the nature of stress [19].

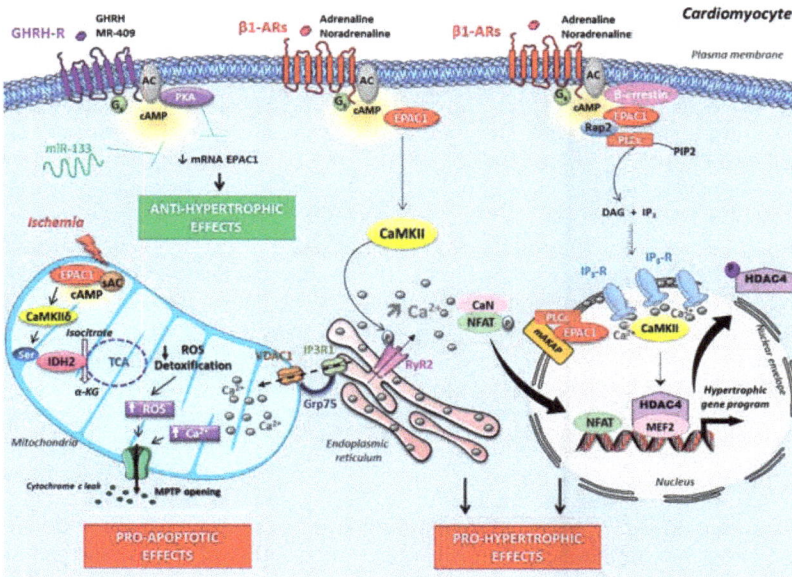

Figure 1. Epac signalosome in cardiac hypertrophy and ischemia. Under adrenergic stimulation, the Epac1–β-arrestin complex is recruited at the $β_1$-AR, and activates a pro-hypertrophic signaling pathway. Epac1 is also scaffolded at the nuclear envelope with phospholipase C (PLC)ε and muscle-specific A-kinase anchoring proteins (mAKAP) to regulate the hypertrophic gene program. In the nuclear/perinuclear region, PLCε increases nuclear Ca^{2+} content via the activation of the perinuclear IP3 receptor (IP3-R). Epac1 hypertrophic signaling also involves CaMKII-dependent phosphorylation of RyR2, leading to Ca^{2+} leak from the sarcoplasmic reticulum and subsequent calcineurin (CaN) activation. The anti-hypertrophic action of the growth hormone-releasing hormone (GHRH) or its agonistic analog, MR-409, involves the protein kinase A (PKA)-dependent inhibition of Epac1 expression. MicroRNA-133 (miR-133) is cardioprotective, and targets several components of $β_1$-AR signaling. In the context of cardiac ischemia, mitochondrial Epac1 (MitEpac1) is activated by cAMP produced by the soluble adenylyl cyclase (sAC), and increases Ca^{2+} overload and ROS accumulation to promote mitochondrial permeability transition pore (MPTP) opening and cardiomyocyte apoptosis. α-KG,α-ketoglutarate; $β_1$-AR, $β_1$-adrenergic receptor; AC, transmembrane adenylyl cyclase; CaMKIIδ, Ca^{2+}/calmodulin-dependent protein kinase II δ-isoform; cAMP, cyclic adenosine monophosphate; DAG, diacylglycerol; GHRH-R, GHRH receptor; GRP75, chaperone glucose-regulated protein 75; HDAC4, histone deacetylase 4; IDH2, isocitrate dehydrogenase 2; IP3, inositol-1,4,5-trisphosphate; IP3R1, IP3 receptor 1; IP3R1, inositol-1,4,5-triphosphate receptor 1; MEF2, myocyte enhancer factor-2; NFAT, nuclear factor of activated T-cells; PIP2, phosphatidylinositol 4,5-biphosphate; ROS, reactive oxygen species; Ser, serine; TCA, tricarboxylic acid cycle; VDAC1, voltage-dependent anion channel 1.

2.2. Role of Epac in Heart Failure and Arrhythmia

Interestingly, Epac1 KO mice show better cardiac contractility (maintenance of the inotropic reserve) and decreased susceptibility to HF in response to different hypertrophic stress conditions (catecholamine infusion or myocardial pressure overload) [14,28]. Further evidence for the cardioprotective effect of Epac1 inhibition came from the recent report that Epac1 deficiency attenuates type 5 adenylyl cyclase-mediated catecholamine stress-induced cardiac dysfunction [35]. It is interesting to note that Epac1 and Epac2 deleted mice are protected from the incidence of atrial and ventricular arrhythmia, respectively, suggesting a specific role of Epac isoforms in cardiac rhythm disorders [28,29]. Conversely, direct pharmacological activation of Epac with the cAMP analogue 8-CPT promotes ventricular arrhythmogenesis in isolated perfused mouse hearts [36]. Such arrhythmogenic features were also observed in rat cardiomyocytes, but after sustained Epac activation [37]. Yet, Brette and colleagues reported that 8-CPT induced an action potential lengthening in rat ventricular myocytes, a process involved in the genesis of arrhythmia by predisposing cardiac myocytes to early after depolarizations and dispersion of repolarization [38].

Mechanistically, few studies demonstrated that mainly Epac1 regulated the expression level of proarrhythmic channels, such as the slow delayed-rectifier potassium K+-current (IKs) subunit potassium voltage-gated channel and transient receptor potential canonical 3 and 4 channels that enhance store-operated Ca^{2+} entry [39,40] (Figure 2). Epac function may also affect susceptibility to arrhythmia via the regulation of gap junction formation [41,42]. Importantly, in isolated ventricular myocytes, activation of Epac with either 8-CPT or β_1-AR induces a spontaneous release of Ca^{2+} from the SR (a process named Ca^{2+} sparks) via the CaMKII-dependent phosphorylation of RyR2 on Serine 2814 or 2815 (depending on the species), thereby causing diastolic Ca^{2+} leak in a PKA-independent manner [29,31–33,43] (Figure 2). Consistent with the localization of Epac2 along T tubules in mouse cardiomyocytes [20], it has been proposed that the increase of ectopic release of Ca^{2+} following Epac2 (and not Epac1) activation by β_1-AR, could be the cause of arrhythmogenic effects in cardiomyocytes [29]. The recent finding that SR Ca^{2+} leak observed upon PDE4 inhibition involves Epac2 suggests that the interaction of PDE4 and Epac2 are critical for coordinating the pro-arrhythmic effect of cAMP [34]. Adding complexity to the matter, another study showed that Epac1 promoted PLB hyperphosphorylation on Serine 16 via PKCε [28]. This could lead to SR Ca^{2+} overload with Ca^{2+} leak and subsequent arrhythmia [28] (Figure 2). Based on the aforementioned studies, the beneficial effect of Epac inhibition seems, therefore, very attractive for the development of novel therapies against HF and arrhythmia. However, few controversies have been reported in the literature. Among them, Yang and colleagues recently reported that pharmacological inhibition of Epac2 with ESI-05 was proarrhythmic in rat [44]. Further pharmacological and genetic studies combining the use of Epac isoform-specific ligands and conditional Epac KO mice are required to better decipher the role of Epac isoforms in cardiac rhythm disorders.

2.3. Role of Mitochondrial Epac in Cardiac Ischemia

Acute myocardial infarction is a leading cause of mortality and morbidity worldwide. Early coronary reperfusion has been established as the best therapeutic strategy to limit infarct size and improve prognosis. However, the process of reperfusion can itself induce cardiomyocyte death, known as myocardial reperfusion injury (I/R), for which there is still no effective therapy [45,46]. Mitochondria have been recognized as playing a central role in both apoptotic and necrotic cell death [47]. Indeed, during I/R injury, cardiomyocyte death is initiated by mitochondrial Ca^{2+} overload and an excessive production of reactive oxygen species (ROS) which trigger the mitochondrial permeability transition pore (MPTP) opening, resulting in mitochondrial depolarization, swelling, and rupture of the external mitochondrial membrane. This leads to the uncoupling of the respiratory chain, and the efflux of cytochrome c and other proapoptotic factors that may induce apoptosis or necrosis [48].

Depending on the nature of the stimulus and the cell type used in the study, Epac may play a proapoptotic or antiapoptotic role [49]. For instance, in neonatal rat cardiomyocytes, Epac cooperates with PKA in the antiapoptotic effects of exendin-4, a glucagon-like peptide-1 receptor agonist [50]. Similarly, activation of both PKA and Epac with cAMP analogues confers cardioprotection against I/R injury in isolated rat heart [51]. Interestingly, it is suggested that long-term feeding of an obesogenic high fat diet renders the myocardium less susceptible to I/R induced injury via Epac-dependent signaling [52]. Yet, recent findings using isolated cardiomyocytes from ischemic rat hearts have implied that the cardioprotective effect induced by urocortin-1 involved the Epac2 pathway [53]. On the contrary, in vivo experiments showed that Epac1 genetic ablation in mice protected against myocardial I/R injury with reduced infarct size and cardiomyocyte apoptosis [54]. Consistent with an earlier finding showing the mitochondrial expression of transfected Epac1 in COS-7 cells [55], Epac1 is expressed in the mitochondrial inner membrane and matrix of cardiomyocytes. A form of Epac1 deleted in its mitochondrial-targeting sequence protects against hypoxia/reoxygenation (a condition mimicking in vivo I/R)-induced cell death, indicating that mitochondrial Epac1 participates in cardiomyocyte death during hypoxic stress [54]. Mechanistic studies demonstrated that during hypoxia/reoxygenation, Epac1 was activated by the type 10 soluble adenylyl cyclase (sAC) to increase mitochondrial Ca^{2+} uptake and ROS production, thereby promoting mitochondrial death signaling, such as MPTP opening, cytochrome c release, and both caspase-9 and -3 activation [54]. However, these results are not in agreement with another study, which reported that direct activation of sAC with HCO_3^- prevented Ca^{2+}-induced MPTP opening through Epac1, suggesting that Epac1 might protect from cardiomyocyte death [56]. The higher amount of cAMP produced in the model of hypoxia/reoxygenation, and subsequent massive increase in mitochondrial ROS and Ca^{2+} levels, could potentially account for the observed differences.

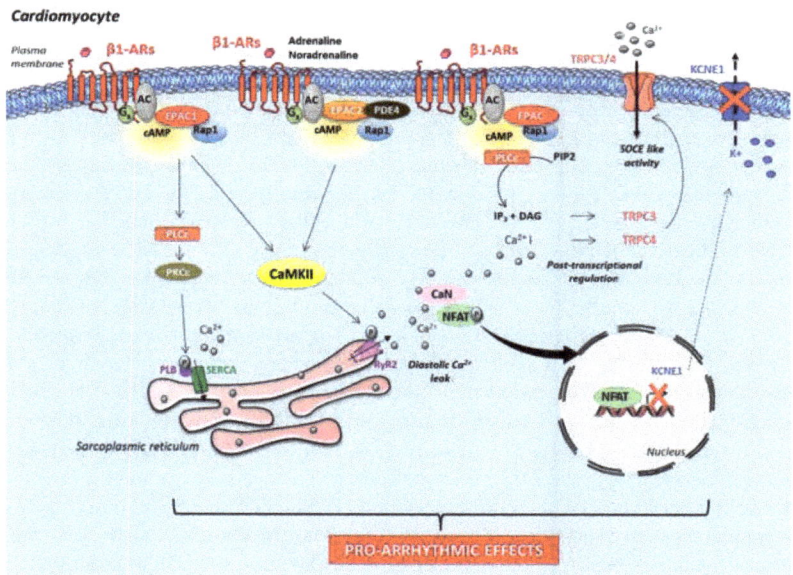

Figure 2. Role of Epac in cardiac arrhythmia. Epac proteins increase the phosphorylation state of the ryanodine receptor 2 (RyR2) via CaMKII, and subsequent Ca^{2+} leak from the sarcoplasmic reticulum (SR) may trigger arrhythmia. Epac1-induced hyperphosphorylation of phospholamban (PLB) may also contribute to the development of arrhythmia and heart failure. In addition, Epac enhances store-operated Ca^{2+} entry (SOCE)-like activity, which is related to an increased amount of functional transient receptor potential canonical (TRPC) 3 (TRCP3) and TRCP4 channels. This additional Ca^{2+} entry pathway in the cardiomyocyte and the downregulation of the potassium voltage-gated channel subfamily E member 1 (KCNE1) participate in the proarrhythmic effect of Epac proteins. β_1-AR, β_1-adrenergic receptor; AC, transmembrane adenylyl cyclase; CaMKII, Ca^{2+}/calmodulin-dependent protein kinase II; cAMP, cyclic adenosine monophosphate; CaN, Calcineurin; DAG, diacylglycerol; IP3, inositol-1,4,5-trisphosphate; P, phosphorylation; PDE4, phosphodiesterase 4; PIP2, phosphatidylinositol 4,5-biphosphate; PKCɛ, protein kinase C epsilon type; PLB, phospholamban; PLCɛ, phospholipase C epsilon type; SERCA, sarcoendoplasmic reticulum calcium transport ATPase.

Interestingly, we found that Epac1 is highly compartmentalized in mitochondria and targets key proteins involved in mitochondrial Ca^{2+} uptake and ROS production. Indeed, firstly, we revealed that Epac1 interrelated with a macromolecular complex composed of the VDAC1 (voltage-dependent anion channel 1), the GRP75 (chaperone glucose-regulated protein 75), and the IP3R1 (inositol-1,4,5-triphosphate receptor 1). This complex localized at the endoplasmic reticulum (ER) junction is considered as a hot spot from Ca^{2+} transfer from the ER to the mitochondria [57]. Under hypoxic condition, Epac1 activation increased the interaction with the VDAC1/GRP75/IP3R1 complex, hence facilitating ER to mitochondrial Ca^{2+} transfer. Epac1-mediated mitochondrial Ca^{2+} overload subsequently provoked MPTP opening, cytochrome c release, and ultimately, cardiomyocyte death [54] (Figure 1). Secondly, our study revealed a key role for Epac1 in the accumulation of mitochondrial ROS production during hypoxia. Surprisingly, we observed that Epac1 imported CaMKII into matrix where they formed a multi-molecular complex with isocitrate dehydrogenase 2 (IDH2), a critical mitochondrial enzyme of the tricarboxylic acid (TCA) cycle involved in ROS detoxification [54]. Mitochondrial Epac1 negatively regulates via the CaMKIIδ-dependent phosphorylation activity of IDH2, and hence, decreases the antioxidant capabilities of the cardiomyocytes during I/R [54] (Figure 1). Altogether, these findings identify Epac1 as a central mechanism for mitochondrial Ca^{2+} entry and ROS production in myocardial cell death, and indicate that mitochondrial-targeted Epac1 inhibition could prevent or reduce myocardial death in the setting of cardiac ischemia.

3. Chronic Obstructive Pulmonary Disease

Chronic obstructive pulmonary disease (COPD) is one major health problem known to increase morbidity and mortality all over the world. It is predicted that COPD will become the third leading cause of death (~8.3 million), and the third leading cause of death by disability until 2030 [58]. Globally, exposure to cigarette smoke (CS) is considered to be the primary cause for COPD. Inhalation of CS causes the release of different cytokines, chemokines, and lipid mediators (such as tumor necrosis factor-α (TNF-α), interleukin 8 (IL-8), transforming growth factor-β (TGF-β) and leukotriene B4) from resident cells in the lung including epithelial cells and alveolar macrophages. Subsequently, these mediators activate inflammatory cells which release large amounts of proteases, including elastase and matrix metalloproteinases (MMPs), into the matrix compartment, thereby triggering the complex process of remodeling, thus leading to obstruction of small airways, emphysema, with enlargement of air spaces and destruction of lung parenchyma, loss of lung elasticity, and closure of small airways, fibrosis, inflammation, mucus hyper-secretion, and pulmonary hypertension. Furthermore, more and more evidence indicates that CS exposure also provokes an oxidant/antioxidant imbalance, which in turn will subsequently induce COPD exacerbations [59,60]. Therefore, the most effective way to prevent the development of COPD is smoke cessation [61,62]. Additionally, other factors including exposure to indoor air pollutions from biomass fuels, particularly in developing countries, occupational dusts, chemicals, and genetics, may also contribute toward disease morbidity and mortality [63,64]. Currently, the pharmacological management of COPD mainly relies on bronchodilator therapy, mainly β2-agonists and anticholinergics, by activating different signaling pathways [65–68]. β2-Agonists induce airway smooth muscle (ASM) cell relaxation through enhanced intracellular cAMP production, whereas anticholinergics or antimuscarinic drugs antagonize muscarinic receptors (M1, M2 and M3) to a certain extent, thus inhibiting ASM contraction, due to the reduction of intracellular Ca^{2+}. PDE4 inhibitors, which mediates cAMP breakdown (see below), are also approved to be used as an add-on treatment for severe COPD patients associated with bronchitis and a history of frequent exacerbations [69]. In addition, anti-inflammatory drugs, such as inhaled glucocorticosteroids, are often used, mainly in patients with frequent exacerbations [70].

3.1. Compartmentalization of cAMP in the Lung

The production of cAMP is initiated by the stimulation of Gs-coupled receptors, such as the β-AR and distinct subset of prostanoid receptors [71]. After receptor ligand binding, ACs are activated by the α subunit of the Gs-protein, thus resulting in cAMP synthesis from adenosine triphosphate (ATP) [72]. Intracellular cAMP levels are tightly controlled by cyclic nucleotide PDEs, which hydrolyze cAMP to 5′-AMP, and thereby terminate its signaling [73]. Membrane clustering of Gs-coupled receptors ACs and PDEs, which are localized in lipid rafts and caveolae, together with cAMP downstream effectors, such as cAMP-gated ion channels, PKA, and Epac, dynamically regulate intracellular cAMP signaling in the lung, including airway relaxation [74,75], reduction of inflammation [76–79], and fibrosis [77,80]. In addition, AKAPs bind directly to PKA and its targeted proteins, and physically tether these multi-protein complexes to specific locations, generating spatiotemporal discrete signaling complexes [81,82], and subsequently controlling specific cellular responses (Figure 3).

Lung

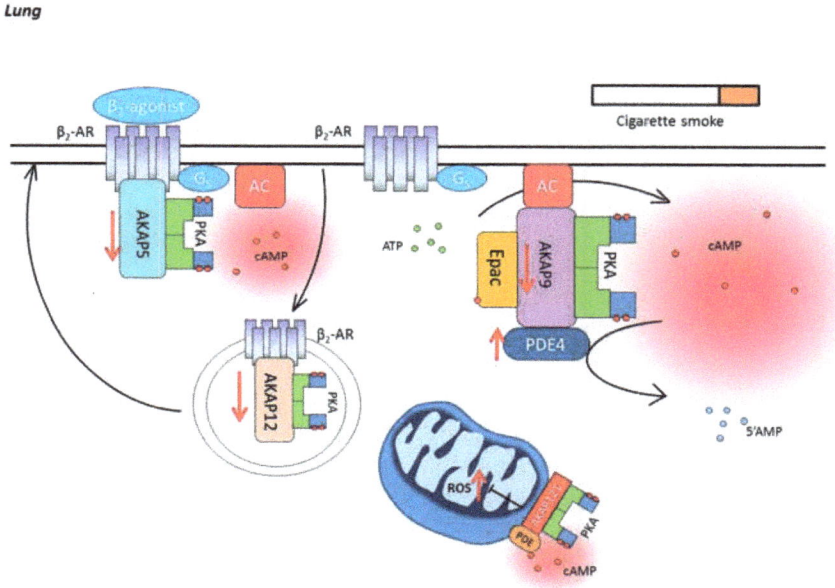

Figure 3. cAMP compartmentalization in COPD. As one of main inducing factors, cigarette smoke (CS) is able to modulate numerous molecular signals in both structural and inflammatory cells in the lung. CS decreases the expressions of A-kinase anchoring protein (AKAP)5 and AKAP12, thus, regulating the effect of β2-agonists on COPD pathological development. Moreover, CS interferes with cAMP compartments by AKAP9, which binds and regulates the function of adenylyl cyclases (ACs). In addition, intracellular cAMP concentration is further decreased by upregulating cAMP hydrolyzing enzyme PDEs expression. β2-AR, β2-adrenergic receptor; AC, transmembrane adenylyl cyclase; cAMP, cyclic adenosine monophosphate; ATP, adenosine triphosphate; PDE4, phosphodiesterase 4; AKAP, A-kinase anchoring protein; PKA, protein kinase A; Epac, exchange protein directly activated by cAMP; ROS, reactive oxygen species.

3.2. Cyclic Nucleotide Phosphodiesterases in COPD

PDEs, which comprise 11 family members and at least 21 isoforms with different splice variants [83], are able to hydrolyze cyclic nucleotides (cAMP and cGMP) to their inactivate 5′ monophosphates within subcellular microdomains, thereby modulating cyclic nucleotide signaling pathways.

PDE4 is the most extensively studied PDE, and it is widely expressed in almost all different kinds of cells in the lung. From a clinical viewpoint, there are dramatic differences in the PDE4 isoforms' expression in inflammatory cells of smokers with COPD, smokers without COPD, and nonsmokers [84].

PDE4A4 was significantly upregulated not only in lung macrophages from COPD patients, but also in peripheral blood monocytes of smokers, together with PDE4B2 [84]. In isolated peripheral blood neutrophils, significantly higher PDE4B and PDE4D, but not PDE4A or PDE4C, mRNA levels could be observed in the COPD patients compared to healthy subjects. Yoon et al. reported the association of a novel PDE4D single nucleotide polymorphism (rs16878037) with COPD from a genome-wide association study [85]. PDE4 is also of importance in other pulmonary diseases, such as asthma. It was shown by Trian et al. that β-agonist isoproterenol-induced cAMP production in asthmatics ASM cells was dramatically decreased due to increased PDE4D expression, rather than an alteration in PDE3A or PDE5A expression [86]. Furthermore, CS, as the primary cause for COPD, was also proven to increase PDE4 isoforms' expression and activity in different experimental settings. Higher PDE4B and PDE4D mRNA levels could be detected after 6 h CS extract exposure in isolated peripheral blood neutrophils [87]. Exposure with CS extract for 24 h upregulated PDE4 activity in differentiated bronchial epithelial cells, with a markedly increased mRNA transcripts for PDE4B, while increments in PDE4A and D transcripts remained below significance [88].

Other PDE family members also attracted the attention of researchers, such as PDE7, which is encoded by PDE7A and PDE7B. PDE7B is expressed predominantly in brain, heart, and liver, but not in lung [89,90]. However, PDE7A, which is widely expressed in airway structural cells, including airway epithelial cells [91], ASM cells and lung fibroblast, and also human proinflammatory and immune cells [92], has particularly drawn attention in the treatment of COPD [93]. It has been shown that the protein expression of PDE7A1 is significantly increased in human monocytes during cell aging [94]. In addition, PDE3A is upregulated in human endobronchial biopsies obtained from patients with asthma, indicating that PDE3 is also involved in the pathogenesis of lung diseases.

3.3. AKAPs in COPD

As one of the most vital pharmaceutical targets in COPD, β$_2$-AR directly interacts with AKAP5 and AKAP12, which modulate either the downstream extracellular signal-regulated protein kinase (ERK)1/2 activation or receptor resensitization [81,94–96]. Therefore, it is believed that AKAP5 and AKAP12 play a pivotal role in modulating the effect of β$_2$-agonists on COPD pathological development. Poppinga et al. showed that less AKAP5 and AKAP12 proteins could be detected in CS-exposed ASM cells, which was also confirmed using lung tissues from COPD patients [97]. Moreover, st-Ht31, which disrupts global AKAP–PKA interactions (see Figure 3), increased the IL-8 secretion induced by CS exposure in human ASM cells, and reduced the suppression of β$_2$-agonist fenoterol through disturbed ERK signaling [97]. On the contrary, AKAP5 and AKAP12 expression were not significantly changed by CS in human bronchial epithelial cells [98], indicating a different regulatory pathway involved other AKAP members in epithelial cells (Figure 3). Indeed, it has been demonstrated that AKAP9, which binds and regulates ACs [99,100], was able to maintain epithelial barrier function [99] (Figure 3). In addition, as a major site for energy generation and reactive oxygen species (ROS) production, mitochondria cAMP compartments was regulated by a set of mitochondrial AKAPs. In particular, AKAP121, tethering PKA to the outer wall of mitochondria, play a pivotal role in mitochondrial function maintenance and keeping the tolerance to oxidative stress in vascular smooth muscle cells [101], indicating a potential protective effect on CS-induced ROS production for future studies (Figure 3).

3.4. Epac in COPD

In addition to PKA, as mentioned earlier, Epac is another downstream effector for cAMP [102]. Epac, which is able to be activated by PKA or cAMP in both a PKA-dependent and -independent manner, has been proven to associate with diverse effectors, thus contributing to numerous cellular processes, including airway relaxation, cytokine secretion, barrier function, cell proliferation, migration, and protein translocation in the lung. Also, it has been demonstrated by Scott et al. that Epac activation by 8-CPT could reverse neutrophils' phagocytic impairment induced experimentally by using β$_2$-agonists, without interfering with RhoA activity [103]. In addition. Epac activation by 8-CPT changed methacholine-induced myosin light chain (MLC) phosphorylation in ASM cells, skewing the balance between RhoA and Rac1 towards Rac1, and thus reducing the phosphorylation of MLC; a process leading to ASM relaxation [75]. In addition, pharmacological activation of Epac attenuated CS extract-induced IL-8 release from human ASM cells by activating the NF-κB inhibitory protein IκBα and inhibiting p65 nuclear translocation, underling the inhibitory effect of Epac on NF-κB activation [104]. Two isoforms, Epac1 and Epac2, are expressed in most lung cell types, among them, ASM, epithelial cells, fibroblasts, and some immune cells [103,105]. Intriguingly, a selective downregulation of Epac1, rather than Epac2, expression was observed in both CS-exposed ASM cells and lung tissue from COPD patients, pointing to distinct intracellular functions and locations of Epac1 and Epac2 [104]. It was further demonstrated that the upregulation of miRNA7 expression in COPD patients was linked to the downregulation of Epac1 [106]. Moreover, the role of Epac1 and Epac2 was further investigated in Epac1(−/−) and Epac2(−/−) mice using an acute and short-term CS exposure model. Compared to wild type mice exposed to CS, Epac1(−/−) mice showed increased MUC5AC and matrix remodeling parameters (TGF-β, collagen I, and fibronectin) in the lung homogenates, however, Epac2(−/−) mice had lower amount of inflammatory cells (total inflammatory cells, macrophages, and neutrophils) in the bronchoalveolar lavage fluid, suggesting that Epac1 was able to inhibit remodeling process, whereas Epac2 primarily increased inflammatory processes [107]. These differences between Epac1 and Epac2 indicate compartmentalized cAMP signaling in the lung, which needs to be further studied in the future.

4. Conclusions and Future Perspectives

Evidence collected over the last decade indicates that Epac and the cAMP signalosome substantially contribute to the development and progression of heart and obstructive lung disorders, as exemplified here by studies focusing on COPD. Traditionally, research focused on PKA as one of the main targets of cAMP. However, recent studies indicated that next to classical signaling pathways, there seem to be substantial role for additional cAMP targets, such as Epac, and for the theme of compartmentalized cAMP signaling. The latter topic involves next to cAMP-elevating receptors (for example the β-ARs), cAMP-producing adenylyl cyclase and cAMP-degrading PDEs, a subset of AKAPs. Particularly, studies on the levels of Epac and PDEs benefit from the recent development of pharmacological tools [13,19,108], suggesting that the therapeutic arsenal to treat chronic disorders of the heart and the lung will be substantially improved in the next decades. Unfortunately, the research on compartments being stabilized and maintained by members of the AKAP superfamily still lacks the development of subtype specific modulators, which will hopefully be the focus of future studies.

In the heart, research over the last years has shown that particularly Epac1 seems to act cardioprotectively with regard to cardiac fibrosis and apoptosis, but that the role of Epac1 seems to be rather distinct, and being largely dependent on the nature of the stress inducer. Such findings nicely reflect the fact that our aging world population requires a vast majority of novel personalized medicine-based drugs [19,71,109]. Distinct roles of Epac1 and Epac2 seemed to emerge in the field of heart failure and arrhythmia, as well as cardiac ischemia. Here, interaction of Epac with members of the AKAP family or PDE subtype, such as PDE4, seem to be leading next to a defined subcellular targeting of Epacs to defined compartments, such as the nucleus and mitochondria. In the lung, it seemed to be that PDEs are crucially involved in the compartmentalization of cAMP next to members of the AKAP family and Epac. Interestingly, it seemed to be that subtypes of PDEs guide cAMP properties in a rather response-specific manner, such as anti-inflammation and bronchodilation. Novel anti-inflammatory drugs are urgently required, as under disease conditions being characterized by an overload of ROS, the golden treatment standard, glucocorticosteroids, are ineffective. Most likely, compartment-specific mode of actions of PDEs are supported by AKAPs and Epac. Future studies should focus on unravelling compartmentalized signaling cues in the heart and lung.

Acknowledgments: The work of F.L. mentioned herein was supported by grants from Institute National de la Santé et de la Recherche Médicale, Fondation pour la Recherche Médicale (Programme "Equipes FRM 2016", No. DEQ20160334892), Fondation de France (No. 00066331), and Université de Toulouse. M.L. is supported by a Ph.D. training grant from Université de Toulouse. The work of M.S. was supported by the Groningen Institute of Pharmacy (GRIP), and the Faculty of Science and Engineering (FSE) of the Univeristy Groningen. H.Z. is supported by the Ubbo Emmius Programme of the University Groningen.

Author Contributions: M.L., H.Z., F.L. and M.S. wrote the manuscript.

Conflicts of Interest: The authors declare no conflict of interest.

References

1. Bers, D.M. Calcium cycling and signaling in cardiac myocytes. *Annu. Rev. Physiol.* **2008**, *70*, 23–49. [CrossRef] [PubMed]

2. Berthouze, M.; Laurent, A.-C.; Breckler, M.; Lezoualc'h, F. New perspectives in cAMP-signaling modulation. *Curr. Heart Fail. Rep.* **2011**, *8*, 159–167. [CrossRef] [PubMed]

3. Bristow, M.R. Treatment of chronic heart failure with β-adrenergic receptor antagonists: A convergence of receptor pharmacology and clinical cardiology. *Circ. Res.* **2011**, *109*, 1176–1194. [CrossRef] [PubMed]

4. El-Armouche, A.; Eschenhagen, T. β-adrenergic stimulation and myocardial function in the failing heart. *Heart Fail. Rev.* **2009**, *14*, 225–241. [CrossRef] [PubMed]

5. Von Lueder, T.G.; Krum, H. New medical therapies for heart failure. *Nat. Rev. Cardiol.* **2015**, *12*, 730–740. [CrossRef] [PubMed]

6. Cohn, J.N.; Levine, T.B.; Olivari, M.T.; Garberg, V.; Lura, D.; Francis, G.S.; Simon, A.B.; Rector, T. Plasma norepinephrine as a guide to prognosis in patients with chronic congestive heart failure. *N. Engl. J. Med.* **1984**, *311*, 819–823. [CrossRef] [PubMed]

7. Hill, J.A.; Olson, E.N. Cardiac plasticity. *N. Engl. J. Med.* **2008**, *358*, 1370–1380. [CrossRef] [PubMed]

8. Métrich, M.; Lucas, A.; Gastineau, M.; Samuel, J.-L.; Heymes, C.; Morel, E.; Lezoualc'h, F. Epac mediates β-adrenergic receptor-induced cardiomyocyte hypertrophy. *Circ. Res.* **2008**, *102*, 959–965. [CrossRef] [PubMed]

9. Ulucan, C.; Wang, X.; Baljinnyam, E.; Bai, Y.; Okumura, S.; Sato, M.; Minamisawa, S.; Hirotani, S.; Ishikawa, Y. Developmental changes in gene expression of Epac and its upregulation in myocardial hypertrophy. *Am. J. Physiol. Heart Circ. Physiol.* **2007**, *293*, H1662–H1672. [CrossRef] [PubMed]

10. Castaldi, A.; Zaglia, T.; Di Mauro, V.; Carullo, P.; Viggiani, G.; Borile, G.; Di Stefano, B.; Schiattarella, G.G.; Gualazzi, M.G.; Elia, L.; et al. MicroRNA-133 modulates the β1-adrenergic receptor transduction cascade. *Circ. Res.* **2014**, *115*, 273–283. [CrossRef] [PubMed]

11. Gesmundo, I.; Miragoli, M.; Carullo, P.; Trovato, L.; Larcher, V.; Di Pasquale, E.; Brancaccio, M.; Mazzola, M.; Villanova, T.; Sorge, M.; et al. Growth hormone-releasing hormone attenuates cardiac hypertrophy and improves heart function in pressure overload-induced heart failure. *Proc. Natl. Acad. Sci. USA* **2017**, *114*, 12033–12038. [CrossRef] [PubMed]

12. Morel, E.; Marcantoni, A.; Gastineau, M.; Birkedal, R.; Rochais, F.; Garnier, A.; Lompré, A.-M.; Vandecasteele, G.; Lezoualc'h, F. cAMP-binding protein Epac induces cardiomyocyte hypertrophy. *Circ. Res.* **2005**, *97*, 1296–1304. [CrossRef] [PubMed]

13. Schwede, F.; Bertinetti, D.; Langerijs, C.N.; Hadders, M.A.; Wienk, H.; Ellenbroek, J.H.; de Koning, E.J.P.; Bos, J.L.; Herberg, F.W.; Genieser, H.-G.; et al. Structure-guided design of selective Epac1 and Epac2 agonists. *PLoS Biol.* **2015**, *13*, e1002038. [CrossRef] [PubMed]

14. Laurent, A.-C.; Bisserier, M.; Lucas, A.; Tortosa, F.; Roumieux, M.; De Régibus, A.; Swiader, A.; Sainte-Marie, Y.; Heymes, C.; Vindis, C.; et al. Exchange protein directly activated by cAMP 1 promotes autophagy during cardiomyocyte hypertrophy. *Cardiovasc. Res.* **2015**, *105*, 55–64. [CrossRef] [PubMed]

15. Bisserier, M.; Blondeau, J.-P.; Lezoualc'h, F. Epac proteins: Specific ligands and role in cardiac remodelling. *Biochem. Soc. Trans.* **2014**, *42*, 257–264. [CrossRef] [PubMed]

16. Courilleau, D.; Bisserier, M.; Jullian, J.-C.; Lucas, A.; Bouyssou, P.; Fischmeister, R.; Blondeau, J.-P.; Lezoualc'h, F. Identification of a tetrahydroquinoline analog as a pharmacological inhibitor of the cAMP-binding protein Epac. *J. Biol. Chem.* **2012**, *287*, 44192–44202. [CrossRef] [PubMed]

17. Monceau, V.; Llach, A.; Azria, D.; Bridier, A.; Petit, B.; Mazevet, M.; Strup-Perrot, C.; To, T.-H.-V.; Calmels, L.; Germaini, M.-M.; et al. Epac contributes to cardiac hypertrophy and amyloidosis induced by radiotherapy but not fibrosis. *Radiother. Oncol. J. Eur. Soc. Ther. Radiol. Oncol.* **2014**, *111*, 63–71. [CrossRef] [PubMed]

18. Cazorla, O.; Lucas, A.; Poirier, F.; Lacampagne, A.; Lezoualc'h, F. The cAMP binding protein Epac regulates cardiac myofilament function. *Proc. Natl. Acad. Sci. USA* **2009**, *106*, 14144–14149. [CrossRef] [PubMed]

19. Lezoualc'h, F.; Fazal, L.; Laudette, M.; Conte, C. Cyclic AMP Sensor EPAC Proteins and Their Role in Cardiovascular Function and Disease. *Circ. Res.* **2016**, *118*, 881–897. [CrossRef] [PubMed]

20. Pereira, L.; Rehmann, H.; Lao, D.H.; Erickson, J.R.; Bossuyt, J.; Chen, J.; Bers, D.M. Novel Epac fluorescent ligand reveals distinct Epac1 vs. Epac2 distribution and function in cardiomyocytes. *Proc. Natl. Acad. Sci. USA* **2015**, *112*, 3991–3996. [CrossRef] [PubMed]

21. Mangmool, S.; Shukla, A.K.; Rockman, H.A. β-Arrestin-dependent activation of Ca^{2+}/calmodulin kinase II after β1-adrenergic receptor stimulation. *J. Cell Biol.* **2010**, *189*, 573–587. [CrossRef] [PubMed]

22. Berthouze-Duquesnes, M.; Lucas, A.; Saulière, A.; Sin, Y.Y.; Laurent, A.-C.; Galés, C.; Baillie, G.; Lezoualc'h, F. Specific interactions between Epac1, β-arrestin2 and PDE4D5 regulate β-adrenergic receptor subtype differential effects on cardiac hypertrophic signaling. *Cell. Signal.* **2013**, *25*, 970–980. [CrossRef] [PubMed]

23. Dodge-Kafka, K.L.; Soughayer, J.; Pare, G.C.; Carlisle Michel, J.J.; Langeberg, L.K.; Kapiloff, M.S.; Scott, J.D. The protein kinase A anchoring protein mAKAP coordinates two integrated cAMP effector pathways. *Nature* **2005**, *437*, 574–578. [CrossRef] [PubMed]

24. Zhang, L.; Malik, S.; Pang, J.; Wang, H.; Park, K.M.; Yule, D.I.; Blaxall, B.C.; Smrcka, A.V. Phospholipase Cε hydrolyzes perinuclear phosphatidylinositol 4-phosphate to regulate cardiac hypertrophy. *Cell* **2013**, *153*, 216–227. [CrossRef] [PubMed]

25. Pereira, L.; Ruiz-Hurtado, G.; Morel, E.; Laurent, A.-C.; Métrich, M.; Domínguez-Rodríguez, A.; Lauton-Santos, S.; Lucas, A.; Benitah, J.-P.; Bers, D.M.; et al. Epac enhances excitation-transcription coupling in cardiac myocytes. *J. Mol. Cell. Cardiol.* **2012**, *52*, 283–291. [CrossRef] [PubMed]

26. Métrich, M.; Laurent, A.-C.; Breckler, M.; Duquesnes, N.; Hmitou, I.; Courillau, D.; Blondeau, J.-P.; Crozatier, B.; Lezoualc'h, F.; Morel, E. Epac activation induces histone deacetylase nuclear export via a Ras-dependent signalling pathway. *Cell. Signal.* **2010**, *22*, 1459–1468. [CrossRef] [PubMed]

27. Ruiz-Hurtado, G.; Morel, E.; Domínguez-Rodríguez, A.; Llach, A.; Lezoualc'h, F.; Benitah, J.-P.; Gomez, A.M. Epac in cardiac calcium signaling. *J. Mol. Cell. Cardiol.* **2013**, *58*, 162–171. [CrossRef] [PubMed]

28. Okumura, S.; Fujita, T.; Cai, W.; Jin, M.; Namekata, I.; Mototani, Y.; Jin, H.; Ohnuki, Y.; Tsuneoka, Y.; Kurotani, R.; et al. Epac1-dependent phospholamban phosphorylation mediates the cardiac response to stresses. *J. Clin. Investig.* **2014**, *124*, 2785–2801. [CrossRef] [PubMed]

29. Pereira, L.; Cheng, H.; Lao, D.H.; Na, L.; van Oort, R.J.; Brown, J.H.; Wehrens, X.H.T.; Chen, J.; Bers, D.M. Epac2 mediates cardiac β1-adrenergic-dependent sarcoplasmic reticulum Ca^{2+} leak and arrhythmia. *Circulation* **2013**, *127*, 913–922. [CrossRef] [PubMed]

30. Kaur, S.; Kong, C.H.T.; Cannell, M.B.; Ward, M.-L. Depotentiation of intact rat cardiac muscle unmasks an Epac-dependent increase in myofilament Ca^{2+} sensitivity. *Clin. Exp. Pharmacol. Physiol.* **2016**, *43*, 88–94. [CrossRef] [PubMed]

31. Lezcano, N.; Mariángelo, J.I.E.; Vittone, L.; Wehrens, X.H.T.; Said, M.; Mundiña-Weilenmann, C. Early effects of Epac depend on the fine-tuning of the sarcoplasmic reticulum Ca^{2+} handling in cardiomyocytes. *J. Mol. Cell. Cardiol.* **2017**, *114*, 1–9. [CrossRef] [PubMed]

32. Oestreich, E.A.; Wang, H.; Malik, S.; Kaproth-Joslin, K.A.; Blaxall, B.C.; Kelley, G.G.; Dirksen, R.T.; Smrcka, A.V. Epac-mediated activation of phospholipase C(epsilon) plays a critical role in β-adrenergic receptor-dependent enhancement of Ca^{2+} mobilization in cardiac myocytes. *J. Biol. Chem.* **2007**, *282*, 5488–5495. [CrossRef] [PubMed]

33. Pereira, L.; Bare, D.J.; Galice, S.; Shannon, T.R.; Bers, D.M. β-Adrenergic induced SR Ca^{2+} leak is mediated by an Epac-NOS pathway. *J. Mol. Cell. Cardiol.* **2017**, *108*, 8–16. [CrossRef] [PubMed]

34. Bobin, P.; Varin, A.; Lefebvre, F.; Fischmeister, R.; Vandecasteele, G.; Leroy, J. Calmodulin kinase II inhibition limits the pro-arrhythmic Ca^{2+} waves induced by cAMP-phosphodiesterase inhibitors. *Cardiovasc. Res.* **2016**, *110*, 151–161. [CrossRef] [PubMed]

35. Cai, W.; Fujita, T.; Hidaka, Y.; Jin, H.; Suita, K.; Prajapati, R.; Liang, C.; Umemura, M.; Yokoyama, U.; Sato, M.; et al. Disruption of Epac1 protects the heart from adenylyl cyclase type 5-mediated cardiac dysfunction. *Biochem. Biophys. Res. Commun.* **2016**, *475*, 1–7. [CrossRef] [PubMed]

36. Hothi, S.S.; Gurung, I.S.; Heathcote, J.C.; Zhang, Y.; Booth, S.W.; Skepper, J.N.; Grace, A.A.; Huang, C.L.-H. Epac activation, altered calcium homeostasis and ventricular arrhythmogenesis in the murine heart. *Pflug. Arch.* **2008**, *457*, 253–270. [CrossRef] [PubMed]

37. Ruiz-Hurtado, G.; Domínguez-Rodríguez, A.; Pereira, L.; Fernández-Velasco, M.; Cassan, C.; Lezoualc'h, F.; Benitah, J.-P.; Gómez, A.M. Sustained Epac activation induces calmodulin dependent positive inotropic effect in adult cardiomyocytes. *J. Mol. Cell. Cardiol.* **2012**, *53*, 617–625. [CrossRef] [PubMed]

38. Brette, F.; Blandin, E.; Simard, C.; Guinamard, R.; Sallé, L. Epac activator critically regulates action potential duration by decreasing potassium current in rat adult ventricle. *J. Mol. Cell. Cardiol.* **2013**, *57*, 96–105. [CrossRef] [PubMed]

39. Aflaki, M.; Qi, X.-Y.; Xiao, L.; Ordog, B.; Tadevosyan, A.; Luo, X.; Maguy, A.; Shi, Y.; Tardif, J.-C.; Nattel, S. Exchange protein directly activated by cAMP mediates slow delayed-rectifier current remodeling by sustained β-adrenergic activation in guinea pig hearts. *Circ. Res.* **2014**, *114*, 993–1003. [CrossRef] [PubMed]

40. Domínguez-Rodríguez, A.; Ruiz-Hurtado, G.; Sabourin, J.; Gómez, A.M.; Alvarez, J.L.; Benitah, J.-P. Proarrhythmic effect of sustained EPAC activation on TRPC3/4 in rat ventricular cardiomyocytes. *J. Mol. Cell. Cardiol.* **2015**, *87*, 74–78. [CrossRef] [PubMed]

41. Duquesnes, N.; Derangeon, M.; Métrich, M.; Lucas, A.; Mateo, P.; Li, L.; Morel, E.; Lezoualc'h, F.; Crozatier, B. Epac stimulation induces rapid increases in connexin43 phosphorylation and function without preconditioning effect. *Pflugers Arch.* **2010**, *460*, 731–741. [CrossRef] [PubMed]

42. Somekawa, S.; Fukuhara, S.; Nakaoka, Y.; Fujita, H.; Saito, Y.; Mochizuki, N. Enhanced functional gap junction neoformation by protein kinase A-dependent and Epac-dependent signals downstream of cAMP in cardiac myocytes. *Circ. Res.* **2005**, *97*, 655–662. [CrossRef] [PubMed]

43. Pereira, L.; Métrich, M.; Fernández-Velasco, M.; Lucas, A.; Leroy, J.; Perrier, R.; Morel, E.; Fischmeister, R.; Richard, S.; Bénitah, J.-P.; et al. The cAMP binding protein Epac modulates Ca^{2+} sparks by a Ca^{2+}/calmodulin kinase signalling pathway in rat cardiac myocytes. *J. Physiol.* **2007**, *583*, 685–694. [CrossRef] [PubMed]

44. Yang, Z.; Kirton, H.M.; Al-Owais, M.; Thireau, J.; Richard, S.; Peers, C.; Steele, D.S. Epac2-Rap1 Signaling Regulates Reactive Oxygen Species Production and Susceptibility to Cardiac Arrhythmias. *Antioxid. Redox Signal.* **2017**, *27*, 117–132. [CrossRef] [PubMed]

45. Heusch, G. Treatment of Myocardial Ischemia/Reperfusion Injury by Ischemic and Pharmacological Postconditioning. *Compr. Physiol.* **2015**, *5*, 1123–1145. [CrossRef] [PubMed]

46. Yellon, D.M.; Hausenloy, D.J. Myocardial reperfusion injury. *N. Engl. J. Med.* **2007**, *357*, 1121–1135. [CrossRef] [PubMed]

47. Murphy, E.; Ardehali, H.; Balaban, R.S.; DiLisa, F.; Dorn, G.W.; Kitsis, R.N.; Otsu, K.; Ping, P.; Rizzuto, R.; Sack, M.N.; et al. Mitochondrial Function, Biology, and Role in Disease: A Scientific Statement From the American Heart Association. *Circ. Res.* **2016**, *118*, 1960–1991. [CrossRef] [PubMed]

48. Ong, S.-B.; Samangouei, P.; Kalkhoran, S.B.; Hausenloy, D.J. The mitochondrial permeability transition pore and its role in myocardial ischemia reperfusion injury. *J. Mol. Cell. Cardiol.* **2015**, *78*, 23–34. [CrossRef] [PubMed]

49. Suzuki, S.; Yokoyama, U.; Abe, T.; Kiyonari, H.; Yamashita, N.; Kato, Y.; Kurotani, R.; Sato, M.; Okumura, S.; Ishikawa, Y. Differential roles of Epac in regulating cell death in neuronal and myocardial cells. *J. Biol. Chem.* **2010**, *285*, 24248–24259. [CrossRef] [PubMed]

50. Mangmool, S.; Hemplueksa, P.; Parichatikanond, W.; Chattipakorn, N. Epac is required for GLP-1R-mediated inhibition of oxidative stress and apoptosis in cardiomyocytes. *Mol. Endocrinol.* **2015**, *29*, 583–596. [CrossRef] [PubMed]

51. Khaliulin, I.; Bond, M.; James, A.F.; Dyar, Z.; Amini, R.; Johnson, J.L.; Suleiman, M.-S. Functional and cardioprotective effects of simultaneous and individual activation of protein kinase A and Epac. *Br. J. Pharmacol.* **2017**, *174*, 438–453. [CrossRef] [PubMed]

52. Edland, F.; Wergeland, A.; Kopperud, R.; Åsrud, K.S.; Hoivik, E.A.; Witsø, S.L.; Æsøy, R.; Madsen, L.; Kristiansen, K.; Bakke, M.; et al. Long-term consumption of an obesogenic high fat diet prior to ischemia-reperfusion mediates cardioprotection via Epac1-dependent signaling. *Nutr. Metab.* **2016**, *13*, 87. [CrossRef] [PubMed]

53. Calderón-Sánchez, E.; Díaz, I.; Ordóñez, A.; Smani, T. Urocortin-1 Mediated Cardioprotection Involves XIAP and CD40-Ligand Recovery: Role of EPAC2 and ERK1/2. *PLoS ONE* **2016**, *11*, e0147375. [CrossRef] [PubMed]

54. Fazal, L.; Laudette, M.; Paula-Gomes, S.; Pons, S.; Conte, C.; Tortosa, F.; Sicard, P.; Sainte-Marie, Y.; Bisserier, M.; Lairez, O.; et al. Multifunctional Mitochondrial Epac1 Controls Myocardial Cell Death. *Circ. Res.* **2017**, *120*, 645–657. [CrossRef] [PubMed]

55. Qiao, J.; Mei, F.C.; Popov, V.L.; Vergara, L.A.; Cheng, X. Cell cycle-dependent subcellular localization of exchange factor directly activated by cAMP. *J. Biol. Chem.* **2002**, *277*, 26581–26586. [CrossRef] [PubMed]

56. Wang, Z.; Liu, D.; Varin, A.; Nicolas, V.; Courilleau, D.; Mateo, P.; Caubere, C.; Rouet, P.; Gomez, A.-M.; Vandecasteele, G.; et al. A cardiac mitochondrial cAMP signaling pathway regulates calcium accumulation, permeability transition and cell death. *Cell Death Dis.* **2016**, *7*, e2198. [CrossRef] [PubMed]

57. Paillard, M.; Tubbs, E.; Thiebaut, P.-A.; Gomez, L.; Fauconnier, J.; Da Silva, C.C.; Teixeira, G.; Mewton, N.; Belaidi, E.; Durand, A.; et al. Depressing mitochondria-reticulum interactions protects cardiomyocytes from lethal hypoxia-reoxygenation injury. *Circulation* **2013**, *128*, 1555–1565. [CrossRef] [PubMed]

58. Available online: http://www.who.int/respiratory/copd/en/ (accessed on 31 January 2018).

59. Antus, B.; Kardos, Z. Oxidative stress in COPD: Molecular background and clinical monitoring. *Curr. Med. Chem.* **2015**, *22*, 627–650. [CrossRef] [PubMed]

60. Kirkham, P.A.; Barnes, P.J. Oxidative Stress in COPD. *Chest* **2013**, *144*, 266–273. [CrossRef] [PubMed]

61. Bergeron, C.; Boulet, L.-P. Structural changes in airway diseases: Characteristics, mechanisms, consequences, and pharmacologic modulation. *Chest* **2006**, *129*, 1068–1087. [CrossRef] [PubMed]

62. Tønnesen, P. Smoking cessation and COPD. *Eur. Respir. Rev.* **2013**, *22*, 37–43. [CrossRef] [PubMed]

63. Boswell-Smith, V.; Spina, D. PDE4 inhibitors as potential therapeutic agents in the treatment of COPD-focus on roflumilast. *Int. J. Chronic Obstr. Pulm. Dis.* **2007**, *2*, 121–129.

64. Pauwels, R.A.; Buist, A.S.; Calverley, P.M.; Jenkins, C.R.; Hurd, S.S. GOLD Scientific Committee Global strategy for the diagnosis, management, and prevention of chronic obstructive pulmonary disease. NHLBI/WHO Global Initiative for Chronic Obstructive Lung Disease (GOLD) Workshop summary. *Am. J. Respir. Crit. Care Med.* **2001**, *163*, 1256–1276. [CrossRef] [PubMed]

65. Dekkers, B.G.J.; Racké, K.; Schmidt, M. Distinct PKA and Epac compartmentalization in airway function and plasticity. *Pharmacol. Ther.* **2013**, *137*, 248–265. [CrossRef] [PubMed]

66. Kabir, E.R.; Morshed, N. Different approaches in the treatment of obstructive pulmonary diseases. *Eur. J. Pharmacol.* **2015**, *764*, 306–317. [CrossRef] [PubMed]

67. López-Campos, J.L.; Calero Acuña, C. What is in the guidelines about the pharmacological treatment of chronic obstructive pulmonary disease? *Expert Rev. Respir. Med.* **2013**, *7*, 43–51. [CrossRef] [PubMed]

68. Qaseem, A.; Wilt, T.J.; Weinberger, S.E.; Hanania, N.A.; Criner, G.; van der Molen, T.; Marciniuk, D.D.; Denberg, T.; Schünemann, H.; Wedzicha, W.; et al. Diagnosis and management of stable chronic obstructive pulmonary disease: A clinical practice guideline update from the American College of Physicians, American College of Chest Physicians, American Thoracic Society, and European Respiratory Society. *Ann. Intern. Med.* **2011**, *155*, 179–191. [CrossRef] [PubMed]

69. Abbott-Banner, K.H.; Page, C.P. Dual PDE3/4 and PDE4 inhibitors: Novel treatments for COPD and other inflammatory airway diseases. *Basic Clin. Pharmacol. Toxicol.* **2014**, *114*, 365–376. [CrossRef] [PubMed]

70. Raissy, H.H.; Kelly, H.W.; Harkins, M.; Szefler, S.J. Inhaled Corticosteroids in Lung Diseases. *Am. J. Respir. Crit. Care Med.* **2013**, *187*, 798–803. [CrossRef] [PubMed]

71. Schmidt, M.; Dekker, F.J.; Maarsingh, H. Exchange Protein Directly Activated by cAMP (epac): A Multidomain cAMP Mediator in the Regulation of Diverse Biological Functions. *Pharmacol. Rev.* **2013**, *65*, 670–709. [CrossRef] [PubMed]

72. Hanoune, J.; Defer, N. Regulation and role of adenylyl cyclase isoforms. *Annu. Rev. Pharmacol. Toxicol.* **2001**, *41*, 145–174. [CrossRef] [PubMed]

73. Omori, K.; Kotera, J. Overview of PDEs and their regulation. *Circ. Res.* **2007**, *100*, 309–327. [CrossRef] [PubMed]

74. Morgan, S.J.; Deshpande, D.A.; Tiegs, B.C.; Misior, A.M.; Yan, H.; Hershfeld, A.V.; Rich, T.C.; Panettieri, R.A.; An, S.S.; Penn, R.B. β-Agonist-mediated relaxation of airway smooth muscle is protein kinase A-dependent. *J. Biol. Chem.* **2014**, *289*, 23065–23074. [CrossRef] [PubMed]

75. Roscioni, S.S.; Maarsingh, H.; Elzinga, C.R.S.; Schuur, J.; Menzen, M.; Halayko, A.J.; Meurs, H.; Schmidt, M. Epac as a novel effector of airway smooth muscle relaxation. *J. Cell. Mol. Med* **2011**, *15*, 1551–1563. [CrossRef] [PubMed]

76. Birrell, M.A.; Maher, S.A.; Dekkak, B.; Jones, V.; Wong, S.; Brook, P.; Belvisi, M.G. Anti-inflammatory effects of PGE2 in the lung: Role of the EP4 receptor subtype. *Thorax* **2015**, *70*, 740–747. [CrossRef] [PubMed]

77. Mata, M.; Sarriá, B.; Buenestado, A.; Cortijo, J.; Cerdá, M.; Morcillo, E.J. Phosphodiesterase 4 inhibition decreases MUC5AC expression induced by epidermal growth factor in human airway epithelial cells. *Thorax* **2005**, *60*, 144–152. [CrossRef] [PubMed]

78. Profita, M.; Chiappara, G.; Mirabella, F.; Di Giorgi, R.; Chimenti, L.; Costanzo, G.; Riccobono, L.; Bellia, V.; Bousquet, J.; Vignola, A.M. Effect of cilomilast (Ariflo) on TNF-α, IL-8, and GM-CSF release by airway cells of patients with COPD. *Thorax* **2003**, *58*, 573–579. [CrossRef] [PubMed]

79. Wyatt, T.A.; Poole, J.A.; Nordgren, T.M.; DeVasure, J.M.; Heires, A.J.; Bailey, K.L.; Romberger, D.J. cAMP-dependent protein kinase activation decreases cytokine release in bronchial epithelial cells. *Am. J. Physiol. Lung Cell. Mol. Physiol.* **2014**, *307*, L643–L651. [CrossRef] [PubMed]

80. Huang, S.; Wettlaufer, S.H.; Hogaboam, C.; Aronoff, D.M.; Peters-Golden, M. Prostaglandin E2 inhibits collagen expression and proliferation in patient-derived normal lung fibroblasts via E prostanoid 2 receptor and cAMP signaling. *Am. J. Physiol. Lung Cell. Mol. Physiol.* **2007**, *292*, L405–L413. [CrossRef] [PubMed]

81. Carnegie, G.K.; Means, C.K.; Scott, J.D. A-Kinase Anchoring Proteins: From protein complexes to physiology and disease. *IUBMB Life* **2009**, *61*, 394–406. [CrossRef] [PubMed]

82. Poppinga, W.J.; Muñoz-Llancao, P.; González-Billault, C.; Schmidt, M. A-kinase anchoring proteins: cAMP compartmentalization in neurodegenerative and obstructive pulmonary diseases. *Br. J. Pharmacol.* **2014**, *171*, 5603–5623. [CrossRef] [PubMed]

83. Page, C.P.; Spina, D. Selective PDE inhibitors as novel treatments for respiratory diseases. *Curr. Opin. Pharmacol.* **2012**, *12*, 275–286. [CrossRef] [PubMed]

84. Barber, R.; Baillie, G.S.; Bergmann, R.; Shepherd, M.C.; Sepper, R.; Houslay, M.D.; Heeke, G.V. Differential expression of PDE4 cAMP phosphodiesterase isoforms in inflammatory cells of smokers with COPD, smokers without COPD, and nonsmokers. *Am. J. Physiol. Lung Cell. Mol. Physiol.* **2004**, *287*, L332–L343. [CrossRef] [PubMed]

85. Yoon, H.-K.; Hu, H.-J.; Rhee, C.-K.; Shin, S.-H.; Oh, Y.-M.; Lee, S.-D.; Jung, S.-H.; Yim, S.-H.; Kim, T.-M. Korean Obstructive Lung Disease (KOLD) Study Group; et al. Polymorphisms in PDE4D are associated with a risk of COPD in non-emphysematous Koreans. *COPD* **2014**, *11*, 652–658. [CrossRef] [PubMed]

86. Trian, T.; Burgess, J.K.; Niimi, K.; Moir, L.M.; Ge, Q.; Berger, P.; Liggett, S.B.; Black, J.L.; Oliver, B.G. β2-Agonist Induced cAMP Is Decreased in Asthmatic Airway Smooth Muscle Due to Increased PDE4D. *PLoS ONE* **2011**, *6*, e20000. [CrossRef] [PubMed]

87. Milara, J.; Lluch, J.; Almudever, P.; Freire, J.; Xiaozhong, Q.; Cortijo, J. Roflumilast N-oxide reverses corticosteroid resistance in neutrophils from patients with chronic obstructive pulmonary disease. *J. Allergy Clin. Immunol.* **2014**, *134*, 314–322.e9. [CrossRef] [PubMed]

88. Milara, J.; Armengot, M.; Bañuls, P.; Tenor, H.; Beume, R.; Artigues, E.; Cortijo, J. Roflumilast N-oxide, a PDE4 inhibitor, improves cilia motility and ciliated human bronchial epithelial cells compromised by cigarette smoke in vitro. *Br. J. Pharmacol.* **2012**, *166*, 2243–2262. [CrossRef] [PubMed]

89. Gardner, C.; Robas, N.; Cawkill, D.; Fidock, M. Cloning and characterization of the human and mouse PDE7B, a novel cAMP-specific cyclic nucleotide phosphodiesterase. *Biochem. Biophys. Res. Commun.* **2000**, *272*, 186–192. [CrossRef] [PubMed]

90. Hetman, J.M.; Soderling, S.H.; Glavas, N.A.; Beavo, J.A. Cloning and characterization of PDE7B, a cAMP-specific phosphodiesterase. *Proc. Natl. Acad. Sci. USA* **2000**, *97*, 472–476. [CrossRef] [PubMed]

91. Fuhrmann, M.; Jahn, H.-U.; Seybold, J.; Neurohr, C.; Barnes, P.J.; Hippenstiel, S.; Kraemer, H.J.; Suttorp, N. Identification and Function of Cyclic Nucleotide Phosphodiesterase Isoenzymes in Airway Epithelial Cells. *Am. J. Respir. Cell Mol. Biol.* **1999**, *20*, 292–302. [CrossRef] [PubMed]

92. Smith, S.J.; Brookes-Fazakerley, S.; Donnelly, L.E.; Barnes, P.J.; Barnette, M.S.; Giembycz, M.A. Ubiquitous expression of phosphodiesterase 7A in human proinflammatory and immune cells. *Am. J. Physiol. Lung Cell. Mol. Physiol.* **2003**, *284*, L279–L289. [CrossRef] [PubMed]

93. Giembycz, M.A.; Smith, S.J. Phosphodiesterase 7A: A new therapeutic target for alleviating chronic inflammation? *Curr. Pharm. Des.* **2006**, *12*, 3207–3220. [CrossRef] [PubMed]

94. Smith, S.J.; Cieslinski, L.B.; Newton, R.; Donnelly, L.E.; Fenwick, P.S.; Nicholson, A.G.; Barnes, P.J.; Barnette, M.S.; Giembycz, M.A. Discovery of BRL 50481 [3-(N,N-dimethylsulfonamido)-4-methyl-nitrobenzene], a Selective Inhibitor of Phosphodiesterase 7: In Vitro Studies in Human Monocytes, Lung Macrophages, and CD8+ T-Lymphocytes. *Mol. Pharmacol.* **2004**, *66*, 1679–1689. [CrossRef] [PubMed]

95. Cong, M.; Perry, S.J.; Lin, F.T.; Fraser, I.D.; Hu, L.A.; Chen, W.; Pitcher, J.A.; Scott, J.D.; Lefkowitz, R.J. Regulation of membrane targeting of the G protein-coupled receptor kinase 2 by protein kinase A and its anchoring protein AKAP79. *J. Biol. Chem.* **2001**, *276*, 15192–15199. [CrossRef] [PubMed]

96. Fraser, I.D.; Cong, M.; Kim, J.; Rollins, E.N.; Daaka, Y.; Lefkowitz, R.J.; Scott, J.D. Assembly of an A kinase-anchoring protein-β2-adrenergic receptor complex facilitates receptor phosphorylation and signaling. *Curr. Biol.* **2000**, *10*, 409–412. [CrossRef]

97. Tao, J.; Malbon, C.C. G-protein-coupled receptor-associated A-kinase anchoring proteins AKAP5 and AKAP12: Differential signaling to MAPK and GPCR recycling. *J. Mol. Signal.* **2008**, *3*, 19. [CrossRef] [PubMed]

98. Poppinga, W.J.; Heijink, I.H.; Holtzer, L.J.; Skroblin, P.; Klussmann, E.; Halayko, A.J.; Timens, W.; Maarsingh, H.; Schmidt, M. A-kinase-anchoring proteins coordinate inflammatory responses to cigarette smoke in airway smooth muscle. *Am. J. Physiol. Lung Cell. Mol. Physiol.* **2015**, *308*, L766–L775. [CrossRef] [PubMed]

99. Oldenburger, A.; Poppinga, W.J.; Kos, F.; de Bruin, H.G.; Rijks, W.F.; Heijink, I.H.; Timens, W.; Meurs, H.; Maarsingh, H.; Schmidt, M. A-kinase anchoring proteins contribute to loss of E-cadherin and bronchial epithelial barrier by cigarette smoke. *Am. J. Physiol. Cell Physiol.* **2014**, *306*, C585–C597. [CrossRef] [PubMed]

100. Li, Y.; Chen, L.; Kass, R.S.; Dessauer, C.W. The A-kinase anchoring protein Yotiao facilitates complex formation between adenylyl cyclase type 9 and the IKs potassium channel in heart. *J. Biol. Chem.* **2012**, *287*, 29815–29824. [CrossRef] [PubMed]

101. Perrino, C.; Feliciello, A.; Schiattarella, G.G.; Esposito, G.; Guerriero, R.; Zaccaro, L.; Del Gatto, A.; Saviano, M.; Garbi, C.; Carangi, R.; et al. AKAP121 downregulation impairs protective cAMP signals, promotes mitochondrial dysfunction, and increases oxidative stress. *Cardiovasc. Res.* **2010**, *88*, 101–110. [CrossRef] [PubMed]

102. de Rooij, J.; Zwartkruis, F.J.; Verheijen, M.H.; Cool, R.H.; Nijman, S.M.; Wittinghofer, A.; Bos, J.L. Epac is a Rap1 guanine-nucleotide-exchange factor directly activated by cyclic AMP. *Nature* **1998**, *396*, 474–477. [CrossRef] [PubMed]

103. Scott, J.; Harris, G.J.; Pinder, E.M.; Macfarlane, J.G.; Hellyer, T.P.; Rostron, A.J.; Conway Morris, A.; Thickett, D.R.; Perkins, G.D.; McAuley, D.F.; et al. Exchange protein directly activated by cyclic AMP (EPAC) activation reverses neutrophil dysfunction induced by β2-agonists, corticosteroids, and critical illness. *J. Allergy Clin. Immunol.* **2016**, *137*, 535–544. [CrossRef] [PubMed]

104. Oldenburger, A.; Roscioni, S.S.; Jansen, E.; Menzen, M.H.; Halayko, A.J.; Timens, W.; Meurs, H.; Maarsingh, H.; Schmidt, M. Anti-inflammatory role of the cAMP effectors Epac and PKA: Implications in chronic obstructive pulmonary disease. *PLoS ONE* **2012**, *7*, e31574. [CrossRef] [PubMed]

105. Grandoch, M.; Roscioni, S.S.; Schmidt, M. The role of Epac proteins, novel cAMP mediators, in the regulation of immune, lung and neuronal function. *Br. J. Pharmacol.* **2010**, *159*, 265–284. [CrossRef] [PubMed]

106. Oldenburger, A.; van Basten, B.; Kooistra, W.; Meurs, H.; Maarsingh, H.; Krenning, G.; Timens, W.; Schmidt, M. Interaction between Epac1 and miRNA-7 in airway smooth muscle cells. *Naunyn Schmiedebergs Arch. Pharmacol.* **2014**, *387*, 795–797. [CrossRef] [PubMed]

107. Oldenburger, A.; Timens, W.; Bos, S.; Smit, M.; Smrcka, A.V.; Laurent, A.-C.; Cao, J.; Hylkema, M.; Meurs, H.; Maarsingh, H.; et al. Epac1 and Epac2 are differentially involved in inflammatory and remodeling processes induced by cigarette smoke. *FASEB J. Off. Publ. Fed. Am. Soc. Exp. Biol.* **2014**, *28*, 4617–4628. [CrossRef] [PubMed]

108. Börner, S.; Schwede, F.; Schlipp, A.; Berisha, F.; Calebiro, D.; Lohse, M.J.; Nikolaev, V.O. FRET measurements of intracellular cAMP concentrations and cAMP analog permeability in intact cells. *Nat. Protoc.* **2011**, *6*, 427–438. [CrossRef] [PubMed]

109. Kinkorová, J. Biobanks in the era of personalized medicine: Objectives, challenges, and innovation. *EPMA J.* **2016**, *7*. [CrossRef] [PubMed]

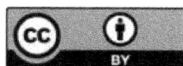

Journal of
Cardiovascular
Development and Disease

MDPI

Review

The Popeye Domain Containing Genes and Their Function as cAMP Effector Proteins in Striated Muscle

Thomas Brand [ORCID]

Cardiovascular Function, National Heart and Lung Institute, Imperial College London,
Imperial Centre for Translational and Experimental Medicine, Rm. 337, Du Cane Road, London W12 0NN, UK;
t.brand@imperial.ac.uk; Tel.: +44-207-594-8744

Received: 27 February 2018; Accepted: 12 March 2018; Published: 13 March 2018

Abstract: The Popeye domain containing (POPDC) genes encode transmembrane proteins, which are abundantly expressed in striated muscle cells. Hallmarks of the POPDC proteins are the presence of three transmembrane domains and the Popeye domain, which makes up a large part of the cytoplasmic portion of the protein and functions as a cAMP-binding domain. Interestingly, despite the prediction of structural similarity between the Popeye domain and other cAMP binding domains, at the protein sequence level they strongly differ from each other suggesting an independent evolutionary origin of POPDC proteins. Loss-of-function experiments in zebrafish and mouse established an important role of POPDC proteins for cardiac conduction and heart rate adaptation after stress. Loss-of function mutations in patients have been associated with limb-girdle muscular dystrophy and AV-block. These data suggest an important role of these proteins in the maintenance of structure and function of striated muscle cells.

Keywords: Popeye domain; cAMP binding; effector protein; cardiac arrhythmia; limb-girdle muscular dystrophy; atrioventricular block

1. Introduction

The second messenger cyclic adenosine $3',5'$-monophosphate (cAMP) activates an evolutionary ancient and universally important intracellular signaling pathway. Several effector proteins have been identified, which bind cAMP with high affinity causing their activation and leading to the execution of a variety of biological activities (Figure 1).

The most important and prominent cAMP effector protein is protein kinase A (PKA), which upon binding of up to four cAMP molecules to the regulatory subunit causes an activation of the catalytic subunits leading to the phosphorylation of many protein substrates. It is estimated that around 350 proteins are phosphorylated in response to β1-adrenergic stimulation, many of which are targeted by PKA [1]. PKA protein substrates are diverse but include proteins regulating energy metabolism, cardiac pacemaking and excitation/contraction coupling. PKA is bound by a number of scaffolding proteins called A kinase anchoring proteins (AKAPs) [2]. In cardiac myocytes, several AKAPs are expressed including D-AKAP1, D-AKAP2, AKAP15/18, AKAP79/150, Yotiao, mAKAPβ, AKAP-Lbc, Gravin and SKIP [3]. AKAPs are responsible to target PKA to specific subcellular domains such as the plasma membrane, transverse (T)-tubules, sarcoplasmatic reticulum, myofilaments and nuclear envelope [2]. AKAP proteins not only bind PKA but also protein substrates and other signaling molecules [2]. Recent data suggest that at physiological cAMP concentrations, dissociation of the PKA holoenzyme does not occur [4]. PKA being bound by different AKAPs in the cell is therefore only able to phosphorylate substrates in its direct vicinity, which enhances specificity and compartmentation of the cellular response.

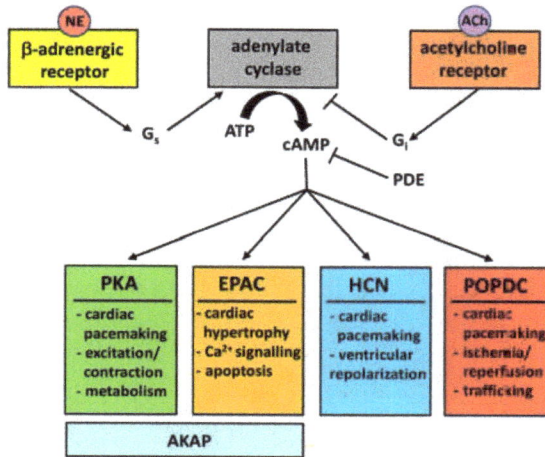

Figure 1. Four cAMP effector proteins are expressed in the heart. Norepinephrine (NE) secreted by sympathetic neurons binds to the β-adrenergic receptor leading to G$_s$ activation and synthesis of cAMP by adenylate cyclase (AC). Acetylcholine (ACh) is secreted by parasympathetic neurons and binds to muscarinergic ACh receptors leading to an activation of G$_i$ causing AC inhibition. The balance of sympathetic and parasympathetic input therefore determines the level of cAMP production. cAMP production in cells is compartmentalized and this is mainly achieved by phoshodiesterases (PDE), which limits cAMP diffusion through degradation. Four effector proteins sense cAMP levels. The best-characterized effector protein is protein kinase A (PKA), which plays a role in cardiac pacemaking, excitation/contraction coupling and cardiac metabolism. The exchange factor directly activated by cAMP (EPAC) has been linked to cardiac hypertrophy, Ca^{2+}-signaling and apoptosis. Often, PKA and EPAC are bound by the same anchor protein (AKAP) along with protein substrates and other enzymes. The hyperpolarization-activated cyclic nucleotide-gated (HCN) channels are important for cardiac pacemaking and ventricular repolarization. Finally, the Popeye domain containing (POPDC) proteins are the most recently identified class of effector proteins and important for cardiac pacemaking, the survival of cardiac myocytes after ischemia/reperfusion and membrane trafficking.

EPAC (exchange factor directly activated by cAMP) is a guanine-nucleotide exchange factors for the Ras-like GTPases, Rap1 and Rap2 [5]. Two EPAC isoforms, EPAC1 and EPAC2 exist in mammals and are thought to modulate Ca^{2+}-homeostasis and hypertrophy in cardiac myocytes [6]. Interestingly, EPAC1 and EPAC2 differ regarding their subcellular localization. EPAC2 is mostly present at the T-tubules and EPAC1 is localized perinuclear [7,8]. EPAC1 is also present in mitochondria and loss of EPAC1 reduces infarct size and cardiomyocyte apoptosis induced by myocardial ischemia/reperfusion injury [9]. EPAC also has pro-arrhythmic effects probably due its ability to decrease potassium currents [10]. Chronic EPAC activation leads to cardiac hypertrophy [11].

Another important effector protein in cardiac myocytes is HCN4, which is a member of the family of hyperpolarization-activated cyclic nucleotide gated channels (HCN). HCN genes encode nonselective voltage-gated cation channels, which are abundantly expressed in cardiac pacemaker cells in the sinoatrial (SAN) and atrioventricular nodes (AVN) but are also present in parts of the ventricular conduction system [12]. Upon binding of cAMP, the HCN4 channel opens more rapidly and completely [13]. This property has led to the assumption that the cAMP-mediated enhancement of HCN channel activity is largely responsible for the increase in heart rate in response to β-adrenergic stimulation. However, the importance of HCN4 in cardiac pacemaking remains controversial [14,15]. Heart rate adaptation in response to adrenergic stimulation remains intact after SAN-specific ablation of the *Hcn4* locus in mice [16]. Moreover, heart rate acceleration in response to adrenergic signaling is unaffected in patients carrying a cAMP-binding site mutation in *HCN4* [17]. To accommodate these facts, it has been proposed that HCN4 may act as a depolarization reserve and its main role may be to counteract parasympathetic slowing of the heart rate [18,19]. In addition to its importance in cardiac pacemaking, HCN channels apparently also have a role in impulse propagation in the SAN and are also essential for ventricular repolarization [20,21]. Importantly, in cardiac hypertrophy, both HCN2 and HCN4 are induced in the ventricular working myocardium causing a prolongation of the cardiac action potential and probably being responsible for the development of cardiac arrhythmia in the hypertrophied ventricle [22].

Although the Popeye domain containing genes were isolated around the same time as EPAC genes [23–26], it took more than a decade to realize that POPDC proteins constitute a novel class of cAMP-effector proteins [27] and an additional four years to demonstrate that cAMP binding is essential for its function [28]. Here we will review the multiple roles of the POPDC gene family in striated muscle biology and disease.

2. The Popeye Gene Family

The POPDC gene family consists of three genes namely *POPDC1* (also known as *BVES*), *POPDC2* and *POPDC3*. In vertebrates, *POPDC1* and *POPDC3* are tandem-organized and in the human genome are present on chromosome 6q21, while *POPDC2* is located on chromosome 3q13.33. [26]. *POPDC1* is the most complex gene with 8 exons, while *POPDC2* and *POPDC3* have only 4 exons. *POPDC1* probably represent the ancestral gene and the other two paralogs were generated through two gene duplication events. The first duplication likely took place at the base of chordate evolution [29]. In support of this view, basic chordates (*Tunicates*, *Cephalochordates*) have two tandem-organized POPDC genes with homologies to *POPDC1* and *POPDC3*. *POPDC2*, which is only found in vertebrates, was probably generated by a second gene duplication event, which probably took place at the base of vertebrate evolution. This view is supported by the fact that *POPDC2* is only present in vertebrates. Moreover, *POPDC2* and *POPDC3* display a similar gene structure and higher similarity at the protein level [30]. The POPDC gene family also evolved independently in invertebrates, where gene duplication events also took place. While molluscs, annelids and dipterans such as *Drosophila* have only a single POPDC gene; many insects have two POPDC genes and some invertebrates (for example the water flea) have multiple POPDC genes. Interestingly, there are also invertebrate species, which lost their POPDC gene during evolution and a prominent example for this is *Caenorhabditis elegans*. Thus, for some species, a lack of POPDC genes is fully compatible with life. We can trace the presence of POPDC genes down to Hydra and the gene family is also found in some protozoan species. We can therefore conclude that POPDC genes have evolved at the base of the animal kingdom. No POPDC genes are found in plants or fungi. Interestingly, the cAMP-binding domain (CNBD) of the bacterial catabolite activator proteins (CAP), also known as catabolite receptor protein (CRP), which are involved in transcriptional regulation of metabolism display the highest similarity of a non-POPDC protein to the Popeye domain.

3. POPDC Proteins

The POPDC proteins are medium-sized transmembrane proteins. They consist of a short extracellular domain (ECD, Figure 2), which in case of POPDC1 has been shown to be subject to N-glycosylation. Potentially, N-glycosylation is more extensive in skeletal muscle and brain than in the heart [31,32]. A consensus sequence for N-glycosylation is also present in the ECD of POPDC2 and POPDC3. POPDC proteins all have three transmembrane domains. In the cytoplasmic part, the conserved Popeye domain is present, which functions as a cAMP-binding domain [27].

The Popeye domain is slightly larger than a typical cyclic nucleotide monophosphate (cNMP)-binding domain (CNBD), suggesting that additional functions other than cAMP-binding reside in the Popeye domain. Indeed, the binding sites of KCNK2 (TREK-1) or CAV3 have been mapped to the Popeye domain of POPDC1 [28,33] (Figure 2). Soon after its discovery, the dimerization of POPDC1 was first described [31,32]. Dimerization is stabilized through disulfide bridge formation. In order to map the sequences, which mediate dimerization, a series of experiments including carboxy-terminal deletions, peptide-mapping and site-directed mutagenesis was utilized [34]. Dimerization appeared to depend on two conserved lysine residues at the end of the Popeye domain. Mutation of the dimerization motif interfered with cell adhesion, and epithelia formation There are probably other sequences in POPDC1 also responsible for dimerization as POPDC1 protein, which lacked these sequences, were still able to homodimerize [37].

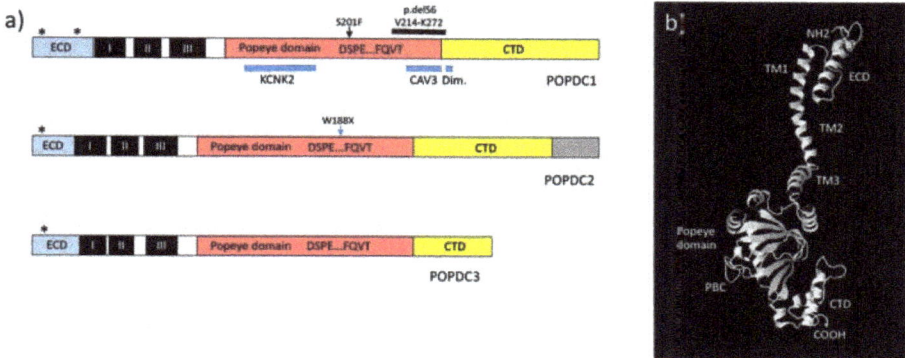

Figure 2. Structure of the Popeye domain containing proteins. (**a**) Schematic structure of the human POPDC isoforms. The three POPDC proteins share a similar protein structure. In each case a 20–40 amino acid long extracellular domain (ECD), which harbors one or two N-glycosylation sites (asterisks) is followed by three transmembrane (TM) domains (I–III, black boxes). The cytoplasmic portion of the POPDC proteins consists of the Popeye domain (red box) and the carboxyterminal domain (CTD, yellow box). The phosphate-binding cassette (PBC), which is thought to bind cAMP, consists of the two tetrapeptides DSPE and FQVT. In case of POPDC1, the locations for the KCNK2 (TREK-1) [28] and CAV3 [33] binding sites and the putative dimerization motif [34] are indicated (blue bars). POPDC2 generates three alternative splice products, which differ in their carboxy-terminus labeled by a grey box. Mutations in POPDC1 and POPDC2, which have been identified in patients with muscle and heart disease are indicated above each protein model. (**b**) 3-D structure of POPDC3. A homology-based structural model was generated with the help of the Phyre 2 algorithm [35]. The resulting structure was visualized with the help of First Glance in JMOL [36].

4. The Popeye Domain Is a Novel cAMP-Binding Domain

It is thought that the main function of the 150 amino acids long Popeye domain is to bind cAMP [27]. The structural prediction of the Popeye domain revealed a similarity to the CNBD of the catalytic subunit of PKA [27]. The structure of the CNBD is categorized as jelly-roll β-barrel fold, which is found in many proteins. However, not all of these proteins bind cyclic nucleotides but other ligands [38]. A conserved feature of the CNBD is the phosphate-binding cassette (PBC), which directly makes contact to cAMP and consists of a short α-helix and a loop located between β-sheets 6 and 7. Two conserved residues found in all PBCs include an arginine, which binds to the phosphate group of cAMP and a glutamate that binds the 2'-OH group of the ribose [39]. Those proteins that share the jelly-roll β-barrel fold structure but lack these arginine and glutamate residues, bind to ligands other than cNMPs. It is, therefore, essential that sufficient experimental evidence will be generated that it is unequivocally established that POPDC proteins bind cAMP despite their lack of a canonical PBC. The non-canonical PBC of the Popeye domain is thought to consist of two conserved sequence motifs (FL/IDSPEW/F) and FQVT/S), which are linked by a non-conserved sequence of variable length [27] (Figure 3).

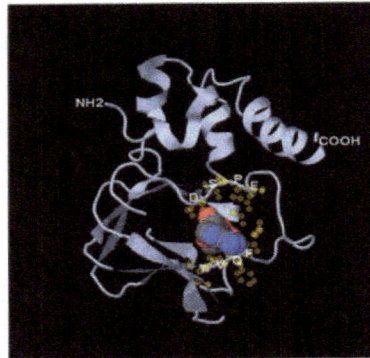

Figure 3. Structure of the Popeye domain. A homology-based structural model of human POPDC1 was generated. A space-filling model of cAMP was placed in the putative phosphate-binding cassette. The DSPE and FQVT motifs, depicted as yellow halos, surround the cAMP molecule and as mutagenesis studies suggest, seem to be directly involved in cAMP-binding.

Several of these evolutionary conserved residues were mutagenized by a charge-to-alanine strategy in POPDC1 and POPDC2 and as expected, the resulting mutant proteins displayed a reduction in the cAMP-binding affinity supporting their involvement in nucleotide-binding [27].

Assays were developed to demonstrate cAMP-binding by POPDC proteins. The first one, is a cAMP agarose precipitation assay, which established cAMP-binding of native POPDC1 protein extracted from the chicken heart [27]. POPDC1 was also precipitated by cGMP agarose and free cGMP was able to elute POPDC1 from cAMP agarose and thus, at this stage it was unclear, whether POPDC1 binds cAMP selectively, or both cyclic nucleotides with equal affinity. The agarose-precipitation assay also established that the three POPDC proteins are all able to bind cAMP [27].

A recombinant POPDC1 protein encompassing the cytoplasmic part of the protein was employed in a competitive radio-ligand binding assay, which established an IC_{50} concentration of 118.4 ± 7.1 nM for cAMP and of 5.27 ± 0.68 µM for cGMP [27]. The approximately 40-fold difference in affinity between cAMP and cGMP is typical for a cAMP-binding protein and similar differences in affinities for both nucleotides have been described for the CNBDs of PKA [40].

A third assay demonstrating cAMP binding was developed based on the interaction of POPDC1 with the two-pore potassium channel KCNK2 (TREK-1) [27]. A bimolecular fluorescence resonance energy transfer (FRET) assay using CFP-tagged POPDC1 and YFP-tagged TREK-1 was utilized. Addition of the β-adrenergic agonist isoproterenol or direct stimulation of adenylate cyclase by forskolin caused a rapid decline of the YFP/CFP ratio with a kinetic, typical for an adenylate cyclase-dependent process [27]. A mutant protein, carrying a mutation in D200, which is one of the residues of the DSPE motif in the PBC of POPDC1 (Figure 3), did not cause any changes in the FRET signal after the addition of isoproterenol. Likewise, nitroprussid, which raises cGMP levels in cells, did not affect the FRET signal, which supports the notion that at physiological concentration levels, POPDC1 protein binds cAMP but not cGMP.

Finally, evidence for cAMP-binding of POPDC proteins stems from the discovery of a POPDC1[S201F] mutation, which is present in patients, which develop a limb-girdle muscular dystrophy (LGMD) phenotype [28]. The serine residue 201 of POPDC1 is part of the PBC and change of serine into phenylalanine is likely to reduce the cAMP-binding affinity. Indeed, measurements of cAMP affinity established a loss of about 50% in case of the mutant protein [28]. Thus, there is ample of experimental and genetic evidence, which establishes the Popeye domain as a novel cAMP-binding domain with a highly divergent protein sequence [28]. However, so far, the molecular characterization mostly dealt with POPDC1 protein and therefore it will be important to extend these experiments also to the other two family members and to determine, whether cyclic nucleotide specificity is the same for each of the POPDC proteins, and whether all three POPDC isoforms bind cAMP with equal affinity.

5. Expression Pattern of POPDC Genes

RNA expression data for the POPDC family members revealed the highest expression level of POPDC genes in striated muscle tissue (Figure 4) [26]. While *POPDC2* is preferentially expressed in the heart, *POPDC1* and *POPDC3* show higher expression levels in skeletal muscle. Of the three genes, *POPDC1* shows a more widespread expression than *POPDC2* and *POPDC3*. In many tissues, *POPDC1* and at least one other POPDC gene is co-expressed. Apart from striated muscle, expression was also observed in smooth muscle cells, neurons, and epithelial cells [41]. Conflicting data have been published for the heart regarding the presence of POPDC1 in non-muscle cell types of the heart. Several studies from my lab revealed an exclusive expression in cardiac myocytes [41–43], while another group reported expression in cardiac myocytes but also presence of POPDC1 in the epicardium and in coronary arteries [25,44,45]. The LacZ reporter gene, which was knocked into *POPDC1* did not reveal a significant expression in any of the non-muscle cell lineages in the adult heart [26,41]. However, a shortcoming of these data is the fact that the LacZ reporter gene may not fully recapitulate the expression domains of the endogenous gene. On the other end, it is equally conceivable that the antibodies employed may be cross-reactive. A thorough investigation of the expression patterns of POPDC genes and proteins in vertebrate embryos and in the adult seems to be required to settle this case.

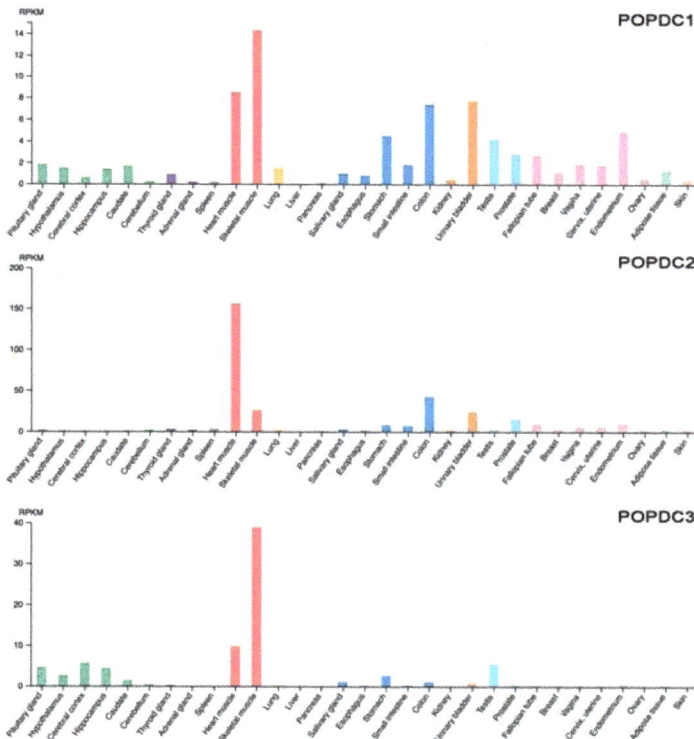

Figure 4. Expression of POPDC genes in the human body. RNA seq data of *POPDC1*, *POPDC2* and *POPDC3* in human tissue. RNA expression is quantified as reads per kilogram per million mapped reads (RPKM). Data were copied from the Human Protein Atlas website [45–48].

Immunolocalization of POPDC proteins revealed an expression at the plasma membrane of isolated cardiac myocytes and a similar pattern was observed in cardiac tissues. POPDC proteins have been described to be present at the lateral membrane, intercalated disks, costameres [33], t-tubules and caveolae [33] (Figure 5). In addition, POPDC1 was also localized to the nuclear envelope [49], and in the nucleoplasm [50]. Plasma membrane localization was also reported for skeletal muscle, however no detailed analysis of the subcellular localization in different membrane compartments has been reported [28]. A recent report, which was looking for novel intercalated disk proteins described a preferential localization of POPDC2 in the intercalated disk of ventricular myocytes of the human and canine heart, arguing for an important function of POPDC2 for electrical cell-to-cell coupling, and impulse propagation [51].

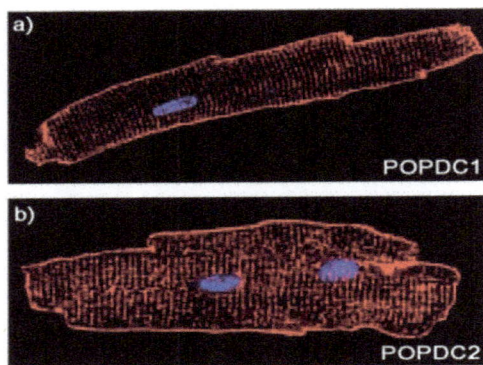

Figure 5. Expression of POPDC1 and POPDC2 in cardiac myocytes. Isolated adult cardiac myocytes were immunostained with (**a**) POPDC1 and (**b**) POPDC2 antibodies, respectively.

6. Animal Models to Define the Function POPDC Genes

In order to define the function of POPDC genes, the *Popdc1* and *Popdc2* genes were ablated in mice by substituting the first coding exon with a LacZ reporter gene [27,52] (Table 1). The resulting homozygous mutants were viable and no embryonic lethality has been reported. Phenotype analysis was guided by the LacZ expression pattern [41]. In the adult mouse heart, *Popdc1* and *Popdc2* are expressed in cardiac myocytes, while no expression in smooth muscle or non-muscle cells is observed [27,41]. *Popdc1* displays higher level of expression in atria than in ventricles, while *Popdc2* is evenly expressed in both chamber types [27]. Both genes display a strong expression in the sinoatrial (SAN) and atrioventricular nodes (AVN) as well as in the ventricular conduction system [27]. The high-level expression of POPDC1 and 2 genes in the cardiac conduction system prompted the investigation of the functional status of it in the null mutant animals. While both *Popdc1* and *Popdc2* null mutants displayed normal heart rhythm at rest, a stress-induced sinus bradycardia developed in response to physical or emotional stress and after β-adrenergic receptor stimulation [27]. ECG analysis revealed the presence of stress-induced sinus pauses. The length of each sinus pause was variable and could be brief or more prolonged. Interestingly, the arrhythmia phenotype developed in both null mutants in an age-dependent manner and was absent in young adults and gradually worsened with increasing age [27]. The phenotype was also present in isolated Langendorff-perfused hearts and a normal cholinergic response was observed after carbachol treatment, which suggests a primary defect in the cardiac pacemaker.

Table 1. Cardiac and skeletal muscle phenotypes in model organism and patients.

Species	Mutation	Heart	Skeletal Muscle	References
mouse	$Popdc1^{-/-}$	stress-induced sinus bradycardia	regeneration defect	[27,50]
		ischemia-reperfusion damage	not analyzed	[33]
	$Popdc2^{-/-}$	Stress-induced sinus bradycardia	not analyzed	[27]
zebrafish	$popdc1$ morphants	AV-block, pericardial effusion	muscular dystrophy	[28]
	$popdc2$ morphants	AV-block, pericardial effusion	muscular dystrophy	[53]
	$popdc1^{S191F}$	AV-block, pericardial effusion	muscular dystrophy	[28]
human	$POPDC1^{S201F}$	2nd degree AV-block	limb-girdle MD	[28]
	$POPDC1^{del56\ V217-K272}$	1st degree AV-block,	limb-girdle MD	[54]
	$POPDC2^{W188X}$	3rd degree AV-block	no known phenotype	[55]

Structural analysis of the sinoatrial node (SAN) morphology revealed significant structural alterations. The SAN is located at the border between vena cava and right atrium and consists of nodal myocytes, which also called spider and spindle cells due to their irregular shape and the long neurite-like cellular extensions [56]. Nodal myocytes are embedded in a rich extracellular matrix and are poorly electrically coupled. In both, *Popdc1* and *Popdc2* null mutants, pacemaker cells displayed a reduced number of cellular extensions, and overall the SAN had a more compact structure. Moreover, a reduction of nodal myocardium was noted in the inferior part of the SAN [27].

The molecular basis of the sinus node dysfunction in *Popdc1* and *Popdc2* null mutants is not well understood. An attractive hypothesis involves a modulatory role of POPDC proteins for the pacemaker current I_f. Therefore, I_f current density and activation time was measured in isolated SAN myocytes from WT and *Popdc2* null mutant mice [27]. Cells of both genotypes were indistinguishable in current density under basal conditions and after superfusion with 8-Br-cAMP. While I_f was not investigated in the *Popdc1* null mutant, therefore an interaction of POPDC1 and HCN4 cannot be excluded, however, the similarity of phenotypes of both *Popdc1* and *Popdc2* null mutants makes it very unlikely that I_f function is modulated by POPDC1.

One of the first POPDC-interacting protein identified in the heart was the potassium channel TWIK-related K$^+$ channel 1 (TREK-1) or KCNK2 [27]. This ion channel is a member of the two-pore domain potassium channel (K$_2$P) family. TREK-1 gating is affected by a large number of stimuli including stretch, pH, temperature, phosphorylation, and is also modulated through the interaction with other proteins [57]. In the presence of POPDC1, TREK-1 produces a twofold higher current in *Xenopus* oocytes [27]. The effect is also observed when POPDC2 or POPDC3 were co-expressed. The doubling of TREK-1 current is probably due to an increase in membrane trafficking as more TREK-1 protein is detected at the cell surface when POPDC proteins are present. The effect of POPDC proteins on TREK-1 is sensitive to cAMP and is lost when cAMP levels were increased after applying the general PDE inhibitor theophylline or 8-Br-cAMP [27,28]. The interaction of POPDC proteins with TREK-1 has been mapped to the Popeye domain by deletion analysis (Figure 2). Based on the interaction of POPDC1 and TREK-1, a bi-molecular Förster-resonance energy transfer (FRET) sensor was constructed. The FRET ratio obtained at baseline decreased after the addition of isoproterenol or forskolin, suggesting that cyclic nucleotide-binding affects the interaction of POPDC1 with TREK-1 [27]. A cardiac specific knockout of *Kcnk2*, which encodes TREK-1, displays a stress-induced sinus bradycardia similar to the one observed in *Popdc1* and *Popdc2* null mutants [58], suggesting that the sinus bradycardia in POPDC mutants may in part be due to an impaired TREK-1 current.

However, it is likely that additional proteins may be involved. Cardiac pacemaking is governed by two oscillatory mechanisms, the membrane clock and the Ca^{2+}-clock [59]. The membrane clock initiates depolarization in response to I_f but also involves the voltage-gated Ca^{2+}-channels. The Ca^{2+}-clock on the other hand is active in late diastole when Ca^{2+} is released from the sarcoplasmatic reticulum by the ryanodine receptors (RyRs) and exchanged for Na$^+$ by NCX, which generates a depolarizing I_{NCX} current. Both clocks are coupled by Ca^{2+}, which enters the cell through the L-type Ca^{2+} channels, which leads to a replenishment of the SR allowing the next pacemaker cycle to be initiated. Interestingly, it was recently reported that the sodium calcium exchanger NCX1 is a POPDC2-interacting protein [60] and the loss of NCX1 causes SAN dysfunction similar to the one observed in POPDC mutants [61]. It seems warranted to thoroughly investigate protein-protein interaction, subcellular localization, and function of proteins of the membrane and Ca^{2+} clocks in the different POPDC mutants.

The impact of ischemia/reperfusion injury was studied in the *Popdc1* null mutant [33]. Langendorff-perfused mutant hearts displayed a significantly lower functional recovery, while infarct size was larger. Isolated cardiac myocytes from *Popdc1* null mutants displayed altered Ca^{2+}-transients and increased vulnerability to oxidative stress. Apparently *Popdc1* is involved in myocyte survival through the suppression of the pro-apoptotic Bcl2 interacting protein 3 (*Bnip3*) gene [62]. While skeletal muscle is not as well studied than cardiac muscle in POPDC null mutants, it has been shown that muscle regeneration is impaired in *Popdc1* null mutants, however, the underlying molecular mechanism has yet to be elucidated [63].

In *Popdc1* null mutant mice, the caveolar compartment is affected and caveolae were fewer in number, however their size was increased [33]. POPDC1 interacts with CAV3 through a consensus sequence present at the end of the Popeye domain (Figure 2). This could have profound effects on cardiac signal transduction given that caveolae in cardiac myocytes are clustering membrane receptors, signaling molecules, protein pumps and ion channels [64]. It has been reported that POPDC2 in human and canine cardiac myocytes are predominantly present at the intercalated disk [51]. The intercalated disk controls electrical coupling between cardiac myocytes and therefore is a major determinant of cardiac conduction. It will be interesting to study the structure and function of the intercalated disk in POPDC2 null mutants and to measure electrical conduction in *Popdc2* null mutants.

Loss-of function experiments were also conducted in zebrafish and morpholino-mediated knockdown of *popdc1* and *popdc2* caused cardiac arrhythmia and muscular dystrophy phenotypes [28,53] (Table 1). The cardiac arrhythmia was already present in the embryo and the severity of the phenotype increased in an age-dependent manner. In young larvae (4 days post-fertilization, dpf) typically a type I AV-block was present. At increasing age total heart block or even non-contracting hearts were also observed. The skeletal muscle phenotype in *popdc1* and *popdc2* morphants was characterized by an impaired formation of the myotendinous junction which probably caused the myofiber rupture, which was seen in both morphants [28,53]. The heart of many *popdc1* and *popdc2* morphants displayed a pericardial effusion, which is thought to indicate myocardial pumping deficiency. However, in the case of *popdc1* morphants, the pericardial effusion could also be based on a defective barrier formation of the skin due to impaired tight junction formation [65]. The molecular basis for the tight junction defect is probably due to abnormal accumulation of tight junction proteins, which is caused by an aberrant localization of atypical protein kinase C (aPKC) [65]. Interestingly, it has been demonstrated that another protein involved in cell contact formation, zonula occludens 1 (ZO1) is a POPDC1-interacting protein [66].

The contact structures between skeletal muscle fibers in the zebrafish tail musculature is formed by the myoseptum or myotendinous junction (MTJ) [67]. The MTJ is a complex structure, which is established by several plasma membrane proteins and various matrix proteins [68,69]. In the *popdc1* and *popdc2* morphants and in the *popdc1*^{S191F} mutant, the MTJ is abnormal in structure and in the *popdc1*^{S191F} mutant lacks the collagen matrix, which probably is essential for the MTJ to withstand the tensile forces of the contracting myofibers. Consistent with this hypothesis, large numbers of hypercontracted myofibers that lost contact to the MTJ are seen in *popdc1* and *popdc2* morphants and the *popdc1*^{S191F} mutant [28,53].

7. Evidence for a Role of POPDC Genes in Human Heart and Skeletal Muscle

The first mutation of *POPDC1* discovered in patients is the recessive *POPDC1*^{S201F} mutation, which was reported to be associated with cardiac arrhythmia and muscular dystrophy [28]. This mutation alters serine 201, which is one of the invariant amino acids present in the putative cAMP binding domain (DSPE motif) (Figure 2, Table 1). The serine residue is substituted by phenylalanine, which may interfere with the cyclic nucleotide gaining access to the PBC. Measurement of the cAMP binding affinity revealed a 50% reduction in case of the mutant protein [28]. Moreover, the S201F mutant caused an increased level of TREK-1 current compared to wildtype (WT) while membrane transport of the channel protein was decreased [28]. This paradoxical finding of decreased membrane transport and increased current may be explained on the basis that PCPDC1 in a complex with TREK-1 protein might be protected from getting inactivated by PKA-dependent phosphorylation [70]. Forced expression of POPDC1^{S201F} in HL1 cells affected the action potential [28]. Three patients from a 3-generation family of Albanian descent carried the POPDC^{S201F} mutation to homozygosity and developed an early onset second-degree AV-block and a late onset limb-girdle muscular dystrophy (LGMD2X, OMIM: #61812) [28]. Serum creatine kinase levels were elevated, and muscle biopsies showed dystrophic changes with increased fiber size variability, increased central nuclei, and a few necrotic fibers. Electron microscopic analysis of skeletal muscle biopsies of one of the patients carrying a POPDC1^{S201F} mutation revealed the presence of membrane discontinuities [28]. Similar discontinuities have been observed in patients with mutations in anoctamine-5 (*ANO5*). While only found in a single patient, these discontinuities are possibly an indication for impaired repair of the muscle plasma membrane [71]. Interestingly, another protein involved in membrane repair, dysferlin, has also been shown to be an interaction partner of POPDC1 [28]. Expression of the *popdc1* disease-associated mutation (S191F) in zebrafish caused similar phenotypes as in the patients. Skeletal muscle from homozygous *popdc1*^{S191F} mutants showed myofibrillar misalignment, aberrant formation of the myotendinous junction, myofiber detachment, and decreased membrane localization of POPDC1 and POPDC2 [28]. Electron microscopy revealed an absence of extracellular matrix at the myotendinous junction. Abnormalities of the zebrafish *popdc1*^{S191} mutant heart also resembled the patient's phenotype displaying an overall reduction in heart rate and stroke volume. Isoproterenol caused an increase in the number of embryos displaying a 2:1 AV block.

Recently, another recessive mutation in *POPDC1* was reported in a consanguineous family of Algerian origin [54]. The splice site mutation (c.816 + 2T > C) affects the splice donor site in intron 8 and may cause skipping of exon 8 resulting in a mutant protein with a predicted loss of 56 amino acids (POPDC1$^{del56\ V217\text{-}K272}$), (Figure 2, Table 1). Two siblings are affected, and both displayed a first-degree atrioventricular (AV)-block, high serum creatine kinase levels and evidence for a mild limb-girdle muscular dystrophy. Immunostaining of biopsies revealed a strong reduction in membrane staining of both, the mutant POPDC1 protein and also of POPDC2. Thus, despite POPDC1^{S201F} and POPDC1$^{del56\ V217\text{-}K272}$ mutations are at different position in the protein they induce a similar pathology and display impaired membrane trafficking [28,54]. The underlying molecular defects require further characterization.

POPDC1 may also contribute to phenotype variability in other LGMDs. Interestingly, heterozygous *POPDC1* mutations were found in patients that also carried Lamin A (*LMNA*) or dysferlin (*DYSF*) mutations. This putative genetic interaction is probably of significance as both proteins, dysferlin and Lamin A also interact at the protein level with PCPDC1.

Patients carrying a recessive *POPDC2* mutation were recently discovered [55]. This mutation (c.563G>A, p.Trp188Stop, POPDC^{W188X}) resulted in the insertion of a premature stop codon at position 188 of *POPDC2*, leading in the protein to a deletion within the putative cAMP binding domain. Even though the FQVT motif of the PBC of POPDC2 was deleted in this mutant, cAMP responsiveness remained unaltered. Likewise, the interaction and modulation of the TREK-1 current remained unaltered. Therefore, currently the pathogenic mechanism is not fully clear. The deletion of part of the Popeye domain and the carboxyterminal domain may influence the kinetics of cAMP binding or could interfere with protein-protein interaction.

8. Conclusions

We recently proposed four working models of how POPDC proteins might modulate proteins in order to mediate cAMP signaling in striated muscle cells [68]. The first model, which is called the *switch model*, proposes that binding of cAMP to POPDC proteins causes an allosteric effect as it was observed for PKA, EPAC and HCN4 [72].

The *switch model* assumes that allostery not only affects POPDC proteins but also interacting proteins. Direct evidence for such a behavior is currently missing. Nonetheless, the TREK-1-POPDC1 FRET assay gives support for the presence of an allosteric effect. Experimental support is present for the *cargo model*, which proposes that POPDC acts on proteins by modulating their membrane trafficking. Strong support for this model comes from the observation that the POPDC1^{S201F} mutant not only affects membrane localization of the mutant protein but also of POPDC2. Similarly, membrane localization of TREK-1 in *Xenopus oocytes* is modulated by POPDC1 and is cAMP-sensitive.

The *shielding model* is a variation of the *switch model* taking into account that POPDC proteins and also some of the interacting proteins are getting phosphorylated in response to βAR activation [1]. It can be envisioned that cAMP binding and phosphorylation of POPDC proteins may lead to conformational changes that may also affect access of PKA or other kinases to their substrates.

Finally, the *sponge model* takes into account that POPDC proteins are abundant in cardiac and skeletal muscle cells and display a complex subcellular localization. POPDC proteins have a high affinity binding site for cAMP, which suggests that these proteins may have a strong impact on cAMP compartmentalization. POPDC proteins may assist adenylate cyclases, phosphodiesterases, and AKAP proteins to create nanodomains of cAMP signaling. Further work is required to confirm or refute these working models.

Acknowledgments: Research in the author's lab was funded through grants of the following funders: British Heart Foundation (BHF) (PG/14/46/30911 and PG/14/83/31128), Medical Research Council (MRC) (MR/J010383/1), the Association Francaise contre le Myopathie (AFM), (project 19469).

Conflicts of Interest: The author declares no conflict of interest.

References

1. Lundby, A.; Andersen, M.N.; Steffensen, A.B.; Horn, H.; Kelstrup, C.D.; Francavilla, C.; Jensen, L.J.; Schmitt, N.; Thomsen, M.B.; Olsen, J.V. In vivo phosphoproteomics analysis reveals the cardiac targets of beta-adrenergic receptor signaling. *Sci. Signal.* **2013**, *6*. [CrossRef] [PubMed]

2. Baldwin, T.A.; Dessauer, C.W. Function of adenylyl cyclase in heart: The AKAP connection. *J. Cardiovasc. Dev. Dis.* **2018**, *5*. [CrossRef] [PubMed]

3. Ercu, M.; Klussmann, E. Roles of A-kinase anchoring proteins and phosphodiesterases in the cardiovascular system. *J. Cardiovasc. Dev. Dis.* **2018**, *5*. [CrossRef] [PubMed]

4. Smith, F.D.; Esseltine, J.L.; Nygren, P.J.; Veesler, D.; Byrne, D.P.; Vonderach, M.; Strashnov, I.; Eyers, C.E.; Eyers, P.A.; Langeberg, L.K.; et al. Local protein kinase A action proceeds through intact holoenzymes. *Science* **2017**, *356*, 1288–1293. [CrossRef] [PubMed]

5. Lezoualc'h, F.; Fazal, L.; Laudette, M.; Conte, C. Cyclic AMP sensor Epac proteins and their role in cardiovascular function and disease. *Circ. Res.* **2016**, *118*, 881–897. [CrossRef] [PubMed]

6. Morel, E.; Marcantoni, A.; Gastineau, M.; Birkedal, R.; Rochais, F.; Garnier, A.; Lompre, A.M.; Vandecasteele, G.; Lezoualc'h, F. cAMP-binding protein Epac induces cardiomyocyte hypertrophy. *Circ. Res.* **2005**, *97*, 1296–1304. [CrossRef] [PubMed]

7. Pereira, L.; Rehmann, H.; Lao, D.H.; Erickson, J.R.; Bossuyt, J.; Chen, J.; Bers, D.M. Novel Epac fluorescent ligand reveals distinct Epac1 vs. Epac2 distribution and function in cardiomyocytes. *Proc. Natl. Acad. Sci. USA* **2015**, *112*, 3991–3996. [CrossRef] [PubMed]

8. Parnell, E.; Smith, B.O.; Yarwood, S.J. The cAMP sensors, Epac1 and Epac2, display distinct subcellular distributions despite sharing a common nuclear pore localisation signal. *Cell. Signal.* **2015**, *27*, 989–996. [CrossRef] [PubMed]

9. Fazal, L.; Laudette, M.; Paula-Gomes, S.; Pons, S.; Conte, C.; Tortosa, F.; Sicard, P.; Sainte-Marie, Y.; Bisserier, M.; Lairez, O.; et al. Multifunctional mitochondrial Epac1 controls myocardial cell death. *Circ. Res.* **2017**, *120*, 645–657. [CrossRef] [PubMed]

10. Brette, F.; Blandin, E.; Simard, C.; Guinamard, R.; Salle, L. EPAC activator critically regulates action potential duration by decreasing potassium current in rat adult ventricle. *J. Mol. Cell. Cardiol.* **2013**, *57*, 96–105. [CrossRef] [PubMed]

11. Metrich, M.; Lucas, A.; Gastineau, M.; Samuel, J.L.; Heymes, C.; Morel, E.; Lezoualc'h, F. Epac mediates β-adrenergic receptor-induced cardiomyocyte hypertrophy. *Circ. Res.* **2008**, *102*, 959–965. [CrossRef] [PubMed]

12. Herrmann, S.; Layh, B.; Ludwig, A. Novel insights into the distribution of cardiac HCN channels: An expression study in the mouse heart. *J. Mol. Cell. Cardiol.* **2011**, *51*, 997–1006. [CrossRef] [PubMed]

13. DiFrancesco, D.; Tortora, P. Direct activation of cardiac pacemaker channels by intracellular cyclic AMP. *Nature* **1991**, *351*, 145–147. [CrossRef] [PubMed]

14. Vinogradova, T.M.; Lyashkov, A.E.; Zhu, W.; Ruknudin, A.M.; Sirenko, S.; Yang, D.; Deo, S.; Barlow, M.; Johnson, S.; Caffrey, J.L.; et al. High basal protein kinase A-dependent phosphorylation drives rhythmic internal Ca^{2+} store oscillations and spontaneous beating of cardiac pacemaker cells. *Circ. Res.* **2006**, *98*, 505–514. [CrossRef] [PubMed]

15. Lakatta, E.G.; Maltsev, V.A.; Vinogradova, T.M. A coupled system of intracellular Ca^{2+} clocks and surface membrane voltage clocks controls the timekeeping mechanism of the heart's pacemaker. *Circ. Res.* **2010**, *106*, 659–673. [CrossRef] [PubMed]

16. Herrmann, S.; Stieber, J.; Stockl, G.; Hofmann, F.; Ludwig, A. HCN4 provides a 'depolarization reserve' and is not required for heart rate acceleration in mice. *EMBO J.* **2007**, *26*, 4423–4432. [CrossRef] [PubMed]

17. Schweizer, P.A.; Duhme, N.; Thomas, D.; Becker, R.; Zehelein, J.; Draguhn, A.; Bruehl, C.; Katus, H.A.; Koenen, M. cAMP sensitivity of HCN pacemaker channels determines basal heart rate but is not critical for autonomic rate control. *Circ. Arrhythm. Electrophysiol.* **2010**, *3*, 542–552. [CrossRef] [PubMed]

18. Kozasa, Y.; Nakashima, N.; Ito, M.; Ishikawa, T.; Kimoto, H.; Ushijima, K.; Makita, N.; Takano, M. HCN4 pacemaker channels attenuate the parasympathetic response and stabilize the spontaneous firing of sinoatrial node. *J. Physiol.* **2018**, *596*, 809–825. [CrossRef] [PubMed]

19. Mesirca, P.; Alig, J.; Torrente, A.G.; Muller, J.C.; Marger, L.; Rollin, A.; Marquilly, C.; Vincent, A.; Dubel, S.; Bidaud, I.; et al. Cardiac arrhythmia induced by genetic silencing of 'funny' (f) channels is rescued by GIRK4 inactivation. *Nat. Commun.* **2014**, *5*, 4664. [CrossRef] [PubMed]

20. Fenske, S.; Krause, S.; Biel, M.; Wahl-Schott, C. The role of HCN channels in ventricular repolarization. *Trends Cardiovasc. Med.* **2011**, *21*, 216–220. [CrossRef] [PubMed]

21. Wahl-Schott, C.; Fenske, S.; Biel, M. HCN channels: New roles in sinoatrial node function. *Curr. Opin. Pharmacol.* **2014**, *15*, 83–90. [CrossRef] [PubMed]

22. Hofmann, F.; Fabritz, L.; Stieber, J.; Schmitt, J.; Kirchhof, P.; Ludwig, A.; Herrmann, S. Ventricular HCN channels decrease the repolarization reserve in the hypertrophic heart. *Cardiovasc. Res.* **2012**, *95*, 317–326. [CrossRef] [PubMed]

23. De Rooij, J.; Zwartkruis, F.J.; Verheijen, M.H.; Cool, R.H.; Nijman, S.M.; Wittinghofer, A.; Bos, J.L. Epac is a Rap1 guanine-nucleotide-exchange factor directly activated by cyclic AMP. *Nature* **1998**, *396*, 474–477. [CrossRef] [PubMed]

24. Kawasaki, H.; Springett, G.M.; Mochizuki, N.; Toki, S.; Nakaya, M.; Matsuda, M.; Housman, D.E.; Graybiel, A.M. A family of cAMP-binding proteins that directly activate Rap1. *Science* **1998**, *282*, 2275–2279. [CrossRef] [PubMed]

25. Reese, D.E.; Zavaljevski, M.; Streiff, N.L.; Bader, D. Bves: A novel gene expressed during coronary blood vessel development. *Dev. Biol.* **1999**, *209*, 159–171. [CrossRef] [PubMed]

26. Andree, B.; Hillemann, T.; Kessler-Icekson, G.; Schmitt-John, T.; Jockusch, H.; Arnold, H.H.; Brand, T. Isolation and characterization of the novel popeye gene family expressed in skeletal muscle and heart. *Dev. Biol.* **2000**, *223*, 371–382. [CrossRef] [PubMed]

27. Froese, A.; Breher, S.S.; Waldeyer, C.; Schindler, R.F.; Nikolaev, V.O.; Rinne, S.; Wischmeyer, E.; Schlueter, J.; Becher, J.; Simrick, S.; et al. Popeye domain containing proteins are essential for stress-mediated modulation of cardiac pacemaking in mice. *J. Clin. Investig.* **2012**, *122*, 1119–1130. [CrossRef] [PubMed]

28. Schindler, R.F.; Scotton, C.; Zhang, J.; Passarelli, C.; Ortiz-Bonnin, B.; Simrick, S.; Schwerte, T.; Poon, K.L.; Fang, M.; Rinne, S.; et al. $POPDC1^{S201F}$ causes muscular dystrophy and arrhythmia by affecting protein trafficking. *J. Clin. Investig.* **2016**, *126*, 239–253. [CrossRef] [PubMed]

29. Tree of the Month: Zebrafish Popeye-Domain-Containing Proteins and Heartbeat Regulation. Available online: http://phylomedb.org/?q=node/659 (accessed on 30 January 2018).

30. Brand, T. The popeye domain-containing gene family. *Cell Biochem. Biophys.* **2005**, *43*, 95–104. [CrossRef]

31. Vasavada, T.K.; DiAngelo, J.R.; Duncan, M.K. Developmental expression of Pop1/Bves. *J. Histochem. Cytochem.* **2004**, *52*, 371–377. [CrossRef] [PubMed]

32. Knight, R.F.; Bader, D.M.; Backstrom, J.R. Membrane topology of Bves/Pop1A, a cell adhesion molecule that displays dynamic changes in cellular distribution during development. *J. Biol. Chem.* **2003**, *278*, 32872–32879. [CrossRef] [PubMed]

33. Alcalay, Y.; Hochhauser, E.; Kliminski, V.; Dick, J.; Zahalka, M.A.; Parnes, D.; Schlesinger, H.; Abassi, Z.; Shainberg, A.; Schindler, R.F.; et al. Popeye domain containing 1 (Popdc1/Bves) is a caveolae-associated protein involved in ischemia tolerance. *PLoS ONE* **2013**, *8*, e71100. [CrossRef] [PubMed]

34. Kawaguchi, M.; Hager, H.A.; Wada, A.; Koyama, T.; Chang, M.S.; Bader, D.M. Identification of a novel intracellular interaction domain essential for Bves function. *PLoS ONE* **2008**, *3*, e2261. [CrossRef] [PubMed]

35. Kelley, L.A.; Mezulis, S.; Yates, C.M.; Wass, M.N.; Sternberg, M.J. The Phyre2 web portal for protein modeling, prediction and analysis. *Nat. Protoc.* **2015**, *10*, 845–858. [CrossRef] [PubMed]

36. First Glance in Jmol. Available online: http://bioinformatics.org/firstglance/fgij/ (accessed on 13 February 2018).

37. Russ, P.K.; Pino, C.J.; Williams, C.S.; Bader, D.M.; Haselton, F.R.; Chang, M.S. Bves modulates tight junction associated signaling. *PLoS ONE* **2011**, *6*, e14563. [CrossRef] [PubMed]

38. Kannan, N.; Wu, J.; Anand, G.S.; Yooseph, S.; Neuwald, A.F.; Venter, J.C.; Taylor, S.S. Evolution of allostery in the cyclic nucleotide binding module. *Genome Biol.* **2007**, *8*, R264. [CrossRef] [PubMed]

39. Berman, H.M.; Ten Eyck, L.F.; Goodsell, D.S.; Haste, N.M.; Kornev, A.; Taylor, S.S. The cAMP binding domain: An ancient signaling module. *Proc. Natl. Acad. Sci. USA* **2005**, *102*, 45–50. [CrossRef] [PubMed]

40. Lorenz, R.; Moon, E.W.; Kim, J.J.; Schmidt, S.H.; Sankaran, B.; Pavlidis, I.V.; Kim, C.; Herberg, F.W. Mutations of PKA cyclic nucleotide-binding domains reveal novel aspects of cyclic nucleotide selectivity. *Biochem. J.* **2017**, *474*, 2389–2403. [CrossRef] [PubMed]

41. Froese, A.; Brand, T. Expression pattern of *Popdc2* during mouse embryogenesis and in the adult. *Dev. Dyn.* **2008**, *237*, 780–787. [CrossRef] [PubMed]

42. Breher, S.S.; Mavridou, E.; Brenneis, C.; Froese, A.; Arnold, H.H.; Brand, T. Popeye domain containing gene 2 (*Popdc2*) is a myocyte-specific differentiation marker during chick heart development. *Dev. Dyn.* **2004**, *229*, 695–702. [CrossRef] [PubMed]

43. Torlopp, A.; Breher, S.S.; Schluter, J.; Brand, T. Comparative analysis of mRNA and protein expression of Popdc1 (Bves) during early development in the chick embryo. *Dev. Dyn.* **2006**, *235*, 691–700. [CrossRef] [PubMed]

44. Wada, A.; Reese, D.; Bader, D. Bves: Prototype of a new class of cell adhesion molecules expressed during coronary artery development. *Development* **2001**, *128*, 2085–2093. [PubMed]

45. Smith, T.K.; Bader, D.M. Characterization of Bves expression during mouse development using newly generated immunoreagents. *Dev. Dyn.* **2006**, *235*, 1701–1708. [CrossRef] [PubMed]

46. The Human Protein Atlas. Available online: https://www.proteinatlas.org/ENSG00000112276-BVES/tissue (accessed on 19 February 2018).

47. The Human Protein Atlas. Available online: https://www.proteinatlas.org/ENSG00000121577-POPDC2/tissue (accessed on 19 February 2018).

48. The Human Protein Atlas. Available online: https://www.proteinatlas.org/ENSG00000132429-POPDC3/tissue (accessed on 19 February 2018).

49. Korfali, N.; Wilkie, G.S.; Swanson, S.K.; Srsen, V.; de Las Heras, J.; Batrakou, D.G.; Malik, P.; Zuleger, N.; Kerr, A.R.; Florens, L.; et al. The nuclear envelope proteome differs notably between tissues. *Nucleus* **2012**, *3*, 552–564. [CrossRef] [PubMed]

50. Schindler, R.; Simrick, S.; Brand, T. Nuclear localization of members of popeye domain containing (Popdc) protein family. *Cardiovasc. Res.* **2012**, *93*, S98.

51. Soni, S.; Raaijmakers, A.J.; Raaijmakers, L.M.; Damen, J.M.; van Stuijvenberg, L.; Vos, M.A.; Heck, A.J.; van Veen, T.A.; Scholten, A. A proteomics approach to identify new putative cardiac intercalated disk proteins. *PLoS ONE* **2016**, *11*, e0152231. [CrossRef] [PubMed]

52. Andrée, B.; Fleige, A.; Arnold, H.H.; Brand, T. Mouse pop1 is required for muscle regeneration in adult skeletal muscle. *Mol. Cell. Biol.* **2002**, *22*, 1504–1512. [CrossRef] [PubMed]

53. Kirchmaier, B.C.; Poon, K.L.; Schwerte, T.; Huisken, J.; Winkler, C.; Jungblut, B.; Stainier, D.Y.; Brand, T. The popeye domain containing 2 (*Popdc2*) gene in zebrafish is required for heart and skeletal muscle development. *Dev. Biol.* **2012**, *363*, 438–450. [CrossRef] [PubMed]

54. Nelson, I.; Beuvin, M.; Ben-Yaou, R.; Masson, C.; Boland, A.; Schindler, R.; Brand, T.; Eymard, B.; Bonne, G. Novel recessive splice site mutation in Popdc1 (Bves) is associated with first-degree atrioventricular block and muscular dystrophy. *Neuromuscul. Disord.* **2017**, *27*, S139–S140. [CrossRef]

55. Rinné, S.; Ortiz-Bonnin, B.; Stallmeyer, B.; Schindler, R.F.R.; Kiper, A.K.; Dittmann, S.; Friedrich, C.; Zumhagen, S.; Simrick, S.L.; Gonzalez, W.; et al. Conduction disorder caused by a mutation in *POPDC2*, a novel modulator of the cardiac sodium channel SCN5A. *Acta Physiol.* **2016**, *216*, 42.

56. Wu, J.; Schuessler, R.B.; Rodefeld, M.D.; Saffitz, J.E.; Boineau, J.P. Morphological and membrane characteristics of spider and spindle cells isolated from rabbit sinus node. *Am. J. Physiol. Regul. Integr. Comp. Physiol.* **2001**, *280*, H1232–H1240. [CrossRef] [PubMed]

57. Honore, E. The neuronal background K2P channels: Focus on TREK1. *Nat. Rev. Neurosci.* **2007**, *8*, 251–261. [CrossRef] [PubMed]

58. Unudurthi, S.D.; Wu, X.; Qian, L.; Amari, F.; Onal, B.; Li, N.; Makara, M.A.; Smith, S.A.; Snyder, J.; Fedorov, V.V.; et al. Two-pore K$^+$ channel TREK-1 regulates sinoatrial node membrane excitability. *J. Am. Heart Assoc.* **2016**, *5*, e002865. [CrossRef] [PubMed]

59. Mangoni, M.E.; Nargeot, J. Genesis and regulation of the heart automaticity. *Physiol. Rev.* **2008**, *88*, 919–982. [CrossRef] [PubMed]

60. Lubelwana Hafver, T.; Wanichawan, P.; Manfra, O.; de Souza, G.A.; Lunde, M.; Martinsen, M.; Louch, W.E.; Mathias Sejersted, O.; Carlson, C.R. Mapping the in vitro interactome of cardiac sodium (Na$^+$)-calcium (Ca^{2+}) exchanger 1 (NCX1). *Proteomics* **2017**, *17*. [CrossRef] [PubMed]

61. Torrente, A.G.; Zhang, R.; Zaini, A.; Giani, J.F.; Kang, J.; Lamp, S.T.; Philipson, K.D.; Goldhaber, J.I. Burst pacemaker activity of the sinoatrial node in sodium-calcium exchanger knockout mice. *Proc. Natl. Acad. Sci. USA* **2015**, *112*, 9769–9774. [CrossRef] [PubMed]

62. Kliminski, V.; Uziel, O.; Kessler-Icekson, G. Popdc1/Bves functions in the preservation of cardiomyocyte viability while affecting Rac1 activity and Bnip3 expression. *J. Cell. Biochem.* **2017**, *118*, 1505–1517. [CrossRef] [PubMed]

63. Andree, B.; Fleige, A.; Hillemann, T.; Arnold, H.H.; Kessler-Icekson, G.; Brand, T. Molecular and functional analysis of popeye genes: A novel family of transmembrane proteins preferentially expressed in heart and skeletal muscle. *Exp. Clin. Cardiol.* **2002**, *7*, 99–103. [PubMed]

64. Harvey, R.D.; Calaghan, S.C. Caveolae create local signalling domains through their distinct protein content, lipid profile and morphology. *J. Mol. Cell. Cardiol.* **2012**, *52*, 366–375. [CrossRef] [PubMed]

65. Wu, Y.C.; Liu, C.Y.; Chen, Y.H.; Chen, R.F.; Huang, C.J.; Wang, I.J. Blood vessel epicardial substance (Bves) regulates epidermal tight junction integrity through atypical protein kinase C. *J. Biol. Chem.* **2012**, *287*, 39887–39897. [CrossRef] [PubMed]

66. Osler, M.E.; Chang, M.S.; Bader, D.M. Bves modulates epithelial integrity through an interaction at the tight junction. *J. Cell Sci.* **2005**, *118*, 4667–4678. [CrossRef] [PubMed]

67. Charvet, B.; Malbouyres, M.; Pagnon-Minot, A.; Ruggiero, F.; Le Guellec, D. Development of the zebrafish myoseptum with emphasis on the myotendinous junction. *Cell Tissue Res.* **2011**, *346*, 439–449. [CrossRef] [PubMed]

68. Charvet, B.; Guiraud, A.; Malbouyres, M.; Zwolanek, D.; Guillon, E.; Bretaud, S.; Monnot, C.; Schulze, J.; Bader, H.L.; Allard, B.; et al. Knockdown of col22a1 gene in zebrafish induces a muscular dystrophy by disruption of the myotendinous junction. *Development* **2013**, *140*, 4602–4613. [CrossRef] [PubMed]

69. Goody, M.F.; Sher, R.B.; Henry, C.A. Hanging on for the ride: Adhesion to the extracellular matrix mediates cellular responses in skeletal muscle morphogenesis and disease. *Dev. Biol.* **2015**, *401*, 75–91. [CrossRef] [PubMed]

70. Brand, T.; Schindler, R. New kids on the block: The popeye domain containing (Popdc) protein family acting as a novel class of cAMP effector proteins in striated muscle. *Cell. Signal.* **2017**, *40*, 156–165. [CrossRef] [PubMed]

J. Cardiovasc. Dev. Dis. **2018**, *5*, 18

71. Magri, F.; Del Bo, R.; D'Angelo, M.G.; Sciacco, M.; Gandossini, S.; Govoni, A.; Napoli, L.; Ciscato, P.; Fortunato, F.; Brighina, E.; et al. Frequency and characterisation of anoctamin 5 mutations in a cohort of italian limb-girdle muscular dystrophy patients. *Neuromuscul. Disord.* **2012**, *22*, 934–943. [CrossRef] [PubMed]
72. Rehmann, H.; Wittinghofer, A.; Bos, J.L. Capturing cyclic nucleotides in action: Snapshots from crystallographic studies. *Nat. Rev. Mol. Cell Biol.* **2007**, *8*, 63–73. [CrossRef] [PubMed]

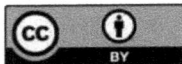

Journal of
Cardiovascular
Development and Disease

MDPI

Review

Using cAMP Sensors to Study Cardiac Nanodomains

Katharina Schleicher [ID] and Manuela Zaccolo *

Department of Physiology, Anatomy and Genetics, University of Oxford, Sherrington Building,
South Parks Road, Oxford OX1 3PT, UK; katharina.schleicher@dpag.ox.ac.uk
* Correspondence: manuela.zaccolo@dpag.ox.ac.uk; Tel.: +44-1865-2725-30

Received: 20 February 2018; Accepted: 9 March 2018; Published: 13 March 2018

Abstract: $3',5'$-cyclic adenosine monophosphate (cAMP) signalling plays a major role in the cardiac myocyte response to extracellular stimulation by hormones and neurotransmitters. In recent years, evidence has accumulated demonstrating that the cAMP response to different extracellular agonists is not uniform: depending on the stimulus, cAMP signals of different amplitudes and kinetics are generated in different subcellular compartments, eliciting defined physiological effects. In this review, we focus on how real-time imaging using fluorescence resonance energy transfer (FRET)-based reporters has provided mechanistic insight into the compartmentalisation of the cAMP signalling pathway and allowed for the precise definition of the regulation and function of subcellular cAMP nanodomains.

Keywords: $3',5'$-cyclic adenosine monophosphate; protein kinase A; fluorescence resonance energy transfer; real-time imaging; compartmentalisation; signalling; cardiac biology; phosphodiesterases; A kinase anchoring proteins

1. Introduction

Cyclic nucleotides, such as $3',5'$-adenosine monophosphate (cAMP), are small molecules used by cells to propagate extracellular information inside the cell and are referred to as second messengers. cAMP is generated by intracellular adenylyl cyclases in response to a first, extracellular message that activates a transmembrane G-protein coupled receptor (GPCR). This second messenger system is used in many types of cells, from prokaryotes to human neurons, and in each cell type its synthesis can be triggered by different extracellular stimuli with different functional outcomes. It is thus imperative to understand how a universal signal like cAMP can be versatile enough to generate cellular effects that are specific to each individual stimulus. This question demands sensitive quantification of the second messenger and accurate comparison of cAMP signal amplitude, dynamics, and subcellular location in response to different extracellular cues.

In the cardiovascular system, the first message that activates the cAMP pathway is provided by a variety of biochemically diverse molecules. These include neurotransmitters, such as adrenaline and noradrenaline; peptide hormones, such as glucagon; and lipid compounds, such as prostaglandins. Each molecule binds to a distinct GPCR, coupling to different kinds of G-proteins with the ability to activate or inhibit cAMP production [1]. Increases in cAMP can activate different families of cAMP-binding proteins. In cardiomyocytes, these include cyclic nucleotide-gated ion channels (CNGC) [2], exchange proteins directly activated by cAMP (Epacs) [3], Popeye domain-containing (POPDC) proteins [4], and protein kinase A (PKA) [5]. The most extensively studied effector molecule of cAMP is PKA. cAMP binding to the regulatory subunit of PKA results in activation of its catalytic subunit. In cardiomyocytes, PKA-mediated phosphorylation modulates ion channels, transmembrane receptors, and regulatory proteins, leading to increased heart rate, increased strength of contraction, and enhanced relaxation. All these effects can improve haemodynamic performance in patients with a failing heart. Consequently, the cAMP signalling pathway is a unique point of interest in the development of treatments for heart failure and congenital heart disease.

Interestingly, not all extracellular stimuli that activate cAMP signalling in the heart increase PKA activity uniformly and to a similar degree throughout the cell. This was first hypothesised on the basis of observations in biochemical fractions of cardiomyocytes, stimulated with either prostaglandins or β-adrenergic receptor agonists [6]. Direct evidence of cAMP compartmentalisation, however, had been difficult to obtain. Clean isolation of cardiomyocyte organelles, to map the heterogenic distribution of cAMP across the cell on a micrometre scale, presents a considerable challenge. Another experimental difficulty is the small molecular size of cAMP itself: cAMP occupies not more than 1.12 nm in a crystal structure in complex with PDE4D (PDB 2PW3) [7], which is more than six times smaller than the $G_s\alpha$ subunit of a heterotrimeric G protein (PDB 1AZT) [8]. A small molecular radius allows for high diffusivity. In a medium with low molecular complexity, such as water, cAMP can reach a diffusion velocity of up to 444 μm^2/s. In molecularly crowded environments, such as the cytoplasm of an adult cardiomyocyte, this can be slowed by more than a factor of ten [9]. Still, assessment of real-time signals in response to cellular stimulation is a considerable challenge when using conventional biochemical methods. To fully understand the conserved and divergent aspects of cAMP signalling downstream of distinct cellular stimuli, temporal and spatial dissection of signalling events is crucial. Live, single cell imaging methods based on fluorescence resonance energy transfer (FRET) provided the means to dissect how cellular signalling occurs in space and time.

Real-time cAMP imaging techniques have greatly enhanced our understanding of the distribution and nature of intracellular cAMP signalling domains. Temporal and spatial resolution of cAMP signalling are among the main advantages that FRET-based imaging methods can offer to the field. In combination with the reversibility of the response and real-time detection of cAMP changes in living cells, this technique has revolutionised our understanding of cAMP signalling in the heart. FRET-based imaging helped replace the coarse definition of cAMP concentration gradients between biochemical fractions with our appreciation of sub-microscopic differences in cAMP signalling at different organelles.

This review gives a brief account of the evolution of FRET-based imaging approaches in the study of cAMP signalling. Different probes have been instrumental in addressing specific aspects of the cAMP signalling pathway and have distinct strengths and weaknesses that are worth considering when designing experiments. We also discuss how several cardiac compartments have been characterised using real-time imaging of cAMP and present specific examples.

2. The Evolution of cAMP Imaging Techniques and Their Contribution to Our Understanding of the Spatio-Temporal Compartmentation of cAMP Signalling

cAMP signalling in cardiac myocytes is compartmentalised. During a signalling event, the cyclic nucleotide is not uniformly distributed through the entire cytoplasm, but it accumulates to a greater or lesser extent in distinct loci within the cell. Due to its physicochemical properties and relatively high diffusivity, this behaviour of cAMP is not intuitive, and the discovery and further analysis of cAMP subcellular compartmentation was a multi-step process that is recounted in the following paragraphs. A single cAMP compartment can be confined to a cellular substructure that involves only a small number of proteins and thus operates on the nanometre scale. Such macromolecular substructures have been termed cAMP nanodomains. cAMP domains contain functionally associated proteins, or signalosomes, which together shape the effect of the cAMP signal within the domain. Signalosomes are usually comprised of cAMP binding proteins, such as PKA and phosphodiesterases (PDEs), as well as their regulators and targets.

cAMP compartmentalisation has a spatial and a temporal dimension. To adequately describe cAMP signalling in cardiomyocytes, the toolkit for cAMP detection and quantification therefore had to evolve considerably from bulk analysis of cAMP content in tissue or cell lysates to targeted, real-time, and quantitative analysis of cAMP nanodomains in living cells (Figure 1). Each of the cAMP sensors described in the following has unique experimental advantages and caveats, including cAMP sensitivity, dynamic range, or sensor biology. This review aims to highlight some of the considerations to take into account when designing an experimental system.

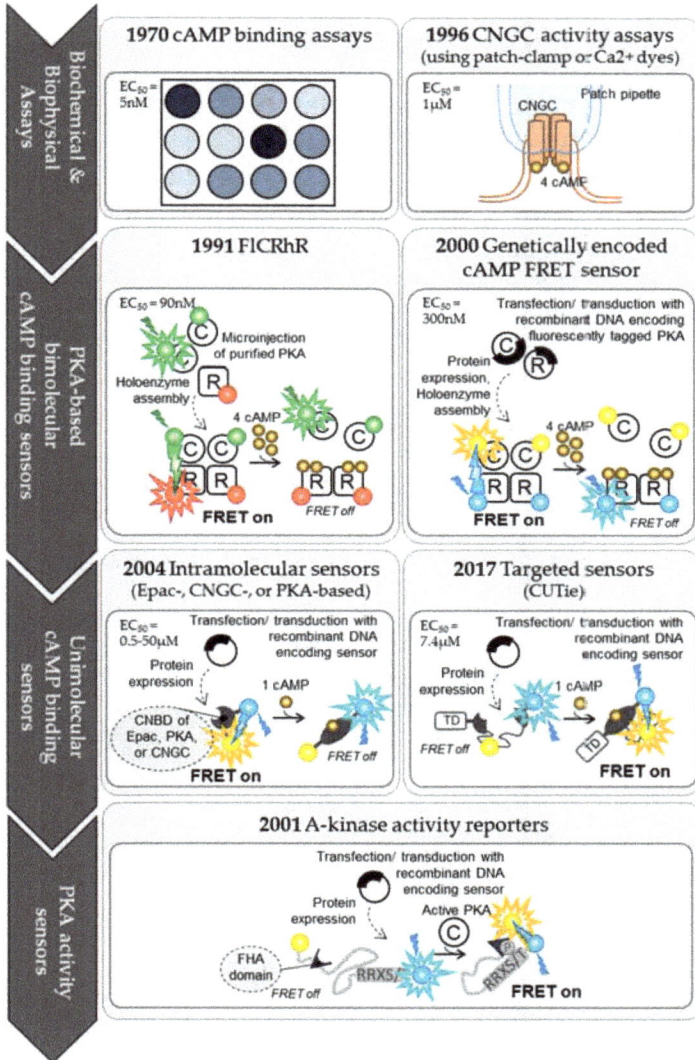

Figure 1. Evolution of cardiac cAMP detection from bulk biochemical analysis to targeted real-time imaging in living cardiomyocytes. In all panels, cAMP molecules are represented by golden spheres; fluorophore molecules are represented by coloured spheres, with the colours indicating their emission spectra. Exposure to light with the excitation spectrum of a fluorophore is represented by a monochrome lightning bolt; emission of fluorescent light is represented by a halo around the fluorophore. Fluorescence transfer is represented by a lightning bolt that originates from the fluorescence donor, which matches the donor in colour and points towards the fluorescence acceptor. EC50 for cAMP is indicated for all cAMP detection systems, as reported in the literature [10–13].

2.1. Biochemical Protein Binding Assays for cAMP

Since the 1970s, detection of cAMP by calibrated amounts of cAMP binding proteins, including cAMP-dependent protein kinase purified from bovine muscle [14] or cAMP-binding antibodies [15,16], has allowed for sensitive and specific quantification of cAMP in tissue lysates, cell lysates, or fractions thereof.

Bulk biochemical quantification of cAMP in membrane and cytosolic fractions from adult rabbit cardiomyocytes revealed that selective stimulation of different families of G-protein coupled receptors elicits distinct cAMP and PKA activation profiles. Concentration of cAMP increases in both the membrane and the cytosolic fraction when β-adrenergic receptors are stimulated with isoproterenol. Meanwhile, stimulation of the prostaglandin receptor with prostaglandin E1 (PGE1) only increases cAMP in the cytosolic fraction [6].

Biochemical cAMP detection in combination with cell fractionation provided first evidence that cAMP signalling in cardiomyocytes is not uniform and that cAMP can be compartmentalised depending on the extracellular stimulus. Biochemical detection can be as sensitive as 1 nM cAMP and is compatible with high throughput screening [17]. However, the technique requires disruption of large numbers of cells. Consequently, it is limited to bulk analysis of a potentially heterogeneous population of cells, and detection of real time dynamics of cAMP is impossible.

2.2. Cyclic Nucleotide Gated Channel (CNGC) Activity Measurements

cAMP can activate non-selective cation channels in the plasma membrane, known as cyclic nucleotide gated channels (CNGC). Activation of these channels leads to a cation current, which can be measured using the patch clamp technique [18]. CNGC activation also triggers an increase in intracellular calcium, which can be quantified with calcium-sensitive dyes [19]. Such measurements of CNGC activity are possible at a single cell level and in living cells; thus, they overcome major limitations of biochemical techniques.

This approach added more detail to the biochemical finding that β-adrenergic and prostaglandin receptors have different effects on membrane and cytosolic cAMP levels, by revealing a temporal dimension: cAMP levels near the surface membrane transiently respond to PGE1 stimulation, while bulk cellular cAMP rises to a steady level in the same time frame [20]. Furthermore, this technique neatly couples cAMP concentration with cardiac physiology. Using patch clamp to measure CNGC-mediated cation currents revealed that β-adrenergic receptors are functionally coupled to nearby Ca^{2+} channels via local elevations of cAMP [21].

While CNGC-based functional assays enabled real-time detection of changes in cAMP concentrations for the first time, CNGC biosensors are restricted to one compartment, the sarcolemma. This precludes studies of other important subcellular structures in cardiomyocytes, such as the sarcomere and sarcoplasmic reticulum. In addition, native CNGCs have comparatively low cAMP/cGMP selectivity [2]. While mutagenesis improves the affinity of the channel to cAMP versus cGMP, the popular E583M single point mutant still retains some affinity for cGMP [22].

2.3. PKA-Based bi-Molecular FRET Sensors

2.3.1. FlCRhR Probes

To create a highly selective probe that can measure cAMP in living cells, Roger Tsien, Susan Taylor, and colleagues made use of the heterotetrameric structure of the cAMP effector PKA [23]. Catalytic and regulatory subunits of PKA were expressed in bacteria as recombinant proteins, and each was tagged with chemical fluorophores of different spectral properties (fluorescein on the catalytic and rhodamine on the regulatory subunits). Upon microinjection into living cells, these labelled subunits form heterotetramers, comprising two catalytic and two regulatory subunits. Their close proximity in the heterotetramer enables fluorescence energy transfer of the fluorescein donor on one of the catalytic subunits to the rhodamine acceptor on one of the regulatory subunits. Thus, if fluorescein is excited with the appropriate excitation wavelength, energy transfer occurs within the heterotetramer, and rhodamine fluorescence emission is detectable. Upon cAMP binding, the heterotetramer dissociates, which leads to release and activation of the catalytic subunit, decrease of fluorescence energy transfer, and a concomitant decrease of rhodamine emission relative to fluorescein emission [23].

Using this probe, intracellular cAMP concentrations were measured in response to short β-adrenergic stimulation of isolated frog ventricular myocytes and correlated to the ensuing calcium transients [24]. This demonstrated that the dynamics of intracellular cAMP concentration and intracellular calcium transients are distinct from each other in response to β-adrenergic stimulation. Thus, the FlCRhR probe constituted an important step towards the dissection of temporal sequences in the cardiac cAMP signalling cascade.

While this technique allowed for specific measurement of cAMP in living cells on a single-cell level, the requirement for production of chemically labelled PKA subunits and microinjection of correctly folded proteins renders it practically challenging. Critically, both the process of microinjection and the non-physiologically high concentrations of PKA catalytic subunits in the cell produce a considerable amount of cytotoxicity that limits the number of cell types that are amenable to this technique.

2.3.2. Genetically Encoded, Tetrameric cAMP FRET Probes

While FlCRhR was an important proof of concept for the use of tetrameric PKA-based FRET in living cells, there was a need to incorporate the probe into a more ubiquitously applicable genetic system. This was generated by tagging the genes for catalytic and regulatory subunits of PKA with the coding sequence for two fluorescent proteins with overlapping emission and excitation spectra. Genetically encoded FRET sensor pairs can be co-transfected into living cells, which leads to their transient expression by the host cell expression system [25]. Similar to the FlCRhR probes, an increase of cAMP leads to dissociation of the PKA heterotetramer and a decrease in energy transfer.

This technique was widely applied to measure changes in intracellular cAMP concentrations in diverse cellular systems. Once expressed, genetically encoded PKA tetramers are compartmentalised by binding to PKA scaffolds called A-Kinase anchoring proteins (AKAPs) [26]. AKAPs can be found in many cardiac subcellular domains proximal to and distal from the sarcolemma, including the T tubules, the sarcoplasmic reticulum, and the Z lines. cAMP measurement with the PKA-based FRET probes revealed that adrenergic stimulation of neonatal rat cardiac myocytes leads to a non-homogeneous increase in cAMP concentrations, providing, for the first time, direct evidence that the activation of β-adrenergic receptors leads to the generation of multiple distinct subcellular cAMP pools. The cAMP domains aligned with AKAP-centred domains, and free diffusion of the second messenger was limited by the activity of phosphodiesterases (PDEs) [26]. The important contribution of different families of PDEs to nanodomain regulation in cardiomyocytes has recently been reviewed elsewhere [27]. Subsequent analysis of the nature of these PDEs revealed that in rat cardiac myocytes, PDE4 is the major cAMP degrading enzyme to shape amplitude and duration of cAMP responses to adrenergic stimulation. Crucially, PDE4 was shown to localise to distinct cardiomyocyte compartments that were different from other PDE isoforms, for example PDE3 [28]. A later study found that the adrenergic cAMP response over Z lines in cardiomyocytes from $PDE4D^{-/-}$ knock out mice, as measured with the tetrameric FRET probe, was higher than in wild-type cardiomyocytes. Critically, $PDE4D^{-/-}$ knock out mice exhibited accelerated progression of heart failure following myocardial infarction and were highly susceptible to cardiac arrhythmias during exercise followed by low-dose epinephrine injection [29].

The ability to measure real-time intracellular cAMP changes in intact, living cells also enabled studies towards understanding the integration of sympathetic and parasympathetic stimulation in cardiomyocyte cAMP signalling [30]. Using this sensor, it was demonstrated directly for the first time that termination of parasympathetic, muscarinic stimulation causes a transient increase in cAMP activity, providing important integrative data on the autonomic control of cardiac function.

J. Cardiovasc. Dev. Dis. **2018**, *5*, 17

Tagged with a peptide sequence that is post-translationally myristoylated and palmitoylated, the PKA-based sensor can be selectively directed to the plasma membrane [31]. In HEK cells, this strategy corroborated the biochemical finding that cAMP levels at the plasma membrane can transiently respond to PGE1 stimulation.

The development of genetically encoded cAMP sensors has strongly facilitated the spatio-temporal dissection of cAMP signalling in cardiomyocytes. However, the multimeric nature of PKA presents several technical limitations for high temporal resolution of intracellular cAMP quantification. As catalytic and regulatory PKA subunits with acceptor and donor fluorophores are transfected and expressed from two different plasmids, equal level of expression cannot be guaranteed. Additionally, each sensor subunit can potentially interact with endogenous PKA subunits, limiting the number of functioning FRET pairs. Both these effects may skew the formation of FRET-competent heterotetramers and make signal termination difficult to assess. As dissociation of the PKA heterotetramer requires cooperative binding of four molecules of cAMP to the two regulatory subunits, sensor kinetics are relatively slow, which may lead to underestimation of cAMP propagation within the cell [32]. PKA tetramers are compartmentalised by binding to AKAPs [26] and/or due to their anisotropic diffusion [24], which limits their applicability to total cytosolic cAMP measurements in cardiomyocytes. Lastly, while the endogenous expression system limits the amount of PKA produced, the tagged catalytic subunits of the sensor retain catalytic activity. This slightly elevated PKA activity can still be toxic in some cell types [33]. However, this remains the only available sensor that can directly report on kinetics of PKA activation in intact cells [34].

2.4. Intramolecular FRET Sensors

To overcome cooperativity and remaining toxicity concerns, single-chain cAMP FRET sensors were developed using the cyclic nucleotide binding domains (CNBDs) obtained from a number of different cAMP binding proteins.

2.4.1. Epac-Based Single-Chain FRET Sensors

Several generations of unimolecular FRET sensors based on exchange protein directly activated by cAMP (Epac) are available to date. Epac is a guanine nucleotide exchange factor (GEF) for Ras-like small GTPases. Binding of cAMP to a unique binding domain induces a conformational change in the inactive Epac protein to expose both the catalytic domain [35] and a targeting domain [36], stimulating GEF activity. In Epac-based sensors, fluorescence donor and acceptor proteins are fused to the N- and C-terminus of either a single cAMP binding domain of human Epac1, a single cAMP binding domain of murine Epac2, full length human Epac1, or truncations of human Epac1 [32,37,38]. While the initial sensors had a limited dynamic range, giving between 10% and 30% FRET change, their range has been significantly improved to over 150% by sequential engineering of both the spectral properties of the FRET pairs and the way they are assembled with the CNBDs [39–41].

The uniform cytosolic distribution, particularly of the sensors based on a single cAMP binding domain, uncoupled the site of cAMP detection from any particular cellular structure and allowed for detection of bulk cytosolic cAMP. However, the site of cAMP detection could be chosen deliberately by fusing these sensors to specific targeting sequences or domains. Directing the sensor to nuclei, mitochondria, or the mitochondrial matrix, for example, allowed for measurement of the dynamic local changes in cAMP concentrations in response to PGE1 or adrenergic stimulation [37], revealing differential dynamics of cAMP signalling in response to the activation of either receptor. Using these sensors coupled to the targeting domain from different PKA isoforms demonstrated that in cardiac myocytes, compartmentalised PKA-RI and PKA-RII respond to distinct, spatially restricted cAMP signals, which leads to phosphorylation of unique subsets of downstream targets [42].

An Epac-based single-chain FRET sensor, in its untargeted form, was used in combination with scanning ion conductance microscopy (SICM). After local receptor stimulation of either β1- or β2-adrenergic receptors, cAMP was found to be differently distributed across the healthy cardiomyocyte membrane. As a consequence of β2-adrenergic receptor redistribution in heart failure, such cAMP compartmentation was altered [43].

Epac-based sensors are versatile and easy to use, but their properties may need to be adjusted to suit a particular cellular system. Some of the Epac-based sensors, including the popular Epac1-camps, have high cAMP sensitivity (ca. 1 µmol/L, [32]). This can lead to fast saturation and limited coverage of the physiological cAMP concentration spectrum, especially in cells with high basal cAMP levels such as cardiomyocytes. Furthermore, the spectral properties of the ECFP/EYFP-containing sensors are relatively sensitive to changes in the intracellular microenvironment, for example intracellular pH [44], which has been improved in later versions of the sensors [41]. However, the critically limiting factor of this system pertains to its molecular design. In all the targeted versions of this sensor [37,42,45–47], the targeting domain is directly attached to one of the fluorophores. This affects the FRET properties that depend on the targeting domain of choice, making direct comparison of cAMP signals detected at different intracellular sites difficult [12].

2.4.2. CNGC-Based Single-Chain FRET Sensors

The sensitivity of Epac-camps sensors to cAMP is a concern in cardiomyocytes with high basal cAMP concentrations, and so a sensor that sandwiches an alternative cyclic nucleotide binding domain between its fluorophores was developed. Here, fluorescence donor and acceptor proteins are fused to the cAMP binding domain of the hyperpolarization-activated, cyclic, nucleotide-gated potassium channel 2 (HCN2) [33].

With this sensor, contributions of different PDE isoforms to cAMP hydrolysis in adult mouse cardiomyocytes after adrenergic stimulation were assessed, which ranked the activity of PDE4 above PDE2 and PDE3 [33]. Measuring cAMP propagation after selective stimulation of β1- and β2-adrenergic receptors indicated that cAMP signals that emanated from β1 receptors propagate over a distance involving multiple sarcomeres in adult cardiomyocytes. In contrast, the cAMP signal on β2 stimulation remained strictly confined [33].

While this sensor addresses some limitations of the Epac-based cAMP sensors in cardiomyocytes, the main issue of comparability between targeted sensors remained unresolved.

2.4.3. PKA-Based Single-Chain FRET Sensors

To minimise potential interference of the targeting domain with FRET, a novel cAMP sensor named CUTie (cAMP Universal Tag for imaging experiments) was developed based on the CNBD of the PKA regulatory subunit IIβ. The unique feature of this new sensor is that CUTie enables fusion of the targeting domain distal to the FRET fluorophore pair. This is attained by fusion of the FRET donor to the C-terminus of the CNBD and insertion of the FRET acceptor in an intra-domain loop of the CNBD, leaving the N-terminus free for the targeting domain. In this configuration, targeting domain and FRET module are physically separated from each other and steric hindrance on the conformational change required for energy transfer is minimised. As a result, the dynamic range of the sensor in different compartments is now comparable [12]. This is not necessarily the case for other reporters that have been targeted to subcellular sites. For studies involving targeted sensors, it is important to keep in mind that their cAMP-binding and spectral properties can be influenced by the targeting domain and its impact on the overall fold of the polypeptide chain. Comparison of the cAMP response at different sites must therefore be interpreted with caution, unless accurate calibration curves are available for the targeted reporters.

The demonstrable independence of the sensor FRET response from the chosen targeting domain, in combination with in-cell calibration techniques, paved the way for accurate quantitation of cAMP concentrations at different compartments of healthy and hypertrophic myocytes. Direct quantitative comparison of cAMP levels obtained with CUTie sensors, targeted to plasmalemma, sarcoplasmic reticulum, or sarcomere, suggested that the size of cAMP subcellular compartments can be sub-microscopic. Importantly, it was observed that the amplitude of the local cAMP signal is independent of the distance from the site of cAMP synthesis. It was also dependent on the activity of phosphodiesterases, indicating that compartmentalisation of cAMP is not simply the result of limited diffusion due to the complex intracellular structure but is an actively regulated phenomenon. The study also showed that the effect of phosphodiesterases is most profound at the sarcomeric nanocompartment. Application of targeted CUTie reporters that were used to compare healthy and diseased hearts revealed that nanodomains can be differentially affected by misregulation of β-adrenergic signalling in heart failure [12]. This highlights the opportunities inherent to selective targeting of cardiac compartments in heart failure therapy. Focussing therapeutic interventions on the compartments that are selectively affected in heart failure may reduce the adverse outcomes of current inotropic agents in long-term treatment [48].

2.5. Single-Wavelength Fluorescent Sensors for cAMP

In cardiomyocytes, cAMP signalling is closely linked to calcium signalling. It is possible to use ECFP/EYFP FRET sensors in combination with Fura-2, a calcium imaging dye with absorption peaks at 340 nm (Ca^{2+}-bound) and 380 nm (Ca^{2+}-free), and follow the activation of both pathways simultaneously [49]. To streamline such multi-colour measurements for off-the-rack microscope setups, several single-wavelength sensors for cAMP have been developed. In Flamindo and Flamindo2, the cAMP binding domain of Epac1 is sandwiched between two halves of the EYFP variant Citrine. Binding of cAMP decreases Citrine fluorescence intensity [50]. In the newly developed cAMPr sensor, circularly permuted GFP is flanked by the full-length catalytic subunit of PKA on one, and a regulatory subunit of PKA lacking the dimerization/docking domain on the other, side. Binding of cAMP separates the PKA subunits and increases GFP fluorescence [51]. Both sensors have been used in combination with calcium sensing dyes, albeit not in cardiomyocytes.

2.6. PKA Activity Sensors

The most extensively studied effector of cAMP in the heart is protein kinase A (PKA) [52]. A family of single-chain FRET sensors was developed to assay PKA-mediated phosphorylation in cells. In these A-kinase activity reporters (AKARs), a phosphorylatable PKA consensus sequence is combined with a phosphate-binding domain into a single polypeptide chain. The two domains of the sensor are flanked by a FRET pair of fluorophores [53]. Phosphorylation of the PKA consensus leads to the interaction of the phosphate-binding domain with the now phosphorylated sequence, which mediates the conformational change necessary for FRET to occur. Since its first conception, the sensor has been optimised in several rounds to give a maximum FRET efficiency of 60% in the latest version [54–56]. An important feature of later versions of this sensor is that it allows for dephosphorylation of the probe. As such, these sensors provide information on both PKA activity, which increases FRET, and phosphatase activity directed against PKA targets, which decreases FRET [54].

Similar to cAMP probes, these sensors are theoretically targetable to any cellular compartment or signalosome. As such, they are useful reporters of the functional effects of cAMP signalling on effector proteins within a pre-defined compartment. Tethering of AKAR reporters to AKAP-binding domains, for example, shortened the response time of the sensor to adenylate cyclase stimulation, whereas tethering to a nuclear localisation sequence prolonged it [53]. This emphasised the importance of proximity in determining which substrates are preferentially phosphorylated by the anchored PKA kinase.

The use of AKAR reporters is extremely effective in real-time quantification of PKA-mediated phosphorylation in a given cellular compartment. It is important to keep in mind that this is an indirect measure of the cAMP signal in this compartment, as signal intensity not only depends on the cAMP concentration but also on the availability of functional PKA to mediate AKAR phosphorylation, and on the level of counteracting phosphatase activity.

3. Cardiac Nanodomains Studied Using FRET-Based cAMP Sensors

Development of genetically encoded cAMP sensors greatly enhanced our ability to describe the biochemical properties of cAMP in living cells through real-time visualisation of cAMP responses. The sensors allowed for more accurate definition of the diffusive properties of the small signalling molecule in a cellular context. Physical barriers in the structurally highly complex adult cardiomyocytes, for example, considerably slow down diffusivity of cAMP compared to the loosely structured neonatal cardiomyocyte [9]. Accurate physiological calibration of the sensors also enabled precise measurement of cAMP binding to cAMP-dependent proteins, such as PKA, in their actual intracellular context [57]. Importantly, genetically encoded cAMP sensors were used to demonstrate, for the first time, that gradients of cAMP are formed within intact cardiac myocytes upon adrenergic stimulation [26]. The possibility to target FRET sensors to distinct subcellular structures makes them an ideal molecular tool for monitoring confined intracellular cAMP nanodomains (Figure 2). cAMP nanodomains often contain a combination of PKA targets and regulators, as well as domain-specific PKA anchoring proteins, PKA itself, and phosphodiesterases. We now know that each nanodomain comprises a unique set of, and combination of, these proteins. PKA targets can be structurally and functionally diverse, including, for example, mechanoenzymes [58], structural proteins [59], regulatory proteins [60], or ion channels [61]. There are at least forty known PKA anchoring proteins, and new ones are still being discovered [62,63]. Depending on the type of regulatory subunit, PKA complexes themselves are targeted to different subcellular sites [64]. Phosphodiesterases are a diverse family of enzymes that can be grouped into 11 families (PDE1-PDE11), with each family often containing distinct variants that are differentially expressed and localised [65]. FRET-based cAMP sensors have been instrumental in detailing the components of signalosomes in different compartments and thus in defining biochemical and physiological effects of local cAMP signalling in cardiomyocytes.

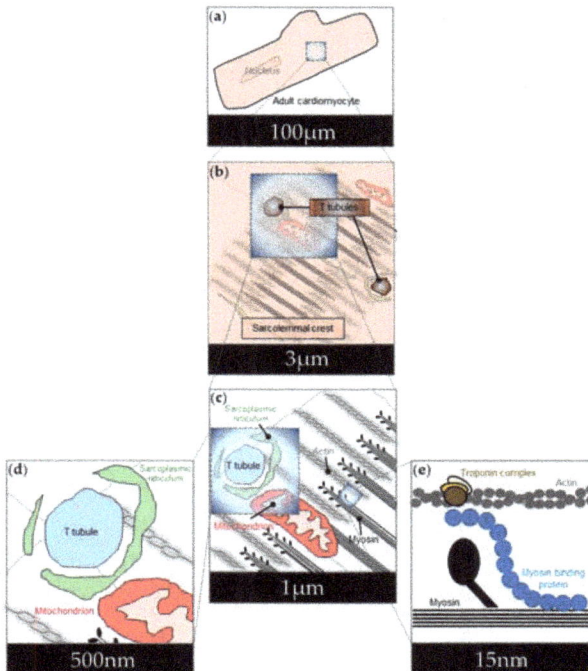

Figure 2. Scales of cAMP signalling domains in adult cardiomyocytes. Continued development of cAMP detection methods improved the resolution of cAMP signal measurement within adult cardiomyocytes. (**a**) Initially, whole-cell and fractionation assays across a 100 µm long adult cardiomyocyte

were performed. (**b**) Later, differences in cAMP concentrations were measured along the sarcolemmal crest and T tubules, which are spread across the membrane roughly every 2 μm. (**c**) Targeted sensors showed differential cAMP signalling between cytosol and mitochondrial matrix, which can be located under 1 μm apart from each other in cardiomyocytes. (**d**) Even differences between mitochondrial outer membrane and matrix, or sarcoplasmic reticulum and T tubules, in cardiomyocytes ca. 100 nm apart, can be detected. (**e**) Future sensors might be able to quantify signalling events within single signalosomes that are few nanometres apart, such as the protein complexes of the sarcomere.

3.1. cAMP Signalling in the Nucleus

Transcriptional regulation of nuclear genes can alter metabolic and developmental programmes, and changes in transcriptional profile are strongly associated with pathological conditions, such as cardiac hypertrophy [66]. Major targets of the cAMP signalling pathway in the nucleus are transcription factors, including the Nuclear factor of activated T-cells (NFAT) and cAMP response element-binding protein (CREB) families, as well as Class II histone deacetylases (HDACs), which regulate gene transcription by increasing the compaction state of DNA. Transcription factors and HDACs can shuttle between nucleus and cytoplasm. Whether cAMP signalling affects them inside the nucleus, outside, or both, is not fully resolved. This is particularly interesting, because G-protein coupled receptors couple predominantly to plasma membrane adenylate cyclases (pmACs), i.e., the primary site of cAMP production after their activation is the plasma membrane. Hence, for nuclear targets of the cAMP pathway, this production site of the second messenger is considerably far removed from their site of activity (Figure 2a). However, there is a soluble adenylate cyclase (sAC) that localises to the nucleus [67,68], raising interesting questions about origin and propagation of cAMP in relation to nuclear signalling.

As detected by Epac-based cAMP FRET sensors targeted with a nuclear localisation sequence (NLS), cAMP concentration in the nucleus increases after stimulation of β-adrenergic or prostaglandin receptors in human embryonic kidney (HEK 293) and airway smooth muscle (ASM) cells [31,37,69]. The increase in cAMP in this compartment reached a plateau after 2 min. However, the increase in cAMP was not immediately followed by an increase in PKA substrate phosphorylation, as measured with the functional PKA sensor AKAR, likewise targeted to the nucleus. Instead, the AKAR response showed a delayed onset of 5–10 min, giving a plateau only after 30 min [37,55]. This delay was inconsistent with activation of resident nuclear PKA by cAMP after β-adrenergic stimulation. It instead favoured a hypothesis that cytoplasmic PKA catalytic subunits, activated in the cytoplasmic compartment, need to translocate to the nucleus to phosphorylate any nuclear targets. In a different study, exclusive nuclear targeting of sAC along with nuclear AKAR revealed that cAMP generated directly in the nucleus of HEK 293 cells can, in fact, activate nuclear PKA immediately after stimulation [70]. Interestingly, even the transmembrane adenylate cyclases can activate nuclear PKA activity much faster, provided PDEs, particularly PDE4, are inhibited, or PKA anchoring to AKAPs is prevented [70].

The direct mechanism of nuclear PKA activation does not seem to be conserved in cardiomyocytes. PDE inhibition in neonatal rat ventricular myocytes does not accelerate nuclear AKAR phosphorylation, despite rapid nuclear cAMP accumulation after co-treatment with adenylate cyclase activators and PDE inhibitors [71]. Disruption of PKA anchoring likewise does not enhance the kinetics of nuclear PKA activity. This suggests that, in cardiomyocytes, translocation from the cytoplasm is the limiting step in nuclear PKA activity. This mechanism may help prevent onset of transcription factor-mediated hypertrophy during transient sympathetic activation.

3.2. cAMP Signalling at the Sarcolemma

The sarcolemma has distinct microscopic domains. T tubules (Figure 2b) reach deep into the cardiomyocyte, increasing its surface area and facilitating rapid delivery of extracellular ions to the core of the cardiomyocyte. Moreover, T tubules contain unique proteins compared to other membrane areas, and they form close contacts with the sarcoplasmic reticulum (Figure 2c,d). Both features cause unique signalling events to take place in T tubular membrane sections. Another smaller membrane compartment, which is best visualised in electron microscopy images, is specialised membrane pits called caveolae. Caveolae, too, increase the membrane surface area and facilitate the formation of signalling complexes.

Using plasma membrane-targeted cAMP sensors, it was established that proximity to the plasma membrane can have a temporal effect on the onset of cAMP signalling. For example, in one study the response time of the Epac-based cAMP sensor ICUE1 targeted to the plasma membrane was 40% reduced over its diffuse cytoplasmic counterpart upon β-adrenergic stimulation [37]. To address the functional effects of such differences in signal initiation, plasma membrane targeted and untargeted AKAR probes were compared in neonatal cardiomyocytes [72]. This study showed that PKA phosphorylation gradients in response to local cAMP production depended predominantly on restricted cAMP diffusion, PDE-mediated cAMP degradation, and PKA-mediated cAMP buffering. Moreover, the different effects of prostaglandins and adrenergic stimulation on cAMP signalling in cardiomyocytes were further described in this study. Prostaglandins stimulated higher PKA activity in the cytosol than at the sarcolemma, whereas β-adrenergic stimulation triggered faster sarcolemmal responses than cytosolic [72].

Not only the agonist, but also the receptor subtype affected the propagation of cAMP in cardiomyocytes. While β1-adrenergic stimulation lead to Epac-based cAMP detection throughout the entire cell, β2-adrenergic stimulation responses were locally confined by an unknown mechanism [33]. β2-adrenergic signalling was similarly confined in human embryonic kidney (HEK 293) cells [40]. Here, β2-adrenergic signalling detected by an untargeted Epac-based sensor, ICUE3, could be amplified by disrupting membrane rafts through cholesterol depletion. In cardiomyocytes, β1-adrenergic receptors can be found in both caveolar and extra-caveolar fractions of the sarcolemma, while prostaglandin receptors are excluded from caveolar fractions. Disruption of caveolae by cholesterol depletion did not lead to significant differences in cytosolic cAMP responses for either of these receptors [73], indicating that the extracaveolar receptor fraction dominates cAMP production in cardiomyocytes. A study combining Epac-based cytosolic cAMP sensors with SICM confirmed that β1-adrenergic receptors can be found across the entire sarcolemma. Yet, β2-adrenergic receptors were exclusively localised to T tubules [43]. Critically, this functional compartmentation is perturbed in failing hearts, leading to loss of the restricted nature of the β2-adrenergic cAMP signal. Later, it was shown using the same technique that caveolin 3 promotes compartmentation of β2-adrenergic cAMP signalling to the T tubules, and overexpression of caveolin 3 in failing cardiomyocytes can partially restore the delocalised signal [74].

Downstream of β1-adrenergic signalling, but not β2-adrenergic signalling, PDE4B-mediated degradation of cAMP is activated in cardiomyocytes [75]. PKA inhibition in wild type, but not PDE4B knock out myocytes, triggered a significant increase of adrenergic receptor generated cAMP levels in the sarcolemmal compartment, indicating that a combination of PKA and PDE4B activity is required to maintain physiological cAMP levels in the β1-receptor domain. These FRET measurements with a plasma membrane-targeted Epac-based sensor thus provided first evidence for a localised, β1-adrenergic receptor-coupled feedback mechanism in cardiomyocytes. This feedback proved essential in the regulation of the amplitude of intracellular calcium currents after adrenergic stimulation. Calcium levels after adrenergic stimulation were higher in PDE4B knock out mice than in controls, which highlights the delicate balance in cAMP production and degradation that healthy cardiomyocytes must maintain in response to sympathetic activation.

3.3. cAMP Signalling at the Mitochondria

In adult cardiomyocytes, mitochondrial fatty acid beta-oxidation is the major source of energy. For this reason, cardiomyocytes are tightly packed with mitochondria (in a healthy heart, about 95% of the heart's ATP production takes place there [76]). This energy is needed to fuel sarcomeric contraction and ATP-dependent ion flux between compartments. Heart failure is associated with significant reductions in mitochondrial respiratory capacity and mitochondrial membrane disruption [77].

cAMP signalling plays important roles in mitochondrial calcium handling, mitochondrial metabolism, and protection against cytochrome c-mediated apoptosis in cardiomyocytes. Close proximity (Figure 2c,d) between cardiomyocyte mitochondria and sarcoplasmic reticulum facilitates calcium-dependent regulation of mitochondrial respiration upon sympathetic activation. Metabolic activity of the muscle cell is thus tightly synchronised with myocyte activation [78–81].

Ischaemia-reperfusion injury of the heart is associated with a dramatic change in mitochondrial morphology. Changes in mitochondrial structure impact their function and have been shown to induce cyotochrome c-dependent cardiomyocyte apoptosis [82]. Interestingly, cAMP signalling after pharmacological β-adrenergic stimulation or stress and exercise could counteract this programme. [83].

To specifically describe mitochondrial cAMP signalling, FRET-sensors were fused to different mitochondrial targeting domains. An Epac-based FRET sensor, fused to the mitochondrial PKA scaffold protein AKAP1, showed a similar FRET response to β-adrenergic stimulation as in the cytosol [37]. AKAP1 binds to the outer mitochondrial membrane and faces the cytosol [84]. The same sensor was targeted to the mitochondrial matrix, using the first 12 amino acids of human cytochrome oxidase c (subunit IV). The matrix-targeted sensor responded to β-adrenergic stimulation, initially suggesting that membrane-generated cAMP can enter mitochondria and activate downstream signalling in the matrix [37]. This view of a continuous cAMP gradient shared between cytosol and mitochondria was contested by observations made with AKAP-targeted PKA activity sensors. Baseline phosphorylation of the sensor was much higher than its cytosolic equivalent, and phosphodiesterase inhibition even enhanced this difference [55]. Therefore, the cytosolic surface of mitochondria seemed to regulate downstream cAMP signalling differently from the cytosol. This was confirmed with a later generation of PKA activity sensors tagged with the OMM-targeting peptide yTOM70 [85]. When PKA-mediated phosphorylation after extracellular signal termination was monitored in this system, phosphorylation at the mitochondria persisted for longer than in the cytosol. The corresponding outer membrane cAMP concentrations, studied with an OMM-targeted Epac-based sensor, on the contrary, mirrored the bulk cytosol. A matrix-targeted sensor, however, was unable to detect cAMP generated at the plasma membrane. Two separate studies showed that cAMP is unable to permeate the inner mitochondrial membrane [45,85], although both groups found evidence for cAMP signalling within the mitochondrial matrix. The discrepancy between the initial study and follow-up research is most likely due to imprecise targeting of the first sensor. While the authors could demonstrate that some of the sensor was indeed localised to the mitochondrial matrix [37], a significant proportion remained cytosolic [37,45]. This provides key learnings for the design of targeted FRET sensors. It highlights the importance of exclusive targeting of the sensor to the compartment of interest.

In contrast to cAMP generated at the sarcolemma, calcium release from the ER or capacitative calcium influx from the extracellular medium could activate the matrix cAMP sensor [45]. The soluble adenylate cyclase activator bicarbonate, similarly, increased both matrix cAMP concentrations [45] and matrix PKA phosphorylation [85]. As a result, cAMP in the matrix is now thought to be generated by a mitochondrial sAC. The cAMP FRET response in the matrix was further increased by panspecific inhibition of phosphodiesterases, suggesting that matrix cAMP is modulated by phosphodiesterases. Functionally, cAMP signalling in the mitochondrial matrix domain enhances mitochondrial metabolism. Activation of sAC or treatment with phosphodiesterase inhibitors increased mitochondrial ATP production, as measured in a mitochondrially-targeted luciferase assay. PKA inhibition reduced mitochondrial ATP production [45].

Using OMM-, and matrix- and untargeted Epac-based sensors, the outer mitochondrial membrane cAMP nanodomain was subsequently dissected further. It was confirmed that this domain on the mitochondrial surface is supplied by plasma membrane adenylate cyclases and is independent of any cAMP generated in the mitochondrial matrix by sAC [86]. Instead of regulating mitochondrial metabolism, this pool of cAMP is involved in regulation of mitochondrial dynamics and protects them from ionomycin-induced apoptosis.

3.4. cAMP Signalling at the Sarcoplasmic Reticulum

The sarcoplasmic reticulum (SR) of mammalian adult cardiomyocytes is a highly differentiated organelle and the main regulator of calcium transients in these cells. Its proximity to cadiomyocyte T tubules (Figure 2c,d) facilitates rapid translation of adrenergic activation in the T tubular membrane compartment to induction of calcium ion (Ca^{2+}) currents from the SR. Cardiac Ca^{2+} homeostasis is vital in maintaining the ability of the cardiomyocyte to contract and relax, as Ca^{2+} is a necessary co-factor for the force-generating module in the sarcomere [87].

Calcium cycling at the SR is heavily regulated by PKA. PKA phosphorylates the channels that release Ca^{2+} from the SR to enable contraction (ryanodine receptors, RyR) [61,88], as well as phospholamban (PLN), a protein that regulates the sarco/endoplasmic reticulum Ca^{2+}-ATPase (SERCA) [89]. Ca^{2+} handling by the SR is often dysfunctional in heart diseases, including heart failure [90].

An Epac-based cAMP sensor, fused to full-length phospholamban using a flexible linker, was used to investigate propagation of adrenergic signals to the SR. The SR compartment was found to be predominantly under β1-adrenergic control [46]. β2-adrenergic signals were not strong enough to produce a cAMP increase at the SERCA microdomain that was detectable with the phospholamban-anchored sensor. β1-adrenergic stimulation, on the other hand, produced a cAMP signal at the SR that even surpassed the cytosolic cAMP signal in amplitude. The robust effect of β1-adrenergic stimulation in the SR compartment was corroborated in rabbit cardiomyocytes using a PKA activity sensor targeted to the SR with only the transmembrane domain of phospholamban [91]. Interestingly, this sensor also detected a small but significant change in PKA activity upon β2-adrenergic stimulation, although this signal was significantly lower than after β1-adrenergic stimulation [91]. This could mean that either cAMP compartmentalisation differs slightly between species or the amplification of the cAMP signal by PKA is necessary to render the signal detectable. Pan-specific adrenergic stimulation induces a rapid and significant increase in both cAMP concentrations and PKA activity at the SR, as measured by a CUTie sensor targeted to the SR with full length AKAP18δ or the phospholamban PKA activity sensor [12,91,92]. Direct pharmacological activation of adenylyl cyclases induced much slower and smaller increases in PKA-mediated phosphorylation at the SR than activation of the cyclase following adrenergic stimulation, raising the question of how the adrenergic signal is more efficiently relayed to the SR compartment [92].

This could be increasingly relevant as transverse aortic constriction (TAC), which causes pressure overload-induced cardiac hypertrophy in the heart, reduces any differences in cAMP between SR and cytosol observed after adrenergic stimulation [46]. Phosphodiesterases act to counterbalance loss of cAMP gradients. The adrenergic cAMP concentration gradient between SR and cytosol can be reduced upon additional inhibition of phosphodiesterases [46]. This was confirmed when cAMP concentrations at the SR were compared to nanodomains at the sarcolemma or sarcomere using CUTie sensors fused to full length AKAP18δ (SR), AKAP79 (sarcolemma), or cardiac troponin I (sarcomere) [12]. While low-level, pan-specific adrenergic stimulation resulted in different concentrations of cAMP in each compartment, this difference was completely abolished by concomitant inhibition of phosphodiesterases. Measurement of PKA activity in the same compartments with a PKA activity sensor fused to the transmembrane domain of phospholamban (SR), a membrane targeting peptide from Kras (sarcolemma), or the C-terminus of troponin T (sarcomere) confirmed differential regulation of these compartments for β2-adrenergic signals [91]. Strikingly, phosphodiesterase inhibition levelled cAMP concentrations, even in diseased hearts, in which adrenergic responses in the SR and sarcomeric compartments were dampened [12]. Differential analysis of the contribution of specific families of phosphodiesterase revealed that their contribution to reducing phosphorylation in the three compartments varies depending on the health of the myocyte [91]. Both of these results emphasise the importance of local phosphodiesterases in shaping cAMP gradients in both normal and disease conditions.

3.5. cAMP Signalling at the Sarcomere

The sarcomere is the proteinaceous force generator within the cardiomyocyte that mediates muscle contraction. It contains more than 600 structural, regulatory, and associated proteins [93]. The main functional units of the sarcomere are interlaced actin and myosin filaments (Figure 2c). The sarcomere contains some of the most-studied PKA targets in the cardiomyocyte (Figure 2e). PKA phosphorylation at the sarcomere increases contractility by enhancing actin-myosin cross-bridge formation by cardiac myosin binding protein [94]. PKA also mediates relaxation via troponin I phosphorylation by reducing the affinity of the troponin complex for Ca^{2+} [60,95]. In doing so, it ensures the speedy recovery of the sarcomere in preparation for the next cycle.

Taking into account the important functional role of PKA activity in sarcomere contraction, it is interesting that this cellular compartment undergoes the smallest change in cAMP in response to adrenergic signalling in healthy cardiomyocytes. Comparing cAMP levels quantified with CUTie sensors targeted to the sarcomere with full length cardiac troponin I to sarcolemmal and SR-targeted sensors, low level adrenergic stimulation generated only about 60% as much cAMP at the sarcomere than at the other compartments [12]. Calibration of the sensor allowed translation of the measured FRET value to PKA activity, and it was estimated that the amount of cAMP measured at the sarcomere with the CUTie sensor would only activate PKA to about 5% of its maximal activation, in which the activity in resting cells was measured to be ca. 3% [12]. This correlates well with measurements in rabbit myocytes using sarcomere-targeted PKA activity sensors [91], in which the sarcomere was shown to be less sensitive to adrenergic stimulation than sarcolemma and sarcoplasmic reticulum. For example, in cells exclusively stimulated through the β2-adrenergic pathway, sarcomeric PKA phosphorylation was barely detectable by FRET, whereas sarcolemma and sarcoplasmic reticulum showed robust responses [91]. Both the mouse and the rabbit studies show that inhibition of PDEs elevates cAMP and PKA signalling at the sarcomere.

3.6. cAMP Signalling at A Kinase Anchoring Proteins (AKAPs)

AKAPS are intracellular scaffolding proteins that provide a platform for the assembly of PKA-containing signalosomes. AKAPs were first discovered in the 1970s and 80s [96] and then catalogued in different tissues using interaction screens with the PKA dimerization/docking domain that contained an AKAP-binding consensus [97,98].

Targeting FRET sensors to distinct AKAPs can be utilised to directly describe cAMP fluctuations around defined PKA signalosomes in cardiomyocytes. CUTie sensors were used to quantitatively compare cAMP concentrations in the vicinity of AKAP79 at the plasma membrane or AKAP18δ at the sarcoplasmic reticulum with cytosolic cAMP concentrations after adrenergic stimulation of cardiomyocytes. These studies revealed that cAMP concentrations around AKAPs can be detectibly higher than in the bulk cytosol [12].

AKAPs interact with PKA through AKAP-binding domains on the regulatory (R) subunits. Of note, different isoforms of R subunits preferentially interact with distinct AKAPs. By tethering Epac-based cAMP reporters to the dimerization/docking domains of RI and RII, it was possible to specifically dissect molecular components that shape cAMP pools around these different PKA isoforms in cardiomyocytes [42]. Both compartments have access to cAMP at similar levels after direct activation of adenylate cyclase. However, β-adrenergic stimulation leads to a stronger increase in cAMP at the PKA-RII containing compartments, whereas glucagon-like peptide, glucagon, and prostaglandins activate cAMP signalling around PKA-RI. These differences were abolished by simultaneous inhibition of all major phosphodiesterases, highlighting their critical role in shaping distinct receptor-mediated cAMP responses. More detailed analysis of the two compartments by combining β-adrenergic receptor stimulation with family-specific phosphodiesterase inhibitors revealed that, while PDE2 inhibition affected cAMP concentrations in both the RI and the RII compartments, PDE3 inhibition only increased cAMP in the RI compartment [99]. Using a targeted PKA activity sensor confirmed that elevated cAMP levels after co-treatment with β agonist and PDE2 inhibitor lead to increased PKA-dependent phosphorylation in the RII compartment versus the RI compartment. This is significant, because PDE2 inhibition in cardiomyocytes that are chronically stimulated with a β agonist prevented their hypertrophic growth through PKA-mediated phosphorylation of NFAT [99]. Phosphorylation inhibits translocation of the transcription factor to the nucleus and thus activation of the hypertrophic gene transcription programme under its control [100,101]. A different study with the RI and RII-targeted cAMP sensors found that crosstalk with other signalling pathways could help shape the cAMP signal in PKA compartments [102]. Local co-stimulation of cyclic GMP signalling after adrenergic stimulation, for example, selectively reduces the cAMP response around PKA-RII, levelling cAMP signal intensity in PKA-RI and PKA-RII compartments. This study highlights the value of FRET-based cAMP detection, not only for describing the cAMP pathway in isolation, but also for addressing signal integration with other simultaneously active pathways in cardiomyocytes.

Genetically encoded, tetrameric PKA-RII containing FRET probes naturally localise to AKAPs in cardiomyocytes. These probes identified a prominent role for PDE2 in shaping the cAMP response to catecholamines [103]. Inhibiting PDE2, while quantifying cAMP with the anchored FRET sensors, suggested tight coupling of PDE2 to the pool of adenylyl cyclases activated by β-adrenergic receptor stimulation. This coupling resulted in a feedback control loop, in which activation of β3-adrenergic receptors counteracted cAMP generation by β1/β2-adrenoceptors.

To dissect the role of AKAPs on cAMP signal compartmentation themselves, cytosolic FRET responses were compared in neonatal cardiac myocytes from wild type and AKAP5 knock out mice [104]. While there was a clear difference in the amount of cAMP detected after selective β1- or β2-adrenergic stimulation in the wild type, AKAP5 knockout myocytes produced equal cytosolic cAMP levels in response to β1- or β2-adrenergic stimulation.

4. Conclusions

The use of FRET-based cAMP and PKA activity sensors has greatly enhanced our understanding of spatial organisation in the cAMP signalling cascade, as well as the mechanisms that generate a uniquely patterned cAMP response through cardiomyocytes as they react to defined stimuli.

Localised FRET sensors have refined our ability to monitor cAMP signalling events. The sensors constantly evolve (Figure 1), thus increasing the resolution of cAMP monitoring around distinct signalosomes (Figure 2). Initial biochemical studies drew attention to the cAMP concentration gradients between sarcolemma and bulk cytosol of adult cardiomyocytes. This was later confirmed by CNGC activity assays and FRET. cAMP measurements with FRET-based probes, especially in combination with other powerful techniques such as SICM, allowed for narrowing down single cAMP signalling domains to individual T-tubules, which are spread across the sarcolemma of adult cardiomyocytes ca. 2 μm apart from each other [43]. Development of targeted sensors first highlighted differences in cytoplasmic and mitochondrial matrix cAMP concentrations [45,85,86], i.e., in compartments that are only few micrometres apart [105]. This was further refined by sensors targeted to different compartments of the mitochondria itself [85,86]. Likewise, sensors targeted to the sarcoplasmic reticulum were unable to detect cAMP generated by β2-adrenergic receptors in the T tubules [46], even though these organelles are juxtaposed a few hundred nanometres apart from each other at the dyadic junction of a cardiomyocyte [106]. Recent data suggests that there are differential responses in cAMP signalling even between the troponin complex and myosin binding protein C [12], which are located only a few nanometres apart from each other within the sarcomere [107].

FRET-based sensors for cAMP and downstream PKA activity have evolved from a highly demanding technique into a universally applicable tool over the last two decades. In the future, fine tuning this approach by targeting sensors to additional compartments, adjusting their sensitivity accordingly, and improving their dynamic range through engineering the fluorophores in a FRET pair will undoubtedly continue to refine our understanding of cAMP-regulated cardiomyocyte compartments.

Acknowledgments: This work was supported by the British Heart Foundation (PG/10/75/28537 and RG/17/6/32944) and the BHF Centre of Research Excellence, Oxford (RE/13/1/30181).

Author Contributions: All authors contributed to the writing of this manuscript. K.S. prepared the figures.

Conflicts of Interest: The authors declare no conflict of interest.

References

1. Salazar, N.C.; Chen, J.; Rockman, H.A. Cardiac GPCRs: GPCR signaling in healthy and failing hearts. *Biochim. Biophys. Acta Biomembr.* **2007**, *1768*, 1006–1018. [CrossRef] [PubMed]

2. Kaupp, U.B.; Seifert, R. Cyclic nucleotide-gated ion channels. *Physiol. Rev.* **2002**, *82*, 769–824. [CrossRef] [PubMed]

3. Schmidt, M.; Dekker, F.J.; Maarsingh, H. Exchange Protein Directly Activated by cAMP (epac): A Multidomain cAMP Mediator in the Regulation of Diverse Biological Functions. *Pharmacol. Rev.* **2013**, *65*, 670–709. [CrossRef] [PubMed]

4. Schindler, R.F.R.; Brand, T. The Popeye domain containing protein family—A novel class of cAMP effectors with important functions in multiple tissues. *Prog. Biophys. Mol. Biol.* **2016**, *120*, 28–36. [CrossRef] [PubMed]

5. Taylor, S.S.; Kim, C.; Cheng, C.Y.; Brown, S.H.J.; Wu, J.; Kannan, N. Signaling through cAMP and cAMP-dependent protein kinase: Diverse strategies for drug design. *Biochim. Biophys. Acta Proteins Proteom.* **2008**, *1784*, 16–26. [CrossRef] [PubMed]

6. Buxton, I.L.O.; Brunton, L.L. Compartments of cyclic AMP and protein kinase in mammalian cardiomyocytes. *J. Biol. Chem.* **1983**, *258*, 10233–10239. [PubMed]

7. Wang, H.; Robinson, H.; Ke, H. The Molecular Basis for Different Recognition of Substrates by Phosphodiesterase Families 4 and 10. *J. Mol. Biol.* **2007**, *371*, 302–307. [CrossRef] [PubMed]

8. Sunahara, R.K.; Tesmer, J.J.; Gilman, A.G.; Sprang, S.R. Crystal structure of the adenylyl cyclase activator Gsα. *Science* **1997**, *278*, 1943–1947. [CrossRef] [PubMed]

9. Richards, M.; Lomas, O.; Jalink, K.; Ford, K.L.; Vaughan-Jones, R.D.; Lefkimmiatis, K.; Swietach, P. Intracellular tortuosity underlies slow cAMP diffusion in adult ventricular myocytes. *Cardiovasc. Res.* **2016**, *110*, 395–407. [CrossRef] [PubMed]

10. Gesellchen, F.; Stangherlin, A.; Surdo, N.; Terrin, A.; Zoccarato, A.; Zaccolo, M. Measuring spatiotemporal dynamics of cyclic AMP signaling in real-time using FRET-based biosensors. *Methods Mol. Biol.* **2011**, *746*, 297–316. [CrossRef] [PubMed]

11. Sprenger, J.U.; Nikolaev, V.O. Biophysical techniques for detection of cAMP and cGMP in living cells. *Int. J. Mol. Sci.* **2013**, *14*, 8025–8046. [CrossRef] [PubMed]

12. Surdo, N.C.; Berrera, M.; Koschinski, A.; Brescia, M.; Machado, M.R.; Carr, C.; Wright, P.; Gorelik, J.; Morotti, S.; Grandi, E.; et al. FRET biosensor uncovers cAMP nano-domains at β-adrenergic targets that dictate precise tuning of cardiac contractility. *Nat. Commun.* **2017**, *8*, 15031. [CrossRef] [PubMed]

13. Horton, J.K.; Martin, R.C.; Kalinka, S.; Cushing, A.; Kitcher, J.P.; O'Sullivan, M.J.; Baxendale, P.M. Enzyme immunoassays for the estimation of adenosine 3′,5′ cyclic monophosphate and guanosine 3′,5′ cyclic monophosphate in biological fluids. *J. Immunol. Methods* **1992**, *155*, 31–40. [CrossRef]

14. Gilman, A.G. A protein binding assay for adenosine 3′:5′-cyclic monophosphate. *Proc. Natl. Acad. Sci. USA* **1970**, *67*, 305–312. [CrossRef] [PubMed]

15. Pradelles, P.; Grassi, J.; Chabardes, D.; Guiso, N. Enzyme Immunoassays of Adenosine Cyclic 3′,5′-Monophosphate and Guanosine Cyclic 3′,5′-Monophosphate Using Acetylcholinesterase. *Anal. Chem.* **1989**, *61*, 447–453. [CrossRef] [PubMed]

16. Steiner, A.L.; Kipnis, D.M.; Utiger, R.; Parker, C. Radioimmunoassay for the measurement of adenosine 3′,5′-cyclic phosphate. *Proc. Natl. Acad. Sci. USA* **1969**, *64*, 367–373. [CrossRef] [PubMed]

17. Boularan, C.; Gales, C. Cardiac cAMP: Production, hydrolysis, modulation and detection. *Front. Pharmacol.* **2015**, *6*, 203. [CrossRef] [PubMed]

18. Rochais, F.; Vandecasteele, G.; Lefebvre, F.; Lugnier, C.; Lum, H.; Mazet, J.L.; Cooper, D.M.F.; Fischmeister, R. Negative feedback exerted by cAMP-dependent protein kinase and cAMP phosphodiesterase on subsarcolemmal cAMP signals in intact cardiac myocytes: An in vivo study using adenovirus-mediated expression of CNG channels. *J. Biol. Chem.* **2004**, *279*, 52095–52105. [CrossRef] [PubMed]

19. Fagan, K.A.; Schaack, J.; Zweifach, A.; Cooper, D.M.F. Adenovirus encoded cyclic nucleotide-gated channels: A new methodology for monitoring cAMP in living cells. *FEBS Lett.* **2001**, *500*, 85–90. [CrossRef]

20. Rich, T.C.; Fagan, K.A.; Tse, T.E.; Schaack, J.; Cooper, D.M.; Karpen, J.W. A uniform extracellular stimulus triggers distinct cAMP signals in different compartments of a simple cell. *Proc. Natl. Acad. Sci. USA* **2001**, *98*, 13049–13054. [CrossRef] [PubMed]

21. Jurevicius, J.; Fischmeister, R. cAMP compartmentation is responsible for a local activation of cardiac Ca^{2+} channels by β-adrenergic agonists. *Proc. Natl. Acad. Sci. USA* **1996**, *93*, 295–299. [CrossRef] [PubMed]

22. Rich, T.C.; Tse, T.E.; Rohan, J.G.; Schaack, J.; Karpen, J.W. In vivo assessment of local phosphodiesterase activity using tailored cyclic nucleotide-gated channels as cAMP sensors. *J. Gen. Physiol.* **2001**, *118*, 63–78. [CrossRef] [PubMed]

23. Adams, S.R.; Harootunian, A.T.; Buechler, Y.J.; Taylor, S.S.; Tsien, R.Y. Fluorescence ratio imaging of cyclic AMP in single cells. *Nature* **1991**, *349*, 694–697. [CrossRef] [PubMed]

24. Goaillard, J.M.; Vincent, P.; Fischmeister, R. Simultaneous measurements of intracellular cAMP and L-type Ca2+ current in single frog ventricular myocytes. *J. Physiol.* **2001**, *530*, 79–91. [CrossRef] [PubMed]

25. Zaccolo, M.; De Giorgi, F.; Cho, C.Y.; Feng, L.; Knapp, T.; Negulescu, P.A.; Taylor, S.S.; Tsien, R.Y.; Pozzan, T. A genetically encoded, fluorescent indicator for cyclic AMP in living cells. *Nat. Cell Biol.* **2000**, *2*, 25–29. [CrossRef] [PubMed]

26. Zaccolo, M.; Pozzan, T. Discrete Microdomains with High Concentration of cAMP in Stimulated Rat Neonatal Cardiac Myocytes. *Science* **2002**, *295*, 1711–1715. [CrossRef] [PubMed]

27. Kokkonen, K.; Kass, D.A. Nanodomain Regulation of Cardiac Cyclic Nucleotide Signaling by Phosphodiesterases. *Annu. Rev. Pharmacol. Toxicol.* **2017**, *57*, 455–479. [CrossRef] [PubMed]

28. Mongillo, M.; McSorley, T.; Evellin, S.; Sood, A.; Lissandron, V.; Terrin, A.; Huston, E.; Hannawacker, A.; Lohse, M.J.; Pozzan, T.; et al. Fluorescence Resonance Energy Transfer Based Analysis of cAMP Dynamics in Live Neonatal Rat Cardiac Myocytes Reveals Distinct Functions of Compartmentalized Phosphodiesterases. *Circ. Res.* **2004**, *95*, 67–75. [CrossRef] [PubMed]

29. Lehnart, S.E.; Wehrens, X.H.T.; Reiken, S.; Warrier, S.; Belevych, A.E.; Harvey, R.D.; Richter, W.; Jin, S.L.C.; Conti, M.; Marks, A.R. Phosphodiesterase 4D deficiency in the ryanodine-receptor complex promotes heart failure and arrhythmias. *Cell* **2005**, *123*, 25–35. [CrossRef] [PubMed]

30. Warrier, S.; Belevych, A.E.; Ruse, M.; Eckert, R.L.; Zaccolo, M.; Pozzan, T.; Harvey, R.D. Beta-adrenergic- and muscarinic receptor-induced changes in cAMP activity in adult cardiac myocytes detected with FRET-based biosensor. *Am. J. Physiol. Cell Physiol.* **2005**, *289*, C455–C461. [CrossRef] [PubMed]

31. Terrin, A.; Di Benedetto, G.; Pertegato, V.; Cheung, Y.F.; Baillie, G.; Lynch, M.J.; Elvassore, N.; Prinz, A.; Herberg, F.W.; Houslay, M.D.; et al. PGE1 stimulation of HEK293 cells generates multiple contiguous domains with different [cAMP]: Role of compartmentalized phosphodiesterases. *J. Cell Biol.* **2006**, *175*, 441–451. [CrossRef] [PubMed]

32. Nikolaev, V.O.; Bünemann, M.; Hein, L.; Hannawacker, A.; Lohse, M.J. Novel single chain cAMP sensors for receptor-induced signal propagation. *J. Biol. Chem.* **2004**, *279*, 37215–37218. [CrossRef] [PubMed]

33. Nikolaev, V.O.; Bünemann, M.; Schmitteckert, E.; Lohse, M.J.; Engelhardt, S. Cyclic AMP imaging in adult cardiac myocytes reveals far-reaching β1-adrenergic but locally confined β2-adrenergic receptor-mediated signaling. *Circ. Res.* **2006**, *99*, 1084–1091. [CrossRef] [PubMed]

34. Koschinski, A.; Zaccolo, M. Activation of PKA in cell requires higher concentration of cAMP than in vitro: Implications for compartmentalization of cAMP signalling. *Sci. Rep.* **2017**, *7*, 14090. [CrossRef] [PubMed]

35. Tsalkova, T.; Blumenthal, D.K.; Mei, F.C.; White, M.A.; Cheng, X. Mechanism of Epac activation. Structural and functional analyses of Epac2 hinge mutants with constitutive and reduced activities. *J. Biol. Chem.* **2009**, *284*, 23644–23651. [CrossRef] [PubMed]

36. Consonni, S.V.; Gloerich, M.; Spanjaard, E.; Bos, J.L. cAMP regulates DEP domain-mediated binding of the guanine nucleotide exchange factor Epac1 to phosphatidic acid at the plasma membrane. *Proc. Natl. Acad. Sci. USA* **2012**, *109*, 3814–3819. [CrossRef] [PubMed]

37. DiPilato, L.M.; Cheng, X.; Zhang, J. Fluorescent indicators of cAMP and Epac activation reveal differential dynamics of cAMP signaling within discrete subcellular compartments. *Proc. Natl. Acad. Sci. USA* **2004**, *101*, 16513–16518. [CrossRef] [PubMed]

38. Ponsioen, B.; Zhao, J.; Riedl, J.; Zwartkruis, F.; van der Krogt, G.; Zaccolo, M.; Moolenaar, W.H.; Bos, J.L.; Jalink, K. Detecting cAMP-induced Epac activation by fluorescence resonance energy transfer: Epac as a novel cAMP indicator. *EMBO Rep.* **2004**, *5*, 1176–1180. [CrossRef] [PubMed]

39. Violin, J.D.; DiPilato, L.M.; Yildirim, N.; Elston, T.C.; Zhang, J.; Lefkowitz, R.J. β2-Adrenergic receptor signaling and desensitization elucidated by quantitative modeling of real time cAMP dynamics. *J. Biol. Chem.* **2008**, *283*, 2949–2961. [CrossRef] [PubMed]

40. DiPilato, L.M.; Zhang, J. The role of membrane microdomains in shaping beta2-adrenergic receptor-mediated cAMP dynamics. *Mol. Biosyst.* **2009**, *5*, 832–837. [CrossRef] [PubMed]

41. Klarenbeek, J.; Goedhart, J.; Van Batenburg, A.; Groenewald, D.; Jalink, K. Fourth-generation Epac-based FRET sensors for cAMP feature exceptional brightness, photostability and dynamic range: Characterization of dedicated sensors for FLIM, for ratiometry and with high affinity. *PLoS ONE* **2015**, *10*, e0122513. [CrossRef] [PubMed]

42. Di Benedetto, G.; Zoccarato, A.; Lissandron, V.; Terrin, A.; Li, X.; Houslay, M.D.; Baillie, G.S.; Zaccolo, M. Protein kinase A type I and type II define distinct intracellular signaling compartments. *Circ. Res.* **2008**, *103*, 836–844. [CrossRef] [PubMed]

43. Nikolaev, V.O.; Moshkov, A.; Lyon, A.R.; Miragoli, M.; Novak, P.; Paur, H.; Lohse, M.J.; Korchev, Y.E.; Harding, S.E.; Gorelik, J.; et al. β2-adrenergic receptor redistribution in heart failure changes cAMP compartmentation. *Science* **2010**, *327*, 1653–1657. [CrossRef] [PubMed]

44. Llopis, J.; McCaffery, J.M.; Miyawaki, A.; Farquhar, M.G.; Tsien, R.Y. Measurement of cytosolic, mitochondrial, and Golgi pH in single living cells with green fluorescent proteins. *Proc. Natl. Acad. Sci. USA* **1998**, *95*, 6803–6808. [CrossRef] [PubMed]

45. Di Benedetto, G.; Scalzotto, E.; Mongillo, M.; Pozzan, T. Mitochondrial Ca^{2+} uptake induces cyclic AMP generation in the matrix and modulates organelle ATP levels. *Cell Metab.* **2013**, *17*, 965–975. [CrossRef] [PubMed]

46. Sprenger, J.U.; Perera, R.K.; Steinbrecher, J.H.; Lehnart, S.E.; Maier, L.S.; Hasenfuss, G.; Nikolaev, V.O. In vivo model with targeted cAMP biosensor reveals changes in receptor-microdomain communication in cardiac disease. *Nat. Commun.* **2015**, *6*, 6965. [CrossRef] [PubMed]

47. Herget, S.; Lohse, M.J.; Nikolaev, V.O. Real-time monitoring of phosphodiesterase inhibition in intact cells. *Cell. Signal.* **2008**, *20*, 1423–1431. [CrossRef] [PubMed]

48. Packer, M.; Carver, J.R.; Rodeheffer, R.J.; Ivanhoe, R.J.; DiBianco, R.; Zeldis, S.M.; Hendrix, G.H.; Bommer, W.J.; Elkayam, U.; Kukin, M.L.; et al. Effect of oral milrinone on mortality in severe chronic heart failure. *N. Engl. J. Med.* **1991**, *325*, 1468–1475. [CrossRef] [PubMed]

49. Harbeck, M.C.; Chepurny, O.; Nikolaev, V.O.; Lohse, M.J.; Holz, G.G.; Roe, M.W. Simultaneous optical measurements of cytosolic Ca^{2+} and cAMP in single cells. *Sci. Signal.* **2006**, *2006*. [CrossRef] [PubMed]

50. Odaka, H.; Arai, S.; Inoue, T.; Kitaguchi, T. Genetically-encoded yellow fluorescent cAMP indicator with an expanded dynamic range for dual-color imaging. *PLoS ONE* **2014**, *9*, e100252. [CrossRef] [PubMed]

51. Hackley, C.R.; Mazzoni, E.O.; Blau, J. cAMPr: A single-wavelength fluorescent sensor for cyclic AMP. *Sci. Signal.* **2018**, *11*, 255–268. [CrossRef] [PubMed]

52. Beavo, J.A.; Brunton, L.L. Cyclic nucleotide research—Still expanding after half a century. *Nat. Rev. Mol. Cell Biol.* **2002**, *3*, 710–718. [CrossRef] [PubMed]

53. Zhang, J.; Ma, Y.; Taylor, S.S.; Tsien, R.Y. Genetically encoded reporters of protein kinase A activity reveal impact of substrate tethering. *Proc. Natl. Acad. Sci. USA* **2001**, *98*, 14997–15002. [CrossRef] [PubMed]

54. Zhang, J.; Hupfeld, C.J.; Taylor, S.S.; Olefsky, J.M.; Tsien, R.Y. Insulin disrupts β-adrenergic signalling to protein kinase a in adipocytes. *Nature* **2005**, *437*, 569–573. [CrossRef] [PubMed]

55. Allen, M.D.; Zhang, J. Subcellular dynamics of protein kinase A activity visualized by FRET-based reporters. *Biochem. Biophys. Res. Commun.* **2006**, *348*, 716–721. [CrossRef] [PubMed]

56. Depry, C.; Allen, M.D.; Zhang, J. Visualization of PKA activity in plasma membrane microdomains. *Mol. Biosyst.* **2011**, *7*, 52–58. [CrossRef] [PubMed]

57. Koschinski, A.; Zaccolo, M. A novel approach combining real-time imaging and the patch-clamp technique to calibrate FRET-based reporters for cAMP in their cellular microenvironment. In *cAMP Signaling: Methods and Protocols*; Humana Press: New York, NY, USA, 2015; pp. 25–40, ISBN 9781493925377.

58. Chang, C.R.; Blackstone, C. Cyclic AMP-dependent protein kinase phosphorylation of Drp1 regulates its GTPase activity and mitochondrial morphology. *J. Biol. Chem.* **2007**, *282*, 21583–21587. [CrossRef] [PubMed]

59. Hartzell, H.C.; Glass, D.B. Phosphorylation of purified cardiac muscle C-protein by purified cAMP-dependent and endogenous Ca^{2+}-calmodulin-dependent protein kinases. *J. Biol. Chem.* **1984**, *259*, 15587–15596. [PubMed]

60. Solaro, R.J.; Moir, A.J.G.; Perry, S.V. Phosphorylation of troponin I and the inotropic effect of adrenaline in the perfused rabbit heart. *Nature* **1976**, *262*, 615–617. [CrossRef] [PubMed]

61. Marx, S.O.; Reiken, S.; Hisamatsu, Y.; Jayaraman, T.; Burkhoff, D.; Rosemblit, N.; Marks, A.R. PKA Phosphorylation Dissociates FKBP12.6 from the Calcium Release Channel (Ryanodine Receptor). *Cell* **2000**, *101*, 365–376. [CrossRef]

62. Burgers, P.P.; van der Heyden, M.A.; Kok, B.; Heck, A.J.; Scholten, A. A systematic evaluation of protein kinase A-A-kinase anchoring protein interaction motifs. *Biochemistry* **2015**, *54*, 11–21. [CrossRef] [PubMed]

63. Welch, E.J.; Jones, B.W.; Scott, J.D. Networking with AKAPs: Context-dependent regulation of anchored enzymes. *Mol. Interv.* **2010**, *10*, 86–97. [CrossRef] [PubMed]

64. Kinderman, F.S.; Kim, C.; von Daake, S.; Ma, Y.; Pham, B.Q.; Spraggon, G.; Xuong, N.H.; Jennings, P.A.; Taylor, S.S. A Dynamic Mechanism for AKAP Binding to RII Isoforms of cAMP-Dependent Protein Kinase. *Mol. Cell* **2006**, *24*, 397–408. [CrossRef] [PubMed]

65. Maurice, D.H.; Ke, H.; Ahmad, F.; Wang, Y.; Chung, J.; Manganiello, V.C. Advances in targeting cyclic nucleotide phosphodiesterases. *Nat. Rev. Drug Discov.* **2014**, *13*, 290–314. [CrossRef] [PubMed]

66. Akazawa, H.; Komuro, I. Roles of cardiac transcription factors in cardiac hypertrophy. *Circ. Res.* **2003**, *92*, 1079–1088. [CrossRef] [PubMed]

67. Zippin, J.H.; Chen, Y.; Nahirney, P.; Kamenetsky, M.; Wuttke, M.S.; Fischman, D.A.; Levin, L.R.; Buck, J. Compartmentalization of bicarbonate-sensitive adenylyl cyclase in distinct signaling microdomains. *FASEB J.* **2003**, *17*, 82–84. [CrossRef] [PubMed]

68. Zippin, J.H.; Farrell, J.; Huron, D.; Kamenetsky, M.; Hess, K.C.; Fischman, D.A.; Levin, L.R.; Buck, J. Bicarbonate-responsive "soluble" adenylyl cyclase defines a nuclear cAMP microdomain. *J. Cell Biol.* **2004**, *164*, 527–534. [CrossRef] [PubMed]

69. Agarwal, S.R.; Miyashiro, K.; Latt, H.; Ostrom, R.S.; Harvey, R.D. Compartmentalized cAMP responses to prostaglandin EP $_2$ receptor activation in human airway smooth muscle cells. *Br. J. Pharmacol.* **2017**, *174*, 2784–2796. [CrossRef] [PubMed]

70. Sample, V.; DiPilato, L.M.; Yang, J.H.; Ni, Q.; Saucerman, J.J.; Zhang, J. Regulation of nuclear PKA revealed by spatiotemporal manipulation of cyclic AMP. *Nat. Chem. Biol.* **2012**, *8*, 375–382. [CrossRef] [PubMed]

71. Yang, J.H.; Polanowska-Grabowska, R.K.; Smith, J.S.; Shields, C.W.; Saucerman, J.J. PKA catalytic subunit compartmentation regulates contractile and hypertrophic responses to β-adrenergic signaling. *J. Mol. Cell. Cardiol.* **2014**, *66*, 83–93. [CrossRef] [PubMed]

72. Saucerman, J.J.; Zhang, J.; Martin, J.C.; Peng, L.X.; Stenbit, A.E.; Tsien, R.Y.; McCulloch, A.D. Systems analysis of PKA-mediated phosphorylation gradients in live cardiac myocytes. *Proc. Natl. Acad. Sci. USA* **2006**, *103*, 12923–12928. [CrossRef] [PubMed]

73. Agarwal, S.R.; MacDougall, D.A.; Tyser, R.; Pugh, S.D.; Calaghan, S.C.; Harvey, R.D. Effects of cholesterol depletion on compartmentalized cAMP responses in adult cardiac myocytes. *J. Mol. Cell. Cardiol.* **2011**, *50*, 500–509. [CrossRef] [PubMed]

74. Wright, P.T.; Nikolaev, V.O.; O'Hara, T.; Diakonov, I.; Bhargava, A.; Tokar, S.; Schobesberger, S.; Shevchuk, A.I.; Sikkel, M.B.; Wilkinson, R.; et al. Caveolin-3 regulates compartmentation of cardiomyocyte beta2-adrenergic receptor-mediated cAMP signaling. *J. Mol. Cell. Cardiol.* **2014**, *67*, 38–48. [CrossRef] [PubMed]

75. Mika, D.; Richter, W.; Westenbroek, R.E.; Catterall, W.A.; Conti, M. PDE4B mediates local feedback regulation of 1-adrenergic cAMP signaling in a sarcolemmal compartment of cardiac myocytes. *J. Cell Sci.* **2014**, *127*, 1033–1042. [CrossRef] [PubMed]

76. Doenst, T.; Nguyen, T.D.; Abel, E.D. Cardiac metabolism in heart failure: Implications beyond atp production. *Circ. Res.* **2013**, *113*, 709–724. [CrossRef] [PubMed]

J. Cardiovasc. Dev. Dis. **2018**, *5*, 17

77. Neubauer, S. The Failing Heart—An Engine Out of Fuel. *N. Engl. J. Med.* **2007**, *356*, 1140–1151. [CrossRef] [PubMed]

78. Rizzuto, R.; Simpson, A.W.M.; Brini, M.; Pozzan, T. Rapid changes of mitochondrial Ca^{2+} revealed by specifically targeted recombinant aequorin. *Nature* **1992**, *358*, 325–327. [CrossRef] [PubMed]

79. Rizzuto, R.; Brini, M.; Murgia, M.; Pozzan, T. Microdomains with high Ca^{2+} close to IP3-sensitive channels that are sensed by neighboring mitochondria. *Science* **1993**, *262*, 744–747. [CrossRef] [PubMed]

80. Rizzuto, R. Close Contacts with the Endoplasmic Reticulum as Determinants of Mitochondrial Ca^{2+} Responses. *Science* **1998**, *280*, 1763–1766. [CrossRef] [PubMed]

81. Jouaville, L.S.; Pinton, P.; Bastianutto, C.; Rutter, G.A.; Rizzuto, R. Regulation of mitochondrial ATP synthesis by calcium: Evidence for a long-term metabolic priming. *Proc. Natl. Acad. Sci. USA* **1999**, *96*, 13807–13812. [CrossRef] [PubMed]

82. Chen, L.; Gong, Q.; Stice, J.P.; Knowlton, A.A. Mitochondrial OPA1, apoptosis, and heart failure. *Cardiovasc. Res.* **2009**, *84*, 91–99. [CrossRef] [PubMed]

83. Cribbs, J.T.; Strack, S. Reversible phosphorylation of Drp1 by cyclic AMP-dependent protein kinase and calcineurin regulates mitochondrial fission and cell death. *EMBO Rep.* **2007**, *8*, 939–944. [CrossRef] [PubMed]

84. Ma, Y.; Taylor, S.S. A molecular switch for targeting between endoplasmic reticulum (ER) and mitochondria: Conversion of a mitochondria-targeting element into an ER-targeting signal in DAKAP1. *J. Biol. Chem.* **2008**, *283*, 11743–11751. [CrossRef] [PubMed]

85. Lefkimmiatis, K.; Leronni, D.; Hofer, A.M. The inner and outer compartments of mitochondria are sites of distinct cAMP/PKA signaling dynamics. *J. Cell Biol.* **2013**, *202*, 453–462. [CrossRef] [PubMed]

86. Monterisi, S.; Lobo, M.J.; Livie, C.; Castle, J.C.; Weinberger, M.; Baillie, G.; Surdo, N.C.; Musheshe, N.; Stangherlin, A.; Gottlieb, E.; et al. PDE2A2 regulates mitochondria morphology and apoptotic cell death via local modulation of cAMP/PKA signalling. *Elife* **2017**, *6*. [CrossRef] [PubMed]

87. Moss, R.L.; Razumova, M.; Fitzsimons, D.P. Myosin crossbridge activation of cardiac thin filaments: Implications for myocardial function in health and disease. *Circ. Res.* **2004**, *94*, 1290–1300. [CrossRef] [PubMed]

88. Wehrens, X.H.T.; Lehnart, S.E.; Reiken, S.; Vest, J.A.; Wronska, A.; Marks, A.R. Ryanodine receptor/calcium release channel PKA phosphorylation: A critical mediator of heart failure progression. *Proc. Natl. Acad. Sci. USA* **2006**, *103*, 511–518. [CrossRef] [PubMed]

89. Ceholski, D.K.; Trieber, C.A.; Holmes, C.F.B.; Young, H.S. Lethal, hereditary mutants of phospholamban elude phosphorylation by protein kinase A. *J. Biol. Chem.* **2012**, *287*, 26596–26605. [CrossRef] [PubMed]

90. Piacentino, V.; Weber, C.R.; Chen, X.; Weisser-Thomas, J.; Margulies, K.B.; Bers, D.M.; Houser, S.R. Cellular basis of abnormal calcium transients of failing human ventricular myocytes. *Circ. Res.* **2003**, *92*, 651–658. [CrossRef] [PubMed]

91. Barbagallo, F.; Xu, B.; Reddy, G.R.; West, T.; Wang, Q.; Fu, Q.; Li, M.; Shi, Q.; Ginsburg, K.S.; Ferrier, W.; et al. Genetically Encoded Biosensors Reveal PKA Hyperphosphorylation on the Myofilaments in Rabbit Heart Failure. *Circ. Res.* **2016**, *119*, 931–943. [CrossRef] [PubMed]

92. Liu, S.; Zhang, J.; Xiang, Y.K. FRET-based direct detection of dynamic protein kinase a activity on the sarcoplasmic reticulum in cardiomyocytes. *Biochem. Biophys. Res. Commun.* **2011**, *404*, 581–586. [CrossRef] [PubMed]

93. Yin, X.; Cuello, F.; Mayr, U.; Hao, Z.; Hornshaw, M.; Ehler, E.; Avkiran, M.; Mayr, M. Proteomics analysis of the cardiac myofilament subproteome reveals dynamic alterations in phosphatase subunit distribution. *Mol. Cell. Proteom.* **2010**, *9*, 497–509. [CrossRef] [PubMed]

94. Kensler, R.W.; Craig, R.; Moss, R.L. Phosphorylation of cardiac myosin binding protein C releases myosin heads from the surface of cardiac thick filaments. *Proc. Natl. Acad. Sci. USA* **2017**, *114*, E1355–E1364. [CrossRef] [PubMed]

95. Ray, K.P.; England, P.J. Phosphorylation of the inhibitory subunit of troponin and its effect on the calcium dependence of cardiac myofibril adenosine triphosphatase. *FEBS Lett.* **1976**, *70*, 11–16. [CrossRef]

96. Scott, J.D.; Santana, L.F. A-Kinase Anchoring Proteins: Getting to the heart of the matter. *Circulation* **2010**, *121*, 1264–1271. [CrossRef] [PubMed]

97. Carr, D.W.; Hausken, Z.E.; Fraser, I.D.C.; Stofko-Hahn, R.E.; Scott, J.D. Association of the type II cAMP-dependent protein kinase with a human thyroid RII-anchoring protein: Cloning and characterization of the RII-binding domain. *J. Biol. Chem.* **1992**, *267*, 13376–13382. [PubMed]

98. Carr, D.W.; Stofko-Hahn, R.E.; Fraser, I.D.C.; Bishop, S.M.; Acott, T.S.; Brennan, R.G.; Scott, J.D. Interaction of the regulatory subunit (RII) of cAMP-dependent protein kinase with RII-anchoring proteins occurs through an amphipathic helix binding motif. *J. Biol. Chem.* **1991**, *266*, 14188–14192. [PubMed]

99. Zoccarato, A.; Surdo, N.C.; Aronsen, J.M.; Fields, L.A.; Mancuso, L.; Dodoni, G.; Stangherlin, A.; Livie, C.; Jiang, H.; Sin, Y.Y.; et al. Cardiac Hypertrophy Is Inhibited by a Local Pool of cAMP Regulated by Phosphodiesterase 2. *Circ. Res.* **2015**, *117*, 707–719. [CrossRef] [PubMed]

100. Sheridan, C.M.; Heist, E.K.; Beals, C.R.; Crabtree, G.R.; Gardner, P. Protein kinase A negatively modulates the nuclear accumulation of NF-ATc1 by priming for subsequent phosphorylation by glycogen synthase kinase-3. *J. Biol. Chem.* **2002**, *277*, 48664–48676. [CrossRef] [PubMed]

101. Molkentin, J.D.; Lu, J.R.; Antos, C.L.; Markham, B.; Richardson, J.; Robbins, J.; Grant, S.R.; Olson, E.N. A calcineurin-dependent transcriptional pathway for cardiac hypertrophy. *Cell* **1998**, *93*, 215–228. [CrossRef]

102. Stangherlin, A.; Gesellchen, F.; Zoccarato, A.; Terrin, A.; Fields, L.A.; Berrera, M.; Surdo, N.C.; Craig, M.A.; Smith, G.; Hamilton, G.; et al. CGMP signals modulate camp levels in a compartment-specific manner to regulate catecholamine-dependent signaling in cardiac myocytes. *Circ. Res.* **2011**, *108*, 929–939. [CrossRef] [PubMed]

103. Mongillo, M.; Tocchetti, C.G.; Terrin, A.; Lissandron, V.; Cheung, Y.F.; Dostmann, W.R.; Pozzan, T.; Kass, D.A.; Paolocci, N.; Houslay, M.D.; et al. Compartmentalized phosphodiesterase-2 activity blunts β-adrenergic cardiac inotropy via an NO/cGMP-dependent pathway. *Circ. Res.* **2006**, *98*, 226–234. [CrossRef] [PubMed]

104. Li, X.; Nooh, M.M.; Bahouth, S.W. Role of AKAP79/150 protein in β1-adrenergic receptor trafficking and signaling in mammalian cells. *J. Biol. Chem.* **2013**, *288*, 33797–33812. [CrossRef] [PubMed]

105. Neary, M.T.; Ng, K.-E.; Ludtmann, M.H.R.; Hall, A.R.; Piotrowska, I.; Ong, S.-B.; Hausenloy, D.J.; Mohun, T.J.; Abramov, A.Y.; Breckenridge, R.A. Hypoxia signaling controls postnatal changes in cardiac mitochondrial morphology and function. *J. Mol. Cell. Cardiol.* **2014**, *74*, 340–352. [CrossRef] [PubMed]

106. Hayashi, T.; Martone, M.E.; Yu, Z.; Thor, A.; Doi, M.; Holst, M.J.; Ellisman, M.H.; Hoshijima, M. Three-dimensional electron microscopy reveals new details of membrane systems for Ca2+ signaling in the heart. *J. Cell Sci.* **2009**, *122*, 1005–1013. [CrossRef] [PubMed]

107. Luther, P.K.; Winkler, H.; Taylor, K.; Zoghbi, M.E.; Craig, R.; Padron, R.; Squire, J.M.; Liu, J. Direct visualization of myosin-binding protein C bridging myosin and actin filaments in intact muscle. *Proc. Natl. Acad. Sci. USA* **2011**, *108*, 11423–11428. [CrossRef] [PubMed]

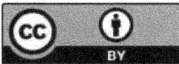

Journal of
Cardiovascular
Development and Disease

MDPI

Review

Imaging of PDE2- and PDE3-Mediated cGMP-to-cAMP Cross-Talk in Cardiomyocytes

Nikoleta Pavlaki [1,2] and Viacheslav O. Nikolaev [1,2,*]

[1] Institute of Experimental Cardiovascular Research, University Medical Center Hamburg-Eppendorf, 20246 Hamburg, Germany; n.pavlaki@uke.de
[2] German Center for Cardiovascular Research (DZHK), Partner Site Hamburg/Kiel/Lübeck, 20246 Hamburg, Germany
* Correspondence: v.nikolaev@uke.de; Tel.: +49-40-7410-51391

Received: 29 December 2017; Accepted: 17 January 2018; Published: 19 January 2018

Abstract: Cyclic nucleotides 3′,5′-cyclic adenosine monophosphate (cAMP) and 3′,5′-cyclic guanosine monophosphate (cGMP) are important second messengers that regulate cardiovascular function and disease by acting in discrete subcellular microdomains. Signaling compartmentation at these locations is often regulated by phosphodiesterases (PDEs). Some PDEs are also involved in the cross-talk between the two second messengers. The purpose of this review is to summarize and highlight recent findings about the role of PDE2 and PDE3 in cardiomyocyte cyclic nucleotide compartmentation and visualization of this process using live cell imaging techniques.

Keywords: cAMP; cGMP; phosphodiesterase; FRET; imaging; cross-talk

1. Introduction

Cyclic nucleotides 3′,5′-cyclic adenosine monophosphate (cAMP) and 3′,5′-cyclic guanosine monophosphate (cGMP) are ubiquitous intracellular second messengers that regulate multiple physiological functions as well as pathological conditions. In cardiomyocytes, there are at least three pathways that normally trigger their production after initial first messenger stimuli: (i) the β-adrenergic pathway for cAMP production, (ii) the nitric oxide, and (iii) the natriuretic peptide (NP) receptor pathways for cGMP synthesis.

1.1. The cAMP and β-Adrenergic Pathway

In healthy cardiomyocytes, sympathetic activation mainly via β-adrenergic receptor (β-AR) signaling leads to the production of cAMP and thereby to increased contractile force (inotropy), heart rate (chronotropy), and cell relaxation (lusitropy) [1]. When a ligand binds to a G protein-coupled receptor (GPCR) located on the plasma membrane, a conformational change occurring in the receptor leads to G-protein activation. Activated G-proteins can in turn, activate or inhibit cAMP-forming enzymes adenylyl cyclases (ACs) which generate cAMP from ATP. Subsequently, cAMP acts in cells via one or more of the following effector proteins:

(a) cAMP-dependent protein kinase (PKA), which is responsible for phosphorylation of several calcium handling proteins involved in cardiac excitation-contraction coupling (ECC) including L-type Ca^{2+} channel (LTCC) at the plasmalemma, phospholamban, and ryanodine receptors at the sarcoplasmic reticulum (SR), myosin-binding protein C, and troponin I at the myofilaments [1,2]. PKA is the main effector protein in the cAMP cascade, while Ca^{2+}-inhibited AC5 and AC6 are the predominant cAMP generating adenylyl cyclases in adult (AC5 and AC6) and fetal (AC6) ventricular cardiac tissue [3];

(b)   exchange proteins directly activated by cAMP (Epac1 and Epac2) [4], which are implicated in pathological cardiomyocyte growth [5,6];

(c)   cyclic nucleotide gated ion channels (CNGCs) including HCN channels located in the sinus node, which regulate the capacity of cardiac cells to initiate spontaneous action potentials (automaticity) [7–9];

(d)   the recently introduced Popeye-domain-containing proteins which affect cardiac pacemaking [10,11].

1.2. NO/sGC/cGMP Pathway

Biosynthesis of cGMP is catalyzed by two discrete guanylyl cyclase (GC) families, one being activated in the presence of nitric oxide (NO) and called soluble guanylyl cyclase (sGC) and the other acting as membrane receptors for natriuretic peptides (NPs), also called particulate guanylyl cyclase (pGC).

NO, alternatively known as "endothelial-derived relaxant factor" (EDRF) [12,13], is produced for example by endothelial cells after acetylcholine administration. It increases cGMP levels, activates cGMP-dependent protein kinase (PKG), and behaves in a way similar to nitrovasodilators [14,15]. Seminal work on the field [16–18] has firmly established that NO is produced by a family of NO biosynthetic enzymes called nitric oxide synthases (NOS). It includes neuronal (NOS-1 or nNOS), inducible (NOS-2 or iNOS), and endothelial nitric oxide synthases (NOS-3 or eNOS) [19], all of which having been detected in heart and vessels [20–24]. iNOS is an inducible biosynthetic enzyme, while eNOS and nNOS are both constitutive and inducible enzymes [25]. NO activates sGC by binding to both heme and non-heme sites [26–28], which leads to the production of cGMP [29] and its subsequent downstream effects [25,30,31].

1.3. NP/pGC/cGMP Pathway

Natriuretic peptides (NPs) constitute important cardiovascular regulators of inotropy and blood pressure [32] with atrial (ANP), brain (BNP), and C-type natriuretic peptides (CNP) being the most well-known ligands. In response to neurohumoral (catecholamines or angiotensin II) or mechanical (e.g., increased myocardial stretch or blood pressure) stimuli [33,34], ANP and BNP are produced and released by the atria and the ventricles of the heart, while CNP is produced mainly by endothelial cells of the vasculature [34].

These NPs can bind and activate several pGCs, two of which are expressed in the heart and exert the majority of their physiological effects. NPR1 (also called NPR-A or GC-A) is the receptor that binds both ANP and BNP with relatively high affinity (ANP > BNP) [35–37]. After ligand binding at its extracellular domain, pGCs undergo a conformational change upon which its intracellular domain generates cGMP [25]. As a widely distributed receptor in the cardiovascular system (heart, vessels, and kidneys), NPR1 regulates blood pressure, exerts antihypertrophic action, and preserves body homeostasis [35–37]. NPR2 (also called NPR-B or GC-B) is the CNP-specific receptor responsible for vascular regeneration and endochondral ossification. It is mainly localized in fibroblasts [38], the sympathetic nervous system [39], and the vascular endothelium and smooth muscle [40] and exerts antihypertrophic effects in cardiomyocytes [41,42].

Both NO/sGC and NP/pGC pathways stimulate cGMP synthesis and participate in the homeostasis of the cardiovascular system via (i) PKG-mediated protein phosphorylation [29–31], (ii) the activation of CNGCs, and (iii) the regulation of PDEs [25]. Physiologically, cGMP binds to specific sites in the regulatory domains of PKG, CNG, or PDE in order to induce conformational changes and downstream effects. Disruption of downstream cascade at any level can initiate pathophysiological effects and may lead to hypertension, atherosclerosis, pulmonary hypertension, hypertrophy, ventricular remodeling, myocardial ischemia, dystrophy-related cardiomyopathies, mitochondrial metabolism, or heart failure [25].

Apart from the classical cyclic nucleotides, cyclic cytidine (cCMP) and cyclic uridine monophosphates (cUMP) have been recently introduced as non-canonical second messengers generated by ACs and

GCs [43,44]. However, available published data provides limited information regarding their effector proteins and physiological significance, so further studies are required to fully elucidate their role in the cardiovascular system.

2. Compartmentation of cAMP and cGMP Signaling

The fact that multiple receptor stimuli can trigger diverse intracellular effects generated via the production of just a few second messengers such as cAMP and cGMP led to a currently accepted theory of cyclic nucleotide compartmentation. Compartmentation refers to the mechanisms by which multiple spatially segregated cAMP/PKA and cGMP/PKG signaling pathways exert different or even opposing functional effects in distinct subcellular microdomains of the same cell [9,45]. It appears to be of critical importance for cardiovascular system, since local cyclic nucleotide actions and the interplay of the cAMP and cGMP signaling pathways have been implicated in physiological functions or pathological conditions.

Several proteins [46–50] contribute to cyclic nucleotide compartmentation, which spatially, temporally, and functionally controls the downstream effects of cyclic nucleotides (extensively studied for cAMP) in the cardiovascular system [25,51–53]. They include (a) GPCRs located in lipid rafts [54,55], at transverse tubules [56] and in non-caveolar membrane domains [57]; (b) ACs and GCs [58,59]; (c) Scaffold proteins [60–62]) such as A-kinase anchoring proteins (AKAPs) [52,63,64] and Calveolin-3 [54,65–67]; (d) physical barriers—e.g., mitochondria, cAMP buffering by PKA, cAMP export [68,69] are some of the mechanisms that create locally confined intracellular domains regulating signaling; and (e), the most prominent and extensively studied of all, the PDE-mediated hydrolysis of cyclic nucleotides, which is of high pharmacological and clinical interest [64,70,71].

PDEs can control cAMP and cGMP compartmentation by providing their local hydrolytic degradation and creating spatial second messenger gradients [72]. Although much fewer scientific data are available on cGMP compartmentation, the role of PDEs in local confinement of cGMP pools has recently been elucidated, especially that of PDE2, PDE5, and PDE9 [25,73]. Furthermore, spatial organization of PKG and GCs in distinct subcellular complexes appears to be another important aspect of cGMP microdomain regulation [74]. It still remains to be established whether, for example, myosin, NPR1, and troponin T could act as PKG scaffolding proteins [75].

Among the relevant experimental evidence, studies on knockout mice do also highlight the importance of the crucial role PDEs play in the cAMP/cGMP signaling pathways and their respective crosstalk [76]. The interplay among the β-adrenergic and NO/cGMP/PKG pathways can be interpreted as a network phenomenon arising from the molecular selectivity of PDEs to cAMP and cGMP [77].

3. Phosphodiesterases (PDEs)

PDEs are the hydrolyzing enzymes that terminate intracellular effects of cyclic nucleotides by their hydrolysis to fine-tune the signaling and to prevent continuous activation of the downstream effector proteins. These cyclic nucleotide-degrading enzymes constitute one of the most important mechanisms, by which cyclic nucleotides are spatially, temporally, and functionally compartmentalized in cardiomyocytes and other cells. Of the 12 PDE families [78,79], there are seven, namely PDE1 [80], PDE2 [81], PDE3 [76], PDE4 [82], PDE5 [83], PDE8 [84], and PDE9 [73] that have been reported to be expressed and active in mammalian cardiomyocytes (Figure 1). They are an integral part of the multimolecular signaling/regulatory complexes, i.e., signalosomes [52,64,76,84]. This review will particularly explore the so-called cGMP-regulated PDEs, especially PDE2 and PDE3, which critically regulate cGMP-to-cAMP cross-talk and cyclic nucleotide actions in cardiomyocyte microdomains.

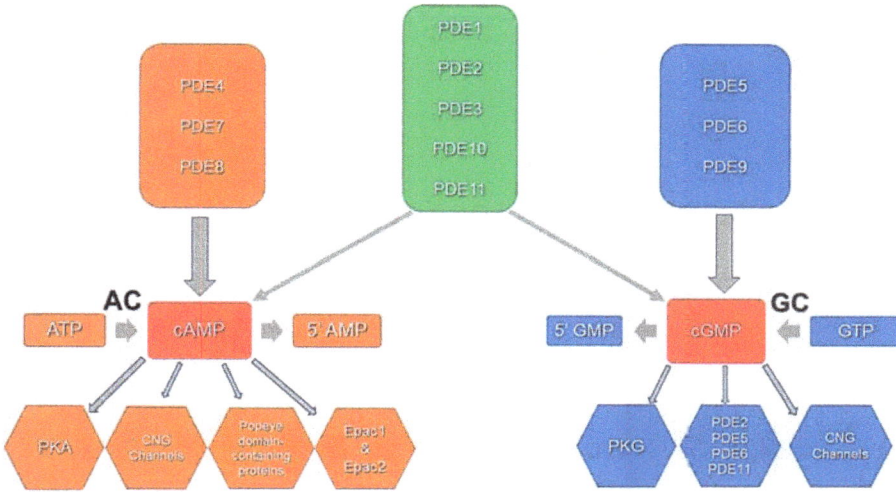

Figure 1. PDE activity, specificity, and cyclic nucleotide effector proteins. PDE4, PDE7, and PDE8 selectively degrade cAMP. PDE5, PDE6, and PDE9 selectively degrade cGMP. PDE1, PDE2, PDE3, PDE10, and PDE11 are dual-specificity phosphodiesterases that hydrolyze both cAMP and cGMP. Downstream effectors include PKA, PKG, Epacs, PDEs, CNG channels and Popeye domain-containing proteins. Adapted from Ahmad et al., 2015 [76].

3.1. Phosphodiesterase 2

PDE2 is a dual-substrate enzyme, which hydrolyzes both cAMP and cGMP with similar maximal rates in bovine adrenal and heart tissues [85]. Only one gene (*Pde2a*) gives rise to three known PDE2A isoforms, which are differentially located in the cytosol, mitochondria, and cellular membranes [58]. It is characteristic of this PDE family that the cGMP-mediated control of cAMP hydrolysis arises, when cGMP binds allosterically to the GAF-B domain of PDE2A, so that cAMP hydrolysis occurs with a 10-fold higher rate [86–88]. In this manner, cGMP via PDE2A is able to negatively regulate cAMP levels [51] and therefore to initiate a negative cGMP-to-cAMP cross-talk [89] (Figure 2). Initially cloned from rat brain [90] and purified from bovine or calf tissues (heart, liver adrenal gland, and platelets) [85,91], the PDE2A protein is also found in endothelial cells, macrophages, and brain [92,93]. Platelet aggregation [94], aldosterone secretion [95], and regulation of calcium channels [96] require PDE2A-mediated hydrolysis of cAMP. Recently, a PDE2A isoform regulating the mitochondrial respiratory chain has been detected, discovering a possible new pathway for the drug-induced control of mitochondrial function [97]. Of particular importance are those studies referring to PDE2A expression in isolated cardiomyocytes and myocardium. In cardiomyocytes, PDE2A together with PDE5 is also involved in the degradation of sGC-synthesized cGMP, whereas pGC-synthesized cGMP is preferentially hydrolyzed by PDE2A [72,98,99].

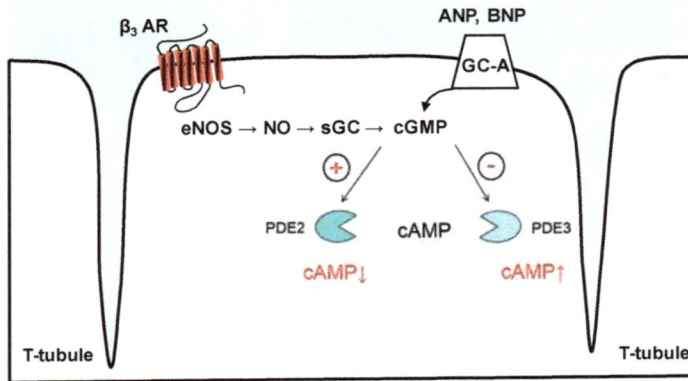

Figure 2. PDE2- and PDE3-mediated cyclic nucleotide crosstalk. cGMP synthesis occurs by pGCs such as GC-A, which serves as a membrane receptor for ANP and BNP, or by NO-activated sGC, e.g., downstream of eNOS and β_3-adrenoreceptor (β_3-AR). Binding of cGMP to PDE2 can allosterically increase its hydrolytic activity, lowering cAMP levels in subcellular microdomains. PDE3 is a "cGMP-inhibited" phosphodiesterase that upon cGMP binding and degradation in the catalytic domain shows reduced rates of cAMP hydrolysis, generating a positive cGMP-to-cAMP cross-talk.

3.2. Phosphodiesterase 3

Another important cGMP-regulated PDE is PDE3. This enzyme hydrolyzes both cAMP and cGMP. Often referred to as cGMP-inhibited PDE, PDE3 shows higher catalytic rates for cAMP but relatively high affinity for cGMP, which acts as a competitive inhibitor of cAMP hydrolysis [100,101]. This creates the so-called positive cGMP-to-cAMP cross-talk (Figure 2). PDE3A and PDE3B are the two PDE3 subfamilies, with the former being abundant in cardiomyocytes, oocytes, vascular smooth muscle and platelets and the latter being expressed in the pancreas, liver, and adipose tissue [100]. PDE3A controls myocardial contractility by interacting with the sarcoplasmic/endoplasmic reticulum calcium ATPase (SERCA2a) [102]. By utilizing their direct positive inotropic effects, PDE3 inhibitors are used for acute treatment of end-stage heart failure (HF) [103], albeit presenting increased mortality as well as incidence of arrhythmias and sudden death after chronic use [104,105]. In contrast, PDE3B seems to be more actively engaged in energy metabolism [106,107], but it can also protect the heart from ischemia/reperfusion injury [108]. Knockout models have revealed that PDE3A, but not PDE3B, exerts inotropic and chronotropic effects after treatment with PDE3 inhibitors [109] because PDE3A regulates SERCA2a activity and subsequent SR Ca^{2+} uptake [102]. By chronically suppressing its expression or action, myocyte apoptosis in vitro [110] or deterioration of ischemia/reperfusion-induced apoptosis and cardiac injury in vivo [111] have been observed. Similarly, disruption of PDE3B interaction with phosphoinositide 3-kinase γ, which can serve as an AKAP, has deleterious effects [112–114] such as arrhythmias [114], necrotic cardiac tissue damage, and fibrosis [112].

PDE3 along with other PDEs constitutes an integral part of cAMP degradation. Evidence suggests that it may also controls cGMP levels [108,115], atrial dynamics, and myocyte ANP release, depending on the involved induction mechanism [72,116]. In terms of cGMP and cAMP pathway interactions, cGMP binding to PDE2 enhances the hydrolytic activity of the enzyme and enables the negative cGMP-to-cAMP cross-talk [75]. Conversely, cGMP binding to the catalytic domains of PDE3 reduced the rate of cAMP degradation, thereby mediating the positive cGMP-to-cAMP cross-talk.

The previously reported experimental data regarding the affinity, specificity, and enzymatic activity of PDE2 and PDE3 can largely explain their crucial role in cGMP/cAMP crosstalk [75].

4. Visualization of Compartmentalized cAMP and cGMP

Initially, the idea of compartmentalized action of cyclic nucleotides was conceived [117] and revealed by several research groups [118–122] with Buxton and Brunton (1983) [122] using classical biochemical methods to show that prostaglandin induces different PKA activity rates in particulate and soluble fractions of cardiac myocytes after cAMP generation. Later on, Jurevicius and Fischmeister (1996) [123], by utilizing a combination of two-barrel microperfusion and whole patch clamp techniques, further confirmed the compartmentation theory in frog ventricular cells, where local application of a β-adrenergic agonist preferentially stimulated the LTCCs close to activated receptors.

To detect cAMP compartmentation in health and disease, multiple techniques have been employed that were only able to detect global concentrations of cyclic nucleotides and required plenty of tissue material [124]. However, biochemical (radio- and enzyme-linked immunoassays) or even electrophysiological approaches (patch-clamp technique), though sensitive and specific, are limited in their capability to record and analyze cyclic nucleotide gradients directly in subcellular microdomains under physiological conditions [124]. Therefore, novel live cell imaging techniques have been developed for the visualization of cyclic nucleotide signaling and its compartmentation in real time with high temporal and spatial resolution [9,124]. Such techniques are mostly based on Förster Resonance Energy Transfer (FRET) biosensors.

FRET biosensors report a non-radiative energy transfer from an excited fluorescent molecule that acts as a donor to a neighboring (located at nm distance) molecule that acts as an acceptor with subsequent fluorescence emission without the direct excitation of the acceptor [125]. Multiple FRET-based biosensors for cGMP [115,126–130] and cAMP [81], and for the activity of the downstream effector proteins such as PKA [131–136], Epac [137–141], or CNG channels [142–144], have been developed and successfully used to visualize cGMP and cAMP gradients [124,145,146]. They can be further combined with other techniques such as scanning ion conductance microscopy (SICM), which can be used to deliver receptor ligands onto defined membrane structures to targeted distinct cAMP or cGMP pools and to study receptor–microdomain interactions. SICM is a non-optical imaging technique that uses a small glass nanopipette to obtain a highly resolved morphological profile of a living cell membrane based on ion current measurement [147–150]. It can also be combined with FRET for more accurate and specific detection of microdomain alterations in health and disease [149,151,152].

5. Imaging of cGMP-to-cAMP Crosstalk via PDE2 and PDE3

Employing FRET for live cell imaging, recent studies have revealed strongly remodeled cAMP/cGMP microdomains and subcellular concentration profiles in various cardiac pathologies, leading among other mechanisms to a putatively enhanced involvement of PDE2 in cAMP/cGMP breakdown and crosstalk compared to the other cardiac PDEs.

As mentioned above, the hydrolytic activity of PDE2 can be allosterically stimulated by cGMP to limit cAMP levels, referred to as a negative cGMP-to-cAMP crosstalk. In cardiomyocytes, cGMP can be produced by either pGC after ANP, BNP, and CNP stimulation or by the NO-dependent sGC. Sources for NO include both synthesis in other cell types (e.g., by endothelial cells) and inside cardiomyocytes, e.g., by β_3-adrenoreceptor (β_3-AR) stimulated pathway, which via inhibitory G-proteins leads to NOS activation (Figure 2). PDE2 hydrolyzes cAMP (e.g., produced in response to the $\beta_{1/2}$-adrenergic agonists such as noradrenaline), but its stimulation can be in turn limited by its cGMP hydrolyzing activity, which increases in importance when cGMP concentration rises [51,89]. It has been suggested that PDE2-dependent cAMP hydrolysis might have a more critical effect on cardiomyocyte function, at least under adrenergic overdrive conditions [81,153,154].

The specific role of PDE2 in orchestrating the cyclic nucleotide compartmentation (i.e., cAMP) was supported by experimental evidence coming from a study that demonstrated that, in neonatal rat ventricular myocytes, activation of PDE2 was ineffective in counteracting the forskolin-mediated rise in intracellular cAMP levels [81]. It could also be inferred that, at least in part, stimulation of PDE2-mediated cAMP hydrolysis occurs via a β_3-AR/eNOS/sGC pathway (Figure 2). On the contrary, evidence from other studies [155–158] showed that PDE2 was effective in blocking intracellular increases of cAMP levels mediated by catecholaminergic activation of β-adrenergic receptors or forskolin-mediated AC activation under hypertrophic conditions. By inhibiting the subsequent inotropic effects, these groups were able to argue for a distinct subcellular localization and activity of PDE2 within cardiomyocytes.

More recently, Mehel and colleagues [155] were able to show that myocardial PDE2 is unregulated in human and experimental heart failure and blocks cAMP increase after acute β-AR stimulation. PDE2 upregulation may act as a counterbalance, neutralizing neurohormonal (i.e., β-adrenergic) hyperactivity typically seen in heart failure [155,159]. Furthermore, specific PDE2 inhibition has restored β-AR-mediated signal in diseased cardiomyocytes, while PDE2 overexpression has completely abolished catecholamine effects and hypertrophy without affecting basal contractility [155]. In addition, cAMP hydrolysis via PDE2 mediated the reduction of aldosterone production in adrenal cells, suggesting beneficial synergy between cardiovascular and renal systems [88]. However, for every experimental study, the limitations dictated by the in vitro acquired results might not reflect the in vivo PDE functions, and further experiments in large animal models are required to fully explore the PDE2 role in heart failure pathophysiology. Nevertheless, the overexpressed PDE2 activity may constitute a potential approach to effectively control the deleterious effects of heart failure, e.g., by augmenting its microdomain-specific actions.

On the other hand, there are also studies in which PDE2 may not necessarily exert beneficial effects, but rather contribute to hypertrophy. In cell-based experiments, another pool of cAMP/PDE2 was found to modulate hypertrophic growth of cardiac myocytes by regulating PKA-dependent phosphorylation of nuclear factors of activated T cells (NFAT) [156]. In this study, Zoccarato and colleagues [156] showed that PDE3 and PDE4 inhibition increase cAMP levels and result in hypertrophy, whereas PDE2 inhibition is antihypertrophic despite an increase in cellular cAMP content. Live cell imaging of intact cardiomyocytes revealed that PDE2 inhibition exerted its antihypertrophic effects by generating a locally confined cAMP microdomain, in which PKA type II plays a significant role by phosphorylating NFAT. These are clearly contradicting reports showing remarkable discrepancies especially in the in vivo actions of cardiac PDE2. Further experimental work is required to fully elucidate this question as well as the role of PDE2 in different subcellular cAMP microdomains. It will be especially important to develop and study a tissue-specific knockout mouse model for PDE2.

Another live cell imaging study has developed the first in vivo model expressing a cAMP biosensor targeted to SERCA2a in transgenic mouse cardiomyocytes [157]. Using FRET imaging, it was able to unveil impaired cAMP signal communication between β_1-AR located at the membrane and sarcoplasmic reticulum microdomains during early heart failure. By inhibiting PDE2, the authors demonstrated its higher contribution to the regulation of local cAMP levels under pathological conditions [157]. These data suggest that PDE2, when locally or globally upregulated, might potentially contribute to cardioprotective effects in certain microdomains.

Moreover, an elegantly-designed study by Perera et al. [158] proved experimentally for the first time that, in early compensated cardiac hypertrophy preceding heart failure, cGMP-sensitive PDE2 and PDE3 were already physically and functionally rearranged between β_1- and β_2-AR-associated cAMP microdomains despite unchanged whole cell expression levels and activities. More specifically, the switch of PDEs from PDE3 to PDE2 at the β_2-AR, accompanied by a reduction of PDE2 at the β_1-AR, led to a turnaround of cAMP cross-talk in a way that, in this pathological setting, the ANP/cGMP signaling pathway by this mechanism could enhance β-AR-mediated cardiac contractility inducing positive inotropic and chronotropic effects following β-AR stimulation (Figure 3). The provided evidence shed light on the poorly understood early microdomain remodeling mechanisms. It has been suggested that, in this way, the heart can compensate for the increased contractility demand under pressure overload [158]. However, our knowledge about microdomain-related contractility mechanisms in early disease is still in its infancy and has to be improved.

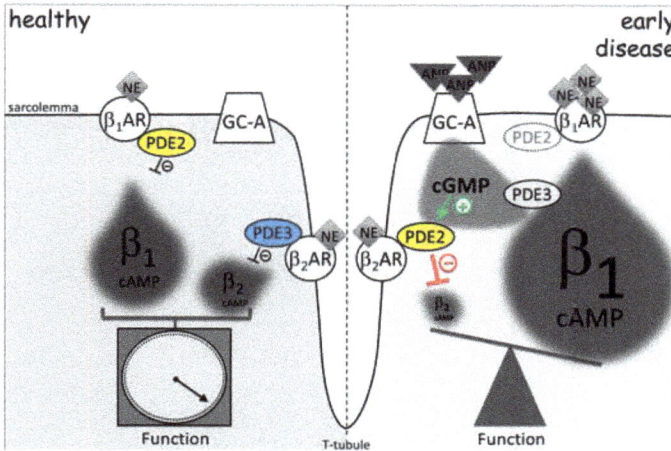

Figure 3. PDE2 and PDE3 redistribution in early cardiac hypertrophy changes cGMP-to-cAMP cross-talk. β_2-AR microdomain is normally controlled by PDE3, while PDE2 is functionally associated with β_1-AR. In disease, redistribution of PDE2 from β_1- to β_2-AR-associated membrane microdomains leads to a decrease of the local β_2-AR-cAMP and to an increase of global β_1-AR-cAMP pool under elevated ANP and cGMP levels observed in hypertrophy. This relocation of cGMP-regulated PDEs leads to a turnaround of cGMP-to-cAMP cross-talk between both β-AR microdomains. By this mechanism, elevated ANP can augment β-adrenoceptor-stimulated contractile function. NE: norepinephrine, the physiological β-AR agonist. Adapted from [158].

The ability of PDE2 to compartmentalize local pools of cAMP has been in part attributed to a much higher speed of cAMP hydrolysis by this PDE as compared to its synthesis by ACs based on FRET imaging in aldosterone producing cells [139]. The most recent finding in regard to cGMP-sensitive cyclic nucleotide compartmentation via PDE2/3 is described in a study using a cardiomyocyte-specific PDE2 transgenic mouse model [159]. In fact, it was shown that endogenous PDE2 contributes to heart rate control under physiological conditions and that PDE2 overexpression protects against arrhythmias and enhances inotropic performance after myocardial infarction [159], providing evidence in support of PDE2 overexpression and highlighting its beneficial role in diseased heart. However, the conclusions from such data obtained from a transgenic mouse model overexpressing this PDE several folds above the endogenous level should be treated with caution since excessive amounts of PDE2 might vanish the boundaries between at least some cAMP microdomains.

Trying to further elucidate the NO/cGMP or NPs/cGMP and cAMP crosstalk, which was also demonstrated in CMs, additional studies utilizing previously developed targeted FRET biosensors [160] and live cell imaging techniques uncovered that the interconnection between cGMP and cAMP in CMs is closely linked to the intracellular locus of regulation [161]. Depending on the recruited cyclase (soluble or particulate) and the associated PDE, cGMP can either augment or inhibit the cAMP levels after catecholamine stimulation and further affect downstream phosphorylation of PKA and contractility. In fact, cGMP can inhibit PDE3 as a competitive substrate for cAMP and allosterically stimulate PDE2A-mediated cAMP hydrolysis [72] locally without largely affecting global cAMP levels in the cell [161]. Induction of cGMP by catecholamine stimulation was found to differentially regulate intracellular cAMP pools that either activate

PKA-RI/PDE3- or PKA-RII/PDE2-associated compartments and provoke opposing effects on local cAMP signals [161]. Low basal cGMP levels (~10–50 nmol/L) which could be detected by FRET in adult cardiomyocytes [115] can even facilitate cGMP hydrolyzing activity of PDE3, while higher (between 200 and 500 nmol/L) cGMP levels can activate PDE2A and inhibit PDE3 towards cAMP hydrolysis [162]. Similarly, NO donors via sGC affect both the PKA-RI and PKA-RII compartments, whereas ANP via pGC limits cGMP action to the PKA-RII compartment only [161]. This evidence supports that cGMP exerts local but not global cAMP control in the cardiomyocyte in neonatal rat ventricular myocytes (NRVMs) when isoproterenol is administered in a microdomain-specific manner [161]. For instance, cGMP diminishes cAMP gradients by PDE2 activity when sGC and ANP/pGC mediate its production, while it augments cAMP gradients by inhibiting PDE3 when sGC does so. It is evident that PDE2 exerts cardioprotective regulation against excessive adrenergic stimulation by interconnecting $\beta_{1/2}$-AR/cAMP and β_3-AR/cGMP pathways [163] and paves the way for further experimental exploration.

Recently, Li and colleagues (2015) [164] showed that PDE2A overexpression blunted BNP-mediated effects by decreasing cGMP production and negatively affecting downstream effectors such as calcium current, intracellular calcium transient, and neurotransmitter release. PDE2A inhibition was also sufficient to reverse the abrogated BNP response. It was also observed that the stellate neurons of the prohypertensive rats express higher PDE2A levels as compared to the normotensive control. These data again underpin the importance of PDE2A upregulation in preventing the BNP-mediated inhibition of sympathetic transmission with subsequent maladaptive changes. Nevertheless, further experimental evidence is required to support whether the BNP-cGMP-PDE2A pathway is actually impaired in hypertensive and heart failure models.

More recently, Meier and colleagues [165] demonstrated the beneficial effect of CNP on β_1- and β_2-adrenoceptor signaling in rat hearts through cGMP-cAMP crosstalk, when PDE3 is inhibited by cGMP. The CNP-mediated interplay of the signaling pathways was unaffected both in healthy and failing hearts, while BNP was not able to regulate similar cAMP-mediated effects in any experimental group. This study analyzed mechanisms of cyclic nucleotide crosstalk, trying to explain the lack of long-term positive effects of natriuretic peptide in therapeutic schemes for heart failure.

In general, the use of family-selective PDE inhibitors and of genetic knock-down or knock-out models is another way to assess the contribution of individual PDE families in the compartmentalization of cAMP signaling pathways in cardiac myocytes [81,134,156,161,166,167]. It would be interesting to generate a tissue-specific PDE2 knock-out mouse line and explore the role of this particular phosphodiesterase in cardiovascular disease. This goal has remained unattainable due to perinatal lethality of global PDE2 knockout mice. The effect of PDE2 overexpression or upregulation e.g., by inflammation, remains to be clarified as to whether it counterbalances or further deteriorates cardiovascular disease in response to pathologic stimuli.

6. Conclusions

In conclusion, cAMP and cGMP signaling pathways as well as their crosstalk offer a high level of intracellular organization and constitute an interesting pharmacological topic in health and disease. The positive or negative cGMP-mediated regulation of cAMP response that occurs in intracellularly confined loci controlled by distinct PDE isoenzymes could potentially pave the way for novel pharmacological approaches in heart failure treatment. Despite the encouraging evidence, there is still a long way to go before we can fully decipher and understand the exact mechanisms by which these distinct molecular effectors maintain homeostasis and induce maladaptive changes in the heart.

Acknowledgments: We thank all members of our group for their support and helpful discussions. The work of our laboratory was supported by the Deutsche Forschungsgemeinschaft (grant NI 1301/3-2 to V.O.N.), the European Research Area Network on Cardiovascular Diseases (ERA-CVD), and the Gertraud und Heinz-Rose Stiftung.

Author Contributions: N.P. and V.O.N. developed the concept and drafted the manuscript.

Conflicts of Interest: The authors declare no conflict of interest.

References

1. Bers, D.M. Calcium cycling and signaling in cardiac myocytes. *Annu. Rev. Physiol.* **2008**, *70*, 23–49. [CrossRef] [PubMed]
2. Bers, D.M. Cardiac excitation-contraction coupling. *Nature* **2002**, *415*, 198–205. [CrossRef] [PubMed]
3. Defer, N.; Best-Belpomme, M.; Hanoune, J. Tissue specificity and physiological relevance of various isoforms of adenylyl cyclase. *Am. J. Physiol. Ren. Physiol.* **2000**, *279*, F400–F416. [CrossRef] [PubMed]
4. De Rooij, J.; Zwartkruis, F.J.; Verheijen, M.H.; Cool, R.H.; Nijman, S.M.; Wittinghofer, A.; Bos, J.L. Epac is a Rap1 guanine-nucleotide-exchange factor directly activated by cyclic AMP. *Nature* **1998**, *396*, 474–477. [CrossRef] [PubMed]
5. Morel, E.; Marcantoni, A.; Gastineau, M.; Birkedal, R.; Rochais, F.; Garnier, A.; Lompre, A.M.; Vandecasteele, G.; Lezoualc'h, F. cAMP-binding protein Epac induces cardiomyocyte hypertrophy. *Circ. Res.* **2005**, *97*, 1296–1304. [CrossRef] [PubMed]
6. Métrich, M.; Lucas, A.; Gastineau, M.; Samuel, J.L.; Heymes, C.; Morel, E.; Lezoualc'h, F. Epac mediates β-adrenergic receptor–induced cardiomyocyte hypertrophy. *Circ. Res.* **2008**, *102*, 959–965. [CrossRef] [PubMed]
7. Wit, A.L.; Rosen, M.R. Pathophysiologic mechanisms of cardiac arrhythmias. *Am. Heart J.* **1983**, *106*, 798–811. [CrossRef]
8. Larsson, H.P. How is the heart rate regulated in the sinoatrial node? Another piece to the puzzle. *J. Gen. Physiol.* **2010**, *88*, 96–107. [CrossRef] [PubMed]
9. Zoccarato, A.; Zaccolo, M. cAMP compartmentalisation and hypertrophy of the heart: "Good" pools of cAMP and "Bad" pools of cAMP coexist in the same cardiac myocyte. In *Microdomains in the Cardiovascular System*; Nikolaev, V.O., Zaccolo, M., Eds.; Springer Nature: Cham, Switzerland, 2017.
10. Froese, A.; Breher, S.S.; Waldeyer, C.; Schindler, R.F.; Nikolaev, V.O.; Rinné, S.; Vauti, F. Popeye domain containing proteins are essential for stress-mediated modulation of cardiac pacemaking in mice. *J. Clin. Investig.* **2012**, *122*. [CrossRef] [PubMed]
11. Schindler, R.F.R.; Brand, T. The Popeye domain containing protein family-A novel class of cAMP effectors with important functions in multiple tissues. *Prog. Biophys. Mol. Biol.* **2016**, *120*, 28–36. [CrossRef] [PubMed]
12. Furchgott, R.F.; Zawadzki, J.V. The obligatory role of endothelial cells in the relaxation of arterial smooth muscle by acetylcholine. *Nature* **1980**, *288*, 373–376. [CrossRef] [PubMed]
13. Cherry, P.D.; Furchgott, R.F.; Zawadski, J.V.; Jothianandan, D. Role of endothelial cells in relaxation of isolated arteries by bradykinin. *Proc. Natl. Acad. Sci. USA* **1982**, *79*, 2106–2110. [CrossRef] [PubMed]
14. Rapoport, R.M.; Draznin, M.B.; Murad, F. Endothelium-dependent relaxation in rat aorta may be mediated through cyclic GMP-dependent protein phosphorylation. *Nature* **1983**, *306*, 174–176. [CrossRef] [PubMed]
15. Rapoport, R.M.; Murad, F. Agonist-induced endothelium-dependent relaxation in rat thoracic aorta may be mediated through cGMP. *Circ. Res.* **1983**, *52*, 352–357. [CrossRef] [PubMed]
16. Furchgott, R.F.; Carvalho, M.H.; Khan, M.T.; Matsunaga, K. Evidence for endothelium-dependent vasodilation of resistance vessels by acetylcholine. *J. Vasc. Res.* **1987**, *24*, 145–149. [CrossRef]
17. Ignarro, L.J.; Buga, G.M.; Wood, K.S.; Byrns, R.E.; Chaudhuri, G. Endothelium-derived relaxing factor produced and released from artery and vein is nitric oxide. *Proc. Natl. Acad. Sci. USA* **1987**, *84*, 9265–9269. [CrossRef] [PubMed]
18. Ignarro, L.J.; Byrns, R.E.; Buga, G.M.; Wood, K.S. Endothelium-derived relaxing factor from pulmonary artery and vein possesses pharmacologic and chemical properties identical to those of nitric oxide radical. *Circ. Res.* **1987**, *61*, 866–879. [CrossRef] [PubMed]
19. Alderton, W.K.; Cooper, C.E.; Knowles, R.G. Nitric oxide synthases: Structure, function and inhibition. *Biochem. J.* **2001**, *357*, 593–615. [CrossRef] [PubMed]
20. Koide, M.; Kawahara, Y.; Nakayama, I.; Tsuda, T.; Yokoyama, M. Cyclic AMP-elevating agents induce an inducible type of nitric oxide synthase in cultured vascular smooth muscle cells. Synergism with the induction elicited by inflammatory cytokines. *J. Biol. Chem.* **1993**, *268*, 24959–24966. [PubMed]

21. Balligand, J.L.; Kobzik, L.; Han, X.; Kaye, D.M.; Belhassen, L.; O'Hara, D.S.; Kelly, R.A.; Smith, T.W.; Michel, T. Nitric oxide-dependent parasympathetic signaling is due to activation of constitutive endothelial (type III) nitric oxide synthase in cardiac myocytes. *J. Biol. Chem.* **1995**, *270*, 14582–14586. [CrossRef] [PubMed]

22. Kurihara, N.; Alfie, M.E.; Sigmon, D.H.; Rhaleb, N.E.; Shesely, E.G.; Carretero, O.A. Role of nNOS in blood pressure regulation in eNOS null mutant mice. *Hypertension* **1998**, *32*, 856–861. [CrossRef] [PubMed]

23. Gyurko, R.; Kuhlencordt, P.; Fishman, M.C.; Huang, P.L. Modulation of mouse cardiac function in vivo by eNOS and ANP. *Am. J. Physiol. Heart Circ. Physiol.* **2000**, *278*, H971–H981. [CrossRef] [PubMed]

24. MacNaul, K.L.; Hutchinson, N.I. Differential expression of iNOS and cNOS mRNA in human vascular smooth muscle cells and endothelial cells under normal and inflammatory conditions. *Biochem. Biophys. Res. Commun.* **1993**, *196*, 1330–1334. [CrossRef] [PubMed]

25. Tsai, E.J.; Kass, D.A. Cyclic GMP signaling in cardiovascular pathophysiology and therapeutics. *Pharmacol. Ther.* **2009**, *122*, 216–238. [CrossRef] [PubMed]

26. Yuen, P.S.; Potter, L.R.; Garbers, D.L. A new form of guanylyl cyclase is preferentially expressed in rat kidney. *Biochemistry* **1990**, *29*, 10872–10878. [CrossRef] [PubMed]

27. Harteneck, C.; Wedel, B.; Koesling, D.; Bo, E. Molecular cloning and expression of a new α-subunit of soluble guanylyl cyclase. Interchangeability of the α-subunits of the enzyme. *FEBS Lett.* **1991**, *292*, 217–222. [PubMed]

28. Behrends, S.; Harteneck, C.; Schultz, G.; Koesling, D. A variant of the α2 subunit of soluble guanylyl cyclase contains an insert homologous to a region within adenylyl cyclases and functions as a dominant negative protein. *J. Biol. Chem.* **1995**, *270*, 21109–21113. [CrossRef] [PubMed]

29. Lee, D.I.; Kass, D.A. Phosphodiesterases and cyclic GMP regulation in heart muscle. *Physiology* **2012**, *27*, 248–258. [CrossRef] [PubMed]

30. Zhao, C.Y.; Greenstein, J.L.; Winslow, R.L. Interaction between phosphodiesterases in the regulation of the cardiac β-adrenergic pathway. *J. Mol. Cell. Cardiol.* **2015**, *88*, 29–38. [CrossRef] [PubMed]

31. Zhao, C.Y.; Greenstein, J.L.; Winslow, R.L. Roles of phosphodiesterases in the regulation of the cardiac cyclic nucleotide cross-talk signaling network. *J. Mol. Cell. Cardiol.* **2016**, *91*, 215–227. [CrossRef] [PubMed]

32. D'souza, S.P.; Davis, M.; Baxter, G.F. Autocrine and paracrine actions of natriuretic peptides in the heart. *Pharmacol. Ther.* **2004**, *101*, 113–129. [CrossRef] [PubMed]

33. De Bold, A.J.; Ma, K.K.Y.; Zhang, Y.; de Bold, M.L.K.; Bensimon, M.; Khoshbaten, A. The physiological and pathophysiological modulation of the endocrine function of the heart. *Can. J. Physiol. Pharmacol.* **2001**, *79*, 705–714. [CrossRef] [PubMed]

34. Kuhn, M. Molecular physiology of membrane guanylyl cyclase receptors. *Physiol. Rev.* **2016**, *96*, 751–804. [CrossRef] [PubMed]

35. Kambayashi, Y.; Nakao, K.; Mukoyama, M.; Saito, Y.; Ogawa, Y.; Shiono, S.; Inouye, K.; Yoshida, N.; Imura, H. Isolation and sequence determination of human brain natriuretic peptide in human atrium. *FEBS Lett.* **1990**, *259*, 341–345. [CrossRef]

36. Mukoyama, M.; Nakao, K.; Saito, Y.; Ogawa, Y.; Hosoda, K.; Suga, S.I.; Shirakami, G.; Jougasaki, M.; Imura, H. Human brain natriuretic peptide, a novel cardiac hormone. *Lancet* **1990**, *335*, 801–802. [CrossRef]

37. Nakao, K.; Itoh, H.; Kambayashi, Y.; Hosoda, K.; Saito, Y.; Yamada, T.; Mukoyama, M.; Arai, H.; Shirakami, G.; Suga, S.I. Rat brain natriuretic peptide. Isolation from rat heart and tissue distribution. *Hypertension* **1990**, *15*, 774–778. [CrossRef] [PubMed]

38. Doyle, D.D.; Upshaw-Earley, J.; Bell, E.L.; Palfrey, H.C. Natriuretic peptide receptor-B in adult rat ventricle is predominantly confined to the nonmyocyte population. *Am. J. Physiol. Heart Circ. Physiol.* **2002**, *282*, H2117–H2123. [CrossRef] [PubMed]

39. Buttgereit, J.; Shanks, J.; Li, D.; Hao, G.; Athwal, A.; Langenickel, T.H.; Wright, H.; da Costa Goncalves, A.C.; Monti, J.; Plehm, R.; et al. C-type natriuretic peptide and natriuretic peptide receptor B signalling inhibits cardiac sympathetic neurotransmission and autonomic function. *Cardiovasc. Res.* **2016**, *112*, 637–644. [CrossRef] [PubMed]

40. Hutchinson, H.G.; Trindade, P.T.; Cunanan, D.B.; Wu, C.F.; Pratt, R.E. Mechanisms of natriuretic-peptide-induced growth inhibition of vascular smooth muscle cells. *Cardiovasc. Res.* **1997**, *35*, 158–167. [CrossRef]

41. Rosenkranz, A.C.; Woods, R.L.; Dusting, G.J.; Ritchie, R.H. Antihypertrophic actions of the natriuretic peptides in adult rat cardiomyocytes: Importance of cyclic GMP. *Cardiovasc. Res.* **2003**, *57*, 515–522. [CrossRef]

42. Tokudome, T.; Horio, T.; Soeki, T.; Mori, K.; Kishimoto, I.; Suga, S.I.; Yoshihara, F.; Kawano, Y.; Kohno, M.; Kangawa, K. Inhibitory effect of C-type natriuretic peptide (CNP) on cultured cardiac myocyte hypertrophy: Interference between CNP and endothelin-1 signaling pathways. *Endocrinology* **2004**, *145*, 2131–2140. [CrossRef] [PubMed]

43. Seifert, R. cCMP and cUMP: Emerging second messengers. *Trends Biochem. Sci.* **2015**, *40*, 8–15. [CrossRef] [PubMed]

44. Seifert, R.; Schneider, E.H.; Bähre, H. From canonical to non-canonical cyclic nucleotides as second messengers: Pharmacological implications. *Pharmacol. Ther.* **2015**, *148*, 154–184. [CrossRef] [PubMed]

45. Zaccolo, M. Spatial control of cAMP signalling in health and disease. *Curr. Opin. Pharmacol.* **2011**, *11*, 649–655. [CrossRef] [PubMed]

46. Saucerman, J.J.; Greenwald, E.C.; Polanowska-Grabowska, R. Mechanisms of cyclic AMP compartmentation revealed by computational models. *J. Gen. Physiol.* **2014**, *143*, 39–48. [CrossRef] [PubMed]

47. Mika, D.; Leroy, J.; Vandecasteele, G.; Fischmeister, R. PDEs create local domains of cAMP signaling. *J. Mol. Cell. Cardiol.* **2012**, *52*, 323–329. [CrossRef] [PubMed]

48. Ziolo, M.T.; Kohr, M.J.; Wang, H. Nitric oxide signaling and the regulation of myocardial function. *J. Mol. Cell. Cardiol.* **2008**, *45*, 625–632. [CrossRef] [PubMed]

49. Fischmeister, R.; Castro, L.R.; Abi-Gerges, A.; Rochais, F.; Jurevičius, J.; Leroy, J.; Vandecasteele, G. Compartmentation of cyclic nucleotide signaling in the heart. *Circ. Res.* **2006**, *99*, 816–828. [CrossRef] [PubMed]

50. Vandecasteele, G.; Rochais, F.; Abi-Gerges, A.; Fischmeister, R. Functional localization of cAMP signalling in cardiac myocytes. *Biochem. Soc. Trans.* **2006**, *34*, 484–488. [CrossRef] [PubMed]

51. Bender, A.T.; Beavo, J.A. Cyclic nucleotide phosphodiesterases: Molecular regulation to clinical use. *Pharmacol. Rev.* **2006**, *58*, 488–520. [CrossRef] [PubMed]

52. Francis, S.H.; Blount, M.A.; Corbin, J.D. Mammalian cyclic nucleotide phosphodiesterases: Molecular mechanisms and physiological functions. *Physiol. Rev.* **2011**, *91*, 651–690. [CrossRef] [PubMed]

53. Keravis, T.; Lugnier, C. Cyclic nucleotide phosphodiesterase (PDE) isozymes as targets of the intracellular signalling network: Benefits of PDE inhibitors in various diseases and perspectives for future therapeutic developments. *Br. J. Pharmacol.* **2012**, *165*, 1288–1305. [CrossRef] [PubMed]

54. Balijepalli, R.C.; Foell, J.D.; Hall, D.D.; Hell, J.W.; Kamp, T.J. Localization of cardiac L-type Ca^{2+} channels to a caveolar macromolecular signaling complex is required for β2-adrenergic regulation. *Proc. Natl. Acad. Sci. USA* **2006**, *103*, 7500–7505. [CrossRef] [PubMed]

55. Pani, B.; Singh, B.B. Lipid rafts/caveolae as microdomains of calcium signalling. *Cell Calcium* **2009**, *45*, 625–633. [CrossRef] [PubMed]

56. Kamp, T.J.; Hell, J.W. Regulation of cardiac L-type calcium channels by protein kinase A and protein kinase C. *Circ. Res.* **2000**, *87*, 1095–1102. [CrossRef] [PubMed]

57. Agarwal, S.R.; Ostrom, R.S.; Harvey, R.D. Membrane Microdomains and cAMP Compartmentation in Cardiac Myocytes. In *Microdomains in the Cardiovascular System*; Nikolaev, V.O., Zaccolo, M., Eds.; Springer: Cham, Switzerland, 2017; pp. 17–35.

58. Guellich, A.; Mehel, H.; Fischmeister, R. Cyclic AMP synthesis and hydrolysis in the normal and failing heart. *Pflügers Arch.* **2014**, *466*, 1163–1175. [CrossRef] [PubMed]

59. Timofeyev, V.; Myers, R.E.; Kim, H.J.; Woltz, R.L.; Sirish, P.; Heiserman, J.P.; Li, N.; Singapuri, A.; Tang, T.; Yarov-Yarovoy, V.; et al. Adenylyl cyclase subtype-specific compartmentalization: Differential regulation of L-type Ca^{2+} current in ventricular myocytes. *Circ. Res.* **2013**, *112*, 1567–1576. [CrossRef] [PubMed]

60. Redden, J.M.; Dodge-Kafka, K.L.; Kapiloff, M.S. Function to Failure: Compartmentalization of Cardiomyocyte Signaling by A-Kinase-Anchoring Proteins. In *Microdomains in the Cardiovascular System*; Nikolaev, V.O., Zaccolo, M., Eds.; Springer: Cham, Switzerland, 2017; pp. 37–57.

61. Schrade, K.; Klussmann, E. Pharmacological approaches for delineating functions of AKAP-based signalling complexes and finding therapeutic targets. In *Microdomains in the Cardiovascular System*; Nikolaev, V.O., Zaccolo, M., Eds.; Springer: Cham, Switzerland, 2017; pp. 59–83.

62. Ghigo, A.; Pirozzi, F.; Li, M.; Hirsch, E. Chatting Second Messengers: PIP3 and cAMP. In *Microdomains in the Cardiovascular System*; Nikolaev, V.O., Zaccolo, M., Eds.; Springer: Cham, Switzerland, 2017; pp. 85–95.

63. Dodge-Kafka, K.L.; Langeberg, L.; Scott, J.D. Compartmentation of cyclic nucleotide signaling in the heart: The role of A-kinase anchoring proteins. *Circ. Res.* **2006**, *98*, 993–1001. [CrossRef] [PubMed]

64. Maurice, D.H.; Ke, H.; Ahmad, F.; Wang, Y.; Chung, J.; Manganiello, V.C. Advances in targeting cyclic nucleotide phosphodiesterases. *Nat. Rev. Drug Discov.* **2014**, *13*, 290–314. [CrossRef] [PubMed]
65. Balijepalli, R.C.; Kamp, T.J. Caveolae, ion channels and cardiac arrhythmias. *Prog. Biophys. Mol. Biol.* **2008**, *98*, 149–160. [CrossRef] [PubMed]
66. Carnegie, G.K.; Means, C.K.; Scott, J.D. A-kinase anchoring proteins: From protein complexes to physiology and disease. *IUBMB Life* **2009**, *61*, 394–406. [CrossRef] [PubMed]
67. Nichols, C.B.; Rossow, C.F.; Navedo, M.F.; Westenbroek, R.E.; Catterall, W.A.; Santana, L.F.; McKnight, G.S. Sympathetic stimulation of adult cardiomyocytes requires association of akap5 with a subpopulation of l-type calcium channels novelty and significance. *Circ. Res.* **2010**, *107*, 747–756. [CrossRef] [PubMed]
68. Cheepala, S.; Hulot, J.S.; Morgan, J.A.; Sassi, Y.; Zhang, W.; Naren, A.P.; Schuetz, J.D. Cyclic nucleotide compartmentalization: Contributions of phosphodiesterases and ATP-binding cassette transporters. *Annu. Rev. Pharmacol. Toxicol.* **2013**, *53*, 231–253. [CrossRef] [PubMed]
69. Sassi, Y.; Abi-Gerges, A.; Fauconnier, J.; Mougenot, N.; Reiken, S.; Haghighi, K.; Kranias, E.G.; Marks, A.R.; Lacampagne, A.; Engelhardt, S.; et al. Regulation of cAMP homeostasis by the efflux protein MRP4 in cardiac myocytes. *FASEB J.* **2012**, *26*, 1009–1017. [CrossRef] [PubMed]
70. Houslay, M.D. Underpinning compartmentalised cAMP signalling through targeted cAMP breakdown. *Trends Biochem. Sci.* **2010**, *35*, 91–100. [CrossRef] [PubMed]
71. Conti, M.; Mika, D.; Richter, W. Cyclic AMP compartments and signaling specificity: Role of cyclic nucleotide phosphodiesterases. *J. Gen. Physiol.* **2014**, *143*, 29–38. [CrossRef] [PubMed]
72. Zaccolo, M.; Movsesian, M.A. cAMP and cGMP signaling cross-talk: Role of phosphodiesterases and implications for cardiac pathophysiology. *Circ. Res.* **2007**, *100*, 1569–1578. [CrossRef] [PubMed]
73. Lee, D.I.; Zhu, G.; Sasaki, T.; Cho, G.S.; Hamdani, N.; Holewinski, R.; Jo, S.H.; Danner, T.; Zhang, M.; Rainer, P.P.; et al. Phosphodiesterase 9A controls nitric-oxide-independent cGMP and hypertrophic heart disease. *Nature* **2015**, *519*, 472–476. [CrossRef] [PubMed]
74. Zhang, M.; Kass, D.A. Phosphodiesterases and cardiac cGMP: Evolving roles and controversies. *Trends Pharmacol. Sci.* **2011**, *32*, 360–365. [CrossRef] [PubMed]
75. Brescia, M.; Zaccolo, M. Modulation of compartmentalised cyclic nucleotide signalling via local inhibition of phosphodiesterase activity. *Int. J. Mol. Sci.* **2016**, *17*. [CrossRef] [PubMed]
76. Ahmad, F.; Muratal, T.; Shimizul, K.; Degerma, E.; Maurice, D.; Manganiello, V. Cyclic nucleotide phosphodiesterases: Important signaling modulators and therapeutic targets. *Oral Dis.* **2015**, *21*, e25–e50. [CrossRef] [PubMed]
77. Zhao, C.Y. Computational modeling of cyclic nucleotide signaling mechanisms in cardiac myocytes. In *Microdomains in the Cardiovascular System*; Nikolaev, V.O., Zaccolo, M., Eds.; Springer Nature: Cham, Switzerland, 2017; pp. 175–213.
78. Conti, M.; Beavo, J. Biochemistry and physiology of cyclic nucleotide phosphodiesterases: Essential components in cyclic nucleotide signaling. *Annu. Rev. Biochem.* **2007**, *76*, 481–511. [CrossRef] [PubMed]
79. Wood, E.R.; Bledsoe, R.; Chai, J.; Daka, P.; Deng, H.; Ding, Y.; Harris-Gurley, S.; Kryn, L.H.; Nartey, E.; Nichols, J.; et al. The role of phosphodiesterase 12 (PDE12) as a negative regulator of the innate immune response and the discovery of antiviral inhibitors. *J. Biol. Chem.* **2015**, *290*, 19681–19696. [CrossRef] [PubMed]
80. Vandeput, F.; Wolda, S.L.; Krall, J.; Hambleton, R.; Uher, L.; McCaw, K.N.; Radwanski, P.B.; Florio, V.; Movsesian, M.A. Cyclic nucleotide phosphodiesterase PDE1C1 in human cardiac myocytes. *J. Biol. Chem.* **2007**, *282*, 32749–32757. [CrossRef] [PubMed]
81. Mongillo, M.; Tocchetti, C.G.; Terrin, A.; Lissandron, V.; Cheung, Y.F.; Dostmann, W.R.; Pozzan, T.; Kass, D.A.; Paolocci, N.; Houslay, M.D.; et al. Compartmentalized phosphodiesterase-2 activity blunts beta-adrenergic cardiac inotropy via an NO/cGMP-dependent pathway. *Circ. Res.* **2006**, *98*, 226–234. [CrossRef] [PubMed]
82. Richter, W.; Xie, M.; Scheitrum, C.; Krall, J.; Movsesian, M.A.; Conti, M. Conserved expression and functions of PDE4 in rodent and human heart. *Basic Res. Cardiol.* **2011**, *106*, 249–262. [CrossRef] [PubMed]
83. Gamanuma, M.; Yuasa, K.; Sasaki, T.; Sakurai, N.; Kotera, J.; Omori, K. Comparison of enzymatic characterization and gene organization of cyclic nucleotide phosphodiesterase 8 family in humans. *Cell Signal. Technol.* **2003**, *15*, 565–574. [CrossRef]
84. Houslay, M.D.; Baillie, G.S.; Maurice, D.H. cAMP-Specific phosphodiesterase-4 enzymes in the cardiovascular system: A molecular toolbox for generating compartmentalized cAMP signaling. *Circ. Res.* **2007**, *100*, 950–966. [CrossRef] [PubMed]

85. Martins, T.J.; Mumby, M.C.; Beavo, J.A. Purification and characterization of a cyclic GMP-stimulated cyclic nucleotide phosphodiesterase from bovine tissues. *J. Biol. Chem.* **1982**, *257*, 1973–1979. [PubMed]

86. Mumby, M.C.; Martins, T.J.; Chang, M.L.; Beavo, J.A. Identification of cGMP-stimulated cyclic nucleotide phosphodiesterase in lung tissue with monoclonal antibodies. *J. Biol. Chem.* **1982**, *257*, 13283–13290. [PubMed]

87. Martinez, S.E.; Wu, A.Y.; Glavas, N.A.; Tang, X.B.; Turley, S.; Hol, W.G.; Beavo, J.A. The two GAF domains in phosphodiesterase 2A have distinct roles in dimerization and in cGMP binding. *Proc. Natl. Acad. Sci. USA* **2002**, *99*, 13260–13265. [CrossRef] [PubMed]

88. Rosman, G.J.; Martins, T.J.; Sonnenburg, W.K.; Beavo, J.A.; Ferguson, K.; Loughney, K. Isolation and characterization of human cDNAs encoding a cGMP-stimulated 3′, 5′-cyclic nucleotide phosphodiesterase. *Gene* **1997**, *191*, 89–95. [CrossRef]

89. Lugnier, C. Cyclic nucleotide phosphodiesterase (PDE) superfamily: A new target for the development of specific therapeutic agents. *Pharmacol. Ther.* **2006**, *109*, 366–398. [CrossRef] [PubMed]

90. Yang, Q.; Paskind, M.; Bolger, G.; Thompson, W.J.; Repaske, D.R.; Cutler, L.S.; Epstein, P.M. A novel cyclic GMP stimulated phosphodiesterase from rat brain. *Biochem. Biophys. Res. Commun.* **1994**, *205*, 1850–1858. [CrossRef] [PubMed]

91. Yamamoto, T.; Manganiello, V.C.; Vaughan, M. Purification and characterization of cyclic GMP-stimulated cyclic nucleotide phosphodiesterase from calf liver. Effects of divalent cations on activity. *J. Biol. Chem.* **1983**, *258*, 12526–12533. [PubMed]

92. Bender, A.T.; Beavo, J.A. Specific localized expression of cGMP PDEs in Purkinje neurons and macrophages. *Neurochem. Int.* **2004**, *45*, 853–857. [CrossRef] [PubMed]

93. Juilfs, D.M.; Soderling, S.; Burns, F.; Beavo, J.A. Cyclic GMP as substrate and regulator of cyclic nucleotide phosphodiesterases (PDEs). In *Reviews of Physiology, Biochemistry and Pharmacology*; Springer: Berlin/Heidelberg, Germany, 1999.

94. Dickinson, N.T.; Haslam, R.J. Activation of cGMP-stimulated phosphodiesterase by nitroprusside limits cAMP accumulation in human platelets: Effects on platelet aggregation. *Biochem. J.* **1997**, *323*, 371–377. [CrossRef] [PubMed]

95. MacFarland, R.T.; Zelus, B.D.; Beavo, J.A. High concentrations of a cGMP-stimulated phosphodiesterase mediate ANP-induced decreases in cAMP and steroidogenesis in adrenal glomerulosa cells. *J. Biol. Chem.* **1991**, *266*, 136–142. [PubMed]

96. Simmons, M.A.; Hartzell, H.C. Role of phosphodiesterase in regulation of calcium current in isolated cardiac myocytes. *Mol. Pharmacol.* **1988**, *33*, 664–671. [PubMed]

97. Acin-Perez, R.; Gatti, D.L.; Bai, Y.; Manfredi, G. Protein phosphorylation and prevention of cytochrome oxidase inhibition by ATP: Coupled mechanisms of energy metabolism regulation. *Cell Metab.* **2011**, *13*, 712–719. [CrossRef] [PubMed]

98. Castro, L.R.; Verde, I.; Cooper, D.M.; Fischmeister, R. Cyclic guanosine monophosphate compartmentation in rat cardiac myocytes. *Circulation* **2006**, *113*, 2221–2228. [CrossRef] [PubMed]

99. Weber, S.; Zeller, M.; Guan, K.; Wunder, F.; Wagner, M.; El-Armouche, A. PDE2 at the crossway between cAMP and cGMP signalling in the heart. *Cell Signal.* **2017**, *38*, 76–84. [CrossRef] [PubMed]

100. Shakur, Y.; Holst, L.S.; Landstrom, T.R.; Movsesian, M.; Degerman, E.; Manganiello, V. Regulation and function of the cyclic nucleotide phosphodiesterase (PDE3) gene family. *Prog. Nucleic Acid Res. Mol. Biol.* **2001**, *66*, 241–277. [PubMed]

101. Degerman, E.; Belfrage, P.; Manganiello, V.C. Structure, localization, and regulation of cGMP-inhibited phosphodiesterase (PDE3). *J. Biol. Chem.* **1997**, *272*, 6823–6826. [CrossRef] [PubMed]

102. Beca, S.; Ahmad, F.; Shen, W.; Liu, J.; Makary, S.; Polidovitch, N.; Sun, J.; Hockman, S.; Chung, Y.W.; Movsenian, M.; et al. Phosphodiesterase type 3A regulates basal myocardial contractility through interacting with sarcoplasmic reticulum calcium ATPase type 2a signaling complexes in mouse heart novelty and significance. *Circ. Res.* **2013**, *112*, 289–297. [CrossRef] [PubMed]

103. McMurray, J.J.; Adamopoulos, S.; Anker, S.D.; Auricchio, A.; Böhm, M.; Dickstein, K.; Jaarsma, T. ESC Guidelines for the diagnosis and treatment of acute and chronic heart failure 2012. *Eur. J. Heart Fail.* **2012**, *14*, 803–869. [CrossRef] [PubMed]

104. Landry, Y.; Gies, J.P. Drugs and their molecular targets: An updated overview. *Fundam. Clin. Pharmacol.* **2008**, *22*, 1–18. [CrossRef] [PubMed]

105. Packer, M.; Carver, J.R.; Rodeheffer, R.J.; Ivanhoe, R.J.; DiBianco, R.; Zeldis, S.M.; Mallis, G.I. Effect of oral milrinone on mortality in severe chronic heart failure. *N. Engl. J. Med.* **1991**, *325*, 1468–1475. [CrossRef] [PubMed]

106. Choi, Y.H.; Park, S.; Hockman, S.; Zmuda-Trzebiatowska, E.; Svennelid, F.; Haluzik, M.; Gavrilova, O.; Ahmad, F.; Pepin, L.; Napolitano, M.; et al. Alterations in regulation of energy homeostasis in cyclic nucleotide phosphodiesterase 3B–null mice. *J. Clin. Investig.* **2006**, *116*, 3240–3251. [CrossRef] [PubMed]

107. Degerman, E.; Ahmad, F.; Chung, Y.W.; Guirguis, E.; Omar, B.; Stenson, L.; Manganiello, V. From PDE3B to the regulation of energy homeostasis. *Curr. Opin. Pharmacol.* **2011**, *11*, 676–682. [CrossRef] [PubMed]

108. Chung, Y.W.; Lagranha, C.; Chen, Y.; Sun, J.; Tong, G.; Hockman, S.C.; Ahmad, F.; Esfahani, S.G.; Bae, D.H.; Polidovitch, N.; et al. Targeted disruption of PDE3B, but not PDE3A, protects murine heart from ischemia/reperfusion injury. *Proc. Natl. Acad. Sci. USA* **2015**, *112*, E2253–E2262. [CrossRef] [PubMed]

109. Sun, B.; Li, H.; Shakur, Y.; Hensley, J.; Hockman, S.; Kambayashi, J.; Manganiello, V.M.; Liu, Y. Role of phosphodiesterase type 3A and 3B in regulating platelet and cardiac function using subtype-selective knockout mice. *Cell Signal.* **2007**, *19*, 1765–1771. [CrossRef] [PubMed]

110. Ding, B.; Abe, J.I.; Wei, H.; Xu, H.; Che, W.; Aizawa, T.; Liu, W.; Molina, C.A.; Sadoshima, J.; Blaxall, B.C.; et al. A positive feedback loop of phosphodiesterase 3 (PDE3) and inducible cAMP early repressor (ICER) leads to cardiomyocyte apoptosis. *Proc. Natl. Acad. Sci. USA* **2005**, *102*, 14771–14776. [CrossRef] [PubMed]

111. Oikawa, M.; Wu, M.; Lim, S.; Knight, W.E.; Miller, C.L.; Cai, Y.; Lu, C.; Blaxall, B.C.; Takeishi, Y.; Abe, J.I.; et al. Cyclic nucleotide phosphodiesterase 3A1 protects the heart against ischemia-reperfusion injury. *J. Mol. Cell. Cardiol.* **2013**, *64*, 11–19. [CrossRef] [PubMed]

112. Patrucco, E.; Notte, A.; Barberis, L.; Selvetella, G.; Maffei, A.; Brancaccio, M.; Marengo, S.; Russo, G.; Azzolino, O.; Rybalkin, S.D.; et al. PI3Kgamma modulates the cardiac response to chronic pressure overload by distinct kinase-dependent and -independent effects. *Cell* **2004**, *118*, 375–387. [CrossRef] [PubMed]

113. Perino, A.; Ghigo, A.; Ferrero, E.; Morello, F.; Santulli, G.; Baillie, G.S.; Damilano, F.; Dunlop, A.J.; Pawson, C.; Walser, R.; et al. Integrating cardiac PIP 3 and cAMP signaling through a PKA anchoring function of p110γ. *Mol. Cell* **2011**, *42*, 84–95. [CrossRef] [PubMed]

114. Ghigo, A.; Perino, A.; Mehel, H.; Zahradníková, A.; Morello, F.; Leroy, J.; Nikolaev, V.O.; Damilano, F.; Cimino, J.; De Luca, E.; et al. Phosphoinositide 3-kinase γ protects against catecholamine-induced ventricular arrhythmia through protein kinase a–mediated regulation of distinct phosphodiesterases. *Circulation* **2012**, *126*, 2073–2083. [CrossRef] [PubMed]

115. Götz, K.R.; Sprenger, J.U.; Perera, R.K.; Steinbrecher, J.H.; Lehnart, S.E.; Kuhn, M.; Gorelik, J.; Balligand, J.L.; Nikolaev, V.O. Transgenic mice for real-time visualization of cGMP in intact adult cardiomyocytes. *Circ. Res.* **2014**, *114*, 1235–1245. [CrossRef] [PubMed]

116. Wen, J.F.; Cui, X.; Jin, J.Y.; Kim, S.M.; Kim, S.Z.; Kim, S.H.; Kim, S.H.; Lee, H.S.; Cho, K.W. High and low gain switches for regulation of camp efflux concentration. *Circ. Res.* **2004**, *94*, 936–943. [CrossRef] [PubMed]

117. Hayes, J.S.; Brunton, L.L. Functional compartments in cyclic nucleotide action. *J. Cycl. Nucleotide Res.* **1982**, *8*, 1–16.

118. Corbin, J.D.; Sugden, P.H.; Lincoln, T.M.; Keely, S.L. Compartmentalization of adenosine 3′: 5′-monophosphate and adenosine 3′: 5′-monophosphate-dependent protein kinase in heart tissue. *J. Biol. Chem.* **1977**, *252*, 3854–3861. [PubMed]

119. Hayes, J.S.; Brunton, L.L.; Brown, J.H.; Reese, J.B.; Mayer, S.E. Hormonally specific expression of cardiac protein kinase activity. *Proc. Natl. Acad. Sci. USA* **1979**, *76*, 1570–1574. [CrossRef] [PubMed]

120. Hayes, J.S.; Brunton, L.L.; Mayer, S.E. Selective activation of particulate cAMP-dependent protein kinase by isoproterenol and prostaglandin E1. *J. Biol. Chem.* **1980**, *255*, 5113–5119. [PubMed]

121. Keely, S.L. Activation of cAMP-dependent protein kinase without a corresponding increase in phosphorylase activity. *Res. Commun. Chem. Pathol. Pharmacol.* **1977**, *18*, 283–290. [PubMed]

122. Buxton, I.L.; Brunton, L.L. Compartments of cyclic AMP and protein kinase in mammalian cardiomyocytes. *J. Biol. Chem.* **1983**, *258*, 10233–10239. [PubMed]

123. Jurevicius, J.; Fischmeister, R. cAMP compartmentation is responsible for a local activation of cardiac Ca^{2+} channels by beta-adrenergic agonists. *Proc. Natl. Acad. Sci. USA* **1996**, *93*, 295–299. [CrossRef] [PubMed]

124. Sprenger, J.U.; Nikolaev, V.O. Biophysical techniques for detection of cAMP and cGMP in Living Cells. *Int. J. Mol. Sci.* **2013**, *14*, 8025–8046. [CrossRef] [PubMed]

125. Förster, T. Zwischenmolekulare energiewanderung und fluoreszenz. *Ann. Phys.* **1948**, *437*, 55–75. [CrossRef]

126. Nikolaev, V.O.; Lohse, M.J. Novel techniques for real-time monitoring of cGMP in living cells. *Handb. Exp. Pharmacol.* **2009**, *191*, 229–243.

127. Honda, A.; Adams, S.R.; Sawyer, C.L.; Lev-Ram, V.; Tsien, R.Y.; Dostmann, W.R. Spatiotemporal dynamics of guanosine 3′, 5′-cyclic monophosphate revealed by a genetically encoded, fluorescent indicator. *Proc. Natl. Acad. Sci. USA* **2001**, *98*, 2437–2442. [CrossRef] [PubMed]

128. Sato, M.; Hida, N.; Ozawa, T.; Umezawa, Y. Fluorescent indicators for cyclic GMP based on cyclic GMP-dependent protein kinase I alpha and green fluorescent proteins. *Anal. Chem.* **2000**, *72*, 5918–5924. [CrossRef] [PubMed]

129. Nikolaev, V.O.; Gambaryan, S.; Lohse, M.J. Fluorescent sensors for rapid monitoring of intracellular cGMP. *Nat. Methods* **2006**, *3*, 23–25. [CrossRef] [PubMed]

130. Niino, Y.; Hotta, K.; Oka, K. Simultaneous live cell imaging using dual FRET sensors with a single excitation light. *PLoS ONE* **2009**, *4*. [CrossRef] [PubMed]

131. Adams, S.R.; Harootunian, A.T.; Buechler, Y.J.; Taylor, S.S.; Tsien, R.Y. Fluorescence ratio imaging of cyclic AMP in single cells. *Nature* **1991**, *349*, 694–697. [CrossRef] [PubMed]

132. Bacskai, B.J.; Hochner, B.; Mahaut-Smith, M.; Adams, S.R.; Kaang, B.K.; Kandel, E.R.; Tsien, R.Y. Spatially resolved dynamics of cAMP and protein kinase A subunits in Aplysia sensory neurons. *Science* **1993**, *260*, 222–226. [CrossRef] [PubMed]

133. Zaccolo, M.; De Giorgi, F.; Cho, C.Y.; Feng, L.; Knapp, T.; Negulescu, P.A.; Taylor, S.S.; Tsien, R.Y.; Pozzan, T. A genetically encoded, fluorescent indicator for cyclic AMP in living cells. *Nat. Cell. Biol.* **2000**, *2*, 25–29. [CrossRef] [PubMed]

134. Zaccolo, M.; Pozzan, T. Discrete microdomains with high concentration of cAMP in stimulated rat neonatal cardiac myocytes. *Science* **2002**, *295*, 1711–1715. [CrossRef] [PubMed]

135. Lehnart, S.E.; Wehrens, X.H.; Reiken, S.; Warrier, S.; Belevych, A.E.; Harvey, R.D.; Richter, W.; Jin, S.L.; Conti, M.; Marks, A.R. Phosphodiesterase 4D deficiency in the ryanodine-receptor complex promotes heart failure and arrhythmias. *Cell* **2005**, *123*, 25–35. [CrossRef] [PubMed]

136. Nikolaev, V.O.; Bünemann, M.; Hein, L.; Hannawacker, A.; Lohse, M.J. Novel single chain cAMP sensors for receptor-induced signal propagation. *J. Biol. Chem.* **2004**, *279*, 37215–37218. [CrossRef] [PubMed]

137. DiPilato, L.M.; Cheng, X.; Zhang, J. Fluorescent indicators of cAMP and Epac activation reveal differential dynamics of cAMP signaling within discrete subcellular compartments. *Proc. Natl. Acad. Sci. USA* **2004**, *101*, 16513–16518. [CrossRef] [PubMed]

138. Ponsioen, B.; Zhao, J.; Riedl, J.; Zwartkruis, F.; van der Krogt, G.; Zaccolo, M.; Moolenaar, W.H.; Bos, J.L.; Jalink, K. Detecting cAMP-induced Epac activation by fluorescence resonance energy transfer: Epac as a novel cAMP indicator. *EMBO Rep.* **2004**, *5*, 1176–1180. [CrossRef] [PubMed]

139. Nikolaev, V.O.; Gambaryan, S.; Engelhardt, S.; Walter, U.; Lohse, M.J. Real-time monitoring of the PDE2 activity of live cells: Hormone-stimulated cAMP hydrolysis is faster than hormone-stimulated cAMP synthesis. *J. Biol. Chem.* **2005**, *280*, 1716–1719. [CrossRef] [PubMed]

140. Calebiro, D.; Nikolaev, V.O.; Gagliani, M.C.; de Filippis, T.; Dees, C.; Tacchetti, C.; Persani, L.; Lohse, M.J. Persistent cAMP-signals triggered by internalized G-protein-coupled receptors. *PLoS Biol.* **2009**, *7*. [CrossRef] [PubMed]

141. Klarenbeek, J.; Goedhart, J.; van Batenburg, A.; Groenewald, D.; Jalink, K. Fourth-generation epac-based FRET sensors for cAMP feature exceptional brightness, photostability and dynamic range: Characterization of dedicated sensors for FLIM, for ratiometry and with high affinity. *PLoS ONE* **2015**, *10*. [CrossRef] [PubMed]

142. Rich, T.C.; Fagan, K.A.; Nakata, H.; Schaack, J.; Cooper, D.M.; Karpen, J.W. Cyclic nucleotide-gated channels colocalize with adenylyl cyclase in regions of restricted cAMP diffusion. *J. Gen. Physiol.* **2000**, *116*, 147–161. [CrossRef] [PubMed]

143. Rich, T.C.; Tse, T.E.; Rohan, J.G.; Schaack, J.; Karpen, J.W. In vivo assessment of local phosphodiesterase activity using tailored cyclic nucleotide-gated channels as cAMP sensors. *J. Gen. Physiol.* **2001**, *118*, 63–78. [CrossRef] [PubMed]

144. Nikolaev, V.O.; Bünemann, M.; Schmitteckert, E.; Lohse, M.J.; Engelhardt, S. Cyclic AMP imaging in adult cardiac myocytes reveals far-reaching beta1-adrenergic but locally confined beta2-adrenergic receptor-mediated signaling. *Circ. Res.* **2006**, *99*, 1084–1091. [CrossRef] [PubMed]

145. Perera, R.K.; Nikolaev, V.O. Compartmentation of cAMP signalling in cardiomyocytes in health and disease. *Acta Physiol.* **2013**, *207*, 650–662. [CrossRef] [PubMed]

146. Bork, N.I.; Nikolaev, V.O. Receptor-cyclic nucleotide microdomains in the heart. In *Microdomains in the Cardiovascular System*; Nikolaev, V.O., Zaccolo, M., Eds.; Springer Nature: Cham, Switzerland, 2017; pp. 3–15.

147. Hansma, P.K.; Drake, B.; Marti, O.; Gould, S.A.; Prater, C.B. The scanning ion-conductance microscope. *Science* **1989**, *243*, 641–643. [CrossRef] [PubMed]

148. Korchev, Y.E.; Bashford, C.L.; Milovanovic, M.; Vodyanoy, I.; Lab, M.J. Scanning ion conductance microscopy of living cells. *Biophys. J.* **1997**, *73*, 653–658. [CrossRef]

149. Nikolaev, V.O.; Moshkov, A.; Lyon, A.R.; Miragoli, M.; Novak, P.; Paur, H.; Lohse, M.J.; Korchev, Y.E.; Harding, S.E.; Gorelik, J. Beta2-adrenergic receptor redistribution in heart failure changes cAMP compartmentation. *Science* **2010**, *327*, 1653–1657. [CrossRef] [PubMed]

150. Miragoli, M.; Moshkov, A.; Novak, P.; Shevchuk, A.; Nikolaev, V.O.; El-Hamamsy, I.; Potter, C.M.; Wright, P.; Kadir, S.H.; Lyon, A.R.; et al. Scanning ion conductance microscopy: A convergent high-resolution technology for multi-parametric analysis of living cardiovascular cells. *J. R. Soc. Interface* **2011**, *8*, 913–925. [CrossRef] [PubMed]

151. Froese, A.; Nikolaev, V.O. Imaging alterations of cardiomyocyte cAMP microdomains in disease. *Front. Pharmacol.* **2015**, *6*. [CrossRef] [PubMed]

152. Berisha, F.; Nikolaev, V.O. Cyclic nucleotide imaging and cardiovascular disease. *Pharmacol. Ther.* **2017**, *175*, 107–115. [CrossRef] [PubMed]

153. Fischmeister, R.; Castro, L.; Abi-Gerges, A.; Rochais, F.; Vandecasteele, G. Species-and tissue-dependent effects of NO and cyclic GMP on cardiac ion channels. *Comp. Biochem. Physiol. A Mol. Integr. Physiol.* **2005**, *142*, 136–143. [CrossRef] [PubMed]

154. Vandecasteele, G.; Verde, I.; Rücker-Martin, C.; Donzeau-Gouge, P.; Fischmeister, R. Cyclic GMP regulation of the L-type Ca^{2+} channel current in human atrial myocytes. *J. Physiol.* **2001**, *533*, 329–340. [CrossRef] [PubMed]

155. Mehel, H.; Emons, J.; Vettel, C.; Wittkopper, K.; Seppelt, D.; Dewenter, M.; Lutz, S.; Sossalla, S.; Maier, L.S.; Lechene, P.; et al. Phosphodiesterase-2 is up-regulated in human failing hearts and blunts beta adrenergic responses in cardiomyocytes. *J. Am. Coll. Cardiol.* **2013**, *62*, 1596–1606. [CrossRef] [PubMed]

156. Zoccarato, A.; Surdo, N.C.; Aronsen, J.M.; Fields, L.A.; Mancuso, L.; Dodoni, G.; Stangherlin, A.; Livie, C.; Jiang, H.; Sin, Y.Y.; et al. Cardiac hypertrophy is inhibited by a local pool of cAMP regulated by phosphodiesterase 2 novelty and significance. *Circ. Res.* **2015**, *117*, 707–719. [CrossRef] [PubMed]

157. Sprenger, J.U.; Perera, R.K.; Steinbrecher, J.H.; Lehnart, S.E.; Maier, L.S.; Hasenfuss, G.; Nikolaev, V.O. In vivo model with targeted cAMP biosensor reveals changes in receptor microdomain communication in cardiac disease. *Nat. Commun.* **2015**, *6*. [CrossRef] [PubMed]

158. Perera, R.K.; Sprenger, J.U.; Steinbrecher, J.H.; Hübscher, D.; Lehnart, S.E.; Abesser, M.; Schuh, K.; El-Armouche, A.; Nikolaev, V.O. Microdomain switch of cGMP-regulated phosphodiesterases leads to ANP-induced augmentation of beta-adrenoceptor-stimulated contractility in early cardiac hypertrophy. *Circ. Res.* **2015**, *116*, 1304–1311. [CrossRef] [PubMed]

159. Vettel, C.; Lindner, M.; Dewenter, M.; Lorenz, K.; Schanbacher, C.; Riedel, M.; Lämmle, S. Phosphodiesterase 2 protects against catecholamine-induced arrhythmia and preserves contractile function after myocardial infarction. *Circ. Res.* **2017**, *120*, 120–132. [CrossRef] [PubMed]

160. Di Benedetto, G.; Zoccarato, A.; Lissandron, V.; Terrin, A.; Li, X.; Houslay, M.D.; Baillie, G.S.; Zaccolo, M. Protein kinase A type I and type II define distinct intracellular signaling compartments. *Circ. Res.* **2008**, *103*, 836–844. [CrossRef] [PubMed]

161. Stangherlin, A.; Gesellchen, F.; Zoccarato, A.; Terrin, A.; Fields, L.A.; Berrera, M.; Surdo, N.C.; Craig, M.A.; Smith, G.; Hamilton, G.; et al. cGMP signals modulate cAMP levels in a compartment-specific manner to regulate catecholamine-dependent signaling in cardiac myocytes. *Circ. Res.* **2011**, *108*, 929–939. [CrossRef] [PubMed]

162. Surapisitchat, J.; Jeon, K.I.; Yan, C.; Beavo, J.A. Differential regulation of endothelial cell permeability by cGMP via phosphodiesterases 2 and 3. *Circ. Res.* **2007**, *101*, 811–818. [CrossRef] [PubMed]

163. Stangherlin, A.; Zaccolo, M. Phosphodiesterases and subcellular compartmentalized cAMP signaling in the cardiovascular system. *Am. J. Physiol. Heart Circ. Physiol.* **2012**, *302*, H379–H390. [CrossRef] [PubMed]

164. Li, D.; Lu, C.J.; Hao, G.; Wright, H.; Woodward, L.; Liu, K.; Vergari, E.; Surdo, N.C.; Herring, N.; Zaccolo, M.; et al. Efficacy of B-type natriuretic peptide is coupled to phosphodiesterase 2A in cardiac sympathetic neurons novelty and significance. *Hypertension* **2015**, *66*, 190–198. [CrossRef] [PubMed]

165. Meier, S.; Andressen, K.W.; Aronsen, J.M.; Sjaastad, I.; Hougen, K.; Skomedal, T.; Osnes, J.B.; Qvigstad, E.; Levy, F.O.; Moltzau, L.R. PDE3 inhibition by C-type natriuretic peptide-induced cGMP enhances cAMP-mediated signaling in both non-failing and failing hearts. *Eur. J. Pharmacol.* **2017**, *812*, 174–183. [CrossRef] [PubMed]

166. Mongillo, M.; McSorley, T.; Evellin, S.; Sood, A.; Lissandron, V.; Terrin, A.; Huston, E.; Hannawacker, A.; Lohse, M.J.; Pozzan, T.; et al. Fluorescence resonance energy transfer–based analysis of cAMP dynamics in live neonatal rat cardiac myocytes reveals distinct functions of compartmentalized phosphodiesterases. *Circ. Res.* **2004**, *95*, 67–75. [CrossRef] [PubMed]

167. Rochais, F.; Abi-Gerges, A.; Horner, K.; Lefebvre, F.; Cooper, D.M.; Conti, M.; Fischmeister, R.; Vandecasteele, G. A specific pattern of phosphodiesterases controls the cAMP signals generated by different Gs-coupled receptors in adult rat ventricular myocytes. *Circ. Res.* **2006**, *98*, 1081–1088. [CrossRef] [PubMed]

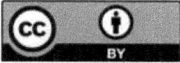

Journal of
Cardiovascular
Development and Disease

MDPI

Review

The Development of Compartmentation of cAMP Signaling in Cardiomyocytes: The Role of T-Tubules and Caveolae Microdomains

Navneet K. Bhogal, Alveera Hasan and Julia Gorelik *

Department of Cardiovascular Sciences, National Heart and Lung Institute, Imperial College London, London W12 0NN, UK; n.bhogal14@imperial.ac.uk (N.K.B.); alveera.hasan13@imperial.ac.uk (A.H.)
* Correspondence: j.gorelik@ic.ac.uk; Tel.: +44-(0)20-7594-2736

Received: 23 February 2018; Accepted: 28 April 2018; Published: 3 May 2018

Abstract: $3'$-$5'$-cyclic adenosine monophosphate (cAMP) is a signaling messenger produced in response to the stimulation of cellular receptors, and has a myriad of functional applications depending on the cell type. In the heart, cAMP is responsible for regulating the contraction rate and force; however, cAMP is also involved in multiple other functions. Compartmentation of cAMP production may explain the specificity of signaling following a stimulus. In particular, transverse tubules (T-tubules) and caveolae have been found to be critical structural components for the spatial confinement of cAMP in cardiomyocytes, as exemplified by beta-adrenergic receptor (β-ARs) signaling. Pathological alterations in cardiomyocyte microdomain architecture led to a disruption in compartmentation of the cAMP signal. In this review, we discuss the difference between atrial and ventricular cardiomyocytes in respect to microdomain organization, and the pathological changes of atrial and ventricular cAMP signaling in response to myocyte dedifferentiation. In addition, we review the role of localized phosphodiesterase (PDE) activity in constraining the cAMP signal. Finally, we discuss microdomain biogenesis and maturation of cAMP signaling with the help of induced pluripotent stem cell-derived cardiomyocytes (iPSC-CMs). Understanding these mechanisms may help to overcome the detrimental effects of pathological structural remodeling.

Keywords: cAMP; phosphodiesterase; FRET; atrial; ventricle; iPSC-CMs; T-tubule; caveolae; development

1. Introduction

The fascination about $3'$-$5'$-cyclic adenosine monophosphate (cAMP), a second messenger molecule, is with its ability to activate multiple signalling pathways having different effects on cellular physiology in many cell types. Cardiomyocytes, in particular, have been studied in detail for the regulation of cAMP production as a result of extracellular stimulation [1,2]. Buxton and Bruton indicated a paradox whereby stimulation of a cell via various receptor pathways provided diverse cellular responses despite generating the same cAMP second messenger [3]. It was further elucidated, that these multiple spatially confined cAMP compartments may be the result of different protein kinase A (PKA) isoforms and other cAMP-sensitive downstream targets having restricted access to cAMP [4]. Studies have since been directed at understanding how these vital compartments of cAMP are maintained within the cell.

The localized synthesis of cAMP by one of 10 different adenylate cyclase (AC) isoforms is crucial in providing initial first step in signalling cascade, however, the manner in which cAMP is compartmentalized within the cell is essential to elicit a specific cellular response.

J. Cardiovasc. Dev. Dis. **2018**, *5*, 25

Saucerman et al. proposed several mechanisms that might be involved in cAMP compartmentalization including: local degradation, physical barriers, and cell shape [5]. There are many factors that come together to give rise to cAMP compartments. In this review, we focus on the role of cardiac microdomains and phosphodiesterases (PDEs).

2. β-Adrenergic Pathway

The heart responds to catecholamines with increases in rate, force of contraction, and speed of relaxation [6]. The main catecholamine-responsive receptors on the surface of cardiac myocytes are β-adrenergic receptors (β-ARs), an important class of G-protein-coupled receptors (GPCR). To generate these responses, β-ARs are coupled to G_s proteins, which activate AC and, thus, induce cAMP production. The cAMP binds to effector proteins including, PKA [7] (preferentiality PKA-RII in the case of β-AR [8]), exchange protein directly activated by cAMP (EPAC) [7], cyclic nucleotide gated ion channels (CNGCs) [9], and Popeye-domain-containing proteins (Popdc) [10]. PKA is the major effector protein and phosphorylates a large number of target proteins which are for example involved in excitation-contraction coupling (ECC) [6].

β-AR stimulation is however more complex. In the late 1960s, Lands et al. studied the activity of sympathomimetic amines in different tissues and concluded that there are two isoforms of β-ARs: $β_1$-AR and $β_2$-AR [11,12]. In the heart, $β_1$-AR is the predominant isoform [12]. The important role of $β_1$-AR for the heart was demonstrated through targeted disruption in mice. The Adrb1 null mutant displayed impaired cardiac performance and prenatal lethality [13]. In contrast, the $β_2$-AR is apparently less important for the heart and more active in the respiratory system [12]. Both receptor types differ in their G-protein coupling, while $β_1$-AR couples only to G_s proteins, $β_2$-AR couples to both G_s and G_i proteins. Adrb2 mutants display normal resting heart rate and blood pressure, but develop hypertension in response to epinephrine infusion or to the cardiovascular stress induced by exercise [14]. Interestingly, human ventricular tissue display a higher expression level of $β_1$-AR in comparison to $β_2$-AR with a ratio of approximately 77:23 [15]. The predominance of $β_1$-AR provides an explanation for the fact that mice lacking $β_2$-AR experience alterations during exercise to their vascular tone and energy metabolism [14], but nothing more fatal. The low cardiac expression level of $β_2$-AR together with its ability to either stimulate (via G_s) or inhibit (via G_i) cAMP synthesis suggests an involvement in the 'fine-tuning' of cardiac contractility. Importantly, $β_2$-AR are thought to have protective effects on cardiac function [16]. In addition to differences in expression level and G-protein coupling, the functional properties of β-ARs can also be affected by their spatial localization at the plasma membrane [16].

An important downstream effector molecule of β-AR signalling is AC. Stimulation of β-AR leads to activation of ACs catalysing the conversion of ATP to cAMP. The two major isoforms of ACs expressed in the heart are AC5 and AC6. Patch clamp recordings of ventricular myocytes from Adcy5 (AC5) and Adcy6 (AC6) knock-out mice, demonstrated the divergent roles of these adenylyl cyclase isoforms [17]. An AC5-mediated increase of the calcium current was recorded from T-tubules, and was mediated by both $β_1$-AR and $β_2$-AR [17]. In contrast, AC6 was shown to interact with $β_1$-AR alone. Interestingly, upon genetic ablation of Adcy5, it was shown that AC5 is protective against cardiac dysfunction in pressure overload induced cardiac hypertrophy [18], thus suggesting that the stimulation of AC5 could potentially be a protective therapeutic approach in heart failure. Introducing AC6 was able to restore the cAMP-generating capacity in a murine cardiomyopathy model [19,20]. The targeted deletion of Adcy6 caused a marked impairment of cAMP synthesis and sarcoplasmic reticulum calcium release [21]. The differing effects on cardiac function upon gene ablation suggests that these AC isoforms provide different functions to the heart.

3. Transverse Axial Tubular System

Important and highly-complex compartments in the cardiac myocyte are the transverse tubules (T-tubules). These deep, penetrative sacrolemmal invaginations are a characteristic of ventricular myocytes, and openings of these tubules can be visualized on the cellular surface in Z-groove structures [22]. These microdomains act as a framework for several ion channels and proteins essential for regulating the strength and synchronicity of each cardiac contraction [23]. These proteins and effector molecules are grouped in specific protein complexes along the plasma membrane [24].

The complexity of the transverse axial tubular (TAT) system has received more attention over the years, due to the presence of axial (also known as longitudinal) elements becoming more apparent [22,25]. The increase in axial elements raises questions of their functional importance. Studying healthy ventricular myocytes have demonstrated that small mammals have a more prominent T-tubular system compared to those from larger mammals [26,27]. Detailed studies in rabbits demonstrated that the diameter of the T-tubules is approximately two-fold wider than in mice [26]. This suggests that the abundant presence of T-tubules seen in mice is likely due to myocyte's requirement to accommodate ECC proteins in order to achieve a proper contractile response. In addition, it is possible that wider T-tubules are able to accommodate the required ECC proteins in fewer structures, which provides an explanation for the patchy tubular system seen in larger animals. These structural differences between species are likely the result of the vast differences in heart rate that exists between small and large mammals; thus, the structure is adjusted to meet the species-specific requirements. Therefore, the regularity and structural environment of these microdomains is crucial for physiological signalling of receptors and ion channels in both atrial and ventricular myocytes [28,29].

It has been long thought that atrial myocytes either lack, or contain only a rudimentary TAT network [30–34]. However, more recently it became evident that atrial myocytes are more diverse. Gadeberg et al. have shown that in atrial myocytes of larger mammals including humans a TAT network is present, with cell size being a determinant for T-tubular density [30]. Interestingly, murine atrial myocytes display a predominantly axial tubular structure, and the diameter of these tubules is wider than in ventricular myocytes [31,32]. Moreover, the most organized atrial myocytes resemble ventricular myocytes with regard to the TAT network.

The atria are structured as two separate "pockets", with the right atrium containing anatomical structures (i.e., crista terminalis and sinoatrial node), which are not present in the left atrium. Yamashita et al. have shown that, although the length to width ratio remains the same, myocytes isolated from the crista terminalis are larger than from pectinate muscle [33]. Therefore, differently structured myocytes may be derived from different atrial regions. Investigations of small mammals also demonstrated the requirement of the TAT structure in the atria and further highlighted the heterogeneous structure in these myocytes [34,35]. Glukhov et al. studied rat atrial myocytes utilizing confocal microscopy with scanning ion conductance microscopy (SICM) to demonstrate the existence of three populations of myocytes: organized, disorganized, and empty cells [34] (Figure 1A). These distinct populations of atrial myocytes have been found in both small and large mammals in multiple independent studies [34–36].

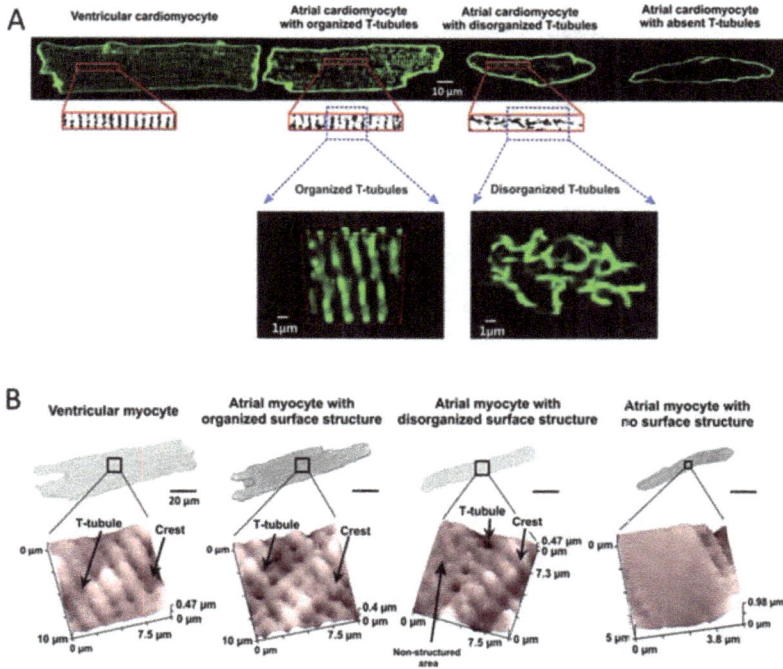

Figure 1. The heterogeneity of myocytes found in the rat heart. (**A**) Representative confocal images of Di-8-ANNEPS-stained myocytes from the atria and the ventricle. Atrial cells were categorized based on the T-tubule organization and density into three distinct subgroups with organized TAT, disorganized TAT and myocytes lacking all T-tubular structure. Parts of images were binarised as shown and used to calculate the density and demonstrate a clear representation of the structural changes between groups; (**B**) Topographical scans of myocytes demonstrating the occurrence of T-tubule opening at the Z-lines of myocytes in relation to their cell size. Arrows indicate T-tubules, crests, and non-structured areas. Adapted from Glukhov et al. 2015 [34].

4. Caveolae

Caveolae are 50–100 nM-wide flask-shaped membrane invaginations. These microdomains are dense in cholesterol and are lined with specialized scaffolding proteins, which are key features distinguishing caveolae from other lipid raft structures [32]. Caveolae are responsible for the spatial organization of signalling proteins, lipid storage, and membrane homeostasis. Although it is well known that the caveolar coat is comprised of oligomers of the scaffolding proteins caveolin and cavin, the process of assembly and recycling of these membrane domains remained debatable for many decades. Recently, Hayer et al. highlighted the multistep process of caveolae assembly [37]. This involves the homo-oligomerisation of caveolin-1 (Cav1) into 8S complexes in the Golgi where they undergo conformational changes and associate with cholesterol, thus assembling into 70S complexes. These newly-assembled caveolin scaffolds are transported to the plasma membrane where they are able to act as functional caveolar domains.

Caveolae have the ability to act as membrane reservoirs allowing the cell to increase its surface area in response to osmotic stress [38–40]. Furthermore, Sinha et al. and others have shown that acute mechanical stress induced by osmotic swelling or stretching, reduced the interaction of caveolin with cavin-1. It increased the concentration of free caveolin proteins at the plasma membrane, thus resulting in a rapid disappearance of caveolae [38,41]. Mohan et al. further elucidated that Cavin-1 regulates caveolae dynamics, by targeting Cavin-3 to caveolae where it interacts with the scaffolding domain of Cav1 [42]. Loss of Cavin-3 resulted in an increase in the long-term stability of caveolae at the plasma membrane, suggesting that it regulates the lifetime of caveolae.

Calaghan et al. studied the dynamic nature of caveolae in response to mechanical stimuli; subjecting adult rat hearts to left ventricular ballooning and the time-dependent effect of stretch on the distribution of caveolin-3 (Cav3) and other caveolar proteins [43]. The authors observed a progressive loss of Cav3 from caveolae, similar to what is seen after chemical disruption of caveolae via cholesterol depletion, thus indicating a mechanotransductive role of caveolae domains in the heart. A key example of caveolae organizing cellular compartmentation of signalling proteins is the interaction of Cav3 with AC5, PDE4B, and PDE4D [17].

5. Microdomains of cAMP Signalling in Healthy Ventricular Myocytes: T-Tubules and Caveolae

Visualization of cAMP signal propagation using flurorescent cAMP sensors has become more sophisticated over recent years, which led to the definition of spatially localized cAMP pools (or nanodomains) [44]. These pools may be located either within a close proximity to receptors and ion channels, or may be distributed throughout the cell. Evidence from adult mouse ventricular myocytes demonstrates the response to stimulation of β_1-AR is a far-reaching cAMP signal, compared with the local response upon stimulation of β_2-AR [44]. The difference in the way G_s-coupled β-ARs compartmentalise cAMP, is linked to two key factors: (i) the localization of the receptor and (ii) the occurrence of cAMP-degrading enzymes.

To identify the different cAMP pools produced by β-ARs, a combination of SICM and Förster resonance energy transfer (FRET) was utilized. SICM identifies specific microdomains (T-tubule and crest) by producing a detailed topographical image of the cell surface (Figure 1B) [34]. β-AR stimulation was then applied locally to adult rat ventricular myocytes, using the SICM nanopipette to a microdomain of interest. cAMP synthesis was measured, using FRET, in response to local (site-specific) stimulation [16,45,46]. This high-tech approach made it possible for Nikolaev et al. to demonstrate that β_1-AR-induced cAMP signalling occurs both at the T-tubule and non-T-tubule areas. In contrast the β_2-AR-induced cAMP response arises from the T-tubules only [16]. In addition, to assessing the cAMP response of β_2-AR irrespective of its coupling to G_i-proteins, PTX was used and caused no difference in cAMP compartmentalisation [44]. The larger diffusion pattern of β_1-AR-cAMP thus explains β_1-ARs' ability to produce such a response, as a result of activating far-reaching proteins involved in ECC.

Caveolae are found in both the T-tubule and the crest membranes in rabbit ventricular myocytes [47]. Caveolae localized at the sarcolemma appear to have a four-fold higher density, compared to those located at the T-tubular membrane [48]. These microdomains act as platforms for the assembly of receptors, signalling components, and their associated targets. They, therefore, undergo dynamic regulation to allow agonist-stimulated receptors to interact efficiently with their respective effectors [49]. Thus the dynamic properties and overall stability of the caveolar microdomains in cardiomyocytes has sparked significant interest over the last decades. Specifically, it is due to these structures being involved in mechanisms responsible for creating distinct β_1- and β_2-AR-dependent cAMP signalling. The distribution and clustering of these GPCRs and their downstream signalling components, within or outside of caveolar domains, are important factors in promoting efficient and accurate functional responses to β-ARs stimulation. Multiple studies report the clustering of β_2-ARs along with its associated signalling elements, including G_s, G_i, AC5, and AC6, and protein kinase A (PKA) within the caveolar membrane fractions [50,51]; which have also been shown to co-immunoprecipitate with Cav3 [24,52]. β_1-AR, on the other hand has been shown to be located in both caveolar and non-caveolar compartments in adult rat ventricular myocytes [51,53]. Thus, a cholesterol/caveolin-3 rich environment is key in building the macromolecular structure, particularly for β_2-AR.

The description of nanodomains of cAMP signalling will be incomplete without mentioning A kinase anchoring proteins (AKAPs), scaffolding proteins which constrain PKA to specific subcellular locations in physical proximity to PKA targets. AKAPs, to a large extent, determine a unique phosphorylation pattern downstream of the kinase. In cells undergoing response to a stimulus, the location of some AKAPs can change, thus altering the functional outcome of cAMP signals. However, the detailed look into the function of AKAPs falls beyond the scope of the present review as it is reviewed extensively elsewhere [54,55].

6. PDEs and cAMP Compartmentation in Ventricular Myocytes

PDEs are a family of enzymes that degrade cyclic nucleotides [56–58]. By acting as functional barriers, they create subcellular cAMP gradients by preventing its free diffusion throughout the cell [59]. They have been divided into 11 families based on their structure, catalytic properties, and their differential affinity for cyclic nuclotides [60,61]. Each family of PDEs has isoforms, which vary according to the following properties: tissue distribution, intracellular localization, and the involvement in cellular signalling. PDE 1–3, 10, and 11 are responsible for degrading both cAMP and cGMP. PDE 4, 7, and 8 are specific for the hydrolysis of cAMP and PDE 5, 6, and 9 are cGMP-specific [62]. It has been shown that blocking all PDEs, using isobutyl-methyl-xanthine (IBMX), after β-AR stimulation leads to changes in physiological response due to the spatial and temporal regulation of cAMP [63,64]. Therefore, this infers that the extensive assortment of PDEs provides routes for cardiomyocytes to modulate cAMP signalling.

The complexity of the various functional abilities of the PDE families is further increased by the concept of cross-talk between cAMP and cGMP pathways. For example, cGMP stimulates PDE2 leading to degradation of both cAMP and cGMP, thus increases in cGMP can alter cAMP hydrolysis. Cyclic GMP can also activate PDE5 and increase the rate of its own degradation [65–68]. PDE3 has dual specificity with a higher catalytic rate for cAMP, therefore, it can be considered as a cGMP-inhibited cAMP-hydrolysing enzyme [65,68].

Compartmentation of cAMP to specific microdomains at the plasma membrane and in the cytoplasm requires a vast variety of PDEs, and their presence or absence in a particular location is also species-specific. To explore the functionality of receptors and enzymes, utilizing genetically-engineered knock-out/overexpression models has become a powerful methodology in cardiovascular research. Employing these methods has determined the vast impact that PDE3 and PDE4 have in cAMP-hydrolytic activity and calcium handling [69]. In addition, it has been highlighted that isoforms of a single family of PDEs can localize to specific compartments. PDE3 has been specifically shown to associate with T-tubule microdomains and with internally-organized sarcoplasmic reticulum structures [63,70]. Investigating the function of PDEs using knock-out mice and inhibitors has collectively provided evidence suggesting each PDE subgroup contains isoforms that have different microdomain locations and functions. The use of mouse knock-out models and selective PDE3 inhibitors have indicated PDE3A to be responsible for chronotropic and inotropic effects [71], whereas PDE3B serves to acutely protect the heart after biomechanical stress [72]. Specifically, PDE3A1 controls the Phospholamban (PLB) and sarcoplasmic reticulum calcium ATPase2 (SERCA2) activity and the re-uptake of calcium in the SR, leading to an increase in cAMP-dependent calcium transients, without affecting L-type calcium channels (LTCCs) [72]. Therefore, Movesesian suggests a PDE3A1-specific inhibitor could potentially improve contractile performance and provide therapy for heart failure (HF) [73].

Unlike PDE3, PDE4 is shown to localize to the sarcolemma [70] and play an important role in cardiomyocytes [74,75]. Although the expression of PDE4 is species-specific, the relative amount of PDE4 compared to overall PDE activity is conserved between humans and rodents. However, the overall cAMP-hydrolytic activity of PDE4 is estimated to be higher in rodents compared to humans [74]. The inhibition of PDE4 was specifically shown to extensively increase cAMP levels. In addition, the PDE4 activity has presented to be specifically enhanced by β-AR stimulation [44,56]. PDE4 has also been demonstrated to be a predominant isoform that hydrolyses cytoplasmic cAMP produced following β_1-AR, but not β_2-AR stimulation [44]. Melsom et al. demonstrated that combined PDE4 and PDE3 inhibition increased the potency of adrenaline on PTX treated β_2-AR [76]. This suggests that it is possible that PDE4 plays a significant role with β_2-ARs. Subgroups of PDE4, mainly: PDE4A, PDE4B, and PDE4D are expressed in the heart (see Conti 2017 [77] for an extensive review on PDE4). Previous studies have shown the importance of PDE4D, in particular through its involvement with the PLB/SERCA2A complex [78], the cardiac ryanodine receptors and the calcium release channel complex [79]. In addition, mice lacking PDE4D develop an age-dependant cardiomyopathy and exercise-induced arrhythmias [79]. Moreover, PDE4D appears to control cAMP levels in subcellular compartments, thus having an impact on myocyte contractility [78].

In addition, PDE2 was shown to hydrolyse cAMP after β-AR stimulation in adult mouse ventricular myocytes. Here, the inhibition of PDE2 releases a higher level of cAMP than that after PDE3 inhibition [44]. Although not extensively studied, measuring cAMP in ventricular myocytes demonstrated that PDE2 affects the regulation of heart rate. Inhibition of PDE2 caused an increased heart rate, while overexpression reduced the heart rate [80], suggesting that the expression levels do not directly relate to functional integrity, and that perhaps a minor PDE2 fraction could play a larger role in specific microdomains.

7. cAMP Compartmentation and PDEs in Atrial Myocytes

In comparison to ventricular myocytes, cAMP compartmentalisation in atrial myocytes remains relatively poorly investigated. The ultrastructural organisation of atrial myocytes differs with ventricular and this suggests differential receptor localization and spatial pools of cAMP leading to unique signaling patterns. So far, to map signalling differences between atrial and ventricular myocytes two major methods have been utilized: electrophysiological methods and expression analysis of β-AR and PDEs. It has now become apparent that in ventricular myocytes caveolae are involved in controlling β-AR signalling [40,43,45,46,48,49,52,53]. Accordingly, an even higher abundance of caveolae in rat atrial myocytes [34] would suggest their important role in the spatial control of cAMP nanodomains in this cell type. Atrial myocytes are thinner and contain less complex TAT networks. Due to their small size, atrial myocytes may not require a complex internal structural architecture. Utilizing methyl-β-cyclodextrin (MβCD)-treated ventricular rat myocytes to disrupt caveolae, β_1-AR has been found in both caveolae and non-caveolae regions, while β_2-AR were confined to the caveolae compartment [53]. It has been demonstrated in human atrial myocytes using the whole-cell voltage-clamp that PDE4 reduces cAMP when combined with either PDE3 inhibition or β-AR stimulation [81]. These earlier studies into atrial myocytes warrant the assumption that although β_1-AR might have a rather similar role to that seen in ventricular myocytes, β2-AR may assume a larger role, due to these receptors being denser, largely because of the increase in caveolar number. To understand the role of PDEs and to establish the principal differences between atrial versus ventricular cardiomyocytes, expression analysis in the mouse right atria (RA) and right ventricle (RV) was performed. PDE2A was shown to be equally expressed across the RA and RV, whereas PDE3B, PDE4B and PDE4D were all expressed at higher levels in the atria [82]. Similar studies have been conducted in rat and human tissue to determine species-specific differences. In contrast to rodent myocytes, human PDE4 is not the predominant subtype regulating cAMP levels. Nevertheless, it was shown that PDE4 inhibition led to the positive inotropic effect of β-AR stimulation, increasing the susceptibility to atrial arrhythmias, and a marked prolongation in cAMP rise [75]. This work is highly suggestive that PDE4 plays a significant role in compartmentation of cAMP. It is possible that PDE4 is more closely associated with caveolae and less with T-tubules, thus explaining why PDE4 has a stronger impact in atrial cells. What would be interesting is to understand how β-AR signalling is propagated in atrial myocytes, and how this impacts the activity of PDEs to compartmentalize cAMP.

8. Failing Myocardium Represents Progressive Reduction in the Complexity of Structure and Receptor Function

Studies in rat ventricular myocytes isolated from failing hearts have shown that the progression of disease causes TAT structure to become more disorganized and diminished [45,83]. In comparison to normal cells, the TAT structure in human chronic unloaded HF also presents a decrease in regularity, and for the first time using 3D imaging, demonstrated a sheet-like T-tubule phenotype [84]. In rats, axial elements were increased during early HF, but reduced as HF progressed [45]. These different tubular structures that are present in failing myocytes are not well characterised. In addition, it is not fully understood what causes the reduced density of the TAT structure.

Lyon et al. have demonstrated that surface structures (Z-grooves) in the human myocardium were lost from the cell surface during HF [85]. A similar study conducted in rats measured the Z-groove index, demonstrating loss of these structures in HF [86]. Hence, it is apparent that the relative changes in the TAT system occur in both large and small animals during HF [27,45,84–88].

The continuous structural adaptation, in response to alterations of mechanical load during HF has become a hallmark of cardiac disease. Patients with severe HF, can be fitted with a left ventricular assist device (LVAD), which reduces the mechanical load to the heart in an attempt to regain cardiac function. Studies on myocytes isolated from such failing hearts have shown that implantation of an LVAD could only be beneficial to those hearts that possess a relatively preserved myocyte TAT structure [84]. In comparison, chronic unloading in rat hearts demonstrated a reduction in the density and regularity of the TAT system, in addition to surface changes [86]. Damage to the heart is inhomogeneous, and so it could be said that TAT density loss would occur to a higher extent in certain regions compared to others. This difference in density would initially be identified by the weak contractility of the heart [36].

Structural adaptations that occur in chronic HF come with a functional price—the relocalization of β-ARs. The change in localization of these receptors generates a modified downstream response. Namely, β$_2$-AR signalling is altered, such that cAMP signalling is seen to spread from both the crest and T-tubule regions, with smaller signalling amplitudes compared to healthy cells [16]. The alterations seen in β$_2$-AR signalling became apparent as early as four weeks post-myocardial infarction (MI) in rats, and progressively worsens over 16 weeks post-MI. It has become evident that as disease progressively worsens, transverse elements are lost and axial elements are gained (Figure 2) [45]. The increase in β$_2$-AR cAMP signalling has been thought to be a compensatory mechanism for decreased β$_1$-AR cAMP signalling [16]. This indicates that a myocyte attempts to maintain orderly signalling, as conditions deteriorates, which as a result changes the dynamics of cellular signalling.

The expression of Cav3 has also been demonstrated to decrease during HF, and this is important for both the TAT system and caveolae [45,89]. The disruption of Cav3 has been shown to be a significant cause of the far-reaching β$_2$-AR-cAMP signals [46]. In support of this, a large portion of β$_2$-ARs have been shown to localize to caveolae [24]. Moreover, it was found that caveolar microdomains, as well as housing β-ARs, also contain LTCCs, a critical ion channels activated by cAMP signalling which regulate ECC. A recent study has suggested that the LTCCs located in caveolae have more impact on hypertrophy than contractile function of the heart [90]. Therefore, it is clear that a better understanding is needed of receptors and ion channel function within caveolae and what impact they have on the contractile function of the heart.

As a result of the breakdown of structural microdomains, PDEs are relocated and they lose connectivity with their native environments; thus losing the capacity to perform their inherent function. PDE4 was shown to lose its influence on the confinement of cAMP during early HF [91]. In agreement with this, Lehnart et al. suggested that deficiency in PDE4D was pro-arrhythmogenic and that it was associated with HF in mice [79]. This is suggestive of the PDE4 isoform being localized in the vicinity of cAMP microdomains during healthy cardiac functionally, allowing for precise cAMP compartmentation. Therefore, when structural microdomains are lost, for example in cardiac hypertrophy, not only are β-ARs relocated and functionally altered, but PDE4 that would normally act as a barrier to cAMP diffusion has locally changed [92]. It is believed that the decompartmentation of PDEs initially compensates for the deficient cAMP synthesis by β-ARs, however, the long-term effects of this leads to a loss of cAMP compartments.

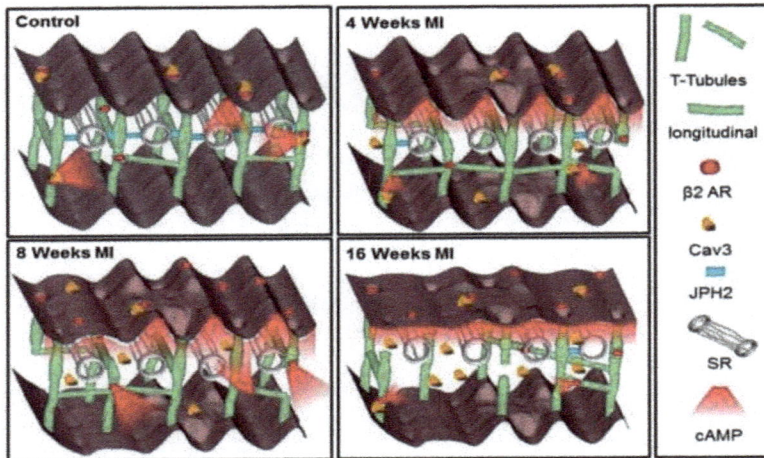

Figure 2. Progressive loss of the t-tubules and the increase of axial (longitudinal) elements of the TAT system demonstrate the change in cAMP signalling in the ventricular myocytes isolated from hearts with myocardial infarction (MI). Focus on the way in which β$_2$-ARs are relocated and become more dispersed throughout the cell. As the disease progressively worsens, the loss of TAT structure deviates further and further away, but still attempts to generate signalling that keeps myocytes functional. Taken from Schobesberger et al., 2017 [45].

PDE2 activity was demonstrated to play a vital role in improving ventricular function. PDE2 is able to provide protective effects under chronic and acute β-AR activation [80]. Whilst the expression of both PDE3 and PDE4 was been shown to be reduced in HF, PDE2 expression was shown to be increased in both animals models and in humans [93]. Therefore, this indicates that cardiac pathophysiology modulates both structure and function of PDEs and the resulting compartmentalization of cAMP. Similar to ventricular cardiomyocytes, the structural architecture of atrial cardiomyocytes is disrupted in disease [70–72]. Glukhov et al. reported that T-tubule structure was diminished in failing rat atrial cardiomyocytes, despite cellular hypertrophy. This was accompanied by a deterioration in structural surface topography [34]. In spite of this finding, atrial myocytes have not been studied sufficiently for conclusions to be made on their function during HF.

Until now, studies on human tissue with persistent atrial fibrillation and HF have shown a decrease in PDE activity, with a selective decrease in PDE4. This has led to the suggestion that PDE4 has a protective role in human atria [75]. It would be interesting to evaluate atrial myocytes structural changes during the HF progression to understand how the TAT structure changes in relation to the caveolae occurrence. This would aid in understanding not only how important Cav3 is to the structure, but how much input caveolae have functionally. Caveolae could be more involved in cellular signalling of atrial versus ventricular myocytes, with resulting changes in PDE compartmentation.

9. Biogenesis and Maturation of Structural Microdomains during Differentiation of Myocytes from Stem Cells

There is an increasing need for the development of effective models of cardiac diseases in order to address the progressive decline in structural and physiological "output" of cardiomyocytes. The use of induced pluripotent stem cell-derived cardiomyocytes (iPSC-CMs) provides an unprecedented opportunity to develop in vitro models of numerous cardiac diseases and for drug discovery to drive the field of personalized medicine. Currently, we face major obstacles in generating cardiomyocytes with precise morphological and functional features resembling healthy adult myocytes, making modelling and understanding of treatments for late-onset diseases more challenging. However, the enthusiasm in the field of cardiac regeneration has been passionately fuelled by recent developments in driving iPSC-CM maturation in order to obtain structurally- and functionally-stable cardiomyocytes.

It has been widely shown that cultured and diseased myocytes undergo rapid T-tubular remodelling; such studies highlight the importance of impaired βAR signalling in cardiac disorders. There is now a particular interest in understanding the developmental processes involved in early cardiomyocytes as many studies have shown that myocytes of failing hearts tend to dedifferentiate into foetal-like phenotypes. On the other hand, the activation of dormant pathways developed early in cellular differentiation has also been suggested [92]. Due to the known challenges in obtaining human embryos for such detailed investigations, many studies resort to the use of iPSC-CMs as an in vitro model of cardiomyogenesis. Below, we discuss the development of cardiac microdomains in early cardiomyocytes and the emergence of β-AR-induced cAMP signalling.

T-tubules are thought to be absent in embryonic and neonatal cardiomyocytes [94] and only begin to develop after birth [95]. It is well understood that cultured and diseased cells rapidly undergo a process of T-tubular remodelling; however, very little is known about the processes involved in T-tubule biogenesis. Understanding the underlying mechanisms of T-tubule formation and correct clustering of ion channels within these microdomains would reveal the key processes required for iPSC-CMs to mature into an adult cardiomyocyte phenotype with functionally-developed membrane structures for efficient ECC machinery.

Multiple membrane scaffolding proteins have been associated with T-tubule biogenesis, such as Cav3, junctophilin-2 (Jph2), and bridging integrator-1 (Bin1). Recent work by Fu et al. indicates that Bin1 assists trafficking and clustering of LTCCs, microdomain organization and T-tubule membrane regulation [96]. Furthermore, they showed that transgenic mice with deletions of these individual genes reveal that the primary t-tubule invaginations still exist [96]. This indicates that a single protein alone is not sufficient for tubulogenesis. Rusconi et al. have developed a mimetic peptide (MP) which functions by modulating the trafficking and life cycle of the LTCC. This study has shown that introducing this peptide successfully restores physiological levels of LTCC in the plasma membrane [97]. This may indicate a potential to drive correct channel localization within the cell membrane. Healthy adult cardiomyocytes are characterized by sarcomeric structures that consist of parallel myofilaments, sarcomeric Z-disk, A-, I-, and H-bands which, altogether, allow for an effective and efficient ECC; therefore, maturation of these structures is pivotal for successfully driving maturation of sarcomeres and T-tubules of early cardiomyocytes. Wang et al. have recently shown that long-term treatment with Puerarin, a traditional Chinese medicine used for the treatment of cardiovascular disease, such as MI, can improve myofibril arrays and significantly enhance T-tubule development in embryonic stem cell-derived cardiomyocytes. The mechanism of action has been suggested through the repression of a specific micro-RNA, miR-22, an important target of Cav3, and the up-regulation of Cav3, Bin1, and Jph2 transcript levels [98]. This strongly supports the role of these proteins in T-tubule biogenesis and stability.

While early myocytes do not have well-developed tubular structures, they possess abundant caveolae structures that may represent sites where receptors and their associated signaling molecules are clustered. Furthermore, it has been suggested that caveolae may be precursors of T-tubules in early cardiomyocytes, or at least fulfil some of the same signalosome functions [99]. Cav3 induces the formation of caveolae, which plays an important role as a cell signaling hub and in the developing T-tubule system. In a recent study maturation of caveolae in human iPSC-CMs, it has been found to be dramatically increased at day 60 in culture and further increased by day 90, as reflected by the *Cav3* gene and protein expressions [100]. Furthermore, a study conducted by Rebiero et al. also addressed the issue of the foetal-like misalignment of iPSC-CM membrane structures. They reported that culturing cells on micropatterns helped mature the alignment of myofibrils and improved contractile activity, calcium flow, cell electrophysiology, as well as T-tubule formation [101]; thus, providing cells with specific mechanical cues may encourage cell maturation.

The positive and negative chronotropic responses to isoproterenol and carbamylcholine demonstrated the presence of functional adrenergic and cholinergic receptors, respectively, in pacemaker cells. A major pathway of the β-AR–dependent chronotropic response is the activation of AC and the consequent rise in cytosolic cAMP and stimulation of PKA. The positive chronotropic effect exerted by forskolin, a direct activator of AC, and by IBMX, a phosphodiesterase inhibitor, suggests that this signalling pathway is already present early in human cardiomyocyte differentiation [102]. Primitive β-AR signalling responses have been detected as early as 13–15 days of differentiation of mouse and human embryonic stem cell-derived cardiomyocytes (ESC-CMs) [92].

Jung et al. further investigated the evolution of the expression and function of the components involved in the βAR signalling pathway in early human iPSC-CMs. It was found that β_2ARs are the primary source of cAMP/PKA signalling in "early" cardiomyocytes; whereas increasing time in culture leads to the β_1-AR dependent cAMP production to increase to 60% rise from day 30 to day 60 [99]. Similarly, Wu et al. reported a dramatic increase in β_2AR gene expression at days 12, 30, and 60 of differentiation, although no significant changes in β_1AR were seen until day 30. Furthermore, with the use of β_1AR- and β_2AR-specific blockers they showed that iPSC-CMs only responded to β_2-AR receptor activation. At day 60, a switch of β-AR subtype dependence was seen, indicating a dynamic regulation of the receptor dependence of the β-AR signalling pathway during maturation of cardiac myocytes. They also highlighted a significant increase in AC expression after day 12 of differentiation, a level comparable to that of adult human left ventricle tissue. In addition, both PDE3A and PDE4D expression rose by day 60 of maturation [103].

The dysregulation of the β-AR pathway is associated with a spectrum of cardiac diseases. For instance, an iPSC model of dilated cardiomyopathy has shown a blunted response to isoproterenol stimulation. Further, epigenetic changes of the PDE genes were found in tissue from a DCM patient and in iPSC-CMs derived from this, leading to an up-regulation of *PDE2A* and *PDE3A* genes [103]. However, these signalling mechanisms have only been minimally investigated, and that too at the whole-cell level. To understand the full functional capacity of these critical regulatory mechanisms in iPSC-CMs, in-depth investigation into how compartmentation can direct these pathways at the subcellular levels remains to be performed.

10. Conclusions

Understanding the detailed organization of cAMP signalling microdomains in mature myocytes of both atria and ventricles will provide an excellent reference point to which immature or failing myocytes are to be compared. Progressive changes in the microdomain structure and function in HF and dedifferentiation may be deconstructed in order to attempt to reverse these changes. The success of this reversal may correlate with the success of inducing maturation of hiPSC-derived myocytes. In particular, the role or assembly of nascent T-tubules within, or in the vicinity of, caveolae needs further investigation. Equally, PDE isoforms, which are specific for different microdomains need to be further characterized.

Author Contributions: J.G., N.K.B., and A.H. developed the concept, drafted, and critically revised the manuscript.

Acknowledgments: We would like to thank Ms Anita Alvarez-Laviada for helpful discussion and correction of the manuscript. We would also like to thank the British Heart Foundation for its generous support (grants FS/14/62/31288, FS/15/65/32036, RM/17/1/33377 and JG12/18/30088).

References

1. Brunton, L.L.; Hayes, J.S.; Mayer, S.E. Hormonally specific phosphorylation of cardiac troponin I and activation of glycogen phosphorylase. *Nature* **1979**, *280*, 78. [CrossRef] [PubMed]
2. Hayes, J.S.; Brunton, L.L.; Brown, J.H.; Reese, J.B.; Mayer, S.E. Hormonally specific expression of cardiac protein kinase activity. *Proc. Natl. Acad. Sci. USA* **1979**, *76*, 1570–1574. [CrossRef] [PubMed]
3. Buxton, I.L.; Brunton, L.L. Compartments of cyclic AMP and protein kinase in mammalian cardiomyocytes. *J. Biol. Chem.* **1983**, *258*, 10233–10239. [PubMed]
4. Steinberg, S.F.; Brunton, L.L. Compartmentation of G protein-coupled signaling pathways in cardiac myocytes. *Annu. Rev. Pharmacol. Toxicol.* **2001**, *41*, 751–773. [CrossRef] [PubMed]
5. Saucerman, J.J.; Greenwald, E.C.; Polanowska-Grabowska, R. Mechanisms of cyclic AMP compartmentation revealed by computational models. *J. Gen. Physiol.* **2014**, *143*, 39–48. [CrossRef] [PubMed]
6. Xiao, R. Beta-adrenergic signaling in the heart: Dual coupling of the beta2-adrenergic receptor to G (s) and G (i) proteins. *Sci. Stke.* **2001**, *104*, re15.
7. Cheng, X.; Ji, Z.; Tsalkova, T.; Mei, F. Epac and PKA: A tale of two intracellular cAMP receptors. *Acta Biochim. Biophys. Sin.* **2008**, *40*, 651–662. [CrossRef] [PubMed]
8. Di Benedetto, G.; Zoccarato, A.; Lissandron, V.; Terrin, A.; Li, X.; Houslay, M.D.; Baillie, G.S.; Zaccolo, M. Protein kinase A type I and type II define distinct intracellular signaling compartments. *Circ. Res.* **2008**, *103*, 836–844. [CrossRef] [PubMed]
9. DiFrancesco, D.; Tortora, P. Direct activation of cardiac pacemaker channels by intracellular cyclic AMP. *Nature* **1991**, *351*, 145. [CrossRef] [PubMed]
10. Froese, A.; Breher, S.S.; Waldeyer, C.; Schindler, R.F.; Nikolaev, V.O.; Rinné, S.; Wischmeyer, E.; Schlueter, J.; Becher, J.; Simrick, S. Popeye domain containing proteins are essential for stress-mediated modulation of cardiac pacemaking in mice. *J. Clin. Investig.* **2012**, *122*, 1119–1130. [CrossRef] [PubMed]
11. Lands, A.M.; Luduena, F.P.; Buzzo, H.J. Differentiation of receptors responsive to isoproterenol. *Life Sci.* **1967**, *6*, 2241–2249. [CrossRef]
12. Lands, A.; ARNOLD, A.; McAuliff, J.P.; Luduena, F.P.; Jun, T.B. Differentiation of receptor systems activated by sympathomimetic amines. *Nature* **1967**, *214*, 597. [CrossRef] [PubMed]
13. Rohrer, D.K.; Desai, K.H.; Jasper, J.R.; Stevens, M.E.; Regula, D.P.; Barsh, G.S.; Bernstein, D.; Kobilka, B.K. Targeted disruption of the mouse beta1-adrenergic receptor gene: developmental and cardiovascular effects. *Proc. Natl. Acad. Sci. USA* **1996**, *93*, 7375–7380. [CrossRef] [PubMed]
14. Chruscinski, A.J.; Rohrer, D.K.; Schauble, E.; Desai, K.H.; Bernstein, D.; Kobilka, B.K. Targeted disruption of the β2 adrenergic receptor gene. *J. Biol. Chem.* **1999**, *274*, 16694–16700. [CrossRef] [PubMed]
15. Bristow, M.R.; Ginsburg, R.; Umans, V.; Fowler, M.; Minobe, W.; Rasmussen, R.; Zera, P.; Menlove, R.; Shah, P.; Jamieson, S. Beta 1-and beta 2-adrenergic-receptor subpopulations in nonfailing and failing human ventricular myocardium: Coupling of both receptor subtypes to muscle contraction and selective beta 1-receptor down-regulation in heart failure. *Circ. Res.* **1986**, *59*, 297–309. [CrossRef] [PubMed]
16. Nikolaev, V.O.; Moshkov, A.; Lyon, A.R.; Miragoli, M.; Novak, P.; Paur, H.; Lohse, M.J.; Korchev, Y.E.; Harding, S.E.; Gorelik, J. β2-adrenergic receptor redistribution in heart failure changes cAMP compartmentation. *Science* **2010**, *327*, 1653–1657. [CrossRef] [PubMed]
17. Timofeyev, V.; Myers, R.E.; Kim, H.J.; Woltz, R.; Sirish, P.; Heiserman, J.; Li, N.; Singapuri, A.; Tang, T.; Yarov-Yarovoy, V. Adenylyl cyclase subtype-specific compartmentalization: Differential regulation of L-type Ca^{2+} current in ventricular myocytes. *Circ. Res.* **2013**, *112*, 1567–1576. [CrossRef] [PubMed]
18. Okumura, S.; Takagi, G.; Kawabe, J.; Yang, G.; Lee, M.; Hong, C.; Liu, J.; Vatner, D.E.; Sadoshima, J.; Vatner, S.F. Disruption of type 5 adenylyl cyclase gene preserves cardiac function against pressure overload. *Proc. Natl. Acad. Sci. USA* **2003**, *100*, 9986–9990. [CrossRef] [PubMed]
19. Roth, D.M.; Gao, M.H.; Lai, N.C.; Drumm, J.; Dalton, N.; Zhou, J.Y.; Zhu, J.; Entrikin, D.; Hammond, H.K. Cardiac-directed adenylyl cyclase expression improves heart function in murine cardiomyopathy. *Circulation* **1999**, *99*, 3099–3102. [CrossRef] [PubMed]
20. Roth, D.M.; Bayat, H.; Drumm, J.D.; Gao, M.H.; Swaney, J.S.; Ander, A.; Hammond, H.K. Adenylyl cyclase increases survival in cardiomyopathy. *Circulation* **2002**, *105*, 1989–1994. [CrossRef] [PubMed]

21. Tang, T.; Gao, M.H.; Lai, N.C.; Firth, A.L.; Takahashi, T.; Guo, T.; Yuan, J.X.; Roth, D.M.; Hammond, H.K. Adenylyl cyclase type 6 deletion decreases left ventricular function via impaired calcium handling. *Circulation* **2008**, *117*, 61–69. [CrossRef] [PubMed]

22. Pinali, C.; Bennett, H.; Davenport, J.B.; Trafford, A.W.; Kitmitto, A. Three-Dimensional Reconstruction of Cardiac Sarcoplasmic Reticulum Reveals a Continuous Network Linking Transverse-TubulesNovelty and Significance: This Organization Is Perturbed in Heart Failure. *Circ. Res.* **2013**, *113*, 1219–1230. [CrossRef] [PubMed]

23. Bers, D.M. Cardiac excitation-contraction coupling. *Nature* **2002**, *415*, 198–205. [CrossRef] [PubMed]

24. Balijepalli, R.C.; Foell, J.D.; Hall, D.D.; Hell, J.W.; Kamp, T.J. Localization of cardiac L-type Ca^{2+} channels to a caveolar macromolecular signaling complex is required for β2-adrenergic regulation. *Proc. Natl. Acad. Sci. USA* **2006**, *103*, 7500–7505. [CrossRef] [PubMed]

25. Wagner, E.; Brandenburg, S.; Kohl, T.; Lehnart, S.E. Analysis of tubular membrane networks in cardiac myocytes from atria and ventricles. *J. Vis. Exp.* **2014**, *92*, 51823. [CrossRef] [PubMed]

26. Kong, C.H.; Rog-Zielinska, E.A.; Orchard, C.H.; Kohl, P.; Cannell, M.B. Sub-microscopic analysis of t-tubule geometry in living cardiac ventricular myocytes using a shape-based analysis method. *J. Mol. Cell. Cardiol.* **2017**, *108*, 1–7. [CrossRef] [PubMed]

27. Heinzel, F.R.; Bito, V.; Volders, P.G.; Antoons, G.; Mubagwa, K.; Sipido, K.R. Spatial and temporal inhomogeneities during Ca^{2+} release from the sarcoplasmic reticulum in pig ventricular myocytes. *Circ. Res.* **2002**, *91*, 1023–1030. [CrossRef] [PubMed]

28. Hanson, M.A.; Cherezov, V.; Griffith, M.T.; Roth, C.B.; Jaakola, V.; Chien, E.Y.; Velasquez, J.; Kuhn, P.; Stevens, R.C. A specific cholesterol binding site is established by the 2.8 Å structure of the human β 2-adrenergic receptor. *Structure* **2008**, *16*, 897–905. [CrossRef] [PubMed]

29. Bhargava, A.; Lin, X.; Novak, P.; Mehta, K.; Korchev, Y.; Delmar, M.; Gorelik, J. Super-resolution Scanning Patch Clamp Reveals Clustering of Functional Ion Channels in Adult Ventricular MyocyteNovelty and Significance. *Circ. Res.* **2013**, *112*, 1112–1120. [CrossRef] [PubMed]

30. Brandenburg, S.; Kohl, T.; Williams, G.S.; Gusev, K.; Wagner, E.; Rog-Zielinska, E.A.; Hebisch, E.; Dura, M.; Didié, M.; Gotthardt, M. Axial tubule junctions control rapid calcium signaling in atria. *J. Clin. Investig.* **2016**, *126*, 3999–4015. [CrossRef] [PubMed]

31. Richards, M.A.; Clarke, J.D.; Saravanan, P.; Voigt, N.; Dobrev, D.; Eisner, D.A.; Trafford, A.W.; Dibb, K.M. Transverse tubules are a common feature in large mammalian atrial myocytes including human. *Am. J. Physiol.-Heart Circ. Physiol.* **2011**, *301*, H1996–H2005. [CrossRef] [PubMed]

32. Gadeberg, H.C.; Bond, R.C.; Kong, C.H.; Chanoit, G.P.; Ascione, R.; Cannell, M.B.; James, A.F. Heterogeneity of T-tubules in pig hearts. *PLoS ONE* **2016**, *11*, e0156862. [CrossRef] [PubMed]

33. Yamashita, T.; Nakajima, T.; Hazama, H.; Hamada, E.; Murakawa, Y.; Sawada, K.; Omata, M. Regional differences in transient outward current density and inhomogeneities of repolarization in rabbit right atrium. *Circulation* **1995**, *92*, 3061–3069. [CrossRef] [PubMed]

34. Glukhov, A.V.; Balycheva, M.; Sanchez-Alonso, J.L.; Ilkan, Z.; Alvarez-Laviada, A.; Bhogal, N.; Diakonov, I.; Schobesberger, S.; Sikkel, M.B.; Bhargava, A. Direct evidence for microdomain-specific localization and remodeling of functional L-type calcium channels in rat and human atrial myocytes. *Circulation* **2015**, *132*, 2372–2384. [CrossRef] [PubMed]

35. Yue, X.; Zhang, R.; Kim, B.; Ma, A.; Philipson, K.D.; Goldhaber, J.I. Heterogeneity of transverse-axial tubule system in mouse atria: Remodeling in atrial-specific Na^+–Ca^{2+} exchanger knockout mice. *J. Mol. Cell. Cardiol.* **2017**, *108*, 50–60. [CrossRef] [PubMed]

36. Frisk, M.; Koivumäki, J.T.; Norseng, P.A.; Maleckar, M.M.; Sejersted, O.M.; Louch, W.E. Variable t-tubule organization and Ca^{2+} homeostasis across the atria. *Am. J. Physiol.-Heart Circ. Physiol.* **2014**, *307*, H609–H620. [CrossRef] [PubMed]

37. Hayer, A.; Stoeber, M.; Bissig, C.; Helenius, A. Biogenesis of caveolae: Stepwise assembly of large caveolin and cavin complexes. *Traffic* **2010**, *11*, 361–382. [CrossRef] [PubMed]

38. Sinha, B.; Köster, D.; Ruez, R.; Gonnord, P.; Bastiani, M.; Abankwa, D.; Stan, R.V.; Butler-Browne, G.; Vedie, B.; Johannes, L. Cells respond to mechanical stress by rapid disassembly of caveolae. *Cell* **2011**, *144*, 402–413. [CrossRef] [PubMed]

39. Kohl, P.; Cooper, P.J.; Holloway, H. Effects of acute ventricular volume manipulation on in situ cardiomyocyte cell membrane configuration. *Prog. Biophys. Mol. Biol.* **2003**, *82*, 221–227. [CrossRef]

40. Kozera, L.; White, E.; Calaghan, S. Caveolae act as membrane reserves which limit mechanosensitive ICl, swell channel activation during swelling in the rat ventricular myocyte. *PLoS ONE* **2009**, *4*, e8312. [CrossRef] [PubMed]

41. Yang, L.; Scarlata, S. Super-resolution Visualization of Caveola Deformation in Response to Osmotic Stress. *J. Biol. Chem.* **2017**, *292*, 3779–3788. [CrossRef] [PubMed]

42. Mohan, J.; Morén, B.; Larsson, E.; Holst, M.R.; Lundmark, R. Cavin3 interacts with cavin1 and caveolin1 to increase surface dynamics of caveolae. *J. Cell. Sci.* **2015**, *128*, 979–991. [CrossRef] [PubMed]

43. Calaghan, S.; Kozera, L.; White, E. Compartmentalisation of cAMP-dependent signalling by caveolae in the adult cardiac myocyte. *J. Mol. Cell. Cardiol.* **2008**, *45*, 88–92. [CrossRef] [PubMed]

44. Nikolaev, V.O.; Bünemann, M.; Schmitteckert, E.; Lohse, M.J.; Engelhardt, S. Cyclic AMP imaging in adult cardiac myocytes reveals far-reaching β1-adrenergic but locally confined β2-adrenergic receptor–mediated signaling. *Circ. Res.* **2006**, *99*, 1084–1091. [CrossRef] [PubMed]

45. Schobesberger, S.; Wright, P.; Tokar, S.; Bhargava, A.; Mansfield, C.; Glukhov, A.V.; Poulet, C.; Buzuk, A.; Monszpart, A.; Sikkel, M. T-tubule remodelling disturbs localized β2-adrenergic signalling in rat ventricular myocytes during the progression of heart failure. *Cardiovasc. Res.* **2017**, *113*, 770–782. [CrossRef] [PubMed]

46. Wright, P.T.; Nikolaev, V.O.; O'Hara, T.; Diakonov, I.; Bhargava, A.; Tokar, S.; Schobesberger, S.; Shevchuk, A.I.; Sikkel, M.B.; Wilkinson, R. Caveolin-3 regulates compartmentation of cardiomyocyte β2-adrenergic receptor-mediated cAMP signaling. *J. Mol. Cell. Cardiol.* **2014**, *67*, 38–48. [CrossRef] [PubMed]

47. Levin, K.R.; Page, E. Quantitative studies on plasmalemmal folds and caveolae of rabbit ventricular myocardial cells. *Circ. Res.* **1980**, *46*, 244–255. [CrossRef] [PubMed]

48. Burton, R.A.; Rog-Zielinska, E.A.; Corbett, A.D.; Peyronnet, R.; Bodi, I.; Fink, M.; Sheldon, J.; Hoenger, A.; Calaghan, S.C.; Bub, G. Caveolae in rabbit ventricular myocytes: distribution and dynamic diminution after cell isolation. *Biophys. J.* **2017**, *113*, 1047–1059. [CrossRef] [PubMed]

49. Harvey, R.D.; Calaghan, S.C. Caveolae create local signalling domains through their distinct protein content, lipid profile and morphology. *J. Mol. Cell. Cardiol.* **2012**, *52*, 366–375. [CrossRef] [PubMed]

50. Rybin, V.O.; Pak, E.; Alcott, S.; Steinberg, S.F. Developmental changes in β2-adrenergic receptor signaling in ventricular myocytes: the role of Gi proteins and caveolae microdomains. *Mol. Pharmacol.* **2003**, *63*, 1338–1348. [CrossRef] [PubMed]

51. Head, B.P.; Patel, H.H.; Roth, D.M.; Lai, N.C.; Niesman, I.R.; Farquhar, M.G.; Insel, P.A. G-protein-coupled receptor signaling components localize in both sarcolemmal and intracellular caveolin-3-associated microdomains in adult cardiac myocytes. *J. Biol. Chem.* **2005**, *280*, 31036–31044 [CrossRef] [PubMed]

52. Calaghan, S.; White, E. Caveolae modulate excitation–contraction coupling and β2-adrenergic signalling in adult rat ventricular myocytes. *Cardiovasc. Res.* **2006**, *69*, 816–824. [CrossRef] [PubMed]

53. Agarwal, S.R.; MacDougall, D.A.; Tyser, R.; Pugh, S.D.; Calaghan, S.C.; Harvey, R.D. Effects of cholesterol depletion on compartmentalized cAMP responses in adult cardiac myocytes. *J. Mol. Cell. Cardiol.* **2011**, *50*, 500–509. [CrossRef] [PubMed]

54. Lefkimmiatis, K.; Zaccolo, M. cAMP signaling in subcellular compartments. *Pharmacol. Ther.* **2014**, *143*, 295–304. [CrossRef] [PubMed]

55. Zaccolo, M. cAMP signal transduction in the heart: understanding spatial control for the development of novel therapeutic strategies. *Br. J. Pharmacol.* **2009**, *158*, 50–60. [CrossRef] [PubMed]

56. Leroy, J.; Abi-Gerges, A.; Nikolaev, V.O.; Richter, W.; Lechêne, P.; Mazet, J.; Conti, M.; Fischmeister, R.; Vandecasteele, G. Spatiotemporal Dynamics of β-Adrenergic cAMP Signals and L-Type Ca^{2+} Channel Regulation in Adult Rat Ventricular Myocytes. *Circ. Res.* **2008**, *102*, 1091–1100. [CrossRef] [PubMed]

57. Mika, D.; Leroy, J.; Vandecasteele, G.; Fischmeister, R. PDEs create local domains of cAMP signaling. *J. Mol. Cell. Cardiol.* **2012**, *52*, 323–329. [CrossRef] [PubMed]

58. Zaccolo, M. Phosphodiesterases and compartmentalized cAMP signalling in the heart. *Eur. J. Cell Biol.* **2006**, *85*, 693–697. [CrossRef] [PubMed]

59. Mongillo, M.; Zaccolo, M. A complex phosphodiesterase system controls beta-adrenoceptor signalling in cardiomyocytes. *Biochem. Soc. Trans.* **2006**, *34*, 510–511. [CrossRef] [PubMed]

60. Conti, M.; Beavo, J. Biochemistry and physiology of cyclic nucleotide phosphodiesterases: Essential components in cyclic nucleotide signaling. *Annu. Rev. Biochem.* **2007**, *76*, 481–511. [CrossRef] [PubMed]

61. Conti, M.; Mika, D.; Richter, W. Cyclic AMP compartments and signaling specificity: Role of cyclic nucleotide phosphodiesterases. *J. Gen. Physiol.* **2014**, *143*, 29–38. [CrossRef] [PubMed]

62. Lomas, O.; Zaccolo, M. Phosphodiesterases maintain signaling fidelity via compartmentalization of cyclic nucleotides. *Physiology* **2014**, *29*, 141–149. [CrossRef] [PubMed]
63. Rapundalo, S.T.; Solaro, R.J.; Kranias, E.G. Inotropic responses to isoproterenol and phosphodiesterase inhibitors in intact guinea pig hearts: Comparison of cyclic AMP levels and phosphorylation of sarcoplasmic reticulum and myofibrillar proteins. *Circ. Res.* **1989**, *64*, 104–111. [CrossRef] [PubMed]
64. Zaccolo, M.; Pozzan, T. Discrete microdomains with high concentration of cAMP in stimulated rat neonatal cardiac myocytes. *Science* **2002**, *295*, 1711–1715. [CrossRef] [PubMed]
65. Francis, S.H.; Blount, M.A.; Corbin, J.D. Mammalian cyclic nucleotide phosphodiesterases: Molecular mechanisms and physiological functions. *Physiol. Rev.* **2011**, *91*, 651–690. [CrossRef] [PubMed]
66. Francis, S.H.; Corbin, J.D. Structure and function of cyclic nucleotide-dependent protein kinases. *Annu. Rev. Physiol.* **1994**, *56*, 237–272. [CrossRef] [PubMed]
67. Stangherlin, A.; Zaccolo, M. Phosphodiesterases and subcellular compartmentalized cAMP signaling in the cardiovascular system. *Am. J. Physiol.-Heart Circ. Physiol.* **2012**, *302*, H379–H390. [CrossRef] [PubMed]
68. Omori, K.; Kotera, J. Overview of PDEs and their regulation. *Circ. Res.* **2007**, *100*, 309–327. [CrossRef] [PubMed]
69. Verde, I.; Vandecasteele, G.; Lezoualc'h, F.; Fischmeister, R. Characterization of the cyclic nucleotide phosphodiesterase subtypes involved in the regulation of the L-type Ca^{2+} current in rat ventricular myocytes. *Br. J. Pharmacol.* **1999**, *127*, 65–74. [CrossRef] [PubMed]
70. Lugnier, C.; Muller, B.; Le Bec, A.; Beaudry, C.; Rousseau, E. Characterization of indolidan-and rolipram-sensitive cyclic nucleotide phosphodiesterases in canine and human cardiac microsomal fractions. *J. Pharmacol. Exp. Ther.* **1993**, *265*, 1142–1151. [PubMed]
71. Sun, B.; Li, H.; Shakur, Y.; Hensley, J.; Hockman, S.; Kambayashi, J.; Manganiello, V.C.; Liu, Y. Role of phosphodiesterase type 3A and 3B in regulating platelet and cardiac function using subtype-selective knockout mice. *Cell. Signal.* **2007**, *19*, 1765–1771. [CrossRef] [PubMed]
72. Beca, S.; Ahmad, F.; Shen, W.; Liu, J.; Makary, S.; Polidovitch, N.; Sun, J.; Hockman, S.; Chung, Y.W.; Movsesian, M. Phosphodiesterase Type 3A Regulates Basal Myocardial Contractility Through Interacting With Sarcoplasmic Reticulum Calcium ATPase Type 2a Signaling Complexes in Mouse HeartNovelty and Significance. *Circ. Res.* **2013**, *112*, 289–297. [CrossRef] [PubMed]
73. Movsesian, M. New pharmacologic interventions to increase cardiac contractility: Challenges and opportunities. *Curr. Opin. Cardiol.* **2015**, *30*, 285–291. [CrossRef] [PubMed]
74. Richter, W.; Xie, M.; Scheitrum, C.; Krall, J.; Movsesian, M.A.; Conti, M. Conserved expression and functions of PDE4 in rodent and human heart. *Basic Res. Cardiol.* **2011**, *106*, 249–262. [CrossRef] [PubMed]
75. Molina, C.E.; Leroy, J.; Richter, W.; Xie, M.; Scheitrum, C.; Lee, I.; Maack, C.; Rucker-Martin, C.; Donzeau-Gouge, P.; Verde, I. Cyclic adenosine monophosphate phosphodiesterase type 4 protects against atrial arrhythmias. *J. Am. Coll. Cardiol.* **2012**, *59*, 2182–2190. [CrossRef] [PubMed]
76. Melsom, C.B.; Hussain, R.I.; Ørstavik, Ø.; Aronsen, J.M.; Sjaastad, I.; Skomedal, T.; Osnes, J.; Levy, F.O.; Krobert, K.A. Non-classical regulation of β1-and β2-adrenoceptor-mediated inotropic responses in rat heart ventricle by the G protein Gi. *Naunyn Schmiedeberg's Arch. Pharmacol.* **2014**, *387*, 1177–1186. [CrossRef] [PubMed]
77. Conti, M. Subcellular Targeting of PDE4 in Cardiac Myocytes and Generation of Signaling Compartments. In *Microdomains in the Cardiovascular System*; Springer: Cham, Switzerland, 2017; pp. 143–160.
78. Beca, S.; Helli, P.B.; Simpson, J.A.; Zhao, D.; Farman, G.P.; Jones, P.; Tian, X.; Wilson, L.S.; Ahmad, F.; Chen, S.W. Phosphodiesterase 4D regulates baseline sarcoplasmic reticulum Ca^{2+} release and cardiac contractility, independently of L-type Ca^{2+} current. *Circ. Res.* **2011**, *109*, 1024–1030. [CrossRef] [PubMed]
79. Lehnart, S.E.; Wehrens, X.H.; Reiken, S.; Warrier, S.; Belevych, A.E.; Harvey, R.D.; Richter, W.; Jin, S.C.; Conti, M.; Marks, A.R. Phosphodiesterase 4D deficiency in the ryanodine-receptor complex promotes heart failure and arrhythmias. *Cell* **2005**, *123*, 25–35. [CrossRef] [PubMed]
80. Vettel, C.; Lindner, M.; Dewenter, M.; Lorenz, K.; Schanbacher, C.; Riedel, M.; Lämmle, S.; Meinecke, S.; Mason, F.E.; Sossalla, S. Phosphodiesterase 2 protects against catecholamine-induced arrhythmia and preserves contractile function after myocardial infarction. *Circ. Res.* **2016**. [CrossRef]
81. Kajimoto, K.; Hagiwara, N.; Kasanuki, H.; Hosoda, S. Contribution of phosphodiesterase isozymes to the regulation of the L-type calcium current in human cardiac myocytes. *Br. J. Pharmacol.* **1997**, *121*, 1549–1556. [CrossRef] [PubMed]
82. Hua, R.; Adamczyk, A.; Robbins, C.; Ray, G.; Rose, R.A. Distinct patterns of constitutive phosphodiesterase activity in mouse sinoatrial node and atrial myocardium. *PLoS ONE* **2012**, *7*, e47652. [CrossRef] [PubMed]

83. Wei, S.; Guo, A.; Chen, B.; Kutschke, W.; Xie, Y.; Zimmerman, K.; Weiss, R.M.; Anderson, M.E.; Cheng, H.; Song, L. T-Tubule Remodeling During Transition From Hypertrophy to Heart Failure Novelty and Significance. *Circ. Res.* **2010**, *107*, 520–531. [CrossRef] [PubMed]

84. Seidel, T.; Navankasattusas, S.; Ahmad, A.; Diakos, N.A.; Xu, W.D.; Tristani-Firouzi, M.; Bonios, M.J.; Taleb, I.; Li, D.Y.; Selzman, C.H. Sheet-Like Remodeling of the Transverse Tubular System in Human Heart Failure Impairs Excitation-Contraction Coupling and Functional Recovery by Mechanical Unloading Clinical Perspective. *Circulation* **2017**, *135*, 1632–1645. [CrossRef] [PubMed]

85. Lyon, A.R.; MacLeod, K.T.; Zhang, Y.; Garcia, E.; Kanda, G.K.; Korchev, Y.E.; Harding, S.E.; Gorelik, J. Loss of T-tubules and other changes to surface topography in ventricular myocytes from failing human and rat heart. *Proc. Natl. Acad. Sci. USA* **2009**, *106*, 6854–6859. [CrossRef] [PubMed]

86. Ibrahim, M.; Al Masri, A.; Navaratnarajah, M.; Siedlecka, U.; Soppa, G.K.; Moshkov, A.; Al-Saud, S.A.; Gorelik, J.; Yacoub, M.H.; Terracciano, C.M. Prolonged mechanical unloading affects cardiomyocyte excitation-contraction coupling, transverse-tubule structure, and the cell surface. *FASEB J.* **2010**, *24*, 3321–3329. [CrossRef] [PubMed]

87. Dibb, K.M.; Clarke, J.D.; Horn, M.A.; Richards, M.A.; Graham, H.K.; Eisner, D.A.; Trafford, A.W. Characterization of an Extensive Transverse Tubular Network in Sheep Atrial Myocytes and its Depletion in Heart FailureCLINICAL PERSPECTIVE. *Circ. Heart Fail.* **2009**, *2*, 482–489. [CrossRef] [PubMed]

88. Crossman, D.J.; Young, A.A.; Ruygrok, P.N.; Nason, G.P.; Baddelely, D.; Soeller, C.; Cannell, M.B. T-tubule disease: Relationship between t-tubule organization and regional contractile performance in human dilated cardiomyopathy. *J. Mol. Cell. Cardiol.* **2015**, *84*, 170–178. [CrossRef] [PubMed]

89. Galbiati, F.; Engelman, J.A.; Volonte, D.; Zhang, X.L.; Minetti, C.; Li, M.; Hou, H.; Kneitz, B.; Edelmann, W.; Lisanti, M.P. Caveolin-3 null mice show a loss of caveolae, changes in the microdomain distribution of the dystrophin-glycoprotein complex, and t-tubule abnormalities. *J. Biol. Chem.* **2001**, *276*, 21425–21433. [CrossRef] [PubMed]

90. Makarewich, C.A.; Correll, R.N.; Gao, H.; Zhang, H.; Yang, B.; Berretta, R.M.; Rizzo, V.; Molkentin, J.D.; Houser, S.R. A Caveolae-Targeted L-Type Ca^{2+} Channel Antagonist Inhibits Hypertrophic Signaling Without Reducing Cardiac Contractility. *Circ. Res.* **2012**, *110*, 669–674. [CrossRef] [PubMed]

91. Sprenger, J.U.; Perera, R.K.; Steinbrecher, J.H.; Lehnart, S.E.; Maier, L.S.; Hasenfuss, G.; Nikolaev, V.O. In vivo model with targeted cAMP biosensor reveals changes in receptor-microdomain communication in cardiac disease. *Nat. Commun.* **2015**, *6*, 6965. [CrossRef] [PubMed]

92. Maltsev, V.A.; Ji, G.J.; Wobus, A.M.; Fleischmann, B.K.; Hescheler, J. Establishment of β-adrenergic modulation of L-type Ca^{2+} current in the early stages of cardiomyocyte development. *Circ. Res.* **1999**, *84*, 136–145. [CrossRef] [PubMed]

93. Mehel, H.; Emons, J.; Vettel, C.; Wittköpper, K.; Seppelt, D.; Dewenter, M.; Lutz, S.; Sossalla, S.; Maier, L.S.; Lechêne, P. Phosphodiesterase-2 is up-regulated in human failing hearts and blunts β-adrenergic responses in cardiomyocytes. *J. Am. Coll. Cardiol.* **2013**, *62*, 1596–1606. [CrossRef] [PubMed]

94. Seki, S.; Nagashima, M.; Yamada, Y.; Tsutsuura, M.; Kobayashi, T.; Namiki, A.; Tohse, N. Fetal and postnatal development of Ca^{2+} transients and Ca^{2+} sparks in rat cardiomyocytes. *Cardiovasc. Res.* **2003**, *58*, 535–548. [CrossRef]

95. Haddock, P.S.; Coetzee, W.A.; Cho, E.; Porter, L.; Katoh, H.; Bers, D.M.; Jafri, M.S.; Artman, M. Subcellular $[Ca^{2+}]_i$ gradients during excitation-contraction coupling in newborn rabbit ventricular myocytes. *Circ. Res.* **1999**, *85*, 415–427. [CrossRef] [PubMed]

96. Fu, Y.; Hong, T. BIN1 regulates dynamic t-tubule membrane. *Biochim. Biophys. Acta (BBA) Mol. Cell Res.* **2016**, *1863*, 1839–1847. [CrossRef] [PubMed]

97. Rusconi, F.; Ceriotti, P.; Miragoli, M.; Carullo, P.; Salvarani, N.; Rocchetti, M.; Di Pasquale, E.; Rossi, S.; Tessari, M.; Caprari, S. Peptidomimetic Targeting of Cavβ2 Overcomes Dysregulation of the L-Type Calcium Channel Density and Recovers Cardiac FunctionClinical Perspective. *Circulation* **2016**, *134*, 534–546. [CrossRef] [PubMed]

98. Wang, L.; Cui, Y.; Tang, M.; Hu, X.; Luo, H.; Hescheler, J.; Xi, J. Puerarin facilitates T-tubule development of murine embryonic stem cell-derived cardiomyocytes. *Cell. Physiol. Biochem.* **2014**, *34*, 383–392. [CrossRef] [PubMed]

99. Carozzi, A.J.; Ikonen, E.; Lindsay, M.R.; Parton, R.G. Role of cholesterol in developing T-Tubules: Analogous mechanisms for T-tubule and caveolae biogenesis. *Traffic* **2000**, *1*, 326–341. [CrossRef] [PubMed]

100. Jung, G.; Fajardo, G.; Ribeiro, A.J.; Kooiker, K.B.; Coronado, M.; Zhao, M.; Hu, D.; Reddy, S.; Kodo, K.; Sriram, K. Time-dependent evolution of functional vs. remodeling signaling in induced pluripotent stem cell-derived cardiomyocytes and induced maturation with biomechanical stimulation. *FASEB J.* **2016**, *30*, 1464–1479. [CrossRef] [PubMed]

101. Ribeiro, A.J.; Ang, Y.; Fu, J.; Rivas, R.N.; Mohamed, T.M.; Higgs, G.C.; Srivastava, D.; Pruitt, B.L. Contractility of single cardiomyocytes differentiated from pluripotent stem cells depends on physiological shape and substrate stiffness. *Proc. Natl. Acad. Sci. USA* **2015**, *112*, 12705–12710. [CrossRef] [PubMed]

102. Kehat, I.; Kenyagin-Karsenti, D.; Snir, M.; Segev, H.; Amit, M.; Gepstein, A.; Livne, E.; Binah, O.; Itskovitz-Eldor, J.; Gepstein, L. Human embryonic stem cells can differentiate into myocytes with structural and functional properties of cardiomyocytes. *J. Clin. Investig.* **2001**, *108*, 407–414. [CrossRef] [PubMed]

103. Wu, H.; Lee, J.; Vincent, L.G.; Wang, Q.; Gu, M.; Lan, F.; Churko, J.M.; Sallam, K.I.; Matsa, E.; Sharma, A. Epigenetic regulation of phosphodiesterases 2A and 3A underlies compromised β-adrenergic signaling in an iPSC model of dilated cardiomyopathy. *Cell Stem Cell* **2015**, *17*, 89–100. [CrossRef] [PubMed]

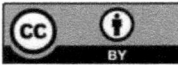

Journal of
Cardiovascular
Development and Disease

MDPI

Review

Polymorphisms/Mutations in A-Kinase Anchoring Proteins (AKAPs): Role in the Cardiovascular System

Santosh V. Suryavanshi *, Shweta M. Jadhav and Bradley K. McConnell *

Department of Pharmacological and Pharmaceutical Sciences, University of Houston College of Pharmacy, Texas Medical Center, Houston, TX 77204, USA; shwetamjadhav@gmail.com
* Correspondence: svsuryavanshi@uh.edu (S.V.S.); bkmcconn@central.uh.edu (B K.M.);
  Tel.: +1-713-743-1220 (S.V.S.); +1-713-743-1218 (B.K.M.)

Received: 5 January 2018; Accepted: 24 January 2018; Published: 25 January 2018

Abstract: A-kinase anchoring proteins (AKAPs) belong to a family of scaffolding proteins that bind to protein kinase A (PKA) by definition and a variety of crucial proteins, including kinases, phosphatases, and phosphodiesterases. By scaffolding these proteins together, AKAPs build a "signalosome" at specific subcellular locations and compartmentalize PKA signaling. Thus, AKAPs are important for signal transduction after upstream activation of receptors ensuring accuracy and precision of intracellular PKA-dependent signaling pathways. Since their discovery in the 1980s, AKAPs have been studied extensively in the heart and have been proven essential in mediating cyclic adenosine monophosphate (cAMP)-PKA signaling. Although expression of AKAPs in the heart is very low, cardiac-specific knock-outs of several AKAPs have a noteworthy cardiac phenotype. Moreover, single nucleotide polymorphisms and genetic mutations in crucial cardiac proteins play a substantial role in the pathophysiology of cardiovascular diseases (CVDs). Despite the significant role of AKAPs in the cardiovascular system, a limited amount of research has focused on the role of genetic polymorphisms and/or mutations in AKAPs in increasing the risk of CVDs. This review attempts to overview the available literature on the polymorphisms/mutations in AKAPs and their effects on human health with a special focus on CVDs.

Keywords: A-kinase anchoring proteins; single nucleotide polymorphisms; genetic mutations; cardiovascular diseases; protein kinase A

---

1. Introduction

The cardiovascular system, which is made up of heart, blood, and blood vessels, is essential for our survival [1]. The human heart provides oxygenated blood to itself and other tissues via a network of blood vessels supplying them with nutrients, and also removes carbon dioxide and other wastes from them. Proper blood circulation is required for effective regulation of these functions. Therefore, the continuous and flawless functioning of the heart becomes a very crucial indicator of normal cardiac physiology. Periodic beatings of the heart are regulated by a plethora of complex intracellular signaling cascades. Similarly, under acute (pregnancy, exercise, etc.) and chronic (pathophysiological stimulations) stress, the heart undergoes physiological and pathophysiological hypertrophy, respectively. Such changes in the anatomy of the heart at the cellular and molecular levels are governed by respective changes in the expression of hypertrophic transcription factors. Expression of essential transcription factors is also regulated by a complex network of intracellular signaling pathways [2,3].

Studying key proteins that are involved in regulating multiple intracellular signaling pathways has always interested cardiovascular scientists across the globe. By participating in the network of several signal transduction processes, these proteins play a central role in cardiac physiology and pathophysiology. A-kinase anchoring proteins (AKAPs) are one such type of proteins that belong to the family of scaffolding proteins. AKAPs have no intrinsic activity of their own, but their crucial function is to bind protein kinase A (PKA) and other signaling proteins [4,5]. PKA-mediated phosphorylation is critical for the physiological functioning of the heart [6]. AKAPs build a "signalosome" at various subcellular locations in the heart and regulate PKA-dependent signaling locally. Similarly, AKAPs speed up the PKA-mediated substrate phosphorylation by bringing all required components into close proximity with each other. Hence, by binding PKA and its substrates in the same scaffold, AKAPs monitor spatial and temporal PKA signaling [7].

AKAPs belong to a class of scaffolding proteins that are structurally not related to each other, but share key structural and/or signaling features. More than 70 AKAPs have been reported so far in humans. To be classified as an AKAP, proteins should have three properties:

(i)   All AKAPs, though structurally different, have 14–18 α-helix amphipathic amino acid sequence that binds to regulatory subunits of PKA.

(ii)   They have a targeting domain that tethers AKAPs to specific subcellular organelles, like mitochondria, the nucleus, and plasma membrane, among others.

(iii)   Lastly, all AKAPs contain multiple binding domains by which they bind to other kinases than PKA, phosphatases, phosphodiesterases, and so on.

As the list of AKAPs is growing, the list of their binding partners is also rising. Hence, at a specific time, AKAPs bind only a subset of their binding partners, which depend on the cellular environment in which they are present [8]. Over the period of the last decade, several AKAPs have been identified in the cardiovascular system. So far, about 17 AKAPs have been discovered in the heart and the list will continue to grow further [9]. Efforts were made to understand the function of individual AKAPs by creating their specific knockouts. To mention a few, our laboratory had developed one such mouse model and has shown that gravin (AKAP12) mutant mice respond better to isoproterenol-induced stimulation than their wild-type counterparts with an improved cardiac profile [10]. Additionally, our unpublished data indicate that AKAP12 scaffolding is crucial for isoproterenol-mediated heart failure, and loss of function of AKAP12 scaffolding can act as a treatment strategy for heart failure [11]. Others have demonstrated that muscle-specific AKAPβ (mAKAPβ) scaffolds crucial signaling proteins around the nuclear envelope of cardiomyocytes that modulate cardiac remodeling. Conditional cardiac-specific deletion of mAKAPβ in adult mice was found to protect the heart from pressure overload and isoproterenol-induced cardiac stress [12]. The AKAP150 scaffold is also one of the promising targets for heart failure treatment. AKAP150 knock-out mice were prone to develop cardiomyopathy under pressure overload and expression of AKAP150 was significantly lower in failing mouse hearts [13].

Despite their importance in cardiac physiology and pathophysiology, there are very limited publications available showing the role of polymorphisms and/or mutations in AKAP in the cardiovascular system. In fact, our laboratory was the first to publish that single nucleotide polymorphisms in mAKAP alter binding propensities of phosphodiesterase4D3 (PDE4D3) and PKA to mAKAP [6]. Therefore, this review will attempt to address all the published literature on polymorphic and mutant AKAP, their role in the cardiovascular system, and their occurrence in other human diseases.

2. Role of AKAPs in Cardiovascular Physiology

AKAPs play a crucial role in human health and disease because of their control over local PKA signaling [3]. As PKA is a cAMP-dependent protein kinase, AKAPs are able to regulate the compartmentalization of cAMP and, therefore, the cAMP/PKA signaling pathway. The cAMP/PKA pathway is ubiquitous and a plethora of biological processes depend on it. Hence, AKAPs have an incomparable contribution in the physiology and pathophysiology of various human diseases [14,15]. In fact, pharmacological targeting of various AKAP-protein interactions has been proved beneficial in cardiovascular diseases, cancer, and other disorders, as shown in animal models of their respective diseases [5,14,16]. To be specific, AKAPs have become very promising drug targets for cardiovascular disease (CVD) due to their role in regulating and coordinating complex cardiac signaling pathways.

The literature on cardiac AKAPs reveals their importance in cardiac health and disease. AKAP-Lbc (AKAP13) is one such AKAP which is a pro-hypertrophic and pro-fibrotic AKAP, where hypertrophy is mediated via interleukin-6 (IL-6) and fibrosis is mediated via the Rho-guanine nucleotide exchange factor, respectively [17,18]. Deletion of AKAP13 in mice exhibited defective cardiac development and embryonic lethality [19]. AKAP150 (AKAP5, AKAP79) has multiple effects on heart function. On one hand, the loss of AKAP150 activates pathological cardiac hypertrophy by interfering with calcium dynamics and myocardial ionotropy, showing that its expression is critical for normal heart function [13]. On the other hand, by activating protein kinase C (PKC), AKAP150 mediates cardiac glucotoxicity [1]. Deletion of AKAP1 (AKAP121, AKAP149) leads to cardiac mitophagy and apoptosis after cardiac insult, thus indicating its role in the mitochondrial function in the heart [20]. mAKAP (AKAP6) is also a pro-hypertrophic AKAP that regulates pathological cardiac hypertrophic signaling pathways by directing the expression of transcription factors nuclear factor of activated T cells, cytoplasmic (NFATc), hypoxia-inducible factor 1 alpha subunit (HIF-1α), myocyte enhancer factor 2D (MEF2D), and histone deacetylase 4 (HDAC4). For this reason, AKAP6 is called the master scaffold for cardiac remodeling [21]. AKAP18 (AKAP15, AKAP7) acts as a nexus of signaling at the sarcoplasmic reticulum by regulating cardiac ionotropy. By binding to both protein phosphatase inhibitor-1 (I-1) and protein phosphatase-1 (PP-1), AKAP18 bi-directionally modulates phospholamban (PLB) phosphorylation and, thus, serves as a crucial regulator of cardiac function [22,23].

Yotiao (AKAP9) is an important AKAP regarding the electrophysiological coupling of the heart. By binding to the potassium channel (KCNQ), this AKAP maintains the slow outward potassium ion current. Specifically, mutations that prevent binding of yotiao and KCNQ result in long QT syndrome [24]. Studies in stem cell-derived cardiomyocytes indicate that AKAP10 (D-AKAP2) is essential in controlling the heart rate and rhythm [25]. Recently, it was shown that AKAP10 is crucial in erythropoietin signaling and heme biosynthesis at the outer mitochondrial membrane [26]. Cardiac phosphoinositide 3-kinase gamma (PI3Kγ) is an AKAP that binds phosphodiesterase3B (PDE3B) and phosphatidylinositol (3,4,5)-trisphosphate (PtdIns(3,4,5)P3) along with PKA regulating cAMP and PtdIns(3,4,5)P3 signaling. The crosstalk between cAMP and PtdIns(3,4,5)P3 is crucial in monitoring β-AR desensitization [27]. The catalytic subunit of PI3Kγ (p110γ) knockout mice exhibited significantly lower PDE3B activity leading to an abrupt increase in cAMP activity. Under stress, p110γ-null mice showed an uncontrolled rise in cAMP with the development of cardiomyopathy [28]. Gravin (AKAP12), on the other hand, is crucial in the β_2-AR desensitization pathway. Our laboratory data revealed that gravin mutant mice performed better under acute isoproterenol stimulation as compared to their wild-type littermates [10]. Overall, these findings strongly suggest the role of AKAPs in cardiac physiology.

3. Polymorphisms/Mutations in AKAPs and CVDs

3.1. DAKAP2 (AKAP10)

Even though AKAPs have been implicated in cardiac disorders, there is a very limited number of publications on the impact of the genetics of AKAPs on CVDs. The first evidence of the direct interaction between polymorphic AKAP and heart disease came in 2003, where the I646V (A to G) polymorphism in D-AKAP2 (AKAP10) was found to be associated with changes in PR interval in the electrocardiography (ECG) of an older population [29]. The PR interval in ECG represents the time starting from the onset of atrial depolarization (the beginning of the P wave) until the onset of ventricular depolarization (the beginning of the QRS complex). It was reported in this study that homozygous valine variants of this old population showed a significantly lower PR intervals (slower atrial depolarization) than individuals who are homozygous for isoleucine. Experimental studies further suggested that this valine variant in AKAP10 had approximately three-fold higher binding to the PKA regulatory subunit RI alpha (PKA-RIα) than with isoleucine. AKAP10 is located in the outer mitochondrial membrane within the cardiomyocyte. Although PKA signaling with respect to AKAP10 is not known, AKAP10 contains a PDZ binding motif which could physically interact with transmembrane receptors and ion channels. Additionally, AKAP10 also contains two regulator of G protein signaling (RGS) domains by which AKAP10 might co-ordinate Gs activation and downstream PKA pathway [29]. Therefore, AKAP10 might scaffold a cardiac ion channel or exchanger. Thus, changes in the localization of PKA-RIα near this region, due to the polymorphic AKAP10, might have a significant impact on phosphorylation states of cardiac ion channel or exchanger leading to modulation of cardiac contraction. [29].

Lower PR intervals in homozygous valine population might be partially due to overactivation of ion channels or exchangers in the heart, and vice versa. Involvement of other possible unknown cell signaling pathways might be possible in the pathophysiology of functional AKAP10 variants. Due to the observed differences in PKA binding and respective changes in ECG due to AKAP10 polymorphism, research from this study showed, for the first time, that functional variants of AKAPs might have direct consequences on the etiology of CVDs. In subsequent studies, it was also shown that the I646V SNP of AKAP10 was common in 122 patients having coronary heart disease, as identified in the Heart and Soul Study (University of California, San Francisco, CA, USA; UCSF) [25]. It was revealed that homozygous carriers of the valine polymorphism had significantly higher heart rates than homozygous isoleucine carriers. Heart rate variability (HRV) and standard deviation of normal-to-normal (SDNN) R-R intervals, where R is the peak of a QRS complex, were found to be significantly lower in these patients. Low HRV and SDNN of R-R intervals are both indicators of sudden cardiac death in patients with some forms of CVDs.

In another study, statistical data revealed that the effects of AKAP10 polymorphisms were independent of age, gender, race, and other heart-related risk parameters [25]. In the same study, and to understand the underlying mechanism, homozygous and heterozygous AKAP10 mutant mice were generated from AKAP10 mutant mouse embryonic stem cells (mESCs) having mutations in AKAP10's PKA binding domain. Both in vivo and in vitro data from this study displayed increased contractile response to cholinergic agonists indicating that AKAP10 variants lead to the increase in vagal nerve sensitivity. Vagal inhibition of the heart was known to reduce pre-disposition to arrhythmia and sudden cardiac death. Hence, changes in vagal nerve sensitivity due to unknown molecular mechanisms contribute to the development of cardiac arrhythmia and death.

Interestingly, it was also found that the 646I allele is exclusively common only in humans, while 15 other non-human animals, including chimpanzees, exhibit valine at 646 [25]. These results were further supported by a larger sample of a healthy middle-aged population of men and women having European ancestry. Association analysis on 1033 unrelated middle-aged men and women showed that participants with homozygous 646V had greater baseline HR and lower HRV values than homozygous 646I individuals. This analysis was done such that the results were not dependent on age, gender, smoking and drinking habits, exercise levels, and blood glucose [30]. In all the studies described above, the valine variant at position 646 was found to be 40% frequent, whereas the isoleucine variant was 60% frequent in all participants. Altogether, these results clearly suggest that the I646V functional variant of AKAP10 affects the sensitivity of heart's pacemaker cells to sympathetic stimulation. In another study of a larger cohort of Japanese individuals, it was revealed that valine at 646 of AKAP10 was significantly associated with higher cases of myocardial infarction (MI) than in people with no history of hypercholesterolemia. The authors concluded that 646V was the risk factor for MI, although the molecular mechanism was not studied [31]. Thus, the AKAP10 I646V variant leads to abrupt heart rate (HR) and HRV changes along with increased risk of MI, possibly making healthy humans susceptible to an increased risk of arrhythmia and sudden cardiac death (Table 1).

In addition to the above-mentioned middle-aged and elderly population studies, the genetics of AKAP10 were also studied in newborns and infants. In polish newborns, 646V homozygous healthy infants showed longer QTc (corrected QT) intervals, but not out of the normal range, than isoleucine homozygous infants, suggesting a possible association between AKAP10 polymorphisms to the QTc interval [32]. Similarly, another study showed significantly higher mean blood pressure (BP) on the day one and the day three post-birth in Polish newborns carrying valine at the 646 position of AKAP10 as compared to isoleucine carriers [33]. Higher cholesterol cord blood concentration was also observed in Polish newborns at the time of birth due to I646V polymorphism in AKAP10. Homozygous valine carrier newborns (GG) had significantly increased levels of cholesterol than heterozygous (AG) and homozygous (AA) isoleucine carriers [34]. Another recent research report identified SNPs in AKAP10 in fetuses with ventricular septal defects and pulmonary stenosis, suggesting AKAP10 as a potential target for these cardiac conditions [35]. These reports suggest that functional AKAP10 variants affect cardiac parameters of newborns and infants, though the underlying molecular mechanisms were not studied. Taken together, AKAP10 polymorphisms play a significant role in increasing the susceptibility of humans of all age groups to develop specific CVDs (Table 1).

3.2. Yotiao (AKAP9)

Pharmacogenomics is a branch of pharmaceutical sciences which comprises studies to understand how genetics affect individual's responses to drugs. Drug-induced prolongation of the QTc interval is a very serious adverse drug reaction causing drug withdrawal [36]. Nearly 1–5% of patients on anti-arrhythmic drug therapy have this severe complication. In one of the studies involving 1351 individuals it was noted that three novel AKAP polymorphisms were related to congenital arrhythmia. SNP in AKAP9 Gln3531Glu was found to be one the novel rare AKAP variants that was observed in congenital arrhythmia cases, which was also highly common in drug-induced Long-QT syndrome (LQTS) (Table 1) [37]. LQTS is one of the inheritable arrhythmia syndromes characterized by prolongation of the QT interval in ECG. LQTS patients undergo syncope, seizures, or cardiac arrest under physical or mental stress [38]. The QT interval indicates the time that is required for the heart muscle to send an electrical impulse through the ventricles and then recharge. LQTS generally occurs due to mutations in cardiac ion channels leading to a defective flow of ions in the heart. If the QT interval is longer than usual, then it will likely lead to a life-threatening ventricular arrhythmia called *torsade de pointes*.

The inheritable S1570L missense mutation in yotiao (AKAP9) was the first report of a disease-causing mutation in an AKAP [39]. Binding of slowly activating delayed rectifier potassium channel alpha subunit (KCNQ1) and yotiao is crucial for delayed rectifier current, which is important during the cardiac cycle of the human heart. Cardiac repolarization is mainly dependent upon rapid and slow delayed-rectifier potassium currents mediated by human ether-a-go-go-related (*hERG*) gene and the *KCNQ1* gene, respectively. KCNQ1 potassium channels become activated after the rapid current in late repolarization phase of the cardiac cycle and both these currents determine the length of action potential duration [40]. Phosphorylation of KCNQ1 is crucial for slow-activating delayed potassium current (I_{Ks}). It was shown that PKA-mediated phosphorylation of KCNQ1 at serine 27 is critical for I_{Ks}. Yotiao (AKAP9) effectively scaffolds PKA and protein phosphatase-1 (PP-1) to KCNQ1, maintaining its phosphorylation levels during upstream receptor activation [41]. The S1570L mutation was found in the KCNQ1-binding domain of yotiao, representing 2% of the clinically-robust LQTS-exhibiting patients. Molecular mechanistic studies showed that this mutation partially inhibits protein-protein interactions of KCNQ1-AKAP9, leading to decreased PKA-mediated phosphorylation of KCNQ1. Decreased phosphorylation of KCNQ1 subsequently resulted in prolonged repolarization of ventricular relaxation due to the elimination of the functional response of I_{Ks} to cAMP. This research displayed a direct link between genetic variants of AKAP and cardiac disease [39]. Furthermore, polymorphisms in AKAP9 were also found to be a modifier of LQTS in the South African population [42]. Four intronic AKAP9 polymorphisms, rs11772585 (C/T), rs7808587 (A/G), rs2282972 (C/T), and rs2961024 (A/C), were studied with or without the presence of the founder mutation, A341V. The rs11772585 T allele, along with the A431V founder mutation, increased the risk of cardiac events by more than two-fold, along with significantly increasing the severity of CVDs. The rs7808587 GG genotype polymorphism increased the risk of developing cardiac events by 74%. Interestingly, the rs2961024 GG genotype increased the QTc interval in the aging population in the absence of A341V mutation while the rs2282972 T allele altered the heart rate and QTc interval [42]. Thus, AKAP9, for the very first time, was shown to modify cardiac disease due to the presence of genetic polymorphisms (Table 1).

3.3. AKAP-Lbc (AKAP13)

Type 2 diabetes (T2D) is a risk factor for coronary artery disease as high blood glucose is known to increase the thickness of the arterial wall. AKAP-Lbc (AKAP13) is a cytoskeleton AKAP that binds to many proteins, including MEK1/2, extracellular signal-regulated kinase-1/2 (ERK1/2), PKCη, and protein kinase D (PKD). The mitogen-activated protein kinase (MAPK) signaling pathway is found to be common in both T2D and coronary artery disease [43]. As AKAP13 binds proteins that are involved in the MAPK pathway, SNPs in AKAP13 were found to be significantly linked with these diseases (Table 1) [43]. Other meta-analysis data on a Genome-Wide Association Study (GWAS) identified SNP in the AKAP13 gene from a Korean population for possible association with high blood pressure [44]. Researchers found that intronic rs11638762 (A/T) SNP in AKAP13, which lies in the GATA-3 binding site, was significantly reproduced in a duplication study done in a completely different group of individuals. AKAP13 scaffolds RhoA along with PKA to mediate activation of Rho family GTPase. Moreover, these GTPases are involved in cardiac hypertrophic signaling and the expression of AKAP13 is upregulated in hypertrophy. Changes in AKAP13 expression were also found to alter the expression of cardiac developmental genes, mainly myocyte enhancer factor 2C [44]. Neonatal death in AKAP10 knock-out mice due to thin-walled heart formation proved that AKAP13 expression is important for the development of the heart. Therefore, the authors hypothesized that the rs11638762 SNP might alter the expression of AKAP13 leading to defective cardiac development, which may have caused alterations in blood pressure levels [44].

3.4. Other AKAPs

Chronic kidney disease is one of the essential risk factors for CVDs. The intronic rs756009 A to G polymorphism in gravin (AKAP12) was associated with a higher risk of chronic kidney disease in Japanese patients with condition that also involves hypertension, diabetes, and high serum cholesterol [45]. However, the underlying molecular mechanisms of this AKAP12 polymorphism on the associated CVD were not studied (Table 1). The obesity-dependent parameters, body mass index (BMI) and waist-hip ratio (WHR), are proven risk factors for T2D and CVD. As such, a GWAS identified that the AKAP6 rs12885467 SNP was significantly associated with higher BMI [46]. Moreover, our unpublished data suggest that mAKAP polymorphisms might make humans more susceptible to cardiovascular diseases by altering cAMP/PKA signaling [47]. Additionally, AKAP7 Gln112Arg and AKAP6 Val839Ala SNPs were reported to be novel rare variants in congenital arrhythmia that were frequently found in drug-induced LQTS [37]. Overall, current evidence on polymorphisms/mutations in AKAPs strongly suggests a significant correlation of genetic variants of AKAPs with the pathophysiology of CVDs.

Table 1. Polymorphisms/mutations in AKAPs and CVDs.

AKAPs	SNPs/Mutations and Heart Disease	Reference
AKAP6	SNP Val839Ala; cardiac arrhythmia	[37]
	SNP rs12885467; higher BMI	[46]
AKAP7	SNP Gln112Arg; cardiac arrhythmia	[37]
AKAP9	SNP Gln3531Glu; cardiac arrhythmia	[37]
	Mutation Ser1570Leu; long-QT syndrome	[39]
	Four SNPs; long-QT Syndrome Type 1	[42]

Table 1. *Cont.*

AKAPs	SNPs/Mutations and Heart Disease	Reference
AKAP10	SNP Ile646Val; decrease in PR interval	[29]
	Mutations; cardiac arrhythmia	[25]
	SNP Ile646Val; myocardial infarction	[31]
	SNP Ile646Val; blood pressure	[33]
	SNP Ile646Val; hypercholesterolemia	[34]
	SNP Ile646Val; heart rate variability	[30]
	SNP Ile646Val; long QTc interval length	[32]
	Copy number variations; ventricular septal defects	[35]
AKAP12	SNP with multiple alleles; chronic kidney disease	[45]
AKAP13	Genetic locus; coronary artery disease	[43]
	SNP; high blood pressure	[44]

4. Polymorphisms/Mutations in AKAPs and Other Human Diseases

4.1. Neurological Disorders

AKAPs have been implicated in human diseases other than CVDs, especially diseases involving the brain, as well as other neurological disorders. Whole exome sequencing analysis of a Chinese family having idiopathic scoliosis (spinal deformity) identified the A2645C mutation in AKAP2 to be inherited in an autosomal dominant fashion [48]. It was also previously shown that disruption of AKAP2 expression, via de novo translocation, may contribute to Kallmann syndrome and bone anomalies [49]. Hence, AKAP2 may have a significant role in the pathogenesis of scoliosis. The K873R SNP in AKAP9 was linked to increased risk of developing schizophrenia in a Spanish population [50]. The AKAP9 SNPs rs144662445 (A/G, I to M) and rs149979685 (C/T, S to L) were found in seven African American Alzheimer's disease patients and replicated successfully in the Alzheimer Disease Genetics Consortium (ADGC) population of 1037 cases and 1869 controls [51]. R3233C and R3832C variants of AKAP9 were identified and found to be prevalent in high-risk autism families [52]. In fact, AKAPs might have an incomparable role in etiology of autism spectrum disorders (ASDs). Single nucleotide polymorphisms in six AKAPs (AKAP7, AKAP10, AKAP11, microtubule-associated protein 2 (MAP2), moesin (MSN), and neurobeachin (NBEA)) were identified with possible association with ASDs. Especially, the SNP rs5918959 near the *MSN* gene displayed genome-wide significance [53]. The DNA copy variants in eight AKAP genes (AKAP5, AKAP8, AKAP9, AKAP10, AKAP13, MAP2, MSN, and NBEA) were also found in individuals with ASDs [53].

In yet other studies, AKAP5, shown to be present in all levels of the human brain, was observed to have a variable copy number in schizophrenia, bipolar disorder, and major depression behavior [54]. AKAP5 is involved in post-synaptic G-protein-coupled receptors (GPCRs)-mediated intracellular signaling which is known to have a role in modulating emotional behavior. Furthermore, studies involving AKAP5 polymorphisms revealed that the P100L polymorphism (rs2230491) affected the behavioral response of its carriers. Proline-carrying individuals had higher behavioral performance and working memory for emotional faces, while the less common leucine carriers exhibited greater control of their anger, but poor control of physical aggression [55,56]. Additional studies in the search of finding molecular mechanisms behind these behavioral changes showed that leucine carriers activated the anterior cingulate cortex (ACC), while proline homozygous individuals activated the orbitofrontal cortex (OFC) in the brain, as identified during emotional evaluation studies [56]. mAKAP (AKAP6) is one of the well-studied AKAPs in the heart. AKAP6 is expressed in cardiac muscle, skeletal muscle, and brain. In addition to its role in the heart, AKAP6 polymorphisms were found in GWAS studies to be related to various other human disorders. The intronic rs2383378 SNP was found to be associated with anorexia nervosa [57] and another intronic rs4296166 SNP was found to increase the risk of developing Alzheimer's disease [58]. The rs17522122 SNP was found to be one of the genetic variants that significantly affect general fluid cognitive functioning in middle and old-age population of 53,949 individuals in the Cohorts for Heart and Aging Research in Genomic Epidemiology (CHARGE) consortium [59]. In a recent study, the rs17522122 T allele (found in UTR-3) SNP was associated with poor performance with respect to episodic memory in older populations, as identified in the Personality And Total Health (PATH) study [60]. Thus, polymorphisms in AKAPs were found to be significantly associated with a plethora of neurological disorders in humans.

4.2. Cancers

Genetic variants of AKAPs have been reported to be very common in the patient populations of various cancers. The whole genome and transcriptome sequencing data have shown that the AKAP2 gene is mutated in gastric and peritoneal metastatic cancer [61]. Yotiao (AKAP9) is a crucial AKAP with an important role in cell cycle progression, centrosome, and cell membrane function. Genetic mutations in AKAP9 are linked to a variety of cancers. Four AKAP9 mutations were associated with gastric cancer and 20 mutations were linked to colorectal cancer [62]. The single nucleotide polymorphisms M463I, 1389G > T and N2792S, 8375A > G in AKAP9 were found to increase the risk of familial breast cancer in German women [63]. The non-synonymous SNP M463I (rs6964587) in AKAP9 was also found to be very an important breast cancer susceptibility polymorphism [64]. The T allele of rs6964587 was frequent in African American, Asian, and European women. The AKAP9 M463I variant was also associated to increase the susceptibility of lung cancer in a large United Kingdom Caucasian population [65]. We previously discussed that the functional polymorphism I646V in D-AKAP2 (AKAP10) has a significant role in the cardiovascular system. In addition, heterozygous and homozygous expression of this valine variant in AKAP10 was also significantly increased in women with colorectal cancer as compared to isoleucine carriers [66]. Additionally, the valine AKAP10 variant carriers were also found to have increased risk of developing familial breast cancer [67]. Furthermore, the AKAP13 K526Q SNP, along with I646V in AKAP10, further augmented the risk for breast cancer [67]. Since AKAP13 plays a crucial scaffolding role in Rho GTPase intracellular signaling, SNPs in this protein may also affect various cancers. The polymorphisms R494W, K526Q, N1086D, and G2461S in AKAP13 were all found in familial breast cancer patients with K526Q having the highest association among all of these SNPs [68]. SNPs in gravin (AKAP12) were also identified to be significantly associated with breast cancer risk and osteosarcoma [69,70]. In conclusion, mutated and/or polymorphic AKAPs have been associated with the increased risk of different types of cancers in humans.

4.3. Other Human Disorders

In addition to neurological diseases and cancers, polymorphic AKAPs were also associated with a few other human disorders. The heterozygous mutation in AKAP4 (887G > A; G296N) was found in men with low sperm motility, a condition known as asthenozoospermia [71]. AKAP4 is a testis-specific AKAP and its removal in mice leads to reduced sperm motility, resulting in infertility. As this mutation was absent in matched control males, this AKAP4 mutation might be the probable cause of male infertility [71]. Another report found that mutations in AKAP4 may cause sperm fibrous sheath dysplasia [72]. In another study, SNPs in the AKAP ezrin were found to increase the risk and development of age-related cataracts [73]. Finally, the AKAP11 genetic locus was identified in the GWAS to be significantly associated with osteoporosis [74]. In summary, genetic variations in AKAPs have also been significantly implicated in other human diseases along with CVDs (Figure 1).

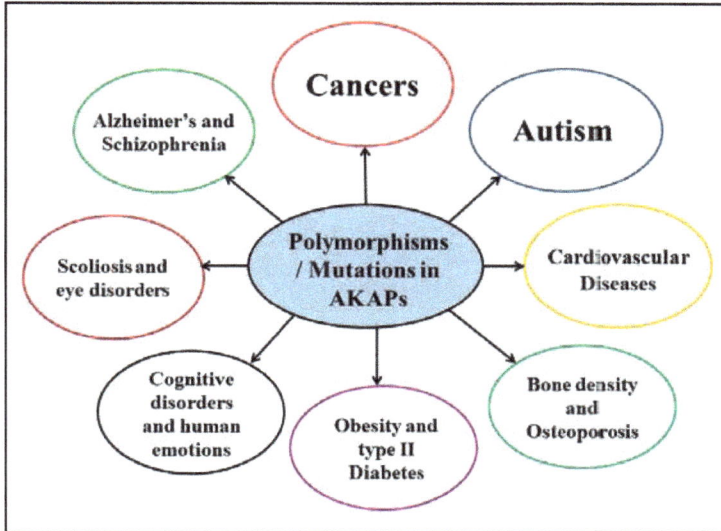

Figure 1. Genetics of AKAPs and human diseases.

5. Conclusions

AKAPs are a group of proteins that scaffold PKA by definition. Along with binding and localizing PKA to specific subcellular compartments, AKAPs also scaffold other proteins in the vicinity of PKA, thus efficiently regulating intracellular PKA-dependent signaling cascades. Additional proteins that AKAPs bind include a variety of other kinases, phosphatases, phosphodiesterases, GPCRs, and signaling proteins. Moreover, AKAPs have been reported to play a pivotal role in both the physiology and the pathophysiology of human diseases. However, the role of genetics in AKAPs with respect to human diseases has been underappreciated, especially in the cardiovascular system where polymorphisms/mutations in AKAPs have been shown to increase the risk of developing various CVDs. Molecular mechanisms behind increasing the risk of CVDs were also studied in certain candidate AKAPs. Similarly, numerous SNPs were identified that increased the susceptibility of individuals to develop cancers, brain disorders, male infertility, and eye disorders. We believe that the majority of the literature only mentions the SNPs and/or mutations in AKAPs with their respective human disorders. However, we think that genetic variants in AKAPs should also be further studied with respect to the molecular mechanisms involved in these disorders. Although very few attempts were made in studying the mechanistic pathways in increasing the risk of developing cardiovascular disease, a substantial amount of additional research should be done with respect to CVDs, as well as other human diseases.

Acknowledgments: This work and open access charges were financed from the National Institutes of Health National Heart, Lung, and Blood Institute (grant R15HL124458 to (B.K.M.)) and a grant from the Robert J. Kleberg, Jr. and Helen C. Kleberg Foundation (to B.K.M.)

Author Contributions: S.V.S. and B.K.M. conceived and designed the outline of the manuscript; S.V.S., S.M.J., and B.K.M. wrote the manuscript; and S.V.S. and S.M.J. prepared the figure and table.

Conflicts of Interest: The authors declare no conflict of interest.

References

1. Diviani, D.; Reggi, E.; Arambasic, M.; Caso, S.; Maric, D. Emerging roles of A-kinase anchoring proteins in cardiovascular pathophysiology. *Biochim. Biophys. Acta* **2016**, *1863*, 1926–1936. [CrossRef] [PubMed]
2. Shimizu, I.; Minamino, T. Physiological and pathological cardiac hypertrophy. *J. Mol. Cell Cardiol.* **2016**, *97*, 245–262. [CrossRef] [PubMed]
3. Rababa'h, A.; Singh, S.; Suryavanshi, S.V.; Altarabsheh, S.E.; Deo, S.V.; McConnell, B.K. Compartmentalization role of A-kinase anchoring proteins (AKAPs) in mediating protein kinase A (PKA) signaling and cardiomyocyte hypertrophy. *Int. J. Mol. Sci.* **2014**, *16*, 218–229. [CrossRef] [PubMed]
4. Li, Z.; Singh, S.; Suryavanshi, S.V.; Ding, W.; Shen, X.; Wijaya, C.S.; Gao, W.D.; McConnell, B.K. Force development and intracellular Ca^{2+} in intact cardiac muscles from gravin mutant mice. *Eur. J. Pharmacol.* **2017**, *807*, 117–126. [CrossRef] [PubMed]
5. Carnegie, G.K.; Means, C.K.; Scott, J.D. A-kinase anchoring proteins: From protein complexes to physiology and disease. *IUBMB Life* **2009**, *61*, 394–406. [CrossRef] [PubMed]
6. Rababa'h, A.; Craft, J.W., Jr.; Wijaya, C.S.; Atrooz, F.; Fan, Q.; Singh, S.; Guillory, A.N.; Katsonis, P.; Lichtarge, O.; McConnell, B.K. Protein kinase A and phosphodiesterase-4D3 binding to coding polymorphisms of cardiac muscle anchoring protein (mAKAP). *J. Mol. Biol.* **2013**, *425*, 3277–3288.
7. Kapiloff, M.S.; Chandrasekhar, K.D. A-kinase anchoring proteins: Temporal and spatial regulation of intracellular signal transduction in the cardiovascular system. *J. Cardiovasc. Pharmacol.* **2011**, *58*, 337–338. [CrossRef] [PubMed]
8. Wong, W.; Scott, J.D. AKAP signalling complexes: Focal points in space and time. *Nat. Rev. Mol. Cell Biol.* **2004**, *5*, 959–970. [CrossRef] [PubMed]
9. Kritzer, M.D.; Li, J.; Dodge-Kafka, K.; Kapiloff, M.S. AKAPs: The architectural underpinnings of local camp signaling. *J. Mol. Cell Cardiol.* **2012**, *52*, 351–358. [CrossRef] [PubMed]
10. Guillory, A.N.; Yin, X.; Wijaya, C.S.; Diaz Diaz, A.C.; Rababa'h, A.; Singh, S.; Atrooz, F.; Sadayappan, S.; McConnell, B.K. Enhanced cardiac function in gravin mutant mice involves alterations in the beta-adrenergic receptor signaling cascade. *PLoS ONE* **2013**, *8*, e74784. [CrossRef] [PubMed]
11. McConnell, B.; Suryavanshi, S.; Fa'ak, F.; Diaz, A.D.; Singh, S. Disruption of gravin's scaffolding protects against isoproterenol induced heart failure. *FASEB J.* **2016**, *30*, 718.
12. Kritzer, M.D.; Li, J.; Passariello, C.L.; Gayanilo, M.; Thakur, H.; Dayan, J.; Dodge-Kafka, K.; Kapiloff, M.S. The scaffold protein muscle A-kinase anchoring protein beta orchestrates cardiac myocyte hypertrophic signaling required for the development of heart failure. *Circ. Heart Fail.* **2014**, *7*, 663–672. [CrossRef] [PubMed]
13. Li, L.; Li, J.; Drum, B.M.; Chen, Y.; Yin, H.; Guo, X.; Luckey, S.W.; Gilbert, M.L.; McKnight, G.S.; Scott, J.D.; et al. Loss of AKAP150 promotes pathological remodelling and heart failure propensity by disrupting calcium cycling and contractile reserve. *Cardiovasc. Res.* **2017**, *113*, 147–159. [CrossRef] [PubMed]
14. Dema, A.; Perets, E.; Schulz, M.S.; Deak, V.A.; Klussmann, E. Pharmacological targeting of AKAP-directed compartmentalized camp signalling. *Cell Signal.* **2015**, *27*, 2474–2487. [CrossRef] [PubMed]
15. Michel, J.J.; Scott, J.D. AKAP mediated signal transduction. *Annu. Rev. Pharmacol. Toxicol.* **2002**, *42*, 235–257. [CrossRef] [PubMed]
16. Troger, J.; Moutty, M.C.; Skroblin, P.; Klussmann, E. A-kinase anchoring proteins as potential drug targets. *Br. J. Pharmacol.* **2012**, *166*, 420–433. [CrossRef] [PubMed]
17. Cavin, S.; Maric, D.; Diviani, D. A-kinase anchoring protein-Lbc promotes pro-fibrotic signaling in cardiac fibroblasts. *Biochim. Biophys. Acta* **2014**, *1843*, 335–345. [CrossRef] [PubMed]
18. Del Vescovo, C.D.; Cotecchia, S.; Diviani, D. A-kinase-anchoring protein-Lbc anchors ikappab kinase beta to support interleukin-6-mediated cardiomyocyte hypertrophy. *Mol. Cell Biol.* **2013**, *33*, 14–27. [CrossRef] [PubMed]
19. Mayers, C.M.; Wadell, J.; McLean, K.; Venere, M.; Malik, M.; Shibata, T.; Driggers, P.H.; Kino, T.; Guo, X.C.; Koide, H.; et al. The rho guanine nucleotide exchange factor AKAP13 (brx) is essential for cardiac development in mice. *J. Biol. Chem.* **2010**, *285*, 12344–12354. [CrossRef] [PubMed]
20. Schiattarella, G.G.; Cattaneo, F.; Pironti, G.; Magliulo, F.; Carotenuto, G.; Pirozzi, M.; Polishchuk, R.; Borzacchiello, D.; Paolillo, R.; Oliveti, M.; et al. AKAP1 deficiency promotes mitochondrial aberrations and exacerbates cardiac injury following permanent coronary ligation via enhanced mitophagy and apoptosis. *PLoS ONE* **2016**, *11*, e0154076. [CrossRef] [PubMed]

21. Passariello, C.L.; Li, J.; Dodge-Kafka, K.; Kapiloff, M.S. mAKAP—A master scaffold for cardiac remodeling. *J. Cardiovasc. Pharmacol.* **2015**, *65*, 218–225. [CrossRef] [PubMed]
22. Redden, J.M.; Dodge-Kafka, K.L. AKAP phosphatase complexes in the heart. *J. Cardiovasc. Pharmacol.* **2011**, *58*, 354–362. [CrossRef] [PubMed]
23. Singh, A.; Redden, J.M.; Kapiloff, M.S.; Dodge-Kafka, K.L. The large isoforms of A-kinase anchoring protein 18 mediate the phosphorylation of inhibitor-1 by protein kinase A and the inhibition of protein phosphatase 1 activity. *Mol. Pharmacol.* **2011**, *79*, 533–540. [CrossRef] [PubMed]
24. Li, Y.; Chen, L.; Kass, R.S.; Dessauer, C.W. The A-kinase anchoring protein Yotiao facilitates complex formation between adenylyl cyclase type 9 and the I_{Ks} potassium channel in heart. *J. Biol. Chem.* **2012**, *287*, 29815–29824. [CrossRef] [PubMed]
25. Tingley, W.G.; Pawlikowska, L.; Zaroff, J.G.; Kim, T.; Nguyen, T.; Young, S.G.; Vranizan, K.; Kwok, P.Y.; Whooley, M.A.; Conklin, B.R. Gene-trapped mouse embryonic stem cell-derived cardiac myocytes and human genetics implicate AKAP10 in heart rhythm regulation. *Proc. Natl. Acad. Sci. USA* **2007**, *104*, 8461–8466. [CrossRef] [PubMed]
26. Chung, J.; Wittig, J.G.; Ghamari, A.; Maeda, M.; Dailey, T.A.; Bergonia, H.; Kafina, M.D.; Coughlin, E.E.; Minogue, C.E.; Hebert, A.S.; et al. Erythropoietin signaling regulates heme biosynthesis. *Elife* **2017**, *6*. [CrossRef] [PubMed]
27. Perrino, C.; Schroder, J.N.; Lima, B.; Villamizar, N.; Nienaber, J.J.; Milano, C.A.; Naga Prasad, S.V. Dynamic regulation of phosphoinositide 3-kinase-γ activity and β-adrenergic receptor trafficking in end-stage human heart failure. *Circulation* **2007**, *116*, 2571–2579. [CrossRef] [PubMed]
28. Perino, A.; Ghigo, A.; Ferrero, E.; Morello, F.; Santulli, G.; Baillie, G.S.; Damilano, F.; Dunlop, A.J.; Pawson, C.; Walser, R.; et al. Integrating cardiac PIP3 and cAMP signaling through a PKA anchoring function of p110γ. *Mol. Cell* **2011**, *42*, 84–95. [CrossRef] [PubMed]
29. Kammerer, S.; Burns-Hamuro, L.L.; Ma, Y.; Hamon, S.C.; Canaves, J.M.; Shi, M.M.; Nelson, M.R.; Sing, C.F.; Cantor, C.R.; Taylor, S.S.; et al. Amino acid variant in the kinase binding domain of dual-specific a kinase-anchoring protein 2: A disease susceptibility polymorphism. *Proc. Natl. Acad. Sci. USA* **2003**, *100*, 4066–4071. [CrossRef] [PubMed]
30. Neumann, S.A.; Tingley, W.G.; Conklin, B.R.; Shrader, C.J.; Peet, E.; Muldoon, M.F.; Jennings, J.R.; Ferrell, R.E.; Manuck, S.B. AKAP10 (i646v) functional polymorphism predicts heart rate and heart rate variability in apparently healthy, middle-aged European-Americans. *Psychophysiology* **2009**, *46*, 466–472. [CrossRef] [PubMed]
31. Nishihama, K.; Yamada, Y.; Matsuo, H.; Segawa, T.; Watanabe, S.; Kato, K.; Yajima, K.; Hibino, T.; Yokoi, K.; Ichihara, S.; et al. Association of gene polymorphisms with myocardial infarction in individuals with or without conventional coronary risk factors. *Int. J. Mol. Med.* **2007**, *19*, 129–141. [CrossRef] [PubMed]
32. Loniewska, B.; Kaczmarczyk, M.; Clark, J.S.; Goracy, I.; Horodnicka-Jozwa, A.; Ciechanowicz, A. Association of functional genetic variants of A-kinase anchoring protein 10 with QT interval length in full-term polish newborns. *Arch. Med. Sci.* **2015**, *11*, 149–154. [CrossRef] [PubMed]
33. Loniewska, B.; Kaczmarczyk, M.; Clark, J.S.; Binczak-Kuleta, A.; Adler, G.; Kordek, A.; Horodnicka-Jozwa, A.; Dawid, G.; Rudnicki, J.; Ciechanowicz, A. Association of 1936a > g in AKAP10 (A-kinase anchoring protein 10) and blood pressure in polish full-term newborns. *Blood Press* **2013**, *22*, 51–56. [CrossRef] [PubMed]
34. Loniewska, B.; Kaczmarczyk, M.; Clark, J.S.; Kordek, A.; Ciechanowicz, A. Polymorphism 1936a > g in the AKAP10 gene (encoding A-kinase-anchoring protein 10) is associated with higher cholesterol cord blood concentration in polish full-term newborns. *J. Perinat. Med.* **2013**, *41*, 205–210. [CrossRef] [PubMed]
35. Fu, F.; Deng, Q.; Lei, T.Y.; Li, R.; Jing, X.Y.; Yang, X.; Liao, C. Clinical application of SNP array analysis in fetuses with ventricular septal defects and normal karyotypes. *Arch. Gynecol. Obstet.* **2017**, *296*, 929–940. [CrossRef] [PubMed]
36. Wilke, R.A.; Lin, D.W.; Roden, D.M.; Watkins, P.B.; Flockhart, D.; Zineh, I.; Giacomini, K.M.; Krauss, R.M. Identifying genetic risk factors for serious adverse drug reactions: Current progress and challenges. *Nat. Rev. Drug Discov.* **2007**, *6*, 904–916. [CrossRef] [PubMed]
37. Ramirez, A.H.; Shaffer, C.M.; Delaney, J.T.; Sexton, D.P.; Levy, S.E.; Rieder, M.J.; Nickerson, D.A.; George, A.L., Jr.; Roden, D.M. Novel rare variants in congenital cardiac arrhythmia genes are frequent in drug-induced torsades de pointes. *Pharmacogenomics J.* **2013**, *13*, 325–329. [CrossRef] [PubMed]

38. Schwartz, P.J.; Crotti, L.; Insolia, R. Long-QT syndrome: From genetics to management. *Circ. Arrhythm. Electrophysiol.* **2012**, *5*, 868–877. [CrossRef] [PubMed]

39. Chen, L.; Marquardt, M.L.; Tester, D.J.; Sampson, K.J.; Ackerman, M.J.; Kass, R.S. Mutation of an A-kinase-anchoring protein causes long-QT syndrome. *Proc. Natl. Acad. Sci. USA* **2007**, *104*, 20990–20995. [CrossRef] [PubMed]

40. Moss, A.J.; Kass, R.S. Long QT syndrome: From channels to cardiac arrhythmias. *J. Clin. Investig.* **2005**, *115*, 2018–2024. [CrossRef] [PubMed]

41. Chen, L.; Sampson, K.J.; Kass, R.S. Cardiac delayed rectifier potassium channels in health and disease. *Card. Electrophysiol. Clin.* **2016**, *8*, 307–322. [CrossRef] [PubMed]

42. De Villiers, C.P.; van der Merwe, L.; Crotti, L.; Goosen, A.; George, A.L., Jr.; Schwartz, P.J.; Brink, P.A.; Moolman-Smook, J.C.; Corfield, V.A. AKAP9 is a genetic modifier of congenital long-QT syndrome type 1. *Circ. Cardiovasc. Genet.* **2014**, *7*, 599–606. [CrossRef] [PubMed]

43. Dong, C.; Tang, L.; Liu, Z.; Bu, S.; Liu, Q.; Wang, Q.; Mai, Y.; Wang, D.W.; Duan, S. Landscape of the relationship between type 2 diabetes and coronary heart disease through an integrated gene network analysis. *Gene* **2014**, *539*, 30–36. [CrossRef] [PubMed]

44. Hong, K.W.; Lim, J.E.; Oh, B. A regulatory SNP in AKAP13 is associated with blood pressure in Koreans. *J. Hum. Genet.* **2011**, *56*, 205–210. [CrossRef] [PubMed]

45. Yoshida, T.; Kato, K.; Yokoi, K.; Oguri, M.; Watanabe, S.; Metoki, N.; Yoshida, H.; Satoh, K.; Aoyagi, Y.; Nozawa, Y.; et al. Association of gene polymorphisms with chronic kidney disease in Japanese individuals. *Int. J. Mol. Med.* **2009**, *24*, 539–547. [PubMed]

46. Horikoshi, M.; Mgi, R.; van de Bunt, M.; Surakka, I.; Sarin, A.P.; Mahajan, A.; Marullo, L.; Thorleifsson, G.; Hgg, S.; Hottenga, J.J.; et al. Discovery and fine-mapping of glycaemic and obesity-related trait loci using high-density imputation. *PLoS Genet.* **2015**, *11*, e1005230. [CrossRef] [PubMed]

47. Suryavanshi, S.; Jadhav, S.; Anderson, K.; Katsonis, P.; Lichtarge, O.; McConnell, B.K. Abstract 24010: Muscle-specific A-kinase anchoring protein polymorphisms pre-dispose humans to cardiovascular diseases by affecting cyclic AMP/PKA signaling. *Circulation* **2017**, *136*, A24010.

48. Li, W.; Li, Y.; Zhang, L.; Guo, H.; Tian, D.; Li, Y.; Peng, Y.; Zheng, Y.; Dai, Y.; Xia, K.; et al. AKAP2 identified as a novel gene mutated in a Chinese family with adolescent idiopathic scoliosis. *J. Med. Genet.* **2016**, *53*, 488–493. [CrossRef] [PubMed]

49. Panza, E.; Gimelli, G.; Passalacqua, M.; Cohen, A.; Gimelli, S.; Giglio, S.; Ghezzi, C.; Sparatore, B.; Heye, B.; Zuffardi, O.; et al. The breakpoint identified in a balanced de novo translocation t(7;9)(p14.1;q31.3) disrupts the A-kinase (PRKA) anchor protein 2 gene (AKAP2) on chromosome 9 in a patient with kallmann syndrome and bone anomalies. *Int. J. Mol. Med.* **2007**, *19*, 429–435. [CrossRef] [PubMed]

50. Suarez-Rama, J.J.; Arrojo, M.; Sobrino, B.; Amigo, J.; Brenlla, J.; Agra, S.; Paz, E.; Brion, M.; Carracedo, A.; Paramo, M.; et al. Resequencing and association analysis of coding regions at twenty candidate genes suggest a role for rare risk variation at AKAP9 and protective variation at nrxn1 in schizophrenia susceptibility. *J. Psychiatr. Res.* **2015**, *66–67*, 38–44. [CrossRef] [PubMed]

51. Logue, M.W.; Schu, M.; Vardarajan, B.N.; Farrell, J.; Bennett, D.A.; Buxbaum, J.D.; Byrd, G.S.; Ertekin-Taner, N.; Evans, D.; Foroud, T.; et al. Two rare AKAP9 variants are associated with Alzheimer's disease in African Americans. *Alzheimer's Dement.* **2014**, *10*, 609–618. [CrossRef] [PubMed]

52. Matsunami, N.; Hensel, C.H.; Baird, L.; Stevens, J.; Otterud, B.; Leppert, T.; Varvil, T.; Hadley, D.; Glessner, J.T.; Pellegrino, R.; et al. Identification of rare DNA sequence variants in high-risk autism families and their prevalence in a large case/control population. *Mol. Autism* **2014**, *5*, 5. [CrossRef] [PubMed]

53. Poelmans, G.; Franke, B.; Pauls, D.L.; Glennon, J.C.; Buitelaar, J.K. AKAPs integrate genetic findings for autism spectrum disorders. *Transl. Psychiatry* **2013**, *3*, e270. [CrossRef] [PubMed]

54. Wilson, G.M.; Flibotte, S.; Chopra, V.; Melnyk, B.L.; Honer, W.G.; Holt, R.A. DNA copy-number analysis in bipolar disorder and schizophrenia reveals aberrations in genes involved in glutamate signaling. *Hum. Mol. Genet.* **2006**, *15*, 743–749. [CrossRef] [PubMed]

55. Richter, S.; Gorny, X.; Machts, J.; Behnisch, G.; Wustenberg, T.; Herbort, M.C.; Munte, T.F.; Seidenbecher, C.I.; Schott, B.H. Effects of AKAP5 pro100leu genotype on working memory for emotional stimuli. *PLoS ONE* **2013**, *8*, e55613. [CrossRef] [PubMed]

56. Richter, S.; Gorny, X.; Marco-Pallares, J.; Kramer, U.M.; Machts, J.; Barman, A.; Bernstein, H.G.; Schule, R.; Schols, L.; Rodriguez-Fornells, A.; et al. A potential role for a genetic variation of AKAP5 in human aggression and anger control. *Front. Hum. Neurosci.* **2011**, *5*, 175. [CrossRef] [PubMed]

57. Wang, K.; Zhang, H.; Bloss, C.S.; Duvvuri, V.; Kaye, W.; Schork, N.J.; Berrettini, W.; Hakonarson, H.; Price Foundation Collaborative Group. A genome-wide association study on common SNPs and rare CNVs in anorexia nervosa. *Mol. Psychiatry* **2011**, *16*, 949–959. [CrossRef] [PubMed]

58. Seshadri, S.; Fitzpatrick, A.L.; Ikram, M.A.; DeStefano, A.L.; Gudnason, V.; Boada, M.; Bis, J.C.; Smith, A.V.; Carassquillo, M.M.; Lambert, J.C.; et al. Genome-wide analysis of genetic loci associated with alzheimer disease. *JAMA* **2010**, *303*, 1832–1840. [CrossRef] [PubMed]

59. Davies, G.; Armstrong, N.; Bis, J.C.; Bressler, J.; Chouraki, V.; Giddaluru, S.; Hofer, E.; Ibrahim-Verbaas, C.A.; Kirin, M.; Lahti, J.; et al. Genetic contributions to variation in general cognitive function: A meta-analysis of genome-wide association studies in the charge consortium (N = 53,949). *Mol Psychiatry* **2015**, *20*, 183–192. [CrossRef] [PubMed]

60. Andrews, S.J.; Das, D.; Anstey, K.J.; Easteal, S. Association of AKAP6 and mir2113 with cognitive performance in a population-based sample of older adults. *Genes Brain Behav.* **2017**, *16*, 472–478. [CrossRef] [PubMed]

61. Zhang, J.; Huang, J.Y.; Chen, Y.N.; Yuan, F.; Zhang, H.; Yan, F.H.; Wang, M.J.; Wang, G.; Su, M.; Lu, G.; et al. Whole genome and transcriptome sequencing of matched primary and peritoneal metastatic gastric carcinoma. *Sci. Rep.* **2015**, *5*, 13750. [CrossRef] [PubMed]

62. Jo, Y.S.; Kim, M.S.; Yoo, N.J.; Lee, S.H. Frameshift mutations of AKAP9 gene in gastric and colorectal cancers with high microsatellite instability. *Pathol. Oncol. Res.* **2016**, *22*, 587–592. [CrossRef] [PubMed]

63. Frank, B.; Wiestler, M.; Kropp, S.; Hemminki, K.; Spurdle, A.B.; Sutter, C.; Wappenschmidt, B.; Chen, X.; Beesley, J.; Hopper, J.L.; et al. Association of a common AKAP9 variant with breast cancer risk: A collaborative analysis. *J. Natl. Cancer Inst.* **2008**, *100*, 437–442. [CrossRef] [PubMed]

64. Milne, R.L.; Burwinkel, B.; Michailidou, K.; Arias-Perez, J.I.; Zamora, M.P.; Menendez-Rodriguez, P.; Hardisson, D.; Mendiola, M.; Gonzalez-Neira, A.; Pita, G.; et al. Common non-synonymous SNPs associated with breast cancer susceptibility: Findings from the breast cancer association consortium. *Hum. Mol. Genet.* **2014**, *23*, 6096–6111. [CrossRef] [PubMed]

65. Rudd, M.F.; Webb, E.L.; Matakidou, A.; Sellick, G.S.; Williams, R.D.; Bridle, H.; Eisen, T.; Houlston, R.S.; Consortium, G. Variants in the *GH-IGF* axis confer susceptibility to lung cancer. *Genome Res.* **2006**, *16*, 693–701. [CrossRef] [PubMed]

66. Wang, M.; Zhang, D.; Wang, R.; Rui, Y.; Zhou, J.; Wang, R.; Zhou, B.; Huang, X.; Yang, L.; Li, Y.; et al. A-kinase anchoring proteins 10 expression in relation to 2073a/g polymorphism and tumor progression in patients with colorectal cancer. *Pathol. Oncol. Res.* **2013**, *19*, 521–527. [CrossRef] [PubMed]

67. Wirtenberger, M.; Schmutzhard, J.; Hemminki, K.; Meindl, A.; Sutter, C.; Schmutzler, R.K.; Wappenschmidt, B.; Kiechle, M.; Arnold, N.; Weber, B.H.; et al. The functional genetic variant ile646val located in the kinase binding domain of the A-kinase anchoring protein 10 is associated with familial breast cancer. *Carcinogenesis* **2007**, *28*, 423–426. [CrossRef] [PubMed]

68. Wirtenberger, M.; Tchatchou, S.; Hemminki, K.; Klaes, R.; Schmutzler, R.K.; Bermejo, J.L.; Chen, B.; Wappenschmidt, B.; Meindl, A.; Bartram, C.R.; et al. Association of genetic variants in the rho guanine nucleotide exchange factor AKAP13 with familial breast cancer. *Carcinogenesis* **2006**, *27*, 593–598. [CrossRef] [PubMed]

69. Kresse, S.H.; Rydbeck, H.; Skarn, M.; Namlos, H.M.; Barragan-Polania, A.H.; Cleton-Jansen, A.M.; Serra, M.; Liestol, K.; Hogendoorn, P.C.; Hovig, E.; et al. Integrative analysis reveals relationships of genetic and epigenetic alterations in osteosarcoma. *PLoS ONE* **2012**, *7*, e48262. [CrossRef] [PubMed]

70. Sun, Y.; Ye, C.; Guo, X.; Wen, W.; Long, J.; Gao, Y.T.; Shu, X.O.; Zheng, W.; Cai, Q. Evaluation of potential regulatory function of breast cancer risk locus at 6q25.1. *Carcinogenesis* **2016**, *37*, 163–168. [CrossRef] [PubMed]

71. Visser, L.; Westerveld, G.H.; Xie, F.; van Daalen, S.K.; van der Veen, F.; Lombardi, M.P.; Repping, S. A comprehensive gene mutation screen in men with asthenozoospermia. *Fertil. Steril.* **2011**, *95*, 1020–1024.e9. [CrossRef] [PubMed]

72. Baccetti, B.; Collodel, G.; Estenoz, M.; Manca, D.; Moretti, E.; Piomboni, P. Gene deletions in an infertile man with sperm fibrous sheath dysplasia. *Hum. Reprod.* **2005**, *20*, 2790–2794. [CrossRef] [PubMed]

73. Lin, Q.; Zhou, N.; Zhang, N.; Zhu, B.; Hu, S.; Zhou, Z.; Qi, Y. Genetic variations and polymorphisms in the ezrin gene are associated with age-related cataract. *Mol. Vis.* **2013**, *19*, 1572–1579. [PubMed]
74. Zhang, L.; Choi, H.J.; Estrada, K.; Leo, P.J.; Li, J.; Pei, Y.F.; Zhang, Y.; Lin, Y.; Shen, H.; Liu, Y.Z.; et al. Multistage genome-wide association meta-analyses identified two new loci for bone mineral density. *Hum. Mol. Genet.* **2014**, *23*, 1923–1933. [CrossRef] [PubMed]

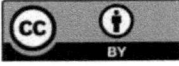

Journal of
*Cardiovascular
Development and Disease*

MDPI

Review

Cyclic Nucleotide-Directed Protein Kinases in Cardiovascular Inflammation and Growth

Nathan A. Holland, Jake T. Francisco, Sean C. Johnson, Joshua S. Morgan, Troy J. Dennis [iD]**, Nishitha R. Gadireddy and David A. Tulis** *[iD]

Department of Physiology, Brody School of Medicine, East Carolina University, 600 Moye Boulevard, Greenville, NC 27834, USA; hollandn17@ecu.edu (N.A.H.); franciscoj13@students.ecu.edu (J.T.F.); johnsonse12@students.ecu.edu (S.C.J.); morganjo15@students.ecu.edu (J.S.M.); dennist15@students.ecu.edu (T.J.D.); gadireddyn16@students.ecu.edu (N.R.G.)
* Correspondence: tulisd@ecu.edu; Tel.: +1-252-744-2771

Received: 3 January 2018; Accepted: 19 January 2018; Published: 23 January 2018

Abstract: Cardiovascular disease (CVD), including myocardial infarction (MI) and peripheral or coronary artery disease (PAD, CAD), remains the number one killer of individuals in the United States and worldwide, accounting for nearly 18 million (>30%) global deaths annually. Despite considerable basic science and clinical investigation aimed at identifying key etiologic components of and potential therapeutic targets for CVD, the number of individuals afflicted with these dreaded diseases continues to rise. Of the many biochemical, molecular, and cellular elements and processes characterized to date that have potential to control foundational facets of CVD, the multifaceted cyclic nucleotide pathways continue to be of primary basic science and clinical interest. Cyclic adenosine monophosphate (cyclic AMP) and cyclic guanosine monophosphate (cyclic GMP) and their plethora of downstream protein kinase effectors serve ubiquitous roles not only in cardiovascular homeostasis but also in the pathogenesis of CVD. Already a major target for clinical pharmacotherapy for CVD as well as other pathologies, novel and potentially clinically appealing actions of cyclic nucleotides and their downstream targets are still being discovered. With this in mind, this review article focuses on our current state of knowledge of the cyclic nucleotide-driven serine (Ser)/threonine (Thr) protein kinases in CVD with particular emphasis on cyclic AMP-dependent protein kinase (PKA) and cyclic GMP-dependent protein kinase (PKG). Attention is given to the regulatory interactions of these kinases with inflammatory components including interleukin 6 signals, with G protein-coupled receptor and growth factor signals, and with growth and synthetic transcriptional platforms underlying CVD pathogenesis. This article concludes with a brief discussion of potential future directions and highlights the importance for continued basic science and clinical study of cyclic nucleotide-directed protein kinases as emerging and crucial controllers of cardiac and vascular disease pathologies.

Keywords: cyclic nucleotide; G protein-coupled receptor; interleukin 6; myocardial infarction; inflammation; protease-activated receptor; protein kinase; Smad3; Stat3; vascular smooth muscle

1. Introduction

Cardiovascular disease (CVD) is a complex and multifaceted class of diseases or disorders of the heart and/or blood vessels and constitutes the number one killer of individuals in the United States [1] and worldwide, accounting for ~18 million (>30%) global deaths annually [2]. Of the many forms of CVD including arterial or venous thromboses, myocarditis, hypertension and valve dysfunction, myocardial infarction (MI) and peripheral or coronary artery disease (PAD, CAD, respectively) represent two of the most significant and account for the vast majority of CVD-related deaths [1]. Notwithstanding significant advances in our understanding of many of the foundational elements underlying CVD realized through extensive basic and clinical investigation, precise and fully effective therapeutic targets have yet to be identified and the prevalence of CVD continues to rise and is expected to afflict ~44% of the US population by the year 2030 [1]. In parallel, the economic burden of CVD, currently estimated over $316 billion per year for direct and indirect costs in the United States alone, is anticipated to surpass $900 billion by 2030 [1]. Undoubtedly, the health and economic impacts of CVD are of utmost significance, and in turn, identification and characterization of key underpinnings in the pathogenesis of CVD in an effort to discern potential therapeutic effectors and/or strategies is most warranted.

In this light, over many years a plethora of bioactive elements and signaling processes has been identified as serving a wide variety of roles in cardiovascular physiology and disease. Of these, the ubiquitous and multifunctional cyclic nucleotide second messenger systems, comprised primarily of purine $3',5'$-cyclic adenosine monophosphate (cyclic AMP) and purine $3',5'$-cyclic guanosine monophosphate (cyclic GMP) and their downstream serine (Ser)/threonine (Thr) protein kinase effectors, serve a multitude of roles in normal vessel physiology and homeostasis and also in the pathogenesis of cardiac and vascular disorders [3]. Of particular interest in cardiovascular tissues are members of the cyclic nucleotide-driven AGC family of Ser/Thr protein kinases: cyclic AMP-dependent protein kinase (PKA), cyclic GMP-dependent protein kinase (PKG), and calcium (Ca^{2+})-activated phospholipid-dependent protein kinase C (PKC) [4]. These robust signaling molecules serve extensive roles in many homeostatic and pathologic processes. Moreover, considering the documented promiscuity and cross-talk amongst protein kinase family members [5–8] and interactions with associated kinases including protein kinase B (PKB/Akt), protein kinase D (PKD), and adenosine monophosphate (AMP)-activated protein kinase (AMPK), the expansion of the biological impact of these kinases is of potential clinical importance in CVD. This review article focuses on our current state of knowledge of the cyclic nucleotide-driven Ser/Thr protein kinases and their related kinase effectors as emerging and important controllers of cardiac and vascular disease pathology [3].

Many functional processes contribute to the development and/or maintenance of CVD depending on the exact nature of the disease or disorder. As mentioned, CVD comprises a large and diverse class, with MI and arterial diseases considered the most critical and clinically significant. In the causation of MI and arterial disease pathologies, primary functional events associated with tissue perfusion include disruption of blood flow or ischemia with ensuing hypoxia and localized acidosis and complications associated with re-establishment of blood flow or re-perfusion injury. Additional contributors to these pathologies can include extensive tissue inflammation, cell necrosis and apoptosis/necroptosis with compromised tissue function, and loss of a quiescent homeostatic phenotype with onset of aberrant cellular growth/wound healing leading to adverse tissue remodeling [6,9,10]. At the biochemical and molecular level, a host of mechanisms underlie these functional changes and include, notably, an array of immune and inflammatory responses, membrane receptor-mediated signals including G protein-coupled receptor (GPCR) and growth factor pathways, and transcriptional platforms for synthetic and proliferative proteins. In this respect, this review article discusses the biological significance of inflammatory interleukin-6 (IL-6) signaling, acidosis-sensitive GPCRs and protease-activated receptors (PARs), synthetic transforming growth factor-β (TGF-β) and its primary Smad-dependent processes, and a transcriptional Smad/FoxO relationship during CVD. Particular attention is then given to the regulatory influence of cyclic nucleotide-directed Ser/Thr protein kinases on these processes as foundational elements of cardiac and vascular pathology. This review concludes with a short synopsis of key findings and highlights the importance for continued basic science and clinical study of cyclic nucleotide-directed protein kinases in CVD.

2. Cyclic Nucleotides and Cyclic Nucleotide-Directed Protein Kinases

As mentioned, the purine-based second messengers cyclic AMP and cyclic GMP are firmly established as essential modulators of wide-ranging cellular functions in mammalian tissues including those in the cardiovascular system. Detailed biomolecular mechanisms for the generation of cyclic

AMP and cyclic GMP have been previously described [7,10–12]. In brief, synthesis of cyclic AMP occurs via multiple processes including stimulation of adenylate cyclase (AC) by direct ligand agonism, by β-adrenergic induction, or by GPCRs coupled to stimulatory G proteins (G$_s$). Following AC stimulation, dephosphorylation of adenosine triphosphate (ATP) yields cyclic AMP and pyrophosphate (PPi). In like fashion, cyclic GMP is synthesized via activation of guanylate cyclase (GC), which can occur by natriuretic peptides (NPs) which activate particulate, membrane-bound GC, or by gaseous ligands such as nitric oxide (NO) or carbon monoxide (CO) which activate soluble GC (sGC). Activated GC then dephosphorylates guanosine triphosphate (GTP) to yield cyclic GMP and PPi. Following synthesis, cyclic AMP and cyclic GMP predominantly exert their effects through respective Ser/Thr AGC kinase family members PKA and PKG [4,5,7,10]. Cyclic AMP can also operate through alternate non-canonical kinase-directed pathways [5], through direct ion current modulation via cyclic nucleotide-gated (CNG) ion channels [13], via binding to Popeye domain-containing (POPDC) proteins [14,15], or through exchange proteins directly activated by cyclic AMP (EPAC) [16,17]. Similarly, cyclic GMP can activate CNG ion channels [13], can act on alternate non-canonical kinases besides PKG and can have kinase-independent effects as well [9]. Cyclic nucleotide signaling can be largely governed by internal localization via scaffolding proteins such as A-kinase anchoring protein for cyclic AMP [18] and inositol 1,4,5-triphosphate (IP$_3$) receptor-associated cGMP kinase substrate (IRAG) and Huntingtin-associated protein 1 (HAP1) for cyclic GMP [19,20]. Lastly, persistence of cyclic AMP and cyclic GMP signals is largely governed by specific phosphodiesterases (PDEs), which cleave their phosphodiester bonds and degrade them into inactive 5'-monophosphates [21]. The schematic in Figure 1 depicts primary routes for synthesis of cyclic AMP and cyclic GMP, their main regulatory modulators, and their respective activation of downstream targets including protein kinase pathways.

Protein kinases have the capacity to serve in a host of physiological and pathophysiological processes and represent one of the most diverse and ubiquitous families in the human genome, constituting ~2% of human genes with over 500 human protein kinases identified thus far [5,22]. Through reversible phosphotransferase-mediated, site-specific (Ser/Thr) phosphorylation of effector proteins, PKA and PKG provoke robust signal transduction cascades with the capacity to control a myriad of intracellular processes. Comprehensive reviews on the mechanisms of action of these protein kinases and others have been published [23,24] and herein only a brief synopsis is provided. In sum, ATP binds to an active site in a conserved catalytic domain (~250 amino acids in length) located between one lobe of N-terminal β-sheets and a second lobe of C-terminal α-helices [25]. Following binding, a set of conserved residues in the catalytic domain transfers the terminal γ-phosphate of ATP to the hydroxyl oxygen of the receiving residue (Ser/Thr) on the target [23,26], after which substrate is released, ADP is removed and phosphorylation-driven activation or inactivation of the downstream effector ensues. This kinase-driven, post-translational, phosphorylation-specific modification of effector proteins then dictates enzyme and protein expression and/or activities and downstream functions including those elemental to cardiac and vascular disease or dysfunction. Uniquely, despite this common mechanism across diverse protein kinases, kinase specificity is imparted by differences in hydrophobicity of surface residues, unique aspects of the active catalytic site and differential kinetics of ATP binding, the overall charge of the enzyme, and presence or absence of anchoring or scaffolding proteins and other accessory proteins along with sub-cellular localization of the kinase.

A caveat must be mentioned when discussing the kinase-mediated impact on target proteins. While Ser/Thr kinases (as well as Tyr kinases) typically act on their preferred residue, they are also attracted to residues flanking their canonical phosphoacceptor site. Among similar substrate family members, the catalytic cleft of these kinases has the capacity to interact with common recognition sequences adjacent to their preferred substrate (Ser/Thr, Tyr), thereby reducing kinase specificity and permitting 'promiscuous' kinase signal transduction. Our research team and others have documented promiscuity and signaling cross-talk for not only the cyclic nucleotide-driven kinases but also for their upstream modes of activation including the second messengers themselves [5–10,27–33]. In this regard, kinase 'cross-talk' affords broad impact of upstream kinase activation but also lends difficulty in determining discrete downstream signaling pathways and effector targets of kinase-mediated events.

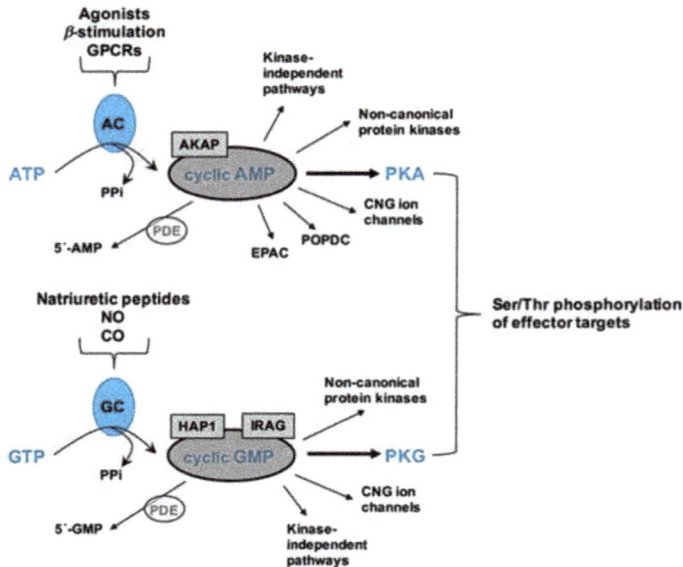

Figure 1. Schematic of cyclic adenosine monophosphate (cyclic AMP) and cyclic guanosine monophosphate (cyclic GMP) signaling. Following activation of adenylate cyclase (AC) by upstream processes including direct ligand agonism, B-adrenergic stimulation, or by stimulatory G protein-coupled receptors (GPCRs), adenosine triphosphate (ATP) is dephosphorylated to yield cyclic AMP and pyrophosphate (PPi). In similar fashion, stimulation of membrane-bound or soluble guanylate cyclase (GC) by natriuretic peptides or gaseous ligands nitric oxide (NO) and/or carbon monoxide (CO), GTP is dephosphorylated to yield cyclic GMP and PPi. Persistence of cyclic nucleotide signaling can be governed by the presence of scaffolding proteins including A-kinase anchoring protein for cyclic AMP or IP$_3$ receptor-associated cGMP kinase substrate (IRAG) and Huntingtin-associated protein 1 (HAP1) for cyclic GMP, and by degradation into inactive 5'-monophosphates by a family of phosphodiesterases (PDEs). Cyclic AMP can operate through kinase-independent pathways, through binding to cyclic nucleotide-gated (CNG) ion channels or Popeye domain-containing proteins (POPDC), via exchange proteins directly activated by cyclic AMP (EPAC), through non-canonical protein kinases or by activation of PKA. In like manner, cyclic GMP can signal through kinase-independent pathways, by binding to CNG ion channels, through non-canonical protein kinases or via PKG. The predominant protein kinases for cyclic AMP and cyclic GMP, PKA, and PKG, can then stimulate Ser/Thr residues on many diverse downstream effector targets to help control normal physiology and homeostasis as well as wide-ranging pathophysiological processes in cardiac and vascular tissues.

It warrants brief mention that in opposition to the Ser/Thr protein kinases a family of dephosphorylating Ser/Thr protein phosphatases (PPs) exists that serves to maintain phosphorylative balance [34,35]. Removal of a phosphate group or groups from Ser/Thr residues by PPs curbs phosphorylation-mediated events in Ser/Thr kinase-targeted proteins and helps to moderate kinase-driven processes. Interestingly, only about 30 Ser/Thr PPs have been identified in the human genome (compared to >400 Ser/Thr protein kinases [5,22,34,35]), which is attributed to their unique combination of homoenzymes from shared catalytic subunits and their large number of regulatory subunits [35]. With respect to cardiovascular physiology and disease, Ser/Thr PPs in addition to their complementary Ser/Thr kinases must be considered for full evaluation of the phosphorylative balance and its potential therapeutic utility [8,36].

From a clinical perspective, mutations in Ser/Thr protein kinases have been linked to human diseases, and protein kinases currently represent a large percentage of all putative protein drug targets [37–40]. In fact, many protein kinases presently serve as discrete targets for use in precision medicine for cardiac and vascular diseases [3] and they likely represent the next major drug development target for diseases and disorders of the cardiovascular system (and others) in the next century [41,42].

3. Vascular Physiology & Pathology

Excellent comprehensive reviews have been published recently that highlight important aspects of blood vessel anatomy and function under homeostatic and pathologic conditions [7,9,43]. In sum, normal arterial anatomy consists of three primary layers: tunica intima, tunica media and tunica externa. A single layer of vascular endothelial cells (VEC) encircle the blood-containing lumen and constitutes the tunica intima. Intimal VECs are normally exposed to laminar shear stress and provide an important interface between flowing thrombogenic blood and the blood vessel wall [43]. In this capacity VECs are responsible for secreting bioactive substances, including the vasodilators NO, CO and prostaglandin I_2 (PGI$_2$) and the vasoconstrictors thromboxane A_2 (TXA$_2$) and angiotensin II (Ang II), that communicate with the underlying vascular smooth muscle (VSM) through the basement membrane in order to control vascular tone [43]. The tunica media, the blood vessel inner layer, contains vascular smooth muscle cells (VSMCs) as well as structural collagen and elastin and is responsible for maintaining normal vascular contraction and dilation. This vessel reactivity, in turn, controls localized intravascular pressures and tissue perfusion [44]. Medial VSMCs are known to be much more plastic than other vessel wall cells because they handle many functions such as contraction and dilation as well as proliferation and extracellular matrix (ECM) synthesis [44]. The outward component of the vessel wall is the tunica externa or adventitia which contains sparse fibroblasts and VSMCs, a vasa vasorum blood supply, and local nerve endings and inflammatory cells spaced throughout the supporting connective tissue [43]. Perivascular adipose tissue located on the outside of the tunica adventitia plays a role in support and anchoring of the vessel yet has also been suggested to serve a role in energy metabolism, regulation of vascular tone, the release of adipokines, and in the storage of free fatty acids and triglycerides [43]. A schematic depicting these key elements in a cross-section of a blood vessel wall is shown in Figure 2.

The predominant overall function of the arterial vasculature is to provide blood flow and nutrients to essential downstream tissues in order to ensure their proper function under homeostatic as well as abnormal conditions. In return, the venous system serves as the conduit for removal of metabolic byproducts and wastes including carbon dioxide for elimination from the body. Based on the amount and functionality of local VSM, most blood vessels have ability to constrict or relax as needed in order to adequately control blood flow and, in turn, to properly supply tissues with blood and nutrients including oxygen as needed per local metabolic demand. In this light, the vasculature provides a basal state of tonic contraction termed vascular tone (or 'myogenic tone' if derived from the VSM itself). In brief, to first summarize vessel contraction, extracellular calcium entry (via voltage-gated, ligand-gated, and/or stretch-activated Ca^{2+} channels) induces intracellular Ca^{2+} levels to rise (via the release of Ca^{2+} from intracellular stores). This elevated intracellular Ca^{2+} then binds to calmodulin and sequentially activates cytosolic Ser/Thr myosin light chain kinase, which then phosphorylates regulatory myosin light chain and activates myosin ATPase activity. This ATPase then initiates actin-myosin cross-bridge formation and cycling and the establishment/maintenance of vessel contraction [10,11]. For vessel relaxation, removal of intracellular Ca^{2+} is the first step and this can occur via re-sequestration back into intracellular stores and/or removal from the cell by Ca^{2+} channels. Following the Law of Mass Action, Ca^{2+} unbinds from calmodulin, myosin light chain kinase activity decreases, myosin phosphatase dephosphorylates myosin light chains, which in turn reduces myosin ATPase activity and muscle tension is decreased. Vascular tone can be regulated by extrinsic (neurohumoral elements, CNS innervation) and intrinsic (VSM-derived, myogenic) elements and so can be determined by numerous influences including competing vasoconstrictor and vasodilator factors and local metabolic demand of downstream tissues in organ- and tissue-specific fashion. Low-level vascular tone results from numerous and differential states of cross-bridge formation that can develop which leads to various contractile states of the VSM including notably a basal steady-state level of contraction (tone). Regarding cyclic nucleotide control of vascular tone, both cyclic AMP/PKA and cyclic GMP/PKG can operate via several mechanisms to reduce intracellular Ca^{2+}, to inhibit myosin light chain phosphorylation, and to stimulate Ca^{2+}-activated potassium channels and promote hyperpolarization, all resulting in reduction in vascular contractility and tone and promotion of vessel relaxation (loss of tone) [10,11].

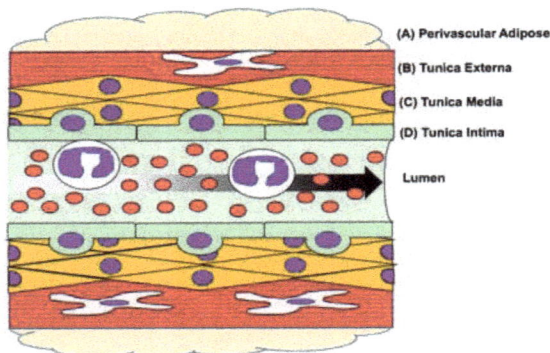

Figure 2. Layers of a blood vessel. Cartoon cross-sectional image of a blood vessel with major layers and cell types depicted. The outermost perivascular fat (**A**) lends support and anchoring for the vessel as well as mediates adipocyte production and influences cellular metabolism. The outermost layer of the vessel proper, the tunica adventitia (**B**); is largely a structural layer of the vessel wall and is comprised of extracellular matrix (ECM) containing resident immune cells, an internal vascular supply (vasa vasorum), sparse nerve endings and fibroblasts. The majority of the arterial vessel wall is comprised of the tunica media (**C**); mostly vascular smooth muscle cells (VSMCs) and ECM. Medial VSMCs are responsible for vasoconstriction and relaxation (i.e., vessel tone) that controls luminal blood flow. The innermost layer of the blood vessel is the tunica intima (**D**) and is comprised of a single layer of vascular endothelial cells (VECs) that surround the lumen of the vessel, that form a critical interface between flowing blood and the vessel wall, and that communicate with the underlying VSMCs to help regulate tone and direct inflammatory responses. Arrow indicates direction of luminal blood flow.

Despite the essential role that our circulatory system plays in normal cardiovascular health, pathological conditions such as vascular disease, dysfunction or injury constitute the number one contributor to CVD [2]. Two primary components in the pathogenesis of vascular disease or injury include overt inflammation of the intimal endothelial lining and abnormal synthesis and growth of medial VSMCs [9,45,46]. In diseased or dysfunctional VECs, production and release of inflammatory cytokines along with increased substrate adhesiveness contribute to the recruitment of leukocytes, which adhere to the (activated) cells, transmigrate and provoke an inflammatory response [47]. In this process, increased expression of vascular cell adhesion molecules, cytokines, and chemokines is essential for the VEC-leukocyte interaction and subsequent inflammation; thus, identification and characterization of molecular mediators and events that regulate VEC inflammation and adhesion is critical. In this light, key VEC inflammatory mediators have been identified including E-selectin, ICAM-I, and VCAM-1 that have potential to serve as therapeutic targets to combat VEC inflammation in the context of CVD [48]. Complementing VEC-driven inflammation is the VSM-dependent proliferative, synthetic 'evolution' phase of CVD pathogenesis [5,9,10,49]. In response to pathologic insult, VSMCs undergo phenotypic switching from homeostatic and contractile to synthetic, migratory and proliferative. This phenotypic conversion is manifested as reduced contractility and a reorganized architecture complete with medial wall remodeling and stenotic neointima development [9,44,50]. This neointimal growth involves fibroblast and cellular accumulation in the perturbed intimal space that results in excessive synthesis and deposition of ECM components and loss of luminal caliber resulting in altered or occluded blood flow [51]. Although vascular remodeling and neointimal formation initially serve as adaptations they can soon progress into uncontrolled, pathologic and self-perpetuating cascades with severe clinical repercussions.

Vessel wall remodeling and neointimal hyperplasia can provoke and serve as a key component of atherogenesis, the process of the build-up of fats and cholesterol (along with numerous cells, matrix components, etc.) in an occlusive plaque on the inner blood vessel wall. Atherosclerosis is the major cause of adverse cardiovascular events including stroke, MI, and peripheral limb ischemia or claudication [1]. Atherosclerosis is multifactorial and complex, combining elements of inflammation and cellular adhesion, VEC dysfunction, formation of reactive oxygen and nitrogen species and oxidative/nitrosative stresses, foam cell development, VSMC migration and proliferation, enhanced ECM development, and formation and evolution of a stenotic plaque within the lumen. If plaque complication and rupture ensue, thrombus formation and adverse cardiovascular events including MI and/or stroke can rapidly develop.

4. Cardiac Physiology & Pathology

The heart is a crucial pump that utilizes the circulatory system to provide the driving force for maintenance of blood pressure and to deliver essential blood flow to target organs. However, any decrement in cardiac function and its ability to serve as a central pump can lead to hypo-perfusion of distal tissues and organs and, in turn, eventuate in organ failure and multi-system dysfunction and ultimately death. In this section, an overview of some general concepts in cardiac physiology and pathology is presented that will be discussed in subsequent sections.

Central to the role of the heart as a pump are several important physiological concepts, and a brief refresher is warranted: chronotropy refers to the generation of pacemaker action potentials in the sinoatrial (SA) node that allow for depolarization of adjacent cells via gap junctions and therefore determines heart rate [52]; SA nodal rate and speed of conduction may by modulated by changes in atrioventricular (AV) nodal depolarization in dromotropy [53]; electrical conduction is converted into mechanical contractility by excitation-contraction coupling via Ca^{2+}-induced Ca^{2+} release [54]; cardiac inotropy describes the force of contraction that results from electrical-mechanical coupling and, when combined with chronotropy and dromotropy, determines cardiac output; and following contraction the rate by which the ventricles relax due to sequestration of Ca^{2+} back into internal stores is known as lusitropy [55].

Structurally, the heart is comprised of several primary cell types. Cardiomyocytes comprise the bulk of the organ and are categorized as either specialized conductive cells [56] or as the cells responsible for myocardial contraction [57]. Fibroblasts are responsible for the structure and maintenance of the cardiac ECM which provides support for the structure of the heart as well as contributing to formation of cardiac valves. VECs and VSMCs comprise the blood vessels within the heart, the coronary circulation [58]. Additionally, resident leukocytes such as macrophages, innate lymphoid cells, and mast cells can be found within the myocardium [59]. Each of these cell types and physiological concepts is critical to maintaining healthy cardiac function. Modulation of both cyclic nucleotide-directed protein kinase signaling and inflammatory processes can be exploited clinically to rescue cardiovascular function in the presence of a pathological state or exacerbation of disease processes such as in myocarditis, myocardial infarction, ischemia-reperfusion (I/R) injury, and the development of heart failure (HF) [3].

Epidemiologic studies indicate CVD as the leading cause of morbidity and mortality in the United States with an estimated 1,255,000 new or recurrent events of myocardial infarction (MI) occur per year [60]. This review will focus primarily on pathologies and sequela related to MI including I/R injury as well as HF due to adverse cardiac remodeling following MI. Current medical opinion divides MI into two distinct categories separated by their underlying etiology, Type 1 and Type 2 [61]. Type 1, or spontaneous, MI is considered the prototypical example of an infarction and is the most common type of MI [62]. As discussed above in vascular pathology, ischemia occurs when a vessel becomes occluded by either a thrombus or less often by an embolus. Commonly, luminal blockages of a coronary artery result paradoxically from normal wound healing and clotting responses gone awry. Coronary thrombosis occurs when a complicated atherosclerotic plaque spontaneously ruptures, and the initial recruitment of platelets to the site of injury begins to block the already narrowed arterial lumen. Ultimately, blood flow to distal portions of the myocardium becomes obstructed.

Although the most common pathological mechanism for initiation of MI, rupture of atherosclerotic plaques are not the only means of inducing myocardial ischemia or MI. When oxygen demand outpaces oxygen supply, such as during strenuous exercise [63] or during coronary vasospasm [64], injury can occur. Myocardial oxygen supply-demand mismatch in the absence of coronary thrombosis is classified as a Type 2 MI and is another leading cause of MI. It is important to note that in Type 1 or Type 2 MI, total luminal occlusion of a coronary artery is not required to induce ischemia because any decrease in coronary flow resulting in inadequate oxygen distribution will result in ischemia and if unresolved ultimately cardiomyocyte death [62]. Although Types 1 and 2 MI are the most common etiologies, there exist several classifications relevant to clinical discrimination of MI. Type 3 MI is an entirely clinical subdivision and reflects sudden cardiac death of unknown etiology, but acute myocardial ischemia is strongly suspected [65]. The gold-standard treatment for Type 1 and Type 2 infarcts is reperfusion by percutaneous coronary intervention (PCI), thrombolysis, or coronary artery bypass grafting (CABG) which has led to two new classifications of Types 4 and 5 MI and indicate iatrogenic origins. Type 4 MI results from PCI or stent placement and involves myocardial ischemia that occurs during the procedure or secondary to vessel restenosis [63,66]. Type 5 MI is very similar to Type 4 except that ischemic complications are secondary to CABG. While most Types 4 and 5 infarcts are due to technical failure that limits resolution of ischemia, some are associated with successful intervention in the face of an excessive inflammatory response to reperfusion.

Ischemia is a condition whereby inadequate blood flow results in inadequate oxygen supply [67]. Mechanisms that ultimately lead to cardiomyocyte death are tied strongly to cellular susceptibility to hypoxia. The myocardium has an incredibly high metabolic demand: making delivery of oxygen by way of the coronary arteries crucial in support of normal cardiac function. Occlusion of one or more coronary arteries leads to ischemia in areas distal to the blockage and, in turn, compromises tissue metabolism and function. Thus, ischemia leads to hypoxic injury in distal tissue, which if left unresolved eventuates in cell/tissue death known as infarct [62]. Hypoxic injury to the myocardium results from an inability to generate sufficient ATP via oxidative phosphorylation causing a shift to anaerobic glycolysis [62]. Anaerobic glycolysis results in intracellular acidosis from the accumulation of intracellular hydrogen ions (H^+), thereby disturbing the sodium (Na^+)/H^+ exchanger [68]. Depletion of available ATP inactivates Na^+/potassium (K^+) ATPase [69]. The combined ionic disturbances result in Na^+ overload. As a result, Na^+-Ca^{2+} exchanger attempts to compensate for the ionic disturbance by pumping Ca^{2+} into the cytoplasm and Na^+ out of the cell. However, the intracellular Ca^{2+} overload induces cardiomyocyte death [62,64,68,69]. The cytosolic oversaturation with Na^+ or Ca^{2+} results in increased cytoplasmic osmolality resulting in cellular edema [64]. Excess Ca^{2+} uptake by cardiac mitochondria induces opening of the mitochondrial permeability transition pore (mPTP) leading to mitochondrial lysis, the release of cytochrome C, and induction of apoptosis [70–72]. Intracellular Ca^{2+} concentration also activates phospholipases that serve to degrade cardiomyocyte cell membranes [68,69]. The cascade of events following an initial ischemic insult, as highlighted above, contribute to cell/tissue death and ultimately the condition of MI. An overview of some of these key elements that serve as foundations for cardiac dysfunction and disease following an ischemic episode is shown in Figure 3.

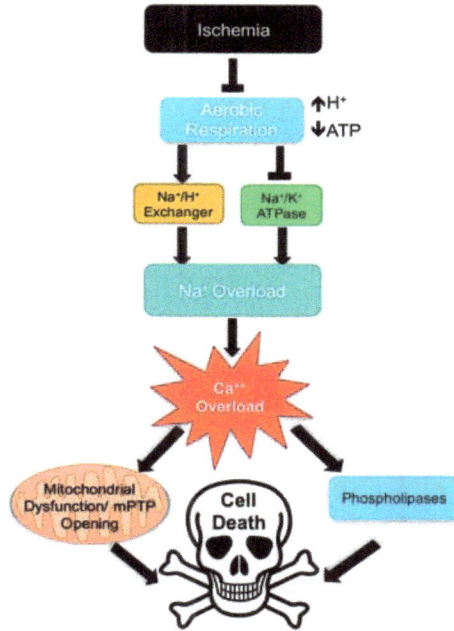

Figure 3. Overview of mechanisms contributing to cell death following ischemia. Ischemia results in ion channel dysfunction following decreased production of ATP and increased hydrogen ion (H+) production leading to cellular acidosis. Ultimately excessive intracellular calcium (Ca^{2+}) triggers activation of phospholipases and the opening of the mitochondrial permeability transition pore (mPTP) in turn inducing cell death.

To salvage myocardial tissue and rescue normal cardiac function it is imperative to rapidly restore coronary blood flow following onset of cardiac dysfunction and/or MI. Clinically, blood flow can be restored through medical interventions such as thrombolytic therapy, PCI, or CABG [73,74]. The goal of MI treatment, restoration of blood flow, however can paradoxically result in further myocardial injury, known as reperfusion injury [68]. Reperfusion injury broadly encompasses several adverse events including arrhythmia, myocardial stunning, and microvascular damage [64,68,69,75,76]. Although the manifestations of reperfusion injury are diverse, in many respects the underlying mechanisms mirror many of the processes witnessed in primary ischemic injury. Complicating the issue of revascularization and reperfusion is the tendency for the aberrant and pathological proliferation of coronary artery VSMCs leading to vascular restenosis through inflammatory processes and growth/remodeling [77,78]. As will be discussed below, data generated over the past decade has also strongly implicated regulatory roles for cyclic nucleotides and their multifunctional protein kinases in these cardiac pathologies [31,36,79–81].

Reactive oxygen species (ROS) play a fundamental role in mediating cardiac reperfusion injury. Surges of oxygen occurring with the restoration of blood flow generate superoxide anion and/or peroxynitrite by cardiomyocyte mitochondria [64,82]. The impact of ROS on reperfusion injury are varied and involve triggering: the activity of protein kinases and subsequent pathways, peroxidation of lipid membranes, apoptosis, and dysfunction in Ca^{2+} handling [82–84]. Ca^{2+} handling in reperfusion injury is influenced by cytosolic influxes in Na^+. Exchange of Na^+ for Ca^{2+} leads to high cytosolic Ca^{2+}, and the overload of Ca^{2+} leads to rigor-type contracture of the myocardium. Rigor-type contraction contributes to the development of myocardial dysfunction. As observed in ischemia, fluctuations in Ca^{2+} released from the sarcoplasmic reticulum stimulate the opening of the mPTP [70–72]. Once the mPTP opens the ionic gradient required for synthesis of ATP rapidly dissipates and water can flood into mitochondria causing swelling [64] and rupture of the mitochondria which triggers apoptosis [68].

Another critical component of reperfusion injury results from leukocyte trafficking to the area of injury which occurs shortly after re-establishment of blood flow [64]. Initially, during reperfusion neutrophils move to areas of ischemia to phagocytose dead tissue, releasing cytokines to further mediate the immune response [64,85,86]. Factors secreted by neutrophils which include ROS, cytokines, and chemokines which promote inflammation may also damage previously viable tissue [68]. Neutrophils obstruct post-capillary venules contributing to microvascular dysfunction [85] which is thought to mediate no-reflow phenomenon associated with reperfusion injury [68,85,87]. Platelets recruited to sites of injury may also contribute to reperfusion injury and microvascular dysfunction by secreting vasoactive thromboxane A_2 and 5-HT. Infiltrating monocytes to the zone of infarction further mediate the inflammatory response to ischemia and reperfusion releasing proteases capable of infarct expansion through proteolysis [68,69,85]. Restoration of flow is required to re-establish oxygenation, so ways to reduce the attendant inflammatory response constitute a significant area of interest in improving recovery from acute ischemic injury.

Following MI the most significant predictor the development of HF is infarct size [88] determined by the death of cardiomyocytes from ischemia or reperfusion injury. Therefore, mitigation of injury size after MI is of chief concern for patient prognosis [89]. The homogeneous cell death pathways triggered by MI lead to release of pro-inflammatory cytokines and danger signals [90], which activate the immune system to respond to the initial cardiac insult clearing the infarcted area of cellular and ECM debris. The initial injury response gives way to a reparative response partially mediated by TGF-β/Smad signaling [91,92], culminating in the formation of a non-contractile scar that significantly diminishes cardiac inotropic capacity and subsequently compromises cardiac output leading to decompensated HF. A cartoon showing an overview of cellular processes during reperfusion and ensuing injury is shown in Figure 4.

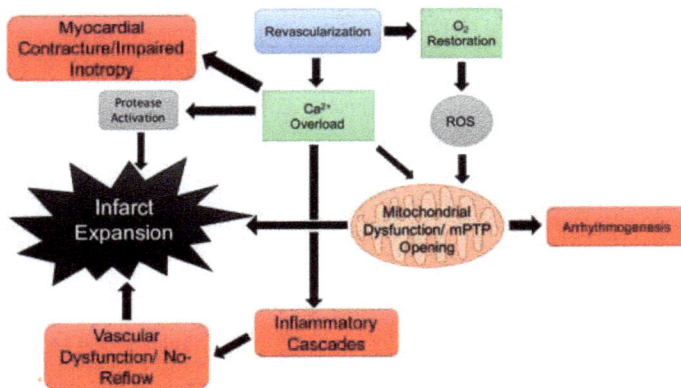

Figure 4. Overview of mechanisms contributing to reperfusion injury. Reperfusion injury results following revascularization and restoration of blood flow to the ischemic myocardium. As with ischemic injury intracellular calcium (Ca^{2+}) overload leads to increased myocardial injury through multiple pathways. Reactive oxygen species (ROS) also contribute to myocardial injury in turn promoting inflammation and altering mitochondrial function.

5. Inflammation & IL-6 Signaling

Inflammation can be broadly defined as a response to stress or injury by the immune system, and the inflammatory response results from complex interactions between immune cells such as leukocytes and molecular mediators such as cytokines and chemokines and the damaged or infected cell. Inflammation serves as a host defense process that ensures timely and adequate disposal of dead or dying cells and/or invading pathogens thereby leading to repair of damaged tissues and paving the way for repair and restoration of tissue and organ function. As discussed, inflammation plays a crucial role in response to bodily insult and is critical to injury repair, particularly in cardiac and vascular tissues. However, perturbations in the typical inflammatory response or unresolved or uncontrolled inflammation plays a pivotal role in the etiology of CVD including but not limited to atherosclerosis [93], MI [94], I/R injury [68], vasculitis [95], neointimal hyperplasia and restenosis [96], hypertension [97], and HF [98].

Cytokines serve as essential proteins that play critical roles in cell-cell communication in response to injury and in the initiation, maintenance, and resolution of inflammation. There is a strong association with elevated levels of circulating cytokines and CVD. In humans with CAD, it has been shown that elevated serum concentrations of IL-1β, TNFα, IL-8, and IL-27 are present during events of unstable angina or are elevated in exacerbations of HF [99,100]. IL-1β and TNFα in addition to IL-18 are responsible for enhanced surface expression of the selectins VCAM-1 and ICAM-1 [101–103], which indicate endothelial activation due to inflammation and may play roles in vascular changes associated with particle exposure and no-reflow phenomenon associated with reperfusion following ischemia [85,104]. IL-1 family cytokines including IL-18 have also been shown to contribute to LV dysfunction [105,106]. TNFα is associated with cardio-depression and dysfunction following MI [107]. IL-2 is a pro-inflammatory cytokine key to T cell differentiation, thereby promoting helper Th1 and Th2 while inhibiting Th17 and T follicular helper cells [108]. Infusion of exogenous IL-2 has been shown to induce heart failure and myocarditis [109,110]. Considering the overall impact on cardiovascular dysfunction directly attributed to pro-inflammatory cytokines in addition to secondary damage from leukocyte recruitment, cytokines play key roles in mediating cardiovascular dysfunction and expansion of cardiac injury.

Interleukin-6 (IL-6) is a pleiotropic cytokine with both pro-inflammatory and anti-inflammatory properties [111–113]. Increased levels of pro-inflammatory IL-6 are associated with atherosclerosis [93], vasculitis [114], MI [94] and HF [115]. Despite the apparent connection between IL-6 and CVD, the IL-6 receptor is only expressed on hepatocytes and in certain leukocytes [116]. The process when IL-6 binds to a membrane-bound IL-6 receptor to induce signal transduction is referred to as classical IL-6 signaling. This limited expression of the IL-6 receptor has traditionally been considered a constraint to the biological significance of classical IL-6 signaling; however, an alternative mechanism by which IL-6 may act directly on the cells of the cardiovascular system has been identified as IL-6 trans-signaling and through this mechanism the biological impact of IL-6 processes are significantly expanded.

Interleukin-6 trans-signaling may serve to override negative feedback mechanisms of classical IL-6 signals in addition to allowing cells without the IL-6 receptor to respond to IL-6. Adding to its biological impact, IL-6 trans-signaling has been implicated in the pathogenesis of conditions including atherosclerosis [117], hemorrhagic trauma [118], and inflammation-based CVD [119]. Over the past decades, much investigation has focused on the role of IL-6 in the pathogenesis of CVD; however, with the recently discovered soluble IL-6 receptor and its trans-signaling mechanism interest has returned to investigating IL-6 in CVD. As a result, this review will focus primarily on the roles IL-6 and trans-signaling in the development or abrogation of CVD.

The interplay and balance of several soluble factors modulate the ability of IL-6 trans-signaling to exert its effects in cardiovascular tissues: a soluble IL-6 receptor (sIL-6R) or soluble glycoprotein 130 (sgp130) act to promote or inhibit IL-6 trans-signaling, respectively. Over time, cardiac injury induces aberrant increases in IL-6 trans-signaling and in turn, mediates adverse cardiac remodeling and exacerbation of HF. Inhibition of IL-6 signal transduction with a blocking IL-6 receptor antibody in a murine model has been shown to ameliorate left ventricular remodeling following MI [120]. Previous work regarding IL-6 biology has focused specifically on classical IL-6 pathways or has sought to attenuate the effects of IL-6 signaling indiscriminately by blocking both classical and trans-signaling through IL-6 receptor blockade. However, this approach neglects the distinct possibility that classical and trans-signaling may play independent biological roles in the cardiovascular injury response. A schematic depicting mechanisms of classical IL-6 signal transduction and IL-6 trans-signaling is shown in Figure 5.

The balance between IL-6 classical and trans-signaling is crucial to physiological function, whereby they have the capacity to produce divergent effects on inflammation and ensuing pathologies [121]. Both mechanisms of IL-6 signaling activate Janus-Kinase (JAK)/Signal Transducer and Activator of Transcription (STAT) pathways, which primarily lead to the activation of STAT3 [122], which has been shown to have cardioprotective effects by acutely promoting cardiomyocyte survival and compensatory hypertrophy [123]. However, prolonged expression of STAT3 has also been demonstrated to negatively impact cardiac function following MI [124].

Of interest, IL-6 signaling may further modulate cardiovascular function by mediating, or getting mediated by, cyclic nucleotide-driven protein kinases. IL-6 signaling has been implicated in decreased cardiac inotropy in adult rat ventricular myocytes mediated by the cyclic GMP/PKG pathway via IL-6 transcriptional upregulation of iNOS [125]. Although IL-6 may induce impaired myocardial function via PKG signals, chronic activation of β-adrenergic receptors, as occurs in HF, can induce IL-6 expression through cyclic AMP/PKA and the induction of STAT3 through IL-6 may induce cardiomyocyte hypertrophy [126], thereby implicating IL-6 signaling in the progression to decompensated HF. However, it remains unclear whether IL-6 classical or trans-signaling is responsible for these observations.

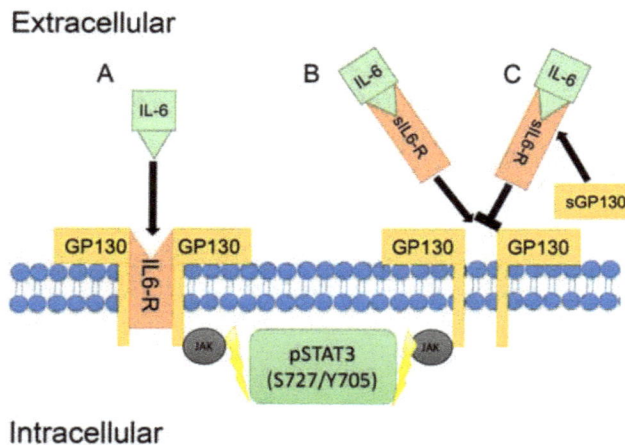

Figure 5. Classical versus interleukin-6/(IL-6) trans-signaling. A simplified schematic depicts classical IL-6 signaling whereby IL-6 binds to membrane-bound IL-6 receptor (IL-6R) initiating signal transduction via glycoprotein 130 (GP130) to increase intracellular STAT3 via JAK (**A**); Alternatively, in (**B**) IL-6 trans-signaling occurs whereby IL-6 binds to soluble IL-6 receptor (sIL-6R) which then complexes to membrane-bound GP130/JAK to initiate STAT3 signal transduction. Inhibition of IL-6 trans-signaling can occur by the decoy soluble GP130 (sGP130) (**C**).

6. Cardiac Physiology/Pathology & Cyclic Nucleotide-Directed Protein Kinases

The complex processes that lead to the development of CVD and particularly MI, I/R injury, can to a certain degree be attenuated or exacerbated by the activity of certain cyclic nucleotide-dependent protein kinases. One such protein kinase responsible for the mitigation of I/R injury is cyclic GMP-driven PKG. Ischemia has been demonstrated to modulate intramyocardial levels of cyclic GMP in multiple animal models, initially increasing cyclic GMP content within the first few minutes of ischemia [127,128]. Furthermore, experimental models of preconditioning prior to an ischemic episode have shown increased myocardial cyclic GMP content compared to tissues exposed to ischemia alone [129]. In the heart, NO is mostly responsible for sGC activation and conversion of GTP to cyclic GMP and subsequent activation of PKG. Ca^{2+} homeostasis can be modulated by PKG interactions with both IP_3 receptors [130] as well as with ryanodine receptors (RyR) [131]. Additionally, Ca^{2+}-sequestering phospholamban can act as a substrate for PKG [132]. Ca^{2+} handling can also be modulated by PKG activity via interaction with L-type Ca^{2+} channels and Ca^{2+}-activated potassium channels, which can all negatively influence cardiac inotropy and chronotropy in addition to reducing VSM tone within the coronary circulation. Cardiac inotropy can also be modulated by interactions of PKG with troponin, thereby decreasing the contractile responsiveness to Ca^{2+} [79,133]. The ability of PKG to modulate cardiac ischemia-reperfusion injury through its actions on thromboxane A_2 receptor and then to inhibit ensuing signal transduction potentially limits platelet activation and aggregation through desensitization [80,134,135], which may ultimately attenuate vascular occlusion due to atherosclerotic rupture or no-reflow phenomenon after reperfusion. Recently and of importance, Frankenreiter and Lukowski and colleagues reported that cyclic GMP and PKG are able to exert cardioprotective effects through stimulation of cardiomyocyte-specific big potassium (BK) channels, demonstrating acute infarct sparing as well as decreased myocardial dysfunction following MI by cyclic GMP/PKG signals [136].

Another critical cyclic nucleotide-directed pathway involved in cardiovascular physiology and pathology involves cyclic AMP-stimulated PKA. As described, PKA is activated by cyclic AMP following its generation from ATP by AC following a variety of mechanisms including catecholamine-mediated stimulation of β-adrenergic receptors [41]. Similar to PKG, PKA has been demonstrated to interact with RyR [137] and L-type Ca^{2+} channels [81,138] to increase cytoplasmic Ca^{2+} concentrations thereby stimulating myocardial contraction while also enhancing Ca^{2+} uptake via phospholamban and increasing cardiac lusitropy [139]. PKA can increase myocardial contraction through phosphorylation of cardiac troponin I (cTnI) inducing accelerated cross-bridge cycling by sensitizing actinomyosin ATPase to Ca^{2+} [140]. Phosphorylation of cardiac myosin binding protein (cMyBP) by PKA induces inotropy by modulating the interaction between thick and thin filaments [141]. Interestingly, hypo-phosphorylation of cMyBP has been demonstrated to be associated with worsening failure HF in animal models [142,143] and in failing hearts in humans [144]. Like PKG, the role of PKA in CVD and particularly MI is multifold and can have direct effects on cardiac function and injury as well as indirect effects that can modulate injury and function which, in many cases, overlap with PKG signaling in apparently antagonistic fashion. While NO ultimately activates downstream PKG and is responsible for decreasing cardiac inotropy, lusitropy, chronopropy, dromotropy, and automaticity, the actions of PKA generally promote cardiac inotropy, lusitropy, chronopropy, dromotropy, and automaticity.

7. G Protein-Coupled Receptor Signaling

The family of GPCRs constitutes the broadest and most diverse group of membrane receptors identified in the human genome that has the capacity to control a myriad of cellular functions. The receptor is integrated into the plasma membrane by seven transmembrane loops, and upon binding of an extracellular agonist a conformational change in the receptor occurs. The cytoplasmic carboxyl tail of the receptor interacts with nearby heterotrimeric (α, β, γ) G proteins, GDP (bound to Gα) is replaced by GTP (which activates stimulatory $Gα_s$), the β and γ subunits dissociate (remaining as a dimer), and intracellular signaling ensues via $Gα_s$-GTP, other Gα subunits, and Gβγ [145]. Both activated Gα subunits and the βγ dimer can interact with numerous membrane proteins to induce broad and diverse signal transduction processes. In fact, activation of a single GPCR can provoke thousands of downstream second messenger signals including commonly AC-mediated cyclic AMP, diacylglycerol and IP_3, and intracellular Ca^{2+}. In opposition to activation by $G\alpha_s$-GTP, stimulation of the inhibitory subunit $_{(i/o)}$ of $G\alpha$ results in inhibition of AC and reduction of cyclic AMP synthesis and downstream PKA signaling [3,7,145]. This complex and highly regulated signal transduction system affords GPCRs the control of innumerable cardiovascular functions and makes GPCRs a critically important target for modern medicinal drugs [146–151].

A unique family of acidosis/pH-sensing heterotrimeric GPCRs has been identified and characterized as extracellular proton sensors and is comprised of G protein-coupled receptor 4 (GPR4), T cell death-associated gene 8 (TDAG8 or GPR65), ovarian cancer G protein-coupled receptor 1 (OGR1 or GPR68), and G protein-coupled receptor G2 accumulation (G2A or GPR132) [152–158]. This family of GPCRs are activated via acidic protonation of histidine residues on the extracellular amino binding domain and signal predominantly through the intracellular subunits $G\alpha_s$ (AC/cyclic AMP stimulation), $G\alpha_{q/11}$ (PLC/DAG/IP_3 and Ca^{2+} stimulation), $G\alpha_{12/13}$ (RhoGEFs/RhoA/Ras stimulation), as well as through the $G\beta\gamma$ subunit (PI3K, GRKs, PLC and Ca^{2+} stimulation) [157]. Obviously, these GPCRs then have the capacity to moderate broad downstream kinases including PKA and PKC as well as MAPKs/ERKs. Cardiovascular tissues and inflammatory cells including leukocytes contain all of these pH-sensing GPCRs, yet interestingly, VECs predominantly express GPR4 [152,158–160] while VSM and cardiomyocytes largely express GPR68 [155,157,161].

During deleterious conditions as found in CVD and other disorders, dysregulated and largely glycolytic anaerobic cellular metabolism occurs which, along with impaired blood perfusion and several other processes, causes acidic byproducts to accumulate, in turn acidifying the local tissue microenvironment. Considering that acidosis is a strong cellular stressor, redundant modes exist for the sensing of extracellular acidosis and the facilitation of downstream signaling and modulation of cellular responses. While it has been theorized that acid-sensing GPCRs may play key roles in the detection of extracellular acidosis and/or in the development or maintenance of cardiovascular pathologies, fundamental mechanisms responsible for the ability of these important GPCRs to moderate cardiovascular dysfunction and their potential interaction with cyclic nucleotide-dependent protein kinases remain to be fully elucidated. Recent work in human umbilical vein endothelial cells (HUVECs) and lung microvascular and pulmonary VECs showed that isocapnia (as found in metabolic acidosis) or hypercapnia (such as respiratory acidosis) independently activate GPR4 to induce broad inflammation characterized by significant upregulation of pro-inflammatory genes including members of the CXC and CCL families of cytokines and chemokines, vascular cell adhesion molecules E-selectin, VCAM1 and ICAM1, members of the TNF and NF-κB signaling systems, elements in the prostaglandin-endoperoxidase synthase family, and transcription factor early growth and stress response genes [159,160]. Using Gene Ontology (GO) Enrichment with the GATHER systems approach [162], the families of acid/GPR4-induced genes correlate with immune, defense and inflammatory responses, consistent with the induction of the inflammatory response through acidosis and GPR4 [160]. It has also been determined that acidic pH induces gene expression of the vascular cell adhesion molecules E-selectin, VCAM1 and ICAM1 and that it does so in cyclic AMP/GPR4-dependent fashion [152,157,159,160]. Complementing these observations, additional work by Yang and colleagues [159,160] showed that acidosis and GPR4, alone or in synergy, significantly increase adhesiveness of monocytes to a confluent VEC monolayer and that this occurs under both static [159] and flow [160] conditions.

Complementing these pro-inflammatory, adhesive characteristics of GPR4, in the original report on GPR68 in human VSMCs [163], acidic pH was found to markedly elevate cyclic AMP (likely occurring via $G\alpha_s/G\alpha_{q/11}$) and to increase intracellular Ca^{2+} and prostacyclin production at an acute time point. In another study the long-term effects of extracellular acidification on GPR68 signals in human VSMCs were examined and the authors observed ability of acidic pH to induce COX-2 signaling, prostacyclin production, MAPK phosphatase, and plasminogen activator inhibitor (PAI-1) [161]; however, many of these results including the observation that acidic pH inhibits cell proliferation were believed to be independent of GPR68 [161]. In line with this theory, acidification has, in general, been reported to influence VSM-mediated vessel dilation and growth [164,165], yet comprehensive documentation of precise involvement of GPR68 (or other pH-sensing GPCRs) in the VSM response to acidosis and/or in pathologic vascular growth is lacking.

The potential role of acidosis/pH-sensing heterotrimeric GPCRs in cardiac disease and dysfunction is emerging. Acidosis is a critical byproduct of many cardiac disease states including ischemia and therefore may be a potential target for the treatment of cardiac disorders. Although GPR4 and GPR68 have been identified primarily in VECs and VSMCs, respectively, whether or not these GPCRs are localized to cardiomyocytes remains unclear. Recent investigations have indicated that experimental MI in a murine model results in greatly increased GPR68 expression in cardiomyocytes within the border zone of the infarcted region 7 days following occlusion [166]. These results concur with preliminary experiments in our own lab that show significant ($p < 0.05$) upregulation of GPR68 protein expression (normalized to total protein; n = 4/group) in mouse cardiac homogenates subjected to a 24 h permanent coronary artery ligation compared to naïve control homogenates (data not shown). It is interesting to note that we have not observed upregulation of GPR68 when myocardial ischemia and acidosis has been corrected by reperfusion (I/R; data not shown). Furthermore Russell et al., provided data suggesting that activation of GPR68 following ischemia was responsible for the upregulation of pro-survival and cardioprotective pathways [166]. GPR4 has also been implicated in mediating outcomes following MI, whereby antagonization of GPR4 was able to completely reduce 28-day mortality following a permanent coronary artery occlusion compared to vehicle controls [167]. Despite both GPR4 and GPR68 having apparent roles in the pathophysiology of cardiac ischemia, it may be that they have opposing roles in cardiomyocytes in the presence of ischemic insult. Of course, it is also possible that in the case of GPR4, there may be no direct effect on cardiomyocytes and the observed reduction in mortality observed following inhibition of GPR4 was due to primary effects on VECs within cardiac circulation and a decreased VEC-mediated inflammatory response. The role of acidosis/pH-sensing heterotrimeric GPCRs in cardiac ischemia with the gold standard therapeutic, reperfusion, has yet to be thoroughly investigated and poses additional questions to how to modulate pH-sensing GPCRs in the treatment of cardiac disease.

Another GPCR family that has the capacity to exert significant biological effects on cardiac and vascular tissues and that are dependent in part on cyclic nucleotide-driven protein kinases are the protease-activated receptors (PARs). Extracellular serine proteases serve pivotal roles in many aspects of cardiovascular homeostasis and physiology yet are also involved in the pathogenesis of cardiac and vascular disorders largely through activation of their respective PARs [168,169]. PARs are proteolytically cleaved and activated by these proteases, thereby revealing a new amino-terminus which acts as an intramolecular ligand leading to sustained receptor activation [170]. Following activation, PARs can be rapidly down-regulated by β-arrestin-mediated desensitization and endocytosis followed by lysosomal targeting and degradation [168–170]. PARs are normally expressed abundantly in platelets and in relatively low levels in VECs and VSMCs and in cardiac myocytes and fibroblasts [168,171,172]. In VECs PARs operate to regulate vascular tone via induction of NO release and subsequent sGC activation and cyclic GMP/PKG induction [168,173], and in stimulated VSM PARs mediate contraction, migration, proliferation, hypertrophy and ECM production which contribute to the development of vascular lesions and CVD pathogenesis [173–175]. Increasing evidence [168,175] supports involvement of PARs in CVD pathophysiology yet their discrete mechanisms have yet to be solidified.

To date four PAR family members have been identified: PAR1, PAR3 and PAR4 are cleaved and activated predominantly by thrombin whereas PAR2 is activated primarily by trypsin and mast cell tryptase [176]. Of these PARs, PAR1 was the first discovered [168] and has since been the most investigated. Early studies identified a role for PAR1 in regulating platelet activation as an underpinning of thrombosis, in turn leading to the creation of Vorapaxar (SCH530348), a selective, competitive antagonist of PAR1. Vorapaxar received FDA approval in 2014 after the Thrombin-Receptor

Antagonist in Secondary Prevention of Atherothrombotic Ischemic Events trial (TRA 2°P-TIMI 50) found it to significantly reduce secondary ischemic events compared to placebo controls [177]. In rat VSMCs, PAR1 was shown to be induced following balloon catheter-induced injury [178] and to be upregulated in a hypertensive model [179]. While PAR1 has been more extensively researched as a key player in cardiovascular pathology, recent evidence that PAR2 also plays a regulatory role. PAR2 has been implicated in mediating inflammatory changes in human VSMCs via interaction with soluble dipeptidyl peptidase 4 (DPP4), a ubiquitously expressed cell-surface protease [172], and apolipoprotein E/PAR2 double knockout mice demonstrated significant decreases in atherosclerotic lesion development and aortic inflammatory cytokine release compared to wild-type controls [180]. Preliminary data generated in our lab show upregulation of both PAR2 and PAR4 protein expression as well as phosphorylated Erk1/2 as an indicator of PAR activity in balloon-injured rat carotid arteries compared to uninjured arteries 30 post-injury (data not shown), and in cultured VSMCs activation of PAR2 or PAR4 show co-dependency following pharmacologic activation or inhibition (data not shown). Indeed, the central role of serine proteases and PARs in cardiac and vascular physiology and pathology warrants continued study as plausible clinical targets against CVD.

Regarding mechanisms of cellular signaling, PARs primarily operate via $G\alpha_{i/o}$ (to inhibit AC and cyclic AMP synthesis), through $G\alpha_{12/13}$ (to activate RhoGEFS/RhoA/Ras) and via $G\alpha_{q/11}$ (to moderate PLC/IP$_3$/DAG and Ca^{2+} signaling), as well as through dissociated G$\beta\gamma$ (to induce PI3K, GRKs, PLC and Ca^{2+} signaling). These processes then lead to modulation of PKA, PKC and MAPK/ERK pathways, in turn eventuating in the regulation of inflammation- and growth-specific functional processes. A schematic depicting a generic pH-sensing GPCR and PAR as well as some of their activated effectors is shown in Figure 6.

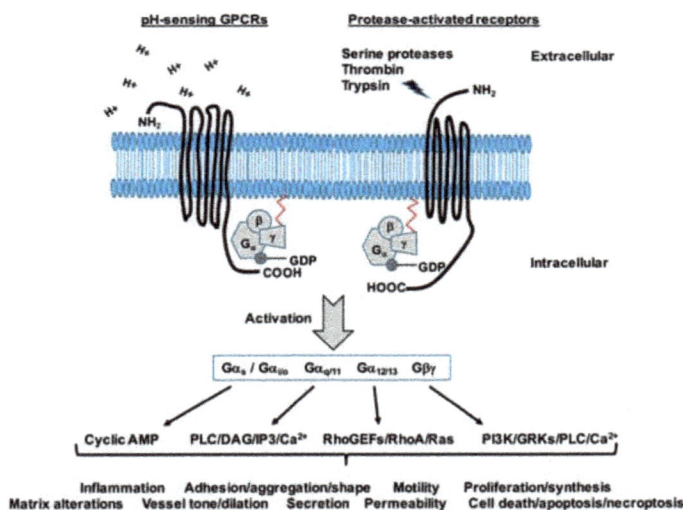

Figure 6. Generalized G protein-coupled receptors: pH-sensing and protease-activated receptors. A schematic depicting a typical pH-sensing GPCR and a protease-activated receptor (PAR) GPCR under non-activated conditions. Both GPCRs are 7 trans-membrane receptors with an extracellular amino terminus and an intracellular carboxyl end associated with G protein subunits. Activation of the pH-sensing GPCR involves extracellular amino terminal histidine sensing of acidic protons (H+) while PAR activation involves cleavage of the extracellular amino terminus by serine proteases, thrombin, trypsin and other agonists and creation of an activating tethered ligand. These GPCRs then stimulate a cascade of G protein-mediated intracellular signals that have the capacity to govern a wide array of inflammation- and growth-regulatory processes in cardiac and vascular tissues.

8. TGF-β/Smad Signaling

The TGF-β superfamily of growth factors are multifunctional cytokines responsible for regulating key developmental and homeostatic cellular functions such as proliferation, differentiation, recognition, apoptosis, adhesion, and migration and have become of major scientific focus over the past several decades [181]. TGF-β can exert its actions in context-specific fashion, sometimes showing different and even opposite effects in varying cell types and environments. Even though non-Smad pathways exist, one primary route through which TGF-β exerts its functions is through the recruitment and phosphorylation of intracellular Smad proteins [181].

In short, TGF-β-dependent Smad signaling is initiated by binding of a TGF-β ligand (existing in three isoforms: TGF-β1, β2, or β3) to a TGF-β type II receptor (TβR-II), thereby causing a TGF-β type I receptor (TβR-I) to co-localize with the TβR-II. While both receptors contain an intracellular Ser/Thr kinase domain, the kinase domain of TβR-II is constitutively active and its phosphorylation is independent of ligand binding. Once the two receptors become associated, the kinase domain of TβR-II phosphorylates the kinase domain of TβR-I and subsequently transmits the signal through phosphorylation of intracellular Smad [182–184]. There are 8 members within the Smad family of proteins that are divided into 3 distinct groups: receptor-regulated Smads (R-Smads), common-mediator Smad (Co-Smad), and inhibitory Smads (I-Smads). The R-Smads (Smads1, 2, 3, 5, and 8, with Smads2 and 3 of primary interest in cardiovascular tissues) are directly phosphorylated by TβR-I and bind with the Co-Smad4 to form a heteromeric complex that can then travel to the nucleus to act as a transcription factor. This process is negatively regulated by inhibitory Smad6 and Smad7 through competing with R-Smads for TβR-I, interacting with Co-Smad4, and/or by initiating the degradation of TGF-β receptors [181].

Recent studies have shown that a correlation exists between the activation of synthetic and growth-promoting TGF-β1, the most abundant and important isoform in the cardiovascular system, and the pathology of CVD [185,186]. Cell-to-cell adhesion through components of the ECM is required for normal growth conditions; however, these adhesive interactions have also been linked to CVD pathogenesis. TGF-β1 is thought to synthesize ECM elements through a Smad3-dependent pathway [187–189]. Considering this correlation between TGF-β1 and CVD, studying its regulation and mechanistic effects on cell proliferation and migration could prove beneficial in combatting CVD pathologies. Past studies involving TGF-β1-directed Smad3 have shown conflicting effects of Smad3, reportedly switching between pro-growth and anti-growth phenotypes depending cell type, concentration, and density [190,191].

The impact of TGF-β signaling on cellular dynamics have been shown at least in part to be regulated by cyclic nucleotide-directed protein kinases. A recent study in fibroblasts showed that pretreatment with cyclic GMP in the presence of TGF-β significantly reduced the amount of phosphorylated Smad3 translocated into the nucleus, in turn limiting its transcriptional capacity [192]. A similar result occurred in pulmonary artery VSMCs where translocation of phosphorylated Smad3 into the nucleus was inhibited by the sequestering of phosphorylated Smad3 to cytosolic β2-tubulin via actions of cyclic GMP-directed PKG [193]. Additionally in this study, treatment with a PDE5 led to an increase in the bioavailability of cyclic GMP/PKG and enhanced its inhibition of Smad3 signaling. Following PDE5 inhibition in cells that were pretreated with TGF-β, fibroblast proliferation and alpha smooth muscle actin (α-SMA) were markedly reduced compared to TGF-β only treatment [194]. These findings indicate that cyclic GMP/PKG act to limit the effects of TGF-β signaling by diverting phosphorylated Smad3 away from the nucleus so that it can no longer act, along with Smad2 and Smad4, as a transcription factor and offer support for cyclic GMP/PKG as a transcriptional regulator of Smad-dependent signal transduction. Figure 7 shows a cartoon of TGF-β/Smad signaling and transcriptional control along with depiction of PKG-mediated cytosolic retention of Smad and suppression of these processes.

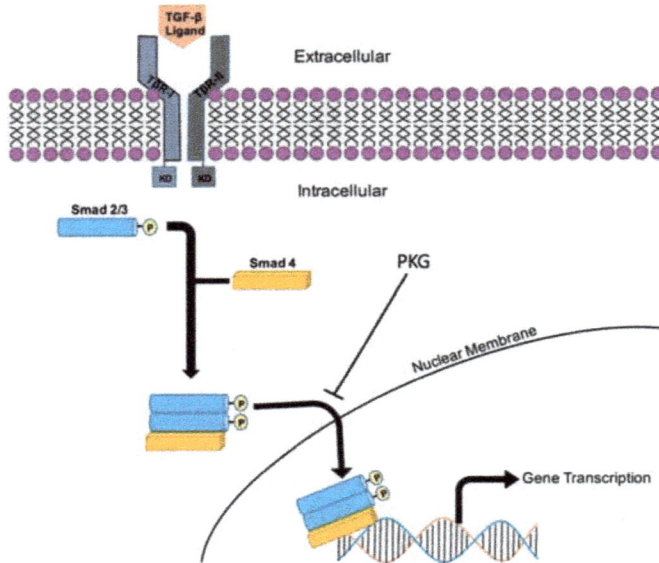

Figure 7. Schematic of transforming growth factor-β (TGF-β) signaling. Binding of an active TGF-β ligand initiates the co-localization of the type II (TβR-II) and type I (TβR-I) TGF-β receptors. The TβR-II remains constitutively phosphorylated and when co-localized phosphorylates the Ser/Thr kinase domain (KD) of the TβR-I. The intracellular signal is subsequently transmitted by phosphorylation of Smad proteins, primarily Smad2/3 in cardiovascular tissues. The phosphorylated Smad proteins combine with Smad4, a common Smad, to form a heterotrimeric complex that can then be shuttled through the nuclear membrane ultimately acting as a transcription factor for inflammatory, synthetic, and growth-promoting genes. The cyclic GMP/PKG system is known to inhibit this pathway by sequestering p-Smad in the cytosol, in turn not allowing it to be shuttled into the nucleus and affect gene transcription.

9. FoxO Transcriptional Signaling

A subgroup of the Forkhead family of transcription factors, Forkhead box O (FoxO) proteins, are characterized by their DNA-binding domain consisting of three α-helices and two loops resembling a butterfly wing motif [195]. Only four mammalian FoxO members are currently known, FoxO1, 3, 4, and 6, and these have been implicated in various cellular processes including cell-cycle regulation, differentiation, apoptosis, and oxidative stress response [196–199]. FoxO transcription factors are tightly regulated by Akt-mediated phosphorylation via the insulin-like growth factor-1 (IGF-1)/phosphatidylinositol-3-kinase (PI3K)/Akt pathway at three conserved amino acid residues [200]. Phosphorylation of FoxO can cause both retention in the cytoplasm or translocation from the nucleus into the cytoplasm, both processes inhibiting it from influencing transcriptional gene regulation and targeting it for degradation [201].

As previously described, VSMC migration and proliferation are key cellular components of CVD. Over the past decades, the impact of FoxO members on cellular dynamics has been studied in relation to CVD pathogenesis. FoxO3a has been implicated in CVD pathology yet the mechanism through which FoxO3 may exacerbate or ameliorate CVD is currently unknown. FoxO3 has been proposed to modulate cell proliferation and cell death pathways [202–204]. Overexpression of FoxO3a was shown to increase gene expression of the cell cycle-dependent kinase inhibitor (CdkI) p27 (Kip1), resulting in cell cycle arrest and attenuation of growth in VSMCs and muscle precursor cells [205,206]. Furthermore, cysteine-rich angiogenic protein 61 (Cyr61), a gene expressed immediately following growth factor stimulation, was inhibited by binding of FoxO3 at the Cyr61 promoter region, illustrating another mechanism by which FoxO3 inhibits vascular cell growth [207].

It has been theorized that a dynamic relationship exists between Smad3 and FoxO3 transcription factors. The gene expression of muscle-specific RING finger-1 (MuRF-1), a ubiquitin ligase, was altered by the levels of FoxO3 and/or Smad3 expression [208]. Smad3 binding to the promoter region of MuRF-1 was shown to increase the abundance of FoxO3 bound to that same promoter region and necessary for optimal FoxO3-induced MuRF-1 gene transcription. Additionally, overexpression of Smad3 increased FoxO3 protein abundance and a synergistic effect was observed on FoxO-induced transcription with co-expression of these transcription factors [208]. In endothelial cells, FoxO and Smad synergistically induced expression of the CdkIs p15Ink4b and p21Cip1 [209,210]. Considering both Smad3 and FoxO transcription factors are implicated in the pathogenesis of CVD, further studies aimed at elucidating Smad3/FoxO3 interactions in VSM could prove beneficial in combatting the etiologies associated with CVD.

While the relationship between elements in FoxO signaling and cyclic nucleotide-directed protein kinases has not been thoroughly investigated, FoxO proteins have been associated with the ability of NO to modulate proliferation and migration in damaged VECs [211]. NO-induced inhibition of cell growth occurs through cyclic GMP and PKG, leading to activation of the PI3K/Atk pathway [212,213]. As a result, FoxO, a downstream phosphorylation target of activated PI3K/Atk, is either maintained in the cytoplasm or, if nuclear, is shuttled into the cytoplasm, in turn targeting it for degradation and preventing its growth-inhibitory, cytostatic effects. Further investigation into the regulation of FoxO proteins, their relationship with growth-promoting synthetic Smads, and their control by cyclic nucleotide-driven protein kinases is necessary to understand the mechanisms underlying growth pathologies in cardiovascular tissues.

10. Summary & Future Directions

Despite ample basic science and translational investigation, CVD remains the major cause of morbidity and mortality in the United States and worldwide, and all estimates suggest an increasing trend in their prevalence over the next several decades. While some authorities suggest that many of the causes behind CVD are preventable, cumulative efforts must continue in order to gain a more thorough understanding of the key elements that serve as the basis for CVD. Only through these endeavors can we hope to better understand crucial aspects of cardiac and vascular pathologies with the aim of expanding our clinical knowledge and therapeutic efficacy. The cyclic nucleotide-driven protein kinase systems represent wide-ranging and multi-functional processes capable of controlling many mechanisms underlying CVD and can serve as current and emerging targets for intervention. Only through expanded knowledge of these many facets of cyclic nucleotide-driven protein kinases and their diverse downstream effectors including their promiscuous 'associated kinases' can we advance our control of these dreaded diseases. In this light, future efforts should be aimed at more completely establishing cyclic nucleotide-driven protein kinases as a therapeutic target to combat and perhaps eliminate CVD, possibly through genetic manipulation/editing or transcriptional control (i.e., Smad/FoxO) of inflammatory/synthetic/growth elements, with pre- and/or post-conditioning interventions [201], or via personalized or precision medicine approaches [3].

Acknowledgments: The authors would like to acknowledge the many investigators who have contributed significantly to the fields of cyclic nucleotide-dependent protein kinases in the cardiovascular sciences but whose works were not cited in this article due to formatting limits. This work was supported by award numbers R01HL81720 and R15HL135699 from the National Heart, Lung, and Blood Institute (NHLBI), National Institutes of Health (NIH), an ECU Brody School of Medicine Seed/Bridge Grant, and a Brody Brothers Endowment Fund Award. This content is solely the responsibility of the authors and does not necessarily represent the official views of the NHLBI, NIH, ECU or the Brody Brothers Endowment Fund.

Author Contributions: Each author (N.A.H., J.T.F., S.C.J., J.S.M., T.J.D., N.R.G., D.A.T.) made substantial conceptual, textual and formatting contributions to this work, and each author approved the final submitted version of this article.

Conflicts of Interest: The authors declare no conflicts of interest.

References

1. Benjamin, E.J.; Blaha, M.J.; Chiuve, S.E.; Cushman, M.; Das, S.R.; Deo, R.; de Ferranti, S.D.; Floyd, J.; Fornage, M.; Gillespie, C.; et al. Heart disease and stroke statistics-2017 update: A report from the American Heart Association. *Circulation* **2017**, *135*, e146–e603. [CrossRef] [PubMed]
2. World Health Organization. Cardiovascular Diseases (CVDs) Fact Sheet. Available online: http://www.who.int/mediacentre/factsheets/fs317/en/ (accessed on 18 December 2017).
3. Tulis, D.A. Novel protein kinase targets in vascular smooth muscle therapeutics. *Curr. Opin. Pharmacol.* **2017**, *33*, 12–16. [CrossRef] [PubMed]
4. Arencibia, J.M.; Pastor-Flores, D.; Bauer, A.F.; Schulze, J.O.; Biondi, R.M. AGC protein kinases: From structural mechanism of regulation to allosteric drug development for the treatment of human diseases. *Biochim. Biophys. Acta* **2013**, *1834*, 1302–1321. [CrossRef] [PubMed]
5. Adderley, S.P.; Joshi, C.N.; Martin, D.N.; Mooney, S.; Tulis, D.A. Multiple kinase involvement in the regulation of vascular growth. In *Advances in Protein Kinases*; Xavier, G.D.S., Ed.; InTech Open Access Publishers: Rijeka, Croatia, 2012; pp. 131–150.
6. Chen, Z.; Zhang, X.; Ying, L.; Dou, D.; Li, Y.; Bai, Y.; Liu, J.; Liu, L.; Feng, H.; Yu, X.; et al. Cimp synthesized by sGC as a mediator of hypoxic contraction of coronary arteries. *Am. J. Physiol.* **2014**, *307*, H328–H336. [CrossRef] [PubMed]
7. Tulis, D.A. Novel cyclic nucleotide signals in the control of pathologic vascular smooth muscle growth. In *Cardiovascular Disease ii*; iCONCEPT Press, Ltd.: Hong Kong, China, 2014; pp. 175–200.
8. Stone, J.D.; Narine, A.; Tulis, D.A. Inhibition of vascular smooth muscle growth via signaling crosstalk between AMP-activated protein kinase and cAMP-dependent protein kinase. *Front. Physiol.* **2012**, *3*, 409. [CrossRef] [PubMed]
9. Holt, D.; Tulis, D. Vascular smooth muscle as a therapeutic target in disease pathology. In *Muscle Cell and Tissue*; Sakuma, K., Ed.; InTech Open Access Publishers: Rijeka, Croatia, 2015; pp. 3–26.
10. Holt, D.; de Castro Brás, L.; Tulis, D. Cyclic nucleotide-driven protein kinase signaling in arterial smooth muscle (patho)physiology. In *Coronary Artery Disease—Causes, Symptoms & Treatments*, 1st ed.; iCONCEPT Press, Ltd.: Hong Kong, China, 2016; ISBN 978-1-922227-92-8.
11. Tulis, D.A. Novel therapies for cyclic GMP control of vascular smooth muscle growth. *Am. J. Ther.* **2008**, *15*, 551–564. [CrossRef] [PubMed]
12. Halls, M.L.; Cooper, D.M. Adenylyl cyclase signalling complexes—Pharmacological challenges and opportunities. *Pharmacol. Ther.* **2017**, *172*, 171–180. [CrossRef] [PubMed]
13. Biel, M.; Michalakis, S. Cyclic nucleotide-gated channels. *Handb. Exp. Pharmacol.* **2009**, 111–136. [CrossRef]
14. Schindler, R.F.; Brand, T. The popeye domain containing protein family—A novel class of cAMP effectors with important functions in multiple tissues. *Prog. Biophys. Mol. Biol.* **2016**, *120*, 28–36. [CrossRef] [PubMed]
15. Brand, T. The popeye domain-containing gene family. *Cell Biochem. Biophys.* **2005**, *43*, 95–103. [CrossRef]
16. Banerjee, U.; Cheng, X. Exchange protein directly activated by cAMP encoded by the mammalian rapgef3 gene: Structure, function and therapeutics. *Gene* **2015**, *570*, 157–167. [CrossRef] [PubMed]
17. Adderley, S.P.; Martin, D.N.; Tulis, D.A. Exchange protein activated by cAMP (Epac) controls migration of vascular smooth muscle cells in concentration- and time-dependent manner. *Arch. Physiol.* **2015**, *2*. [CrossRef]
18. Langeberg, L.K.; Scott, J.D. A-kinase-anchoring proteins. *J. Cell Sci.* **2005**, *118*, 3217–3220. [CrossRef] [PubMed]
19. Corradini, E.; Burgers, P.P.; Plank, M.; Heck, A.J.; Scholten, A. Huntingtin-associated protein 1 (hap1) is a cGMP-dependent kinase anchoring protein (gkap) specific for the cGMP-dependent protein kinase ibeta isoform. *J. Biol. Chem.* **2015**, *290*, 7887–7896. [CrossRef] [PubMed]
20. Casteel, D.E.; Zhang, T.; Zhuang, S.; Pilz, R.B. cGMP-dependent protein kinase anchoring by IRAG regulates its nuclear translocation and transcriptional activity. *Cell. Signal.* **2008**, *20*, 1392–1399. [CrossRef] [PubMed]
21. Adderley, S.P.; Joshi, C.N.; Martin, D.N.; Tulis, D.A. Phosphodiesterases regulate BAY 41-2272-induced VASP phosphorylation in vascular smooth muscle cells. *Front. Pharmacol.* **2012**, *3*, 10. [CrossRef] [PubMed]

22. Manning, G.; Whyte, D.B.; Martinez, R.; Hunter, T.; Sudarsanam, S. The protein kinase complement of the human genome. *Science* **2002**, *298*, 1912–1934. [CrossRef] [PubMed]

23. Ubersax, J.A.; Ferrell, J.E., Jr. Mechanisms of specificity in protein phosphorylation. *Nat. Rev. Mol. Cell Biol.* **2007**, *8*, 530–541. [CrossRef] [PubMed]

24. Khalil, R.A. *Regulation of Vascular Smooth Muscle Function*; Morgan & Claypool Life Sciences: San Rafael, CA, USA, 2010.

25. Knighton, D.R.; Zheng, J.H.; Ten Eyck, L.F.; Ashford, V.A.; Xuong, N.H.; Taylor, S.S.; Sowadski, J.M. Crystal structure of the catalytic subunit of cyclic adenosine monophosphate-dependent protein kinase. *Science* **1991**, *253*, 407–414. [CrossRef] [PubMed]

26. Francis, S.H.; Corbin, J.D. Structure and function of cyclic nucleotide-dependent protein kinases. *Annu. Rev. Physiol.* **1994**, *56*, 237–272. [CrossRef] [PubMed]

27. Worner, R.; Lukowski, R.; Hofmann, F.; Wegener, J.W. cGMP signals mainly through cAMP kinase in permeabilized murine aorta. *Am. J. Physiol.* **2007**, *292*, H237–H244. [CrossRef] [PubMed]

28. Stone, J.D.; Holt, A.W.; Shaver, P.R.; Vuncannon, J.R.; Tulis, D.A. AMP-activated protein kinase inhibits arterial smooth muscle cell proliferation in vasodilator-stimulated phosphoprotein-dependent manner. *J. Non-Inv. Vasc. Investig.* **2016**, *1*. [CrossRef]

29. Mendelev, N.N.; Williams, V.S.; Tulis, D.A. Antigrowth properties of BAY 41-2272 in vascular smooth muscle cells. *J. Cardiovasc. Pharmacol.* **2009**, *53*, 121–131. [CrossRef] [PubMed]

30. Joshi, C.N.; Martin, D.N.; Fox, J.C.; Mendelev, N.N.; Brown, T.A.; Tulis, D.A. The soluble guanylate cyclase stimulator BAY 41-2272 inhibits vascular smooth muscle growth through the cAMP-dependent protein kinase and cGMP-dependent protein kinase pathways. *J. Pharmacol. Exp. Ther.* **2011**, *339*, 394–402. [CrossRef] [PubMed]

31. Holt, A.W.; Martin, D.N.; Shaver, P.R.; Adderley, S.P.; Stone, J.D.; Joshi, C.N.; Francisco, J.T.; Lust, R.M.; Weidner, D.A.; Shewchuk, B.M.; et al. Soluble guanylyl cyclase-activated cyclic GMP-dependent protein kinase inhibits arterial smooth muscle cell migration independent of VASP-serine 239 phosphorylation. *Cell. Signal.* **2016**, *28*, 1364–1379. [CrossRef] [PubMed]

32. Desch, M.; Schinner, E.; Kees, F.; Hofmann, F.; Seifert, R.; Schlossmann, J. Cyclic cytidine 3′,5′-monophosphate (cCMP) signals via cGMP kinase i. *FEBS Lett.* **2010**, *584*, 3979–3984. [CrossRef] [PubMed]

33. Beste, K.Y.; Seifert, R. CCMP, cUMP, cTMP, cIMP and cXMP as possible second messengers: Development of a hypothesis based on studies with soluble guanylyl cyclase alpha(1)beta(1). *Biol. Chem.* **2013**, *394*, 261–270. [CrossRef] [PubMed]

34. Sun, H.; Wang, Y. Novel Ser/Thr protein phosphatases in cell death regulation. *Physiology* **2012**, *27*, 43–52. [CrossRef] [PubMed]

35. Shi, Y. Serine/threonine phosphatases: Mechanism through structure. *Cell* **2009**, *139*, 468–484. [CrossRef] [PubMed]

36. Stone, J.D.; Narine, A.; Shaver, P.R.; Fox, J.C.; Vuncannon, J.R.; Tulis, D.A. AMP-activated protein kinase inhibits vascular smooth muscle cell proliferation and migration and vascular remodeling following injury. *Am. J. Physiol.* **2013**, *304*, H369–H381. [CrossRef] [PubMed]

37. Wang, P.; Liu, Z.; Chen, H.; Ye, N.; Cheng, X.; Zhou, J. Exchange proteins directly activated by cAMP (Epacs): Emerging therapeutic targets. *Bioorg. Med. Chem. Lett.* **2017**, *27*, 1633–1639. [CrossRef] [PubMed]

38. Lahiry, P.; Torkamani, A.; Schork, N.J.; Hegele, R.A. Kinase mutations in human disease: Interpreting genotype-phenotype relationships. *Nat. Rev. Genet.* **2010**, *11*, 60–74. [CrossRef] [PubMed]

39. Kompa, A.R.; Krum, H. Protein kinases as cardiovascular therapeutic targets *Lancet* **2014**, *384*, 1162–1164. [CrossRef]

40. Kini, S.G.; Garg, V.; Prasanna, S.; Rajappan, R.; Mubeen, M. Protein kinases as drug targets in human and animal diseases. *Curr. Enzym. Inhib.* **2017**, *13*, 99–106. [CrossRef]

41. Dhalla, N.S.; Muller, A.L. Protein kinases as drug development targets for heart disease therapy. *Pharmaceuticals* **2010**, *3*, 2111–2145. [CrossRef] [PubMed]

42. Cohen, P. Protein kinases—The major drug targets of the twenty-first century? *Nat. Rev. Drug Discov.* **2002**, *1*, 309–315. [CrossRef] [PubMed]

43. Wang, D.; Wang, Z.; Zhang, L.; Wang, Y. Roles of cells from the arterial vessel wall in atherosclerosis. *Mediat. Inflamm.* **2017**, *2017*. [CrossRef] [PubMed]

44. Wang, G.; Jacquet, L.; Karamariti, E.; Xu, Q. Origin and differentiation of vascular smooth muscle cells. *J. Physiol.* **2015**, *593*, 3013–3030. [CrossRef] [PubMed]

45. Libby, P.; Ridker, P.M.; Maseri, A. Inflammation and atherosclerosis. *Circulation* **2002**, *105*, 1135–1143. [CrossRef] [PubMed]

46. Rocha, V.Z.; Libby, P. Obesity, inflammation, and atherosclerosis. *Nat. Rev. Cardiol.* **2009**, *6*, 399–409. [CrossRef] [PubMed]

47. Muller, W.A. Leukocyte-endothelial-cell interactions in leukocyte transmigration and the inflammatory response. *Trends Immunol.* **2003**, *24*, 327–334. [CrossRef]

48. Sughrue, M.E.; Mehra, A.; Connolly, E.S., Jr.; D'Ambrosio, A.L. Anti-adhesion molecule strategies as potential neuroprotective agents in cerebral ischemia: A critical review of the literature. *Inflamm. Res.* **2004**, *53*, 497–508. [CrossRef] [PubMed]

49. Ross, R. The pathogenesis of atherosclerosis: A perspective for the 1990s. *Nature* **1993**, *362*, 801–809. [CrossRef] [PubMed]

50. Tian, D.Y.; Jin, X.R.; Zeng, X.; Wang, Y. Notch signaling in endothelial cells: Is it the therapeutic target for vascular neointimal hyperplasia? *Int. J. Mol. Sci.* **2017**, *18*, 1615. [CrossRef] [PubMed]

51. Collins, M.J.; Li, X.; Lv, W.; Yang, C.; Protack, C.D.; Muto, A.; Jadlowiec, C.C.; Shu, C.; Dardik, A. Therapeutic strategies to combat neointimal hyperplasia in vascular grafts. *Expert Rev. Cardiovasc. Ther.* **2012**, *10*, 635–647. [CrossRef] [PubMed]

52. Fukuta, H.; Little, W.C. The cardiac cycle and the physiologic basis of left ventricular contraction, ejection, relaxation, and filling. *Heart Fail. Clin.* **2008**, *4*, 1–11. [CrossRef] [PubMed]

53. Tveito, A.; Lines, G.T. A condition for setting off ectopic waves in computational models of excitable cells. *Math. Biosci.* **2008**, *213*, 141–150. [CrossRef] [PubMed]

54. Fabiato, A. Calcium-induced release of calcium from the cardiac sarcoplasmic reticulum. *Am. J. Physiol.* **1983**, *245*, C1–C14. [CrossRef] [PubMed]

55. Katz, A.M. Influence of altered inotropy and lusitropy on ventricular pressure-volume loops. *J. Am. Coll. Cardiol.* **1988**, *11*, 438–445. [CrossRef]

56. Miquerol, L.; Beyer, S.; Kelly, R.G. Establishment of the mouse ventricular conduction system. *Cardiovasc. Res.* **2011**, *91*, 232–242. [CrossRef] [PubMed]

57. Eisner, D.A.; Caldwell, J.L.; Kistamas, K.; Trafford, A.W. Calcium and excitation-contraction coupling in the heart. *Circ. Res.* **2017**, *121*, 181–195. [CrossRef] [PubMed]

58. Hinton, R.B.; Yutzey, K.E. Heart valve structure and function in development and disease. *Annu. Rev. Physiol.* **2011**, *73*, 29–46. [CrossRef] [PubMed]

59. Gentek, R.; Hoeffel, G. The innate immune response in myocardial infarction, repair, and regeneration. *Adv. Exp. Med. Biol.* **2017**, *1003*, 251–272. [PubMed]

60. Roger, V.L.; Go, A.S.; Lloyd-Jones, D.M.; Adams, R.J.; Berry, J.D.; Brown, T.M.; Carnethon, M.R.; Dai, S.; de Simone, G.; Ford, E.S.; et al. Heart disease and stroke statistics—2011 update: A report from the American Heart Association. *Circulation* **2011**, *123*, e18–e209. [CrossRef] [PubMed]

61. Mihatov, N.; Januzzi, J.L., Jr.; Gaggin, H.K. Type 2 myocardial infarction due to supply-demand mismatch. *Trends Cardiovasc. Med.* **2017**, *27*, 408–417. [CrossRef] [PubMed]

62. Burke, A.P.; Virmani, R. Pathophysiology of acute myocardial infarction. *Med. Clin. N. Am.* **2007**, *91*, 553–572. [CrossRef] [PubMed]

63. Montecucco, F.; Carbone, F.; Schindler, T.H. Pathophysiology of st-segment elevation myocardial infarction: Novel mechanisms and treatments. *Eur. Heart J.* **2016**, *37*, 1268–1283. [CrossRef] [PubMed]

64. Moens, A.L.; Claeys, M.J.; Timmermans, J.P.; Vrints, C.J. Myocardial ischemia/reperfusion-injury, a clinical view on a complex pathophysiological process. *Int. J. Cardiol.* **2005**, *100*, 179–190. [CrossRef] [PubMed]

65. Chapman, A.R.; Adamson, P.D.; Mills, N.L. Assessment and classification of patients with myocardial injury and infarction in clinical practice. *Heart* **2017**, *103*, 10–18. [CrossRef] [PubMed]

66. Thygesen, K.; Alpert, J.S.; Jaffe, A.S.; Simoons, M.L.; Chaitman, B.R.; White, H.D. Third universal definition of myocardial infarction. *Circulation* **2012**, *126*, 2020–2035. [CrossRef] [PubMed]

67. Sicari, R.; Cortigiani, L. The clinical use of stress echocardiography in ischemic heart disease. *Cardiovasc. Ultrasound* **2017**, *15*, 7. [CrossRef] [PubMed]

68. Kalogeris, T.; Baines, C.P.; Krenz, M.; Korthuis, R.J. Ischemia/reperfusion. *Compr. Physiol.* **2016**, 113–170. [CrossRef] [PubMed]

69. Kalogeris, T.; Baines, C.P.; Krenz, M.; Korthuis, R.J. Cell biology of ischemia/reperfusion injury. *Int. Rev. Cell Mol. Biol.* **2012**, *298*, 229–317. [PubMed]

70. Ong, S.B.; Samangouei, P.; Kalkhoran, S.B.; Hausenloy, D.J. The mitochondrial permeability transition pore and its role in myocardial ischemia reperfusion injury. *J. Mol. Cell. Cardiol.* **2015**, *78*, 23–34. [CrossRef] [PubMed]

71. Di Lisa, F.; Menabo, R.; Canton, M.; Barile, M.; Bernardi, P. Opening of the mitochondrial permeability transition pore causes depletion of mitochondrial and cytosolic nNAD+ and is a causative event in the death of myocytes in postischemic reperfusion of the heart. *J. Biol. Chem.* **2001**, *276*, 2571–2575. [CrossRef] [PubMed]

72. Abdallah, Y.; Kasseckert, S.A.; Iraqi, W.; Said, M.; Shahzad, T.; Erdogan, A.; Neuhof, C.; Gunduz, D.; Schluter, K.D.; Tillmanns, H.; et al. Interplay between Ca2+ cycling and mitochondrial permeability transition pores promotes reperfusion-induced injury of cardiac myocytes. *J. Cell. Mol. Med.* **2011**, *15*, 2478–2485. [CrossRef] [PubMed]

73. Hausenloy, D.J.; Botker, H.E.; Engstrom, T.; Erlinge, D.; Heusch, G.; Ibanez, B.; Kloner, R.A.; Ovize, M.; Yellon, D.M.; Garcia-Dorado, D. Targeting reperfusion injury in patients with ST-segment elevation myocardial infarction: Trials and tribulations. *Eur. Heart J.* **2016**, *38*, 935–941. [CrossRef] [PubMed]

74. Abdi, S.; Rafizadeh, O.; Peighambari, M.; Basiri, H.; Bakhshandeh, H. Evaluation of the clinical and procedural predictive factors of no-reflow phenomenon following primary percutaneous coronary intervention. *Res. Cardiovasc. Med.* **2015**, *4*, e25414. [CrossRef]

75. Nattel, S.; Maguy, A.; Le Bouter, S.; Yeh, Y.H. Arrhythmogenic ion-channel remodeling in the heart: Heart failure, myocardial infarction, and atrial fibrillation. *Physiol. Rev.* **2007**, *87*, 425–456. [CrossRef] [PubMed]

76. Yellon, D.M.; Hausenloy, D.J. Myocardial reperfusion injury. *N. Engl. J. Med.* **2007**, *357*, 1121–1135. [PubMed]

77. Tellides, G.; Pober, J.S. Inflammatory and immune responses in the arterial media. *Circ. Res.* **2015**, *116*, 312–322. [CrossRef] [PubMed]

78. Jin, R.; Xiao, A.Y.; Song, Z.; Yu, S.; Li, J.; Cui, M.Z.; Li, G. Platelet cd40 mediates leukocyte recruitment and neointima formation after arterial denudation injury in atherosclerosis-prone mice. *Am. J. Pathol.* **2018**, *188*, 252–263. [CrossRef] [PubMed]

79. Hammond, J.; Balligand, J.L. Nitric oxide synthase and cyclic GMP signaling in cardiac myocytes: From contractility to remodeling. *J. Mol. Cell. Cardiol.* **2012**, *52*, 330–340. [CrossRef] [PubMed]

80. Lucas, K.A.; Pitari, G.M.; Kazerounian, S.; Ruiz-Stewart, I.; Park, J.; Schulz, S.; Chepenik, K.P.; Waldman, S.A. Guanylyl cyclases and signaling by cyclic GMP. *Pharmacol. Rev.* **2000**, *52*, 375–414. [PubMed]

81. Kamp, T.J.; Hell, J.W. Regulation of cardiac L-type calcium channels by protein kinase A and protein kinase C. *Circ. Res.* **2000**, *87*, 1095–1102. [CrossRef] [PubMed]

82. Kalogeris, T.; Bao, Y.; Korthuis, R.J. Mitochondrial reactive oxygen species: A double edged sword in ischemia/reperfusion vs. preconditioning. *Redox Biol.* **2014**, *2*, 702–714. [CrossRef] [PubMed]

83. Perrelli, M.G.; Pagliaro, P.; Penna, C. Ischemia/reperfusion injury and cardioprotective mechanisms: Role of mitochondria and reactive oxygen species. *World J. Cardiol.* **2011**, *3*, 186–200. [CrossRef] [PubMed]

84. Webster, K.A. Mitochondrial membrane permeabilization and cell death during myocardial infarction: Roles of calcium and reactive oxygen species. *Future Cardiol.* **2012**, *8*, 863–884. [CrossRef] [PubMed]

85. Butler, M.J.; Chan, W.; Taylor, A.J.; Dart, A.M.; Duffy, S.J. Management of the no-reflow phenomenon. *Pharmacol. Ther.* **2011**, *132*, 72–85. [CrossRef] [PubMed]

86. Pell, V.R.; Chouchani, E.T.; Murphy, M.P.; Brookes, P.S.; Krieg, T. Moving forwards by blocking back-flow: The yin and yang of MI therapy. *Circ. Res.* **2016**, *118*, 898–906. [CrossRef] [PubMed]

87. Jiao, Q.; Ke, Q.; Li, W.; Jin, M.; Luo, Y.; Zhang, L.; Yang, D.; Zhang, X. Effect of inflammatory factor-induced cyclo-oxygenase expression on the development of reperfusion-related no-reflow phenomenon in acute myocardial infarction. *Clin. Exp. Pharmacol. Physiol.* **2015**, *42*, 162–170. [CrossRef] [PubMed]

88. Maskali, F.; Franken, P.R.; Poussier, S.; Tran, N.; Vanhove, C.; Boutley, H.; Le Gall, H.; Karcher, G.; Zannad, F.; Lacolley, P.; et al. Initial infarct size predicts subsequent cardiac remodeling in the rat infarct model: An in vivo serial pinhole gated spect study. *J. Nuclear Med.* **2006**, *47*, 337–344.

89. Selker, H.P.; Udelson, J.E.; Ruthazer, R.; D'Agostino, R.B.; Nichols, M.; Ben-Yehuda, O.; Eitel, I.; Granger, C.B.; Jenkins, P.; Maehara, A.; et al. Relationship between therapeutic effects on infarct size in acute myocardial infarction and therapeutic effects on 1-year outcomes: A patient-level analysis of randomized clinical trials. *Am. Heart J.* **2017**, *188*, 18–25. [CrossRef] [PubMed]

90. Frangogiannis, N.G. The immune system and the remodeling infarcted heart: Cell biological insights and therapeutic opportunities. *J. Cardiovasc. Pharmacol.* **2014**, *63*, 185–195. [CrossRef] [PubMed]

91. Stefanon, I.; Valero-Munoz, M.; Fernandes, A.A.; Ribeiro, R.F., Jr.; Rodriguez, C.; Miana, M.; Martinez-Gonzalez, J.; Spalenza, J.S.; Lahera, V.; Vassallo, P.F.; et al. Left and right ventricle late remodeling following myocardial infarction in rats. *PLoS ONE* **2013**, *8*, e64986. [CrossRef] [PubMed]

92. Dobaczewski, M.; Chen, W.; Frangogiannis, N.G. Transforming growth factor (TGF)-beta signaling in cardiac remodeling. *J. Mol. Cell. Cardiol.* **2011**, *51*, 600–606. [CrossRef] [PubMed]

93. Ridker, P.M. From c-reactive protein to interleukin-6 to interleukin-1: Moving upstream to identify novel targets for atheroprotection. *Circ. Res.* **2016**, *118*, 145–156. [CrossRef] [PubMed]

94. Anderson, D.R.; Poterucha, J.T.; Mikuls, T.R.; Duryee, M.J.; Garvin, R.P.; Klassen, L.W.; Shurmur, S.W.; Thiele, G.M. Il-6 and its receptors in coronary artery disease and acute myocardial infarction. *Cytokine* **2013**, *62*, 395–400. [CrossRef] [PubMed]

95. Dejaco, C.; Brouwer, E.; Mason, J.C.; Buttgereit, F.; Matteson, E.L.; Dasgupta, B. Giant cell arteritis and polymyalgia rheumatica: Current challenges and opportunities. *Nat. Rev. Rheumatol.* **2017**, *13*, 578–592. [CrossRef] [PubMed]

96. Chaabane, C.; Otsuka, F.; Virmani, R.; Bochaton-Piallat, M.L. Biological responses in stented arteries. *Cardiovasc. Res.* **2013**, *99*, 353–363. [CrossRef] [PubMed]

97. Didion, S.P. Cellular and oxidative mechanisms associated with interleukin-6 signaling in the vasculature. *Int. J. Mol. Sci.* **2017**, *18*, 2563. [CrossRef] [PubMed]

98. Von Haehling, S.; Schefold, J.C.; Lainscak, M.; Doehner, W.; Anker, S.D. Inflammatory biomarkers in heart failure revisited: Much more than innocent bystanders. *Heart Fail. Clin.* **2009**, *5*, 549–560. [CrossRef] [PubMed]

99. Jafarzadeh, A.; Nemati, M.; Rezayati, M.T. Serum levels of interleukin (il)-27 in patients with ischemic heart disease. *Cytokine* **2011**, *56*, 153–156. [CrossRef] [PubMed]

100. Heinisch, R.H.; Zanetti, C.R.; Comin, F.; Fernandes, J.L.; Ramires, J.A.; Serrano, C.V., Jr. Serial changes in plasma levels of cytokines in patients with coronary artery disease. *Vasc. Health Risk Manag.* **2005**, *1*, 245–250. [PubMed]

101. Hattori, Y.; Akimoto, K.; Murakami, Y.; Kasai, K. Pyrrolidine dithiocarbamate inhibits cytokine-induced vcam-1 gene expression in rat cardiac myocytes. *Mol. Cell. Biochem.* **1997**, *177*, 177–181. [CrossRef] [PubMed]

102. Marcos-Ramiro, B.; Garcia-Weber, D.; Millan, J. TNF-induced endothelial barrier disruption: Beyond actin and rho. *Thromb. Haemost.* **2014**, *112*, 1088–1102. [CrossRef] [PubMed]

103. Bhat, O.M.; Uday Kumar, P.; Harishankar, N.; Ravichandaran, L.; Bhatia, A.; Dhawan, V. Interleukin-18-induced cell adhesion molecule expression is associated with feedback regulation by PPAR-gamma and Nf-kappa-b in apo e-/- mice. *Mol. Cell. Biochem.* **2017**, *428*, 119–128. [CrossRef] [PubMed]

104. Frangogiannis, N.G.; Smith, C.W.; Entman, M.L. The inflammatory response in myocardial infarction. *Cardiovasc. Res.* **2002**, *53*, 31–47. [CrossRef]

105. Pomerantz, B.J.; Reznikov, L.L.; Harken, A.H.; Dinarello, C.A. Inhibition of caspase 1 reduces human myocardial ischemic dysfunction via inhibition of IL-18 and IL-1beta. *Proc. Natl. Acad. Sci. USA* **2001**, *98*, 2871–2876. [CrossRef] [PubMed]

106. Van Tassell, B.W.; Raleigh, J.M.; Abbate, A. Targeting interleukin-1 in heart failure and inflammatory heart disease. *Curr. Heart Fail. Rep.* **2015**, *12*, 33–41. [CrossRef] [PubMed]

107. Berthonneche, C.; Sulpice, T.; Boucher, F.; Gouraud, L.; de Leiris, J.; O'Connor, S.E.; Herbert, J.M.; Janiak, P. New insights into the pathological role of TNF-alpha in early cardiac dysfunction and subsequent heart failure after infarction in rats. *Am. J. Physiol.* **2004**, *287*, H340–H350.

108. Meng, X.; Yang, J.; Dong, M.; Zhang, K.; Tu, E.; Gao, Q.; Chen, W.; Zhang, C.; Zhang, Y. Regulatory t cells in cardiovascular diseases. *Nat. Rev. Cardiol.* **2016**, *13*, 167–179. [CrossRef] [PubMed]

109. Chow, S.; Cove-Smith, L.; Schmitt, M.; Hawkins, R. High-dose interleukin 2-induced myocarditis: Can myocardial damage reversibility be assessed by cardiac MRI? *J. Immunother.* **2014**, *37*, 304–308. [CrossRef] [PubMed]

110. Thavendiranathan, P.; Verhaert, D.; Kendra, K.L.; Raman, S.V. Fulminant myocarditis owing to high-dose interleukin-2 therapy for metastatic melanoma. *Br. J. Radiol.* **2011**, *84*, e99–e102. [CrossRef] [PubMed]

111. Fontes, J.A.; Rose, N.R.; Cihakova, D. The varying faces of IL-6: From cardiac protection to cardiac failure. *Cytokine* **2015**, *74*, 62–68. [CrossRef] [PubMed]

112. Kanda, T.; Takahashi, T. Interleukin-6 and cardiovascular diseases. *Jpn. Heart J.* **2004**, *45*, 183–193. [CrossRef] [PubMed]

113. Mihara, M.; Hashizume, M.; Yoshida, H.; Suzuki, M.; Shiina, M. IL-6/IL-6 receptor system and its role in physiological and pathological conditions. *Clin. Sci.* **2012**, *122*, 143–159. [CrossRef] [PubMed]

114. Ninan, J.V.; Lester, S.; Hill, C.L. Giant cell arteritis: Beyond temporal artery biopsy and steroids. *Intern. Med. J.* **2017**, *47*, 1228–1240. [CrossRef] [PubMed]

115. Tsutamoto, T.; Hisanaga, T.; Wada, A.; Maeda, K.; Ohnishi, M.; Fukai, D.; Mabuchi, N.; Sawaki, M.; Kinoshita, M. Interleukin-6 spillover in the peripheral circulation increases with the severity of heart failure, and the high plasma level of interleukin-6 is an important prognostic predictor in patients with congestive heart failure. *J. Am. Coll. Cardiol.* **1998**, *31*, 391–398. [CrossRef]

116. Lesina, M.; Kurkowski, M.U.; Ludes, K.; Rose-John, S.; Treiber, M.; Kloppel, G.; Yoshimura, A.; Reindl, W.; Sipos, B.; Akira, S.; et al. Stat3/Socs3 activation by IL-6 transsignaling promotes progression of pancreatic intraepithelial neoplasia and development of pancreatic cancer. *Cancer Cell* **2011**, *19*, 456–469. [CrossRef] [PubMed]

117. Schuett, H.; Oestreich, R.; Waetzig, G.H.; Annema, W.; Luchtefeld, M.; Hillmer, A.; Bavendiek, U.; von Felden, J.; Divchev, D.; Kempf, T.; et al. Transsignaling of interleukin-6 crucially contributes to atherosclerosis in mice. *Arterioscler. Thromb. Vasc. Biol.* **2012**, *32*, 281–290. [CrossRef] [PubMed]

118. Yang, S.; Hu, S.; Choudhry, M.A.; Rue, L.W., 3rd; Bland, K.I.; Chaudry, I.H. Anti-rat soluble IL-6 receptor antibody down-regulates cardiac IL-6 and improves cardiac function following trauma-hemorrhage. *J. Mol. Cell. Cardiol.* **2007**, *42*, 620–630. [CrossRef] [PubMed]

119. Jones, S.A.; Horiuchi, S.; Topley, N.; Yamamoto, N.; Fuller, G.M. The soluble interleukin 6 receptor: Mechanisms of production and implications in disease. *FASEB J.* **2001**, *15*, 43–58. [CrossRef] [PubMed]

120. Kobara, M.; Noda, K.; Kitamura, M.; Okamoto, A.; Shiraishi, T.; Toba, H.; Matsubara, H.; Nakata, T. Antibody against interleukin-6 receptor attenuates left ventricular remodelling after myocardial infarction in mice. *Cardiovasc. Res.* **2010**, *87*, 424–430. [CrossRef] [PubMed]

121. Rose-John, S. IL-6 trans-signaling via the soluble IL-6 receptor: Importance for the pro-inflammatory activities of IL-6. *Int. J. Biol. Sci.* **2012**, *8*, 1237–1247. [CrossRef] [PubMed]

122. Huang, M.; Yang, D.; Xiang, M.; Wang, J. Role of interleukin-6 in regulation of immune responses to remodeling after myocardial infarction. *Heart Fail. Rev.* **2014**, *20*, 25–38. [CrossRef] [PubMed]

123. Haghikia, A.; Stapel, B.; Hoch, M.; Hilfiker-Kleiner, D. Stat3 and cardiac remodeling. *Heart Fail. Rev.* **2011**, *16*, 35–47. [CrossRef] [PubMed]

124. Hilfiker-Kleiner, D.; Shukla, P.; Klein, G.; Schaefer, A.; Stapel, B.; Hoch, M.; Muller, W.; Scherr, M.; Theilmeier, G.; Ernst, M.; et al. Continuous glycoprotein-130-mediated signal transducer and activator of transcription-3 activation promotes inflammation, left ventricular rupture, and adverse outcome in subacute myocardial infarction. *Circulation* **2010**, *122*, 145–155. [CrossRef] [PubMed]

125. Yu, X.W.; Liu, M.Y.; Kennedy, R.H.; Liu, S.J. Both cgmp and peroxynitrite mediate chronic interleukin-6-induced negative inotropy in adult rat ventricular myocytes. *J. Physiol.* **2005**, *566*, 341–353. [CrossRef] [PubMed]

126. Szabo-Fresnais, N.; Lefebvre, F.; Germain, A.; Fischmeister, R.; Pomerance, M. A new regulation of IL-6 production in adult cardiomyocytes by beta-adrenergic and IL-1 beta receptors and induction of cellular hypertrophy by IL-6 trans-signalling. *Cell. Signal.* **2010**, *22*, 1143–1152. [CrossRef] [PubMed]

127. Depre, C.; Hue, L. Cyclic gmp in the perfused rat heart. Effect of ischaemia, anoxia and nitric oxide synthase inhibitor. *FEBS Lett.* **1994**, *345*, 241–245. [CrossRef]

128. Penna, C.; Cappello, S.; Mancardi, D.; Raimondo, S.; Rastaldo, R.; Gattullo, D.; Losano, G.; Pagliaro, P. Post-conditioning reduces infarct size in the isolated rat heart: Role of coronary flow and pressure and the nitric oxide/cgmp pathway. *Basic Res. Cardiol.* **2006**, *101*, 168–179. [CrossRef] [PubMed]

129. Lochner, A.; Genade, S.; Tromp, E.; Opie, L.; Moolman, J.; Thomas, S.; Podzuweit, T. Role of cyclic nucleotide phosphodiesterases in ischemic preconditioning. *Mol. Cell. Biochem.* **1998**, *186*, 169–175. [CrossRef] [PubMed]

130. Burley, D.S.; Ferdinandy, P.; Baxter, G.F. Cyclic GMP and protein kinase-g in myocardial ischaemia-reperfusion: Opportunities and obstacles for survival signaling. *Br. J. Pharmacol.* **2007**, *152*, 855–869. [CrossRef] [PubMed]

131. Takasago, T.; Imagawa, T.; Furukawa, K.; Ogurusu, T.; Shigekawa, M. Regulation of the cardiac ryanodine receptor by protein kinase-dependent phosphorylation. *J. Biochem.* **1991**, *109*, 163–170. [CrossRef] [PubMed]

132. Mattiazzi, A.; Mundina-Weilenmann, C.; Guoxiang, C.; Vittone, L.; Kranias, E. Role of phospholamban phosphorylation on Thr17 in cardiac physiological and pathological conditions. *Cardiovasc. Res.* **2005**, *68*, 366–375. [CrossRef] [PubMed]

133. Layland, J.; Li, J.M.; Shah, A.M. Role of cyclic GMP-dependent protein kinase in the contractile response to exogenous nitric oxide in rat cardiac myocytes. *J. Physiol.* **2002**, *540*, 457–467. [CrossRef] [PubMed]

134. Bauer, J.; Ripperger, A.; Frantz, S.; Ergun, S.; Schwedhelm, E.; Benndorf, R.A. Pathophysiology of isoprostanes in the cardiovascular system: Implications of isoprostane-mediated thromboxane a2 receptor activation. *Br. J. Pharmacol.* **2014**, *171*, 3115–3131. [CrossRef] [PubMed]

135. Chigaev, A.; Smagley, Y.; Sklar, L.A. Nitric oxide/cGMP pathway signaling actively down-regulates alpha4beta1-integrin affinity: An unexpected mechanism for inducing cell de-adhesion. *BMC Immunol.* **2011**, *12*, 28. [CrossRef] [PubMed]

136. Frankenreiter, S.; Bednarczyk, P.; Kniess, A.; Bork, N.I.; Straubinger, J.; Koprowski, P.; Wrzosek, A.; Mohr, E.; Logan, A.; Murphy, M.P.; et al. cGMP-elevating compounds and ischemic conditioning provide cardioprotection against ischemia and reperfusion injury via cardiomyocyte-specific BK channels. *Circulation* **2017**, *136*, 2337–2355. [CrossRef] [PubMed]

137. Bovo, E.; Huke, S.; Blatter, L.A.; Zima, A.V. The effect of PKA-mediated phosphorylation of ryanodine receptor on SR Ca(2+) leak in ventricular myocytes. *J. Mol. Cell. Cardiol.* **2017**, *104*, 9–16. [CrossRef] [PubMed]

138. Najafi, A.; Sequeira, V.; Helmes, M.; Bollen, I.A.; Goebel, M.; Regan, J.A.; Carrier, L.; Kuster, D.W.; Van Der Velden, J. Selective phosphorylation of PKA targets after beta-adrenergic receptor stimulation impairs myofilament function in mybpc3-targeted hcm mouse model. *Cardiovasc. Res.* **2016**, *110*, 200–214. [CrossRef] [PubMed]

139. Chu, G.; Kranias, E.G. Functional interplay between dual site phospholamban phosphorylation: Insights from genetically altered mouse models. *Basic Res. Cardiol.* **2002**, *97* (Suppl. 1), I43–I48. [CrossRef] [PubMed]

140. Pi, Y.; Zhang, D.; Kemnitz, K.R.; Wang, H.; Walker, J.W. Protein kinase C and A sites on troponin I regulate myofilament Ca2+ sensitivity and ATPase activity in the mouse myocardium. *J. Physiol.* **2003**, *552*, 845–857. [CrossRef] [PubMed]

141. Callaghan, N.I. Beta-adrenergic augmentation of cardiac contractility is dependent on PKA-mediated phosphorylation of myosin-binding protein c and troponin i. *J. Physiol.* **2016**, *594*, 4707–4708. [CrossRef] [PubMed]

142. Rosas, P.C.; Liu, Y.; Abdalla, M.I.; Thomas, C.M.; Kidwell, D.T.; Dusio, G.F.; Mukhopadhyay, D.; Kumar, R.; Baker, K.M.; Mitchell, B.M.; et al. Phosphorylation of cardiac myosin-binding protein-c is a critical mediator of diastolic function. *Circulation* **2015**, *8*, 582–594. [CrossRef] [PubMed]

143. Wilson, K.; Guggilam, A.; West, T.A.; Zhang, X.; Trask, A.J.; Cismowski, M.J.; de Tombe, P.; Sadayappan, S.; Lucchesi, P.A. Effects of a myofilament calcium sensitizer on left ventricular systolic and diastolic function in rats with volume overload heart failure. *Am. J. Physiol.* **2014**, *307*, H1605–H1617. [CrossRef] [PubMed]

144. Kooij, V.; Holewinski, R.J.; Murphy, A.M.; Van Eyk, J.E. Characterization of the cardiac myosin binding protein-c phosphoproteome in healthy and failing human hearts. *J. Mol. Cell. Cardiol.* **2013**, *60*, 116–120. [CrossRef] [PubMed]

145. Li, J.; Ning, Y.; Hedley, W.; Saunders, B.; Chen, Y.; Tindill, N.; Hannay, T.; Subramaniam, S. The molecule pages database. *Nature* **2002**, *420*, 716–717. [CrossRef] [PubMed]

146. Rosenbaum, D.M.; Rasmussen, S.G.; Kobilka, B.K. The structure and function of G-protein-coupled receptors. *Nature* **2009**, *459*, 356–363. [CrossRef] [PubMed]

147. Overington, J.P.; Al-Lazikani, B.; Hopkins, A.L. How many drug targets are there? *Nat. Rev. Drug Discov.* **2006**, *5*, 993–996. [CrossRef] [PubMed]

148. Santos, R.; Ursu, O.; Gaulton, A.; Bento, A.P.; Donadi, R.S.; Bologa, C.G.; Karlsson, A.; Al-Lazikani, B.; Hersey, A.; Oprea, T.I.; et al. A comprehensive map of molecular drug targets. *Nat. Rev. Drug Discov.* **2017**, *16*, 19–34. [CrossRef] [PubMed]

149. Schoneberg, T.; Schulz, A.; Biebermann, H.; Hermsdorf, T.; Rompler, H.; Sangkuhl, K. Mutant G-protein-coupled receptors as a cause of human diseases. *Pharmacol. Ther.* **2004**, *104*, 173–206. [CrossRef] [PubMed]

150. Insel, P.A.; Tang, C.M.; Hahntow, I.; Michel, M.C. Impact of GPCRs in clinical medicine: Monogenic diseases, genetic variants and drug targets. *Biochim. Biophys. Acta* **2007**, *1768*, 994–1005. [CrossRef] [PubMed]

151. Cook, J.L. G protein-coupled receptors as disease targets: Emerging paradigms. *Ochsner J.* **2010**, *10*, 2–7. [PubMed]

152. Justus, C.R.; Dong, L.; Yang, L.V. Acidic tumor microenvironment and pH-sensing G protein-coupled receptors. *Front. Physiol.* **2013**, *4*, 354. [CrossRef] [PubMed]

153. Ludwig, M.G.; Vanek, M.; Guerini, D.; Gasser, J.A.; Jones, C.E.; Junker, U.; Hofstetter, H.; Wolf, R.M.; Seuwen, K. Proton-sensing G-protein-coupled receptors. *Nature* **2003**, *425*, 93–98. [CrossRef] [PubMed]

154. Ishii, S.; Kihara, Y.; Shimizu, T. Identification of T cell death-associated gene 8 (TDAG8) as a novel acid sensing G-protein-coupled receptor. *J. Biol. Chem.* **2005**, *280*, 9083–9087. [CrossRef] [PubMed]

155. Tomura, H.; Mogi, C.; Sato, K.; Okajima, F. Proton-sensing and lysolipid-sensitive G-protein-coupled receptors: A novel type of multi-functional receptors. *Cell. Signal.* **2005**, *17*, 1466–1476. [CrossRef] [PubMed]

156. Okajima, F. Regulation of inflammation by extracellular acidification and proton-sensing GPCRs. *Cell. Signal.* **2013**, *25*, 2263–2271. [CrossRef] [PubMed]

157. Sanderlin, E.J.; Justus, C.R.; Krewson, E.K.; Li, V.Y. Emerging roles for the pH-sensing G protein-coupled receptors in response to acidotic stress. *Cell Health Cytoskelet.* **2015**, *2015*, 99–109.

158. Yang, L.V.; Radu, C.G.; Roy, M.; Lee, S.; McLaughlin, J.; Teitell, M.A.; Iruela-Arispe, M.L.; Witte, O.N. Vascular abnormalities in mice deficient for the G protein-coupled receptor GPR4 that functions as a pH sensor. *Mol. Cell. Biol.* **2007**, *27*, 1334–1347. [CrossRef] [PubMed]

159. Chen, A.; Dong, L.; Leffler, N.R.; Asch, A.S.; Witte, O.N.; Yang, L.V. Activation of GPR4 by acidosis increases endothelial cell adhesion through the cAMP/Epac pathway. *PLoS ONE* **2011**, *6*, e27586. [CrossRef] [PubMed]

160. Dong, L.; Li, Z.; Leffler, N.R.; Asch, A.S.; Chi, J.T.; Yang, L.V. Acidosis activation of the proton-sensing GPR4 receptor stimulates vascular endothelial cell inflammatory responses revealed by transcriptome analysis. *PLoS ONE* **2013**, *8*, e61991. [CrossRef] [PubMed]

161. Liu, J.P.; Komachi, M.; Tomura, H.; Mogi, C.; Damirin, A.; Tobo, M.; Takano, M.; Nochi, H.; Tamoto, K.; Sato, K.; et al. Ovarian cancer G protein-coupled receptor 1-dependent and -independent vascular actions to acidic pH in human aortic smooth muscle cells. *Am. J. Physiol.* **2010**, *299*, H731–H742. [CrossRef] [PubMed]

162. Chang, J.T.; Nevins, J.R. Gather: A systems approach to interpreting genomic signatures. *Bioinformatics* **2006**, *22*, 2926–2933. [CrossRef] [PubMed]

163. Tomura, H.; Wang, J.Q.; Komachi, M.; Damirin, A.; Mogi, C.; Tobo, M.; Kon, J.; Misawa, N.; Sato, K.; Okajima, F. Prostaglandin i(2) production and cAMP accumulation in response to acidic extracellular pH through OGR1 in human aortic smooth muscle cells. *J. Biol. Chem.* **2005**, *280*, 34458–34464. [CrossRef] [PubMed]

164. Guan, J.; Wu, X.; Arons, E.; Christou, H. The p38 mitogen-activated protein kinase pathway is involved in the regulation of heme oxygenase-1 by acidic extracellular pH in aortic smooth muscle cells. *J. Cell. Biochem.* **2008**, *105*, 1298–1306. [CrossRef] [PubMed]

165. Rios, E.J.; Fallon, M.; Wang, J.; Shimoda, L.A. Chronic hypoxia elevates intracellular pH and activates Na+/H+ exchange in pulmonary arterial smooth muscle cells. *Am. J. Physiol. Lung Cell. Mol. Physiol.* **2005**, *289*, L867–L874. [CrossRef] [PubMed]

166. Russell, J.L.; Goetsch, S.C.; Aguilar, H.R.; Coe, H.; Luo, X.; Liu, N.; van Rooij, E.; Frantz, D.E.; Schneider, J.W. Regulated expression of pH sensing G protein-coupled receptor-68 identified through chemical biology defines a new drug target for ischemic heart disease. *ACS Chem. Biol.* **2012**, *7*, 1077–1083. [CrossRef] [PubMed]

167. Fukuda, H.; Ito, S.; Watari, K.; Mogi, C.; Arisawa, M.; Okajima, F.; Kurose, H.; Shuto, S. Identification of a potent and selective GPR4 antagonist as a drug lead for the treatment of myocardial infarction. *ACS Med. Chem. Lett.* **2016**, *7*, 493–497. [CrossRef] [PubMed]

168. Hirano, K. The roles of proteinase-activated receptors in the vascular physiology and pathophysiology. *Arterioscler. Thromb. Vasc. Biol.* **2007**, *27*, 27–36. [CrossRef] [PubMed]

169. Leger, A.J.; Covic, L.; Kuliopulos, A. Protease-activated receptors in cardiovascular diseases. *Circulation* **2006**, *114*, 1070–1077. [CrossRef] [PubMed]

170. Coughlin, S.R. Thrombin signalling and protease-activated receptors. *Nature* **2000**, *407*, 258–264. [CrossRef] [PubMed]

171. Lee, H.; Hamilton, J.R. Physiology, pharmacology, and therapeutic potential of protease-activated receptors in vascular disease. *Pharmacol. Ther.* **2012**, *134*, 246–259. [CrossRef] [PubMed]

172. Wronkowitz, N.; Gorgens, S.W.; Romacho, T.; Villalobos, L.A.; Sanchez-Ferrer, C.F.; Peiro, C.; Sell, H.; Eckel, J. Soluble dpp4 induces inflammation and proliferation of human smooth muscle cells via protease-activated receptor 2. *Biochim. Biophys. Acta* **2014**, *1842*, 1613–1621. [CrossRef] [PubMed]

173. Macfarlane, S.R.; Seatter, M.J.; Kanke, T.; Hunter, G.D.; Plevin, R. Proteinase-activated receptors. *Pharmacol. Rev.* **2001**, *53*, 245–282. [PubMed]

174. Steinberg, S.F. The cardiovascular actions of protease-activated receptors. *Mol. Pharmacol.* **2005**, *67*, 2–11. [CrossRef] [PubMed]

175. Alberelli, M.A.; De Candia, E. Functional role of protease activated receptors in vascular biology. *Vasc. Pharmacol.* **2014**, *62*, 72–81. [CrossRef] [PubMed]

176. Coelho, A.M.; Ossovskaya, V.; Bunnett, N.W. Proteinase-activated receptor-2: Physiological and pathophysiological roles. *Curr. Med. Chem. Cardiovasc. Hematol. Agents* **2003**, *1*, 61–72. [CrossRef] [PubMed]

177. Gryka, R.J.; Buckley, L.F.; Anderson, S.M. Vorapaxar: The current role and future directions of a novel protease-activated receptor antagonist for risk reduction in atherosclerotic disease. *Drugs R D* **2017**, *17*, 65–72. [CrossRef] [PubMed]

178. Wilcox, J.N.; Rodriguez, J.; Subramanian, R.; Ollerenshaw, J.; Zhong, C.; Hayzer, D.J.; Horaist, C.; Hanson, S.R.; Lumsden, A.; Salam, T.A.; et al. Characterization of thrombin receptor expression during vascular lesion formation. *Circ. Res.* **1994**, *75*, 1029–1038. [CrossRef] [PubMed]

179. Ku, D.D.; Dai, J. Expression of thrombin receptors in human atherosclerotic coronary arteries leads to an exaggerated vasoconstrictory response in vitro. *J. Cardiovasc. Pharmacol.* **1997**, *30*, 649–657. [CrossRef] [PubMed]

180. Zuo, P.; Zuo, Z.; Zheng, Y.; Wang, X.; Zhou, Q.; Chen, L.; Ma, G. Protease-activated receptor-2 deficiency attenuates atherosclerotic lesion progression and instability in apolipoprotein e-deficient mice. *Front. Pharmacol.* **2017**, *8*, 647. [CrossRef] [PubMed]

181. Shi, Y.; Massague, J. Mechanisms of TGF-beta signaling from cell membrane to the nucleus. *Cell* **2003**, *113*, 685–700. [CrossRef]

182. Massague, J.; Attisano, L.; Wrana, J.L. The TGF-beta family and its composite receptors. *Trends Cell Biol.* **1994**, *4*, 172–178. [CrossRef]

183. Kingsley, D.M. The TGF-beta superfamily: New members, new receptors, and new genetic tests of function in different organisms. *Genes Dev.* **1994**, *8*, 133–146. [CrossRef] [PubMed]

184. Wrana, J.L.; Attisano, L.; Wieser, R.; Ventura, F.; Massague, J. Mechanism of activation of the TGF-beta receptor. *Nature* **1994**, *370*, 341–347. [CrossRef] [PubMed]

185. Annes, J.P.; Munger, J.S.; Rifkin, D.B. Making sense of latent TGFbeta activation. *J. Cell Sci.* **2003**, *116*, 217–224. [CrossRef] [PubMed]

186. Javelaud, D.; Mauviel, A. Mammalian transforming growth factor-betas: Smad signaling and physio-pathological roles. *Int. J. Biochem. Cell Biol.* **2004**, *36*, 1161–1165. [CrossRef]

187. Gonzalez, D.; Contreras, O.; Rebolledo, D.L.; Espinoza, J.P.; van Zundert, B.; Brandan, E. Als skeletal muscle shows enhanced TGF-beta signaling, fibrosis and induction of fibro/adipogenic progenitor markers. *PLoS ONE* **2017**, *12*, e0177649. [CrossRef] [PubMed]

188. Luo, T.; Nocon, A.; Fry, J.; Sherban, A.; Rui, X.; Jiang, B.; Xu, X.J.; Han, J.; Yan, Y.; Yang, Q.; et al. AMPK activation by metformin suppresses abnormal extracellular matrix remodeling in adipose tissue and ameliorates insulin resistance in obesity. *Diabetes* **2016**, *65*, 2295–2310. [CrossRef] [PubMed]

189. Rodriguez-Vita, J.; Sanchez-Galan, E.; Santamaria, B.; Sanchez-Lopez, E.; Rodrigues-Diez, R.; Blanco-Colio, L.M.; Egido, J.; Ortiz, A.; Ruiz-Ortega, M. Essential role of TGF-beta/Smad pathway on statin dependent vascular smooth muscle cell regulation. *PLoS ONE* **2008**, *3*, e3959. [CrossRef] [PubMed]

190. Rodriguez-Vita, J.; Sanchez-Lopez, E.; Esteban, V.; Ruperez, M.; Egido, J.; Ruiz-Ortega, M. Angiotensin ii activates the smad pathway in vascular smooth muscle cells by a transforming growth factor-beta-independent mechanism. *Circulation* **2005**, *111*, 2509–2517. [CrossRef] [PubMed]

191. Hneino, M.; Bouazza, L.; Bricca, G.; Li, J.Y.; Langlois, D. Density-dependent shift of transforming growth factor-beta-1 from inhibition to stimulation of vascular smooth muscle cell growth is based on unconventional regulation of proliferation, apoptosis and contact inhibition. *J. Vasc. Res.* **2009**, *46*, 85–97. [CrossRef] [PubMed]

192. Schinner, E.; Wetzl, V.; Schramm, A.; Kees, F.; Sandner, P.; Stasch, J.P.; Hofmann, F.; Schlossmann, J. Inhibition of the TGFbeta signalling pathway by cGMP and cGMP-dependent kinase i in renal fibrosis. *FEBS Open Bio* **2017**, *7*, 550–561. [CrossRef] [PubMed]

193. Gong, K.; Xing, D.; Li, P.; Hilgers, R.H.; Hage, F.G.; Oparil, S.; Chen, Y.F. cGMP inhibits TGF-beta signaling by sequestering Smad3 with cytosolic beta2-tubulin in pulmonary artery smooth muscle cells. *Mol. Endocrinol.* **2011**, *25*, 1794–1803. [CrossRef] [PubMed]

194. Gong, W.; Yan, M.; Chen, J.; Chaugai, S.; Chen, C.; Wang, D. Chronic inhibition of cyclic guanosine monophosphate-specific phosphodiesterase 5 prevented cardiac fibrosis through inhibition of transforming growth factor beta-induced smad signaling. *Front. Med.* **2014**, *8*, 445–455. [CrossRef] [PubMed]

195. Obsil, T.; Obsilova, V. Structure/function relationships underlying regulation of foxo transcription factors. *Oncogene* **2008**, *27*, 2263–2275. [CrossRef] [PubMed]

196. Carlsson, P.; Mahlapuu, M. Forkhead transcription factors: Key players in development and metabolism. *Dev. Biol.* **2002**, *250*, 1–23. [CrossRef] [PubMed]

197. Lehmann, O.J.; Sowden, J.C.; Carlsson, P.; Jordan, T.; Bhattacharya, S.S. Fox's in development and disease. *Trends Genet.* **2003**, *19*, 339–344. [CrossRef]

198. Greer, E.L.; Brunet, A. Foxo transcription factors at the interface between longevity and tumor suppression. *Oncogene* **2005**, *24*, 7410–7425. [CrossRef] [PubMed]

199. Van der Horst, A.; Burgering, B.M. Stressing the role of FOXO proteins in lifespan and disease. *Nat. Rev. Mol. Cell Biol.* **2007**, *8*, 440–450. [CrossRef] [PubMed]

200. Stitt, T.N.; Drujan, D.; Clarke, B.A.; Panaro, F.; Timofeyva, Y.; Kline, W.O.; Gonzalez, M.; Yancopoulos, G.D.; Glass, D.J. The IGF-1/pPI3K/Akt pathway prevents expression of muscle atrophy-induced ubiquitin ligases by inhibiting FOXO transcription factors. *Mol. Cell* **2004**, *14*, 395–403. [CrossRef]

201. Brunet, A.; Bonni, A.; Zigmond, M.J.; Lin, M.Z.; Juo, P.; Hu, L.S.; Anderson, M.J.; Arden, K.C.; Blenis, J.; Greenberg, M.E. Akt promotes cell survival by phosphorylating and inhibiting a forkhead transcription factor. *Cell* **1999**, *96*, 857–868. [CrossRef]

202. Loebel, M.; Holzhauser, L.; Hartwig, J.A.; Shukla, P.C.; Savvatis, K.; Jenke, A.; Gast, M.; Escher, F.; Becker, S.C.; Bauer, S.; et al. The forkhead transcription factor FOXO3 negatively regulates natural killer cell function and viral clearance in myocarditis. *Eur. Heart J.* **2017**. [CrossRef] [PubMed]

203. Zhou, L.; Li, R.; Liu, C.; Sun, T.; Htet Aung, L.H.; Chen, C.; Gao, J.; Zhao, Y.; Wang, K. Foxo3a inhibits mitochondrial fission and protects against doxorubicin-induced cardiotoxicity by suppressing mief2. *Free Radic. Biol. Med.* **2017**, *104*, 360–370. [CrossRef] [PubMed]

204. Elmadhun, N.Y.; Sabe, A.A.; Lassaletta, A.D.; Chu, L.M.; Sellke, F.W. Metformin mitigates apoptosis in ischemic myocardium. *J. Surg. Res.* **2014**, *192*, 50–58. [CrossRef] [PubMed]

205. Park, K.W.; Kim, D.H.; You, H.J.; Sir, J.J.; Jeon, S.I.; Youn, S.W.; Yang, H.M.; Skurk, C.; Park, Y.B.; Walsh, K.; et al. Activated forkhead transcription factor inhibits neointimal hyperplasia after angioplasty through induction of p27. *Arterioscler. Thromb. Vasc. Biol.* **2005**, *25*, 742–747. [CrossRef] [PubMed]

206. Rathbone, C.R.; Booth, F.W.; Lees, S.J. Foxo3a preferentially induces p27kip1 expression while impairing muscle precursor cell-cycle progression. *Muscle Nerve* **2008**, *37*, 84–89. [CrossRef] [PubMed]

207. Lee, H.Y.; Chung, J.W.; Youn, S.W.; Kim, J.Y.; Park, K.W.; Koo, B.K.; Oh, B.H.; Park, Y.B.; Chaqour, B.; Walsh, K.; et al. Forkhead transcription factor Foxo3a is a negative regulator of angiogenic immediate early gene cyr61, leading to inhibition of vascular smooth muscle cell proliferation and neointimal hyperplasia. *Circ. Res.* **2007**, *100*, 372–380. [CrossRef] [PubMed]

208. Bollinger, L.M.; Witczak, C.A.; Houmard, J.A.; Brault, J.J. Smad3 augments FoxO3-induced MuRF-1 promoter activity in a DNA-binding-dependent manner. *Am. J. Physiol. Cell Physiol.* **2014**, *307*, C278–C287. [CrossRef] [PubMed]

209. Seoane, J.; Le, H.V.; Shen, L.; Anderson, S.A.; Massague, J. Integration of Smad and forkhead pathways in the control of neuroepithelial and glioblastoma cell proliferation. *Cell* **2004**, *117*, 211–223. [CrossRef]

210. Gomis, R.R.; Alarcon, C.; Nadal, C.; Van Poznak, C.; Massague, J. C/EBPbeta at the core of the TGFbeta cytostatic response and its evasion in metastatic breast cancer cells. *Cancer Cell* **2006**, *10*, 203–214. [CrossRef] [PubMed]

211. Borniquel, S.; Garcia-Quintans, N.; Valle, I.; Olmos, Y.; Wild, B.; Martinez-Granero, F.; Soria, E.; Lamas, S.; Monsalve, M. Inactivation of FoxO3a and subsequent downregulation of PGC-1 alpha mediate nitric oxide-induced endothelial cell migration. *Mol. Cell. Biol.* **2010**, *30*, 4035–4044. [CrossRef] [PubMed]

212. Kawasaki, K.; Smith, R.S., Jr.; Hsieh, C.M.; Sun, J.; Chao, J.; Liao, J.K. Activation of the phosphatidylinositol 3-kinase/protein kinase Akt pathway mediates nitric oxide-induced endothelial cell migration and angiogenesis. *Mol. Cell. Biol.* **2003**, *23*, 5726–5737. [CrossRef] [PubMed]

213. Denninger, J.W.; Marletta, M.A. Guanylate cyclase and the NO/cGMP signaling pathway. *Biochim. Biophys. Acta* **1999**, *1411*, 334–350. [CrossRef]

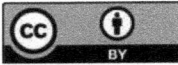

Journal of
*Cardiovascular
Development and Disease*

MDPI

Review

cGMP Signaling and Vascular Smooth Muscle Cell Plasticity

Moritz Lehners †, Hyazinth Dobrowinski †, Susanne Feil and Robert Feil *

Interfaculty Institute of Biochemistry, University of Tübingen, 72076 Tübingen, Germany;
moritz.lehners@uni-tuebingen.de (M.L.); hyazinth.dobrowinski@uni-tuebingen.de (H.D.);
susanne.feil@uni-tuebingen.de (S.F.)
* Correspondence: robert.feil@uni-tuebingen.de; Tel.: +49-7071-2973350
† These authors contributed equally to this work.

Received: 14 March 2018; Accepted: 16 April 2018; Published: 19 April 2018

Abstract: Cyclic GMP regulates multiple cell types and functions of the cardiovascular system. This review summarizes the effects of cGMP on the growth and survival of vascular smooth muscle cells (VSMCs), which display remarkable phenotypic plasticity during the development of vascular diseases, such as atherosclerosis. Recent studies have shown that VSMCs contribute to the development of atherosclerotic plaques by clonal expansion and transdifferentiation to macrophage-like cells. VSMCs express a variety of cGMP generators and effectors, including NO-sensitive guanylyl cyclase (NO-GC) and cGMP-dependent protein kinase type I (cGKI), respectively. According to the traditional view, cGMP inhibits VSMC proliferation, but this concept has been challenged by recent findings supporting a stimulatory effect of the NO-cGMP-cGKI axis on VSMC growth. Here, we summarize the relevant studies with a focus on VSMC growth regulation by the NO-cGMP-cGKI pathway in cultured VSMCs and mouse models of atherosclerosis, restenosis, and angiogenesis. We discuss potential reasons for inconsistent results, such as the use of genetic versus pharmacological approaches and primary versus subcultured cells. We also explore how modern methods for cGMP imaging and cell tracking could help to improve our understanding of cGMP's role in vascular plasticity. We present a revised model proposing that cGMP promotes phenotypic switching of contractile VSMCs to VSMC-derived plaque cells in atherosclerotic lesions. Regulation of vascular remodeling by cGMP is not only an interesting new therapeutic strategy, but could also result in side effects of clinically used cGMP-elevating drugs.

Keywords: cyclic guanosine $3'$-$5'$ monophosphate; nitric oxide; vascular smooth muscle cells; cGMP-dependent protein kinase type I; atherosclerosis; cell plasticity; transdifferentiation; cell fate mapping; imaging

1. Introduction

Cyclic guanosine $3'$-$5'$ monophosphate (cGMP) is a versatile intracellular signaling molecule present in many cell types. It controls numerous physiological processes, from cell contractility, secretion, and permeability to cell differentiation, growth, and survival [1,2]. In mammals, two types of guanylyl cyclases (GCs) have been identified that can generate cGMP from GTP: intracellular NO-sensitive GCs ("soluble" GCs or NO-GCs) [3] and transmembrane GCs ("particulate" GCs or pGCs), such as GC-A, GC-B, and GC-C [4]. The activity of NO-GC is stimulated by the gaseous signaling molecule NO, which is generated by NO synthases (NOSs) [5]. Several pGCs are receptors for peptide hormones. GC-A binds atrial and B-type natriuretic peptide (ANP, BNP), GC-B binds C-type natriuretic peptide (CNP), and GC-C is stimulated by guanylin and uroguanylin [4]. Levels of cGMP are also controlled by cGMP-hydrolyzing phosphodiesterases (PDEs), such as PDE5. The effects of cGMP are mediated by its binding to three classes of cGMP effector proteins: cyclic nucleotide-gated (CNG) cation channels, cGMP-dependent protein kinases (cGKs, also known as PKGs), and cGMP-regulated PDEs [6–8]. While CNG channels play a more restricted role in the sensory system, many tissues and cell types express PDEs and cGKs.

Cardiovascular diseases are frequently linked to dysfunctions in vascular smooth muscle cells (VSMCs). VSMCs express various components of the cGMP signaling cascade [3,4,9]. They can generate cGMP in response to NO and natriuretic peptides via NO-GCs and pGCs, respectively, and they express PDEs that degrade cGMP (e.g., PDE5) or cAMP (e.g., PDE3). An interesting aspect is that cAMP hydrolysis by PDE3 is inhibited in the presence of high concentrations of cGMP [7,10]. This inhibition of PDE3 enables crosstalk between cGMP and cAMP signaling in VSMCs in that an increase of cGMP can also result in an elevation of cAMP. A major cGMP effector in VSMCs is cGK type I (cGKI, also known as PKG1), which is encoded by the *prkg1* gene and belongs to the Ser/Thr protein kinase family. cGKI comprises an N-terminal regulatory domain with two cGMP-binding sites and a C-terminal catalytic domain. Two cGKI isoforms are known, cGKIα and cGKIβ, and both are expressed in VSMCs. However, whether cGKIα and cGKIβ have specific functions in vivo is not clear [11,12].

In vascular biology, the classical effects of NO and natriuretic peptides are vasodilation and regulation of blood flow. It is well-accepted that these acute effects are beneficial and mediated by activation of GCs and the cGMP-cGKI pathway in VSMCs [8,9]. NO and natriuretic peptides also have long-term effects on vascular diseases, such as atherosclerosis and restenosis. However, as previously summarized by us [13] and others [14,15], it is still debated whether the cGMP-cGKI axis is involved and, if so, whether it has a positive or negative impact on vascular remodeling and disease. In this review, we will focus on recent in vivo studies that identified a previously unknown form of VSMC plasticity in the context of atherosclerosis and indicate a stimulatory role of the NO-cGMP-cGKI pathway on the growth/survival and phenotypic switching of VSMCs in atherosclerotic plaques. We will also discuss potential reasons for the apparent discrepancy of these studies with a number of studies that reported an anti-proliferative effect of NO, cGMP, or cGKI in VSMCs. Furthermore, we will outline how the use of innovative technologies, such as cGMP imaging and cell tracking, could help to further clarify the role of cGMP in vascular plasticity in the future.

2. Role of VSMCs in Physiology and Pathophysiology

2.1. Vasodilation via the NO-cGMP-cGKI Pathway

VSMCs are contractile cells that regulate blood flow and their abnormalities contribute to a range of diseases [16]. Numerous studies have demonstrated that activation of the cGMP-cGKI axis in VSMCs leads to vasodilation [9]. The canonical NO-cGMP-cGKI pathway for vasodilation is depicted in Figure 1a. It comprises generation of NO in the endothelium via endothelial NOS (eNOS) followed by diffusion of NO into VSMCs in the vascular media, where NO-GC is stimulated to generate cGMP. The increased cGMP concentration activates cGKI, which triggers relaxation of VSMCs, likely by phosphorylating several substrate proteins, whose identity has not been completely established [8,11]. Note that vascular NO can also be derived from non-endothelial sources, such as neuronal NOS (nNOS) in neurons or inducible NOS (iNOS) in inflammatory cells [5]. It is generally assumed that activation of the cGMP pathway also dilates resistance-type blood vessels and, thus, lowers blood pressure. Indeed, mouse mutants with impaired NO-GC activity show an elevated basal blood pressure [17–20]. In contrast, the analysis of cGKI knockout mice indicated that cGKI is not required for basal blood pressure homeostasis, but mediates blood pressure drops in response to the administration of NO-releasing drugs [21,22]. These findings suggest that NO-GC-derived cGMP regulates blood pressure, but the contribution of the cGMP-cGKI downstream pathway to endogenous mechanisms that control blood pressure under basal conditions is probably less important than previously thought.

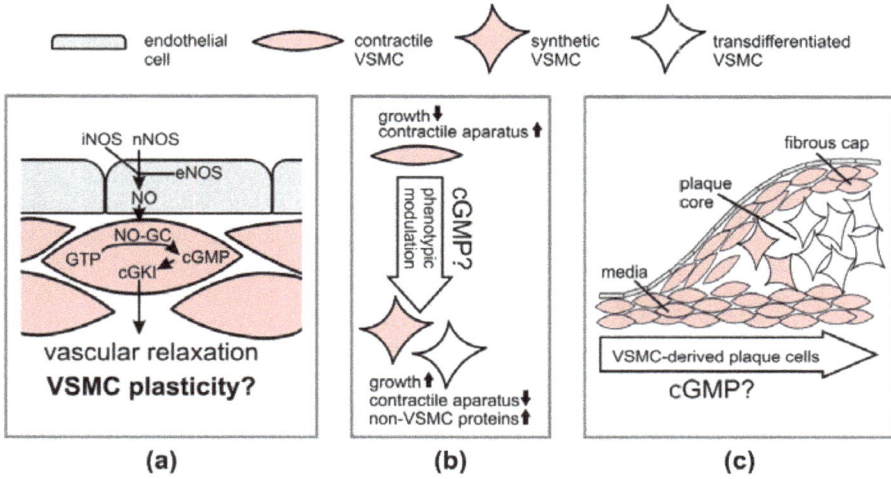

Figure 1. cGMP signaling and vascular smooth muscle cell (VSMC) plasticity. (**a**) The canonical NO-cGMP-cGKI pathway in the vessel wall; (**b**) Concept of VSMC plasticity and (**c**) VSMC-derived cells and VSMC transdifferentiation in atherosclerotic plaques and potential role of cGMP. Note that monocyte-derived macrophages and other plaque cells are not shown. For further explanations, see main text. eNOS, endothelial NO synthase; iNOS, inducible NO synthase; nNOS, neuronal NO synthase.

2.2. VSMCs in Vascular Diseases

In addition to blood flow regulation, VSMCs are involved in vascular remodeling during vascular diseases, such as atherosclerosis and restenosis. "Contractile" VSMCs with low proliferative activity and abundant contractile protein expression adapt to the disease situation by changing to highly proliferative "synthetic" cells that have low contractility and produce large amounts of extracellular matrix [23] (Figure 1b). Thus, VSMCs display a remarkable ability to modulate their phenotype in response to changing internal and external stimuli in the context of vascular disease, a process also referred to as phenotypic plasticity. Before discussing the effects of cGMP signaling on vascular plasticity and disease, we will briefly outline the general role of VSMCs in atherosclerosis and restenosis.

2.2.1. Atherosclerosis

Atherosclerosis leads to myocardial infarction and stroke and is the major cause of death in the western world. It is a chronic inflammatory condition that results from complex interactions of modified lipoproteins and various cell types, including monocyte-derived macrophages and cells of the vessel wall [24–26]. How each particular cell type contributes to the development of an atherosclerotic lesion is not completely understood [27–30]. One unsolved issue is the role of mature VSMCs that reside in the vascular media [31,32]. It is well-known that medial VSMCs generate VSMCs that retain contractile protein expression and cover the plaque on its luminal side forming the so-called fibrous cap (Figure 1c). Fibrous cap VSMCs are thought to stabilize the plaque by synthesis of extracellular matrix proteins and, thus, to be beneficial. On the other hand, it was a long-standing matter of debate whether medial VSMCs also contribute to the makeup of the plaque core region, which was assumed to contain mainly monocyte-derived lipid-loaded macrophages, also known as foam cells [33]. Fifteen years ago, we established a Cre/lox-based genetic inducible fate mapping system to track medial VSMCs during atherogenesis in mice. Surprisingly, our initial lineage tracing studies identified a large

J. Cardiovasc. Dev. Dis. **2018**, *5*, 20

number of VSMC-derived cells in the core region of atherosclerotic plaques [34,35] and some of them were positively stained for the macrophage marker Mac-2 [34]. These in vivo findings were also consistent with data from cultured VSMCs [36] and led us to put forward the hypothesis that VSMCs can transdifferentiate to macrophage-like cells during atherogenesis [34]. In line with our hypothesis, immunostainings of human plaque sections revealed that some intimal cells co-express markers of smooth muscle cells and macrophages, suggesting the existence of a VSMC–macrophage chimeric cell type in human lesions [37,38]. In 2014, we could indeed demonstrate by definitive lineage tracing and co-staining of VSMC-derived plaque cells with smooth muscle and macrophage markers that medial VSMCs can undergo clonal expansion and convert to macrophage-like cells that have lost classic smooth muscle marker expression and make up a major component of advanced atherosclerotic lesions [39]. This study, as well as the results of other groups that have used similar experimental approaches and reached similar conclusions [40–43], provide strong in vivo evidence for a major role of VSMC plasticity in atherosclerosis and call for a revised look at the pathogenesis of this devastating disease [33,44]. According to the new model, mature VSMCs that are present in the media of the non-atherosclerotic vessel wall possess the potential to become activated during plaque development and transdifferentiate to macrophage-like cells and perhaps also to other cells that reside within the lesion and have lost expression of VSMC markers (Figure 1c). Interestingly, the VSMC-derived plaque cells have a clonal origin in the vascular media and can make up a major fraction of the intimal cells [39,42,43]. It is likely that previous studies that were based on immunostaining of plaque cells for smooth muscle markers have vastly underestimated the role of VSMC plasticity in atherosclerosis.

2.2.2. Restenosis

Advanced atherosclerotic lesions or plaque rupture can result in occlusion of blood vessels and severe restriction of blood flow [26]. The common approach to restore blood flow in these stenotic vessels is balloon angioplasty or the use of vascular stents. However, these intra-arterial interventions may disrupt normal blood vessel integrity and lead to a long-term risk of restenosis, i.e., the remodeling and eventual re-occlusion of treated arteries. Restenosis is characterized by the formation of a so-called neointima that consists mainly of VSMCs. The exact mechanism of restenosis is still unclear. It involves an inflammatory response and activation of quiescent medial VSMCs with subsequent proliferation and extracellular matrix deposition, thereby forming a neointima [45]. Recent lineage tracing data showed that, similar to atherosclerosis, the neointima is formed by clonal expansion of a small number of medial VSMCs. However, in contrast to the core of atherosclerotic lesions, VSMCs in the neointima exist in a largely contractile and smooth muscle marker-positive state [42]. These findings suggest that neointimal VSMCs may resemble the phenotype of fibrous cap VSMCs in plaques and that the extent of VSMC transdifferentiation is less pronounced in restenosis than in atherosclerosis.

Taken together, vascular remodeling in atherosclerosis and restenosis shows interesting similarities and differences with respect to the behavior of VSMCs. While clonal VSMC expansion is involved in both diseases, VSMC transdifferentiation to other cell types seems to contribute to the formation of atherosclerotic lesions, but not neointima, in the setting of restenosis. Considering the crucial role of VSMC phenotypic plasticity in these vascular diseases, a better understanding of the underlying signaling mechanisms will help to develop novel therapeutic approaches. As discussed in the following sections, shifting the VSMC phenotype from potentially detrimental macrophage-like cells to beneficial fibrous cap cells with drugs that target the NO-cGMP-cGKI signaling pathway in VSMCs could be a novel strategy to treat atherosclerosis.

3. cGMP and VSMC Plasticity in Cell Culture

It has long been known that VSMCs grown in vitro lose properties associated with the contractile phenotype (e.g., expression of contractile proteins) and gain "synthetic" features (e.g., proliferation and extensive synthesis of extracellular matrix) [46,47] (Figure 1b). This process is called phenotypic switching or modulation and takes place already during primary culture (e.g., in cells isolated from the aorta, plated

J. Cardiovasc. Dev. Dis. **2018**, *5*, 20

on plastic dishes, and grown for 3–7 days) and is further enhanced by subculturing (passaging) of primary VSMCs [48]. Under certain conditions, the loss of contractile marker proteins can be accompanied by expression of marker proteins for other cell types. For instance, after cholesterol loading, cultured VSMCs can modulate to macrophage-like cells [36,49]. Thus, cultured VSMCs appear to provide a useful cell model to study VSMC plasticity, including the process of VSMC-to-macrophage transdifferentiation.

Studies with cultured VSMCs have linked components of the cGMP signaling pathway to VSMC proliferation and marker protein expression, indicating a role of cGMP in phenotypic switching of VSMCs. In particular, the mechanism and therapeutic relevance of cGMP-regulated VSMC plasticity via the NO-cGMP-cGKI axis has been intensively investigated over the past few decades [9,13,15,35,50–52]. However, it is still debated if stimulation of this cascade inhibits or promotes the growth of VSMCs. In this section, we will summarize previous data obtained with cultured VSMCs and provide explanations for the seemingly contradicting results.

A general problem in cGMP research is the lack of highly specific activators and inhibitors of pathway components, in particular for use in experiments with intact cells [53]. Many studies with VSMCs applied cGKI activators and inhibitors, but few of them determined the actual efficiency and specificity of the compounds used in the respective experiments. For instance, "cGKI-specific" cGMP analogues may have effects independent of cGKI [54,55]. KT5823, which was frequently used as cGKI-specific inhibitor, might stimulate rather than inhibit cGKI in intact cells [56]; Rp-PET-8-Br-cGMP, which is considered one of the most permeable, selective, and potent cGKI inhibitors, was demonstrated to be a partial agonist of cGKIα rather than an antagonist [57]; and another frequently used cGKI inhibitor, DT-2, was shown to lose its specificity in intact cells [58]. One way to tackle the problems associated with the pharmacological manipulation of cGMP signaling in VSMCs is to combine these tools with genetic deletion or RNA knockdown models of the NO-cGMP-cGKI pathway.

Data obtained with subcultured VSMCs indicated that activation of the NO-cGMP pathway promotes a shift of VSMCs towards the contractile phenotype reflected by reduced proliferation and/or increased contractile marker protein expression [15]. For example, Garg and Hassid [59] showed that NO donors and the membrane-permeable cGMP analogue 8-Br-cGMP (which activates cGKI and other cGMP effectors) reduced the proliferation of subcultured rat aortic smooth muscle cells (RASMCs). Similar results were obtained by application of YC-1 [60], a stimulator of NO-GC [61–63]. After adenoviral expression of cGKI in subcultured RASMCs, Chiche et al. confirmed this observation and, in addition, showed an increase in apoptosis after enhancing cGMP signaling [64]. As the overexpression of cGKI in subcultured VSMCs led to increased contractile protein expression (e.g., SM-MHC, calponin), a role for cGKI in maintaining a differentiated/contractile phenotype was postulated [52,65,66].

In contrast to the results obtained with subcultured VSMCs, studies with primary VSMCs revealed a stimulation of VSMC growth and survival by the NO-cGMP-cGKI pathway. Hassid and colleagues demonstrated that the growth-promoting effect of fibroblast growth factor 2 on primary RASMCs was potentiated by NO/cGMP [67]. Interestingly, they did not detect this growth potentiation with cells of higher passages. Another study reported an activation of the mitogen-activated protein kinase pathway (commonly known to be pro-proliferative) by cGMP analogues in freshly isolated RASMCs [68]. We observed a growth-promoting effect of 8-Br-cGMP in primary VSMCs from mouse aorta, and by comparing cGKI-expressing and cGKI-deficient VSMCs, we were able to prove that growth stimulation by cGMP was mediated by cGKI [35]. In the same study, we demonstrated opposing concentration-dependent effects of NO on the growth of primary VSMCs. While a low concentration (0.5 µM) of the NO donor diethylenetriamine NONOate (DETA-NO) enhanced proliferation via a cGKI-dependent pathway, high concentrations of DETA-NO (100 µM) strongly reduced VSMC growth independent of cGKI. A cGMP-independent, anti-proliferative effect of NO in VSMCs was also observed by other groups [50,69]. In sum, there is strong evidence that low/physiological NO concentrations promote VSMC growth via the cGMP-cGKI axis, whereas high/pathophysiological concentrations of NO inhibit VSMC growth in a cGMP/cGKI-independent manner.

Based on the previous studies, it appears that cGMP promotes the growth and survival of primary VSMCs, while it inhibits subcultured VSMCs. Indeed, Weinmeister and colleagues [70] demonstrated that the relatively strong cGKI-dependent growth-promoting effect of 8-Br-cGMP in primary VSMCs (to ≈200–300% of control cells without cGMP) was lost after the first passage and even reversed to a weak growth inhibition in later passages (to ≈90% of control cells without cGMP). These observations imply that passaging of VSMCs results in functional changes of the endogenous NO-cGMP-cGKI signaling pathway and/or more general alterations of the cells' growth response. Considering the relative magnitudes of cGMP-mediated growth effects, the strong growth stimulation observed in primary VSMCs might be (patho-)physiologically more relevant than the weak inhibition detected in subcultured cells.

Weinmeister et al. [70] also addressed the mechanism underlying growth stimulation of primary VSMCs via the cGMP-cGKI pathway. It was mainly due to a higher efficiency of cell adhesion in the presence of elevated cGMP, while proliferation and apoptosis played minor roles. A known substrate of cGKI that is involved in cell adhesion is the small GTPase RhoA [71,72]. Phosphorylation by cGKI stabilizes RhoA in an inactive cytosolic RhoA-GTP/GDI complex [73,74]. Indeed, the RhoA/Rho kinase signaling pathway was suppressed by activation of the cGMP-cGKI pathway in VSMCs. This led to activation of β_1/β_3 integrins and enhanced adhesion of primary VSMCs [70].

Recently, Segura-Puimedon and colleagues [50] analyzed the phenotype of VSMCs from knockout mice lacking the α1 subunit of the cGMP-generating NO-GC. Compared to wild-type VSMCs, NO-GC knockout cells showed less proliferation and migration and increased expression of contractile marker proteins. These data are in line with the results obtained with cGKI knockout VSMCs [35]. Together, these in vitro studies support a model in which increased NO-cGMP-cGKI signaling promotes the growth and survival of VSMCs and stimulates their modulation towards a synthetic phenotype (Figure 1b).

4. cGMP and Vascular Diseases

The critical role of NO and natriuretic peptides in the cardiovascular system has been known for a long time. NO-releasing organic nitrates have been used for the treatment of angina pectoris for more than a century. Novel functions of cGMP and clinical applications of cGMP-based drugs are continuously being discovered [75,76]. Indeed, drugs that increase cGMP concentration have emerged as one of the most successful areas in recent drug development and clinical pharmacology [77,78]. For example, the PDE5 inhibitor sildenafil is used for erectile dysfunction, the GC-C agonist linaclotide for chronic idiopathic constipation and irritable bowel syndrome, and recently a combination drug consisting of valsartan (an angiotensin II receptor blocker) and sacubitril, which inhibits the ANP-/BNP-degrading endopeptidase neprilysin, was approved for use in heart failure [79]. The NO-GC stimulator riociguat is used for several forms of pulmonary hypertension [80]. Currently, a plethora of preclinical and clinical studies are testing NO-GC stimulators and activators for their therapeutic potential in various diseases, including heart failure, aortic valve calcification, achalasia, and fibrosis [75,78,80].

The clinical data is supported by genetic association studies, which have implicated dysfunctions of the cGMP signaling cascade in hypertension, coronary artery disease, and myocardial infarction in humans [81]. Importantly, even subtle changes due to genetic variants in components of this pathway (e.g., NO-GC, ANP, BNP; PDEs) significantly influence blood pressure and cardiovascular disease risk [82–86]. Interestingly, genetic mutations in NO-GC or cGKI found in humans are causally associated with altered vascular structure and remodeling [87,88]. However, the effects of genetic polymorphisms on the expression level and/or enzymatic activity of the respective proteins are not always known and, because the genetic alterations are present in all cells of the body, it is difficult to identify the causative cell type(s) (e.g., endothelial cells, platelets, VSMCs, etc.). Although it is commonly thought that the net effect of cGMP signaling on cardiovascular disease is protective, it is conceivable that an increase of cGMP in different cell types can have different, and even opposing, effects on disease progression. In particular, the in vivo relevance of vascular plasticity regulated by the NO-cGMP-cGKI cascade is not completely understood.

In recent years, knockout mouse models for NOS, NO-GC, and cGKI have been established. Table 1 summarizes the vascular phenotypes of the respective mouse mutants. Conventional null mutants that lack the β1 subunit of NO-GC [89] or cGKI [22] "chronically" in all cells have a strongly reduced life span limiting their use for long-term experiments, such as the analysis of atherosclerosis. Another drawback of conventional knockout technology is the fact that the gene mutation is present in all cells, making it difficult to assign a phenotype to a specific cell type. To circumvent problems associated with global gene knockouts, time- and tissue-specific mutagenesis utilizing the Cre/lox recombination system can be performed [90], and conditional alleles of NO-GC [89] and cGKI [91] have been generated.

Table 1. Genetic mouse models of NO-cGMP-cGKI signaling and their vascular phenotypes.

Gene	Mouse Model	Effect of Mutation on Vascular Remodeling	References
eNOS	Null mutation	Enhanced atherosclerosis on ApoE$^{-/-}$ [1] background	[92–94]
		Enhanced neointima formation after vascular injury	[95–97]
		Impaired angiogenesis	[98–100]
nNOS	Null mutation	Enhanced atherosclerosis on ApoE$^{-/-}$ background	[101]
		Enhanced neointima formation after vascular injury	[102]
iNOS	Null mutation	Reduced atherosclerosis on ApoE$^{-/-}$ background	[103,104]
		Reduced neointima formation after vascular injury	[105]
		Reduced pathological neovascularization in the ischemic retina	[106]
NO-GC α1-subunit	Null mutation	Reduced atherosclerosis on ApoE$^{-/-}$ background	[50]
		Reduced neointima formation after vascular injury in male mice	[107]
NO-GC β1-subunit	Smooth muscle-specific knockout (tamoxifen-inducible)	Reduced arteriogenesis in hindlimb ischemia model	[108]
	Null mutation	Reduced arteriogenesis in hindlimb ischemia model	[108]
cGKI	Smooth muscle-specific knockout (tamoxifen-inducible)	Reduced atherosclerosis on ApoE$^{-/-}$ background	[35]
	Smooth muscle-specific knockout	No effect on neointima formation after vascular injury	[51]
	Null mutation	Reduced angiogenesis	[109,110]

[1] Apolipoprotein E (ApoE).

4.1. Role of cGMP in Atherosclerosis

Several genetic mouse studies investigated the role of NO-cGMP signaling for the development of atherosclerotic plaques, a process strongly dependent on VSMC plasticity. Interestingly, the phenotypes of NOS knockout mice indicated an ambivalent role of NO in atherosclerosis (Table 1). While NO generated by eNOS [92,94] and nNOS [101] was atheroprotective, NO synthesized by iNOS, which is upregulated under inflammatory conditions and generates high amounts of NO, promoted atherosclerosis [103,104]. Interestingly, publications on the effects of pharmacological activation of NO-GC on atherosclerosis are scarce [62]. One study reported that the NO-GC stimulator YC-1 prevents foam cell formation and atherosclerosis [111]. The opposing effects of NO might be related to the different spatiotemporal profile (cell types, time) and quantity of NO generation by eNOS/nNOS versus iNOS [112]. These results are also consistent with in vitro data showing that NO can promote and inhibit VSMC growth via cGMP-dependent and cGMP-independent pathways, respectively (see Section 3, "cGMP and VSMC Plasticity in Cell Culture"). Clearly, the interpretation of in vivo knockout phenotypes is complicated if the gene mutation is present in all cells and/or the mutant mice display multiple phenotypes that could influence each other. For instance, eNOS-deficient mice are also hypertensive and it is debated whether or not this may be another reason for their enhanced atherosclerosis independent of a potential direct effect of NO on VSMC plasticity [92,93].

Using an inducible smooth muscle-specific cGKI knockout model that was combined with genetic tracking of VSMC fate during plaque development, we demonstrated that the cGMP-cGKI axis in VSMCs promotes the growth of atherosclerotic lesions [35]. After postnatal ablation of cGKI in VSMCs, mutant mice developed smaller plaques. In these plaques, cells derived from cGKI-deficient VSMCs were almost exclusively located in the media but not the plaque core region. In contrast, cells derived from wild-type VSMCs were found in both the vascular media and inside the plaque. These cell-fate mapping data indicated that cGKI is involved in the development of VSMC-derived plaque cells, which were later identified as macrophage-like cells (see Section 2, "Role of VSMCs in Physiology and Pathophysiology"). Thus, it is tempting to speculate that cGMP-cGKI signaling promotes smooth muscle-to-macrophage transdifferentiation in atherosclerosis (Figure 1c).

In line with a pro-atherogenic role of the NO-cGMP-cGKI signaling cascade, Segura-Puimedon and colleagues recently demonstrated that deletion of the α1 subunit of NO-GC led to a reduced size of atherosclerotic plaques [50]. Their in vitro and in vivo results clearly confirm and further extend the atherosclerosis data obtained with cGKI mouse mutants [35]. Together, these studies suggest that the activated NO-cGMP-cGKI pathway promotes the phenotypic switching of VSMCs from a contractile/quiescent phenotype to a synthetic/proliferative state including macrophage-like plaque cells. It is important to note that cGMP-dependent plaque growth is not necessarily an unfavorable process. Indeed, the cGMP-mediated increase in lesion size is associated with an altered plaque composition, which may or may not stabilize the plaque. These questions as well as the role of NO-GC and cGKI in multiple cell types involved in atherosclerosis (e.g., VSMCs, endothelial cells, platelets, immune cells) should be further addressed in future studies with conditional knockout mice.

4.2. Role of cGMP in Restenosis

Paralleling the effects of NOS-derived NO in atherosclerosis, studies using knockout models in the setting of restenosis (Table 1) demonstrated vasculoprotective effects of eNOS [95–97] and nNOS [102] and a vasculoproliferative effect of iNOS [105]. The dual role of NO in vascular remodeling might be the reason why NO-releasing drugs, to our knowledge, have not been reported to exert beneficial effects on atherosclerosis or restenosis. In contrast to the strong in vivo evidence supporting a role of the NO-cGMP-cGKI axis in atherosclerosis, data proving an influence of this signaling pathway on the development of neointima during restenosis are scarce. Adenoviral transduction of the constitutively active kinase domain of cGKI led to an attenuated formation of neointima in vascular injury models of rat and swine [113]. It is important to note that this kinase construct is not regulated by cGMP and lacks the N-terminus, which is responsible for substrate specificity [8,9]. In the same study, the transduction of the full-length cGKIβ isoform did not affect the formation of neointima. Lukowski and colleagues showed that smooth muscle-specific ablation of cGKI and treatment of wild-type mice with the PDE5 inhibitor sildenafil had no significant effect on restenosis in various models of vascular injury, except for a slight reduction of neointima formation in a short vessel segment of cGKI mutants after wire injury of the carotid artery [51].

Pharmacological approaches applying the NO-GC stimulator YC-1 [114,115] or the NO-GC activator cinaciguat [116] indicated a vasculoprotective role of NO-GC activation in rat models of restenosis. It is, however, not clear whether these effects were related to drug action on VSMCs and/or other cell types. It should be considered that pharmacological activation of NO-GC can exert hypotensive [61,62,117] and anti-inflammatory effects [111,118], which could influence restenosis. Furthermore, YC-1 is known to have cGMP-independent effects [62,117]. In contrast to the pharmacological studies, Vermeersch et al. reported that NO-GC might promote restenosis based on their finding that global knockout of the NO-GC α1 subunit resulted in a reduction of neointima formation in male mice [107]. Together with the analysis of cGKI mouse mutants, these genetic knockout studies suggest that the NO-cGMP-cGKI cascade is not critically involved in the regulation of VSMC growth during restenosis. If at all, this

J. Cardiovasc. Dev. Dis. **2018**, *5*, 20

pathway may slightly promote rather than inhibit neointima formation, which points to the same direction as the growth-promoting effect of cGMP during atherosclerosis. However, the effects of cGMP on restenosis appear relatively weak and it is unlikely that the effects of NO on restenosis are mediated by the cGMP-cGKI pathway. Presumably, the spatiotemporal profile, the amount of NO synthesized, and the source of its production after vascular injury result in the activation of alternative mechanisms, such as redox regulation of target proteins [119]. The preclinical evidence summarized above also indicates that the contribution of cGKI-mediated mechanisms to vascular remodeling is context-specific, and arguably more important in atherosclerosis than in restenosis. A disease-specific role of the cGMP-cGKI axis is plausible considering our hypothesis that this pathway acts on smooth muscle-to-macrophage transdifferentiation (see above, this section), a process that seems to contribute to the formation of atherosclerotic lesions, but not neointima in the setting of restenosis (see Section 2, "Role of VSMCs in Physiology and Pathophysiology").

4.3. Role of cGMP in Angiogenesis

Another process influenced by the phenotypic plasticity of VSMCs is the formation of blood vessels. It is known that NO induces postnatal neovascularization through both angiogenesis (the development of new blood vessels derived from existing vessels) and vasculogenesis (blood vessel formation de novo from progenitor cells), but the respective mechanisms are still unclear [112]. Hindlimb ischemia is a common model to investigate blood vessel formation during pathological conditions, as angiogenesis is the natural response to restore blood supply after ischemia. In this model, the pro-angiogenic effect of NO was demonstrated by using a NOS inhibitor [120] or eNOS knockout models with impaired NO generation [100] (Table 1). Pro-angiogenic effects of eNOS [98,99] and iNOS [106] were also observed in other models of neovascularization. A recent study identified NO-GC as a component of cGMP-mediated angiogenesis [108]. By comparison of ischemia-induced angiogenesis in global, endothelial-, and smooth muscle-specific NO-GC β1 knockout mice, the authors showed that NO-GC expression in VSMCs, but not endothelial cells, improved neovascularization. In line with the role of NO and NO-GC, several studies also suggested a pro-angiogenic function for cGKI. Yamahara and colleagues reported that angiogenesis in response to hindlimb ischemia was increased in mice that overexpressed cGKIα, while it was significantly reduced in heterozygous cGKI knockout mice [110]. Aicher et al. confirmed the pro-angiogenic cGKI effects observed by Yamahara using a cGKIα leucine zipper mutant unable to interact with downstream targets [109]. Furthermore, this study reported reduced blood vessel formation of cGKI-null mutants in a disc neovascularization model. Moreover, Senthilkumar and colleagues proposed a cGKI-dependent pro-angiogenic effect of sildenafil [121]. Taken together, these studies strongly suggest a pro-angiogenic function of the NO-cGMP-cGKI pathway.

5. Limitations and Future Directions

Clearly, the present data call for more studies on the mechanisms and therapeutic relevance of cGMP-regulated vascular remodeling. These studies should address how cGMP signaling affects VSMC phenotype and vice versa. The relevance of cGMP-triggered VSMC transdifferentiation should be analyzed in detail as well as the effects of cGMP on other cell types involved in vascular disease, such as endothelial cells, platelets, and immune cells. To answer these and other interesting questions, it will be instrumental to monitor the spatiotemporal profile of cGMP signals generated in living vascular cells and tissues, and to track the cells' fate after endogenous or pharmacological modulation of the cGMP pathway.

A major obstacle in drawing a complete picture of cGMP signaling in VSMCs is their phenotypic heterogeneity. It is likely that the initial state of a VSMC influences the effect of cGMP on it. Therefore, it is important to investigate cGMP signaling at the single-cell level. To some extent, this is possible by classical immunostainings of VSMC populations in cell culture or tissue sections for cGMP, "marker" proteins, or other proteins of interest. However, this method does not allow one to follow dynamic changes and it is limited by the availability of specific antibodies. With the development of genetically-encoded fluorescent cGMP sensors, it is now possible to visualize cGMP in living cells by fluorescence microscopy [122,123]. Recently, we have generated transgenic mice expressing the cGMP indicator cGi500 [124] either ubiquitously or in specific cell types [125]. The cGMP sensor mice are a convenient source to isolate sensor-expressing primary cells [122,125] and tissues [126,127] for ex vivo cGMP imaging, or they can be used directly for intravital cGMP imaging in vivo [128]. Thus, it is possible to monitor dynamic cGMP changes in real time in individual VSMCs in culture or in a living tissue/animal under close-to-native conditions. In contrast to conventional end point cGMP assays, which measure cGMP in cell/tissue extracts, the cGMP sensor mice allow for monitoring of cGMP levels in single cells in response to multiple stimulations [122,125]. This will help to correlate cGMP responses elicited by different cGMP-elevating agents with the phenotypic state of individual VSMCs and, thereby, deepen our understanding of the role of cGMP in phenotypic plasticity. Furthermore, the cGMP-modulating effects of PDE inhibitors or other substances can be investigated at the single-cell level as was recently shown for neurons [129]. Besides this, spatiotemporal differences of cGMP signals can be analyzed in intact tissues, which has already provided new insights about cGMP signaling in the cochlea [126] and oocytes [127].

It is increasingly recognized that previous studies have underestimated the importance of VSMC phenotypic plasticity in atherosclerosis and the impact a single VSMC can have on disease progression. With the use of genetic cell-fate mapping, it was shown that individual medial VSMCs can expand clonally and transdifferentiate to macrophage-like cells in atherosclerotic plaques. These studies also showed that classification of cell types exclusively via immunostainings for "specific" marker proteins, which they might lose or gain during phenotypic switching, can lead to misinterpretations concerning the cells' origin. We anticipate that genetic lineage tracing will continue to discover new aspects of VSMC plasticity in vascular diseases, such as conversion to bone-like cells and other cells. Recently, a new mouse model for cell tracking with positron emission tomography (PET) was described [130]. This cell tracking mouse allows for non-invasive imaging of specific cell types by PET and should further improve data quality with a reduction in the number of animals needed. Importantly, we can now track VSMCs over time in an individual living animal without the need to sacrifice it. In the future, combining cGMP imaging and VSMC tracking will help to improve our understanding of cGMP's role in VSMC plasticity in vivo.

6. Conclusions

The cGMP signaling pathway has a strong impact on human cardiovascular physiology and pathophysiology and is an attractive drug target to tackle an array of major human diseases. As discussed in this review article, in vitro and in vivo data support an important role of the NO-cGMP-cGKI axis in vascular remodeling, particularly in the context of atherosclerosis and angiogenesis. It is likely that many of these effects are related to stimulation of VSMC growth and plasticity by this signaling pathway (Figure 1b). A major future challenge is to evaluate the relevance of cGMP-regulated vascular plasticity for human health and disease. Preclinical studies strongly support the notion that the cGMP-cGKI axis increases VSMC growth and survival. Similar growth/survival-promoting effects of cGMP have been reported in other cell types, including cardiomyocytes [131–134], hematopoietic [135] and vascular [109] progenitor cells, stroma cells in the bone marrow [136], erythrocytes [137], platelets [138], osteoblasts [139], sensory hair cells [140], and melanoma cells [141]. Thus, we propose that stimulation of cell growth and survival by cGMP is a common mechanism in many cell types and tissues. The growth-promoting effects of cGMP could be highly relevant for pharmacotherapies. Inhibition of the cGMP-cGKI pathway could be a novel strategy to treat proliferative diseases, such as atherosclerosis and cancer. Stimulation of this pathway might counteract cell degeneration and death in settings such as heart attack, stroke, or noise-induced hearing loss. However, cGMP-elevating drugs used in clinics might also have unwanted side effects related to stimulation of cell growth and survival. Indeed, two recent clinical studies reported that use of PDE5 inhibitors in men is linked to a modest increase in melanoma risk [142,143]. We [141] and others [144] discovered a growth-promoting cGMP pathway in melanoma cells that might provide a mechanistic basis for this clinical finding [145]. In the future, it will be interesting to evaluate the effects of cGMP-modulating drugs on atherosclerosis and other diseases that are associated with cell growth and plasticity.

Acknowledgments: The authors would like to thank Michael Paolillo for reading the manuscript as well as the current and past members of the Feil laboratory for critical discussions. We apologize to all our colleagues whose work could not be cited due to space limitations. The work in the authors' laboratory is supported by the Fund for Science, Karl Helmut Eberle Stiftung, European Research Area Network on Cardiovascular Diseases (ERA-CVD), and Deutsche Forschungsgemeinschaft (FOR 2060 projects FE 438/5-2 and FE 438/6-2, KFO 274 projects FE 438/7-1 and FE 438/8-2).

Author Contributions: All authors contributed to the conceptual drafting, writing, and editing of this manuscript.

Conflicts of Interest: The authors declare no conflict of interest.

References

1. Beavo, J.A.; Brunton, L.L. Cyclic nucleotide research—Still expanding after half a century. *Nat. Rev. Mol. Cell Biol.* **2002**, *3*, 710–718. [CrossRef] [PubMed]
2. Kemp-Harper, B.; Feil, R. Meeting report: cGMP matters. *Sci. Sign.* **2008**, *1*, pe2. [CrossRef] [PubMed]
3. Friebe, A.; Koesling, D. The function of NO-sensitive guanylyl cyclase: What we can learn from genetic mouse models. *Nitric Oxide* **2009**, *21*, 149–156. [CrossRef] [PubMed]
4. Kuhn, M. Molecular physiology of membrane guanylyl cyclase receptors. *Physiol. Rev.* **2016**, *96*, 751–804. [CrossRef] [PubMed]
5. Forstermann, U.; Sessa, W.C. Nitric oxide synthases: Regulation and function. *Eur. Heart J.* **2012**, *33*, 829–837. [CrossRef] [PubMed]
6. Biel, M.; Michalakis, S. Cyclic nucleotide-gated channels. In *cGMP: Generators, Effectors and Therapeutic Implications*; Schmidt, H.H.H.W., Hofmann, F., Stasch, J.-P., Eds.; Springer: Berlin/Heidelberg, Germany, 2009; pp. 111–136.
7. Francis, S.H.; Blount, M.A.; Corbin, J.D. Mammalian cyclic nucleotide phosphodiesterases: Molecular mechanisms and physiological functions. *Physiol. Rev.* **2011**, *91*, 651–690. [CrossRef] [PubMed]
8. Hofmann, F.; Feil, R.; Kleppisch, T.; Schlossmann, J. Function of cGMP-dependent protein kinases as revealed by gene deletion. *Physiol. Rev.* **2006**, *86*, 1–23. [CrossRef] [PubMed]
9. Feil, R.; Lohmann, S.M.; de Jonge, H.; Walter, U.; Hofmann, F. Cyclic GMP-dependent protein kinases and the cardiovascular system: Insights from genetically modified mice. *Circ. Res.* **2003**, *93*, 907–916. [CrossRef] [PubMed]
10. Aizawa, T.; Wei, H.; Miano, J.M.; Abe, J.; Berk, B.C.; Yan, C. Role of phosphodiesterase 3 in NO/cGMP-mediated antiinflammatory effects in vascular smooth muscle cells. *Circ. Res.* **2003**, *93*, 406–413. [CrossRef] [PubMed]
11. Surks, H.K. cGMP-dependent protein kinase i and smooth muscle relaxation: A tale of two isoforms. *Circ. Res.* **2007**, *101*, 1078–1080. [CrossRef] [PubMed]
12. Weber, S.; Bernhard, D.; Lukowski, R.; Weinmeister, P.; Worner, R.; Wegener, J.W.; Valtcheva, N.; Feil, S.; Schlossmann, J.; Hofmann, F.; et al. Rescue of cGMP kinase I knockout mice by smooth muscle specific expression of either isozyme. *Circ. Res.* **2007**, *101*, 1096–1103. [CrossRef] [PubMed]
13. Feil, R.; Feil, S.; Hofmann, F. A heretical view on the role of NO and cGMP in vascular proliferative diseases. *Trends Mol. Med.* **2005**, *11*, 71–75. [CrossRef] [PubMed]
14. Kemp-Harper, B.; Schmidt, H.H.H.W. cGMP in the vasculature. In *cGMP: Generators, Effectors and Therapeutic Implications*; Schmidt, H.H.H.W., Hofmann, F., Stasch, J.-P., Eds.; Springer: Berlin/Heidelberg, Germany, 2009; pp. 447–467.
15. Lincoln, T.M.; Wu, X.; Sellak, H.; Dey, N.; Choi, C.S. Regulation of vascular smooth muscle cell phenotype by cyclic GMP and cyclic GMP-dependent protein kinase. *Front. Biosci.* **2006**, *11*, 356–367. [CrossRef] [PubMed]
16. Somlyo, A.P.; Somlyo, A.V. Signal transduction and regulation in smooth muscle. *Nature* **1994**, *372*, 231–236. [CrossRef] [PubMed]
17. Buys, E.S.; Sips, P.; Vermeersch, P.; Raher, M.J.; Rogge, E.; Ichinose, F.; Dewerchin, M.; Bloch, K.D.; Janssens, S.; Brouckaert, P. Gender-specific hypertension and responsiveness to nitric oxide in sGCα1 knockout mice. *Cardiovasc. Res.* **2008**, *79*, 179–186. [CrossRef] [PubMed]

18. Groneberg, D.; Konig, P.; Wirth, A.; Offermanns, S.; Koesling, D.; Friebe, A. Smooth muscle-specific deletion of nitric oxide-sensitive guanylyl cyclase is sufficient to induce hypertension in mice. *Circulation* **2010**, *121*, 401–409. [CrossRef] [PubMed]

19. Mergia, E.; Friebe, A.; Dangel, O.; Russwurm, M.; Koesling, D. Spare guanylyl cyclase NO receptors ensure high NO sensitivity in the vascular system. *J. Clin. Investig.* **2006**, *116*, 1731–1737. [CrossRef] [PubMed]

20. Thoonen, R.; Cauwels, A.; Decaluwe, K.; Geschka, S.; Tainsh, R.E.; Delanghe, J.; Hochepied, T.; De Cauwer, L.; Rogge, E.; Voet, S.; et al. Cardiovascular and pharmacological implications of haem-deficient NO-unresponsive soluble guanylate cyclase knock-in mice. *Nat. Commun.* **2015**, *6*, 8482. [CrossRef] [PubMed]

21. Koeppen, M.; Feil, R.; Siegl, D.; Feil, S.; Hofmann, F.; Pohl, U.; de Wit, C. cGMP-dependent protein kinase mediates NO- but not acetylcholine-induced dilations in resistance vessels in vivo. *Hypertension* **2004**, *44*, 952–955. [CrossRef] [PubMed]

22. Pfeifer, A.; Klatt, P.; Massberg, S.; Ny, L.; Sausbier, M.; Hirneiss, C.; Wang, G.X.; Korth, M.; Aszodi, A.; Andersson, K.E.; et al. Defective smooth muscle regulation in cGMP kinase I-deficient mice. *EMBO J.* **1998**, *17*, 3045–3051. [CrossRef] [PubMed]

23. Owens, G.K.; Kumar, M.S.; Wamhoff, B.R. Molecular regulation of vascular smooth muscle cell differentiation in development and disease. *Physiol. Rev.* **2004**, *84*, 767–801. [CrossRef] [PubMed]

24. Libby, P.; Ridker, P.M.; Hansson, G.K. Progress and challenges in translating the biology of atherosclerosis. *Nature* **2011**, *473*, 317–325. [CrossRef] [PubMed]

25. Moore, K.J.; Tabas, I. Macrophages in the pathogenesis of atherosclerosis. *Cell* **2011**, *145*, 341–355. [CrossRef] [PubMed]

26. Ross, R. Atherosclerosis—An inflammatory disease. *N. Engl. J. Med.* **1999**, *340*, 115–126. [CrossRef] [PubMed]

27. Doherty, T.M.; Shah, P.K.; Rajavashisth, T.B. Cellular origins of atherosclerosis: Towards ontogenetic endgame? *FASEB J.* **2003**, *17*, 592–597. [CrossRef] [PubMed]

28. Gomez, D.; Owens, G.K. Smooth muscle cell phenotypic switching in atherosclerosis. *Cardiovasc. Res.* **2012**, *95*, 156–164. [CrossRef] [PubMed]

29. Iwata, H.; Manabe, I.; Nagai, R. Lineage of bone marrow-derived cells in atherosclerosis. *Circ. Res.* **2013**, *112*, 1634–1647. [CrossRef] [PubMed]

30. Moore, K.J.; Sheedy, F.J.; Fisher, E.A. Macrophages in atherosclerosis: A dynamic balance. *Nat. Rev. Immunol.* **2013**, *13*, 709–721. [CrossRef] [PubMed]

31. Nguyen, A.T.; Gomez, D.; Bell, R.D.; Campbell, J.H.; Clowes, A.W.; Gabbiani, G.; Giachelli, C.M.; Parmacek, M.S.; Raines, E.W.; Rusch, N.J.; et al. Smooth muscle cell plasticity: Fact or fiction? *Circ. Res.* **2013**, *112*, 17–22. [CrossRef] [PubMed]

32. Tang, Z.; Wang, A.; Wang, D.; Li, S. Smooth muscle cells: To be or not to be? Response to Nguyen et al. *Circ. Res.* **2013**, *112*, 23–26. [CrossRef] [PubMed]

33. Bennett, M.R.; Sinha, S.; Owens, G.K. Vascular smooth muscle cells in atherosclerosis. *Circ. Res.* **2016**, *118*, 692–702. [CrossRef] [PubMed]

34. Feil, S.; Hofmann, F.; Feil, R. SM22α modulates vascular smooth muscle cell phenotype during atherogenesis. *Circ. Res.* **2004**, *94*, 863–865. [CrossRef] [PubMed]

35. Wolfsgruber, W.; Feil, S.; Brummer, S.; Kuppinger, O.; Hofmann, F.; Feil, R. A proatherogenic role for cGMP-dependent protein kinase in vascular smooth muscle cells. *Proc. Natl. Acad. Sci. USA* **2003**, *100*, 13519–13524. [CrossRef] [PubMed]

36. Rong, J.X.; Shapiro, M.; Trogan, E.; Fisher, E.A. Transdifferentiation of mouse aortic smooth muscle cells to a macrophage-like state after cholesterol loading. *Proc. Natl. Acad. Sci. USA* **2003**, *100*, 13531–13536. [CrossRef] [PubMed]

37. Allahverdian, S.; Chehroudi, A.C.; McManus, B.M.; Abraham, T.; Francis, G.A. Contribution of intimal smooth muscle cells to cholesterol accumulation and macrophage-like cells in human atherosclerosis. *Circulation* **2014**, *129*, 1551–1559. [CrossRef] [PubMed]

38. Andreeva, E.R.; Pugach, I.M.; Orekhov, A.N. Subendothelial smooth muscle cells of human aorta express macrophage antigen in situ and in vitro. *Atherosclerosis* **1997**, *135*, 19–27. [CrossRef]

39. Feil, S.; Fehrenbacher, B.; Lukowski, R.; Essmann, F.; Schulze-Osthoff, K.; Schaller, M.; Feil, R. Transdifferentiation of vascular smooth muscle cells to macrophage-like cells during atherogenesis. *Circ. Res.* **2014**, *115*, 662–667. [CrossRef] [PubMed]

40. Shankman, L.S.; Gomez, D.; Cherepanova, O.A.; Salmon, M.; Alencar, G.F.; Haskins, R.M.; Swiatlowska, P.; Newman, A.A.; Greene, E.S.; Straub, A.C.; et al. KLF4-dependent phenotypic modulation of smooth muscle cells has a key role in atherosclerotic plaque pathogenesis. *Nat. Med.* **2015**, *21*, 628–637. [CrossRef] [PubMed]

41. Albarran-Juarez, J.; Kaur, H.; Grimm, M.; Offermanns, S.; Wettschureck, N. Lineage tracing of cells involved in atherosclerosis. *Atherosclerosis* **2016**, *251*, 445–453. [CrossRef] [PubMed]

42. Chappell, J.; Harman, J.L.; Narasimhan, V.M.; Yu, H.; Foote, K.; Simons, B.D.; Bennett, M.R.; Jorgensen, H.F. Extensive proliferation of a subset of differentiated, yet plastic, medial vascular smooth muscle cells contributes to neointimal formation in mouse injury and atherosclerosis models. *Circ. Res.* **2016**, *119*, 1313–1323. [CrossRef] [PubMed]

43. Jacobsen, K.; Lund, M.B.; Shim, J.; Gunnersen, S.; Fuchtbauer, E.M.; Kjolby, M.; Carramolino, L.; Bentzon, J.F. Diverse cellular architecture of atherosclerotic plaque derives from clonal expansion of a few medial SMCs. *JCI Insight* **2017**, *2*. [CrossRef] [PubMed]

44. Swirski, F.K.; Nahrendorf, M. Do vascular smooth muscle cells differentiate to macrophages in atherosclerotic lesions? *Circ. Res.* **2014**, *115*, 605–606. [CrossRef] [PubMed]

45. Marx, S.O.; Totary-Jain, H.; Marks, A.R. Vascular smooth muscle cell proliferation in restenosis. *Circ. Cardiovasc. Interv.* **2011**, *4*, 104–111. [CrossRef] [PubMed]

46. Chamley-Campbell, J.; Campbell, G.R.; Ross, R. The smooth muscle cell in culture. *Physiol. Rev.* **1979**, *59*, 1–61. [CrossRef] [PubMed]

47. Owens, G.K. Regulation of differentiation of vascular smooth muscle cells. *Physiol. Rev.* **1995**, *75*, 487–517. [CrossRef] [PubMed]

48. Worth, N.F.; Rolfe, B.E.; Song, J.; Campbell, G.R. Vascular smooth muscle cell phenotypic modulation in culture is associated with reorganisation of contractile and cytoskeletal proteins. *Cell Motil. Cytoskel.* **2001**, *49*, 130–145. [CrossRef] [PubMed]

49. Vengrenyuk, Y.; Nishi, H.; Long, X.; Ouimet, M.; Savji, N.; Martinez, F.O.; Cassella, C.P.; Moore, K.J.; Ramsey, S.A.; Miano, J.M.; et al. Cholesterol loading reprograms the microRNA-143/145-myocardin axis to convert aortic smooth muscle cells to a dysfunctional macrophage-like phenotype. *Arterioscler. Thromb. Vasc. Biol.* **2015**, *35*, 535–546. [CrossRef] [PubMed]

50. Segura-Puimedon, M.; Mergia, E.; Al-Hasani, J.; Aherrahrou, R.; Stoelting, S.; Kremer, F.; Freyer, J.; Koesling, D.; Erdmann, J.; Schunkert, H.; et al. Proatherosclerotic effect of the alpha1-subunit of soluble guanylyl cyclase by promoting smooth muscle phenotypic switching. *Am. J. Pathol.* **2016**, *186*, 2220–2231. [CrossRef] [PubMed]

51. Lukowski, R.; Weinmeister, P.; Bernhard, D.; Feil, S.; Gotthardt, M.; Herz, J.; Massberg, S.; Zernecke, A.; Weber, C.; Hofmann, F.; et al. Role of smooth muscle cGMP/cGKI signaling in murine vascular restenosis. *Arterioscler. Thromb. Vasc. Biol.* **2008**, *28*, 1244–1250. [CrossRef] [PubMed]

52. Dey, N.B.; Foley, K.F.; Lincoln, T.M.; Dostmann, W.R. Inhibition of cGMP-dependent protein kinase reverses phenotypic modulation of vascular smooth muscle cells. *J. Cardiovasc. Pharmacol.* **2005**, *45*, 404–413. [CrossRef] [PubMed]

53. Butt, E. cGMP-dependent protein kinase modulators. In *cGMP: Generators, Effectors and Therapeutic Implications*; Schmidt, H.H.H.W., Hofmann, F., Stasch, J.-P., Eds.; Springer: Berlin/Heidelberg, Germany, 2009; pp. 409–421.

54. Gambaryan, S.; Geiger, J.; Schwarz, U.R.; Butt, E.; Begonja, A.; Obergfell, A.; Walter, U. Potent inhibition of human platelets by cGMP analogs independent of cGMP-dependent protein kinase. *Blood* **2004**, *103*, 2593–2600. [CrossRef] [PubMed]

55. Marshall, S.J.; Senis, Y.A.; Auger, J.M.; Feil, R.; Hofmann, F.; Salmon, G.; Peterson, J.T.; Burslem, F.; Watson, S.P. Gpib-dependent platelet activation is dependent on src kinases but not MAP kinase or cGMP-dependent kinase. *Blood* **2004**, *103*, 2601–2609. [CrossRef] [PubMed]

56. Burkhardt, M.; Glazova, M.; Gambaryan, S.; Vollkommer, T.; Butt, E.; Bader, B.; Heermeier, K.; Lincoln, T.M.; Walter, U.; Palmetshofer, A. KT5823 inhibits cGMP-dependent protein kinase activity in vitro but not in intact human platelets and rat mesangial cells. *J. Biol. Chem.* **2000**, *275*, 33536–33541. [CrossRef] [PubMed]

57. Valtcheva, N.; Nestorov, P.; Beck, A.; Russwurm, M.; Hillenbrand, M.; Weinmeister, P.; Feil, R. The commonly used cGMP-dependent protein kinase type I (cGKI) inhibitor Rp-8-Br-PET-cGMPS can activate cGKI in vitro and in intact cells. *J. Biol. Chem.* **2009**, *284*, 556–562. [CrossRef] [PubMed]

58. Gambaryan, S.; Butt, E.; Kobsar, A.; Geiger, J.; Rukoyatkina, N.; Parnova, R.; Nikolaev, V.O.; Walter, U. The oligopeptide DT-2 is a specific PKG I inhibitor only in vitro, not in living cells. *Br. J. Pharmacol.* **2012**, *167*, 826–838. [CrossRef] [PubMed]

59. Garg, U.C.; Hassid, A. Nitric oxide-generating vasodilators and 8-bromo-cyclic guanosine monophosphate inhibit mitogenesis and proliferation of cultured rat vascular smooth muscle cells. *J. Clin. Investig.* **1989**, *83*, 1774–1777. [CrossRef] [PubMed]

60. Tulis, D.A.; Bohl Masters, K.S.; Lipke, E.A.; Schiesser, R.L.; Evans, A.J.; Peyton, K.J.; Durante, W.; West, J.L.; Schafer, A.I. YC-1-mediated vascular protection through inhibition of smooth muscle cell proliferation and platelet function. *Biochem. Biophys. Res. Commun.* **2002**, *291*, 1014–1021. [CrossRef] [PubMed]

61. Evgenov, O.V.; Pacher, P.; Schmidt, P.M.; Hasko, G.; Schmidt, H.H.; Stasch, J.P. NO-independent stimulators and activators of soluble guanylate cyclase: Discovery and therapeutic potential. *Nat. Rev. Drug Discov.* **2006**, *5*, 755–768. [CrossRef] [PubMed]

62. Stasch, J.P.; Pacher, P.; Evgenov, O.V. Soluble guanylate cyclase as an emerging therapeutic target in cardiopulmonary disease. *Circulation* **2011**, *123*, 2263–2273. [CrossRef] [PubMed]

63. Follmann, M.; Griebenow, N.; Hahn, M.G.; Hartung, I.; Mais, F.J.; Mittendorf, J.; Schafer, M.; Schirok, H.; Stasch, J.P.; Stoll, F.; et al. The chemistry and biology of soluble guanylate cyclase stimulators and activators. *Angew. Chem. Int. Ed. Engl.* **2013**, *52*, 9442–9462. [CrossRef] [PubMed]

64. Chiche, J.D.; Schlutsmeyer, S.M.; Bloch, D.B.; de la Monte, S.M.; Roberts, J.D., Jr.; Filippov, G.; Janssens, S.P.; Rosenzweig, A.; Bloch, K.D. Adenovirus-mediated gene transfer of cGMP-dependent protein kinase increases the sensitivity of cultured vascular smooth muscle cells to the antiproliferative and pro-apoptotic effects of nitric oxide/cGMP. *J. Biol. Chem.* **1998**, *273*, 34263–34271. [CrossRef] [PubMed]

65. Boerth, N.J.; Dey, N.B.; Cornwell, T.L.; Lincoln, T.M. Cyclic GMP-dependent protein kinase regulates vascular smooth muscle cell phenotype. *J. Vasc. Res.* **1997**, *34*, 245–259. [CrossRef] [PubMed]

66. Choi, C.; Sellak, H.; Brown, F.M.; Lincoln, T.M. cGMP-dependent protein kinase and the regulation of vascular smooth muscle cell gene expression: Possible involvement of ELK-1 sumoylation. *Am. J. Physiol. Heart Circ. Physiol.* **2010**, *299*, H1660–H1670. [CrossRef] [PubMed]

67. Hassid, A.; Arabshahi, H.; Bourcier, T.; Dhaunsi, G.S.; Matthews, C. Nitric oxide selectively amplifies FGF-2-induced mitogenesis in primary rat aortic smooth muscle cells. *Am. J. Physiol.* **1994**, *267*, H1040–H1048. [CrossRef] [PubMed]

68. Komalavilas, P.; Shah, P.K.; Jo, H.; Lincoln, T.M. Activation of mitogen-activated protein kinase pathways by cyclic GMP and cyclic GMP-dependent protein kinase in contractile vascular smooth muscle cells. *J. Biol. Chem.* **1999**, *274*, 34301–34309. [CrossRef] [PubMed]

69. Ignarro, L.J.; Buga, G.M.; Wei, L.H.; Bauer, P.M.; Wu, G.; del Soldato, P. Role of the arginine-nitric oxide pathway in the regulation of vascular smooth muscle cell proliferation. *Proc. Natl. Acad. Sci. USA* **2001**, *98*, 4202–4208. [CrossRef] [PubMed]

70. Weinmeister, P.; Lukowski, R.; Linder, S.; Traidl-Hoffmann, C.; Hengst, L.; Hofmann, F.; Feil, R. Cyclic guanosine monophosphate-dependent protein kinase I promotes adhesion of primary vascular smooth muscle cells. *Mol. Biol. Cell* **2008**, *19*, 4434–4441. [CrossRef] [PubMed]

71. Ridley, A.J.; Hall, A. The small GTP-binding protein rho regulates the assembly of focal adhesions and actin stress fibers in response to growth factors. *Cell* **1992**, *70*, 389–399. [CrossRef]

72. Burridge, K.; Wennerberg, K. Rho and Rac take center stage. *Cell* **2004**, *116*, 167–179. [CrossRef]

73. Rolli-Derkinderen, M.; Sauzeau, V.; Boyer, L.; Lemichez, E.; Baron, C.; Henrion, D.; Loirand, G.; Pacaud, P. Phosphorylation of serine 188 protects RhoA from ubiquitin/proteasome-mediated degradation in vascular smooth muscle cells. *Circ. Res.* **2005**, *96*, 1152–1160. [CrossRef] [PubMed]

74. Sauzeau, V.; Le Jeune, H.; Cario-Toumaniantz, C.; Smolenski, A.; Lohmann, S.M.; Bertoglio, J.; Chardin, P.; Pacaud, P.; Loirand, G. Cyclic GMP-dependent protein kinase signaling pathway inhibits RhoA-induced Ca^{2+} sensitization of contraction in vascular smooth muscle. *J. Biol. Chem.* **2000**, *275*, 21722–21729. [CrossRef] [PubMed]

75. Friebe, A.; Sandner, P.; Schmidtko, A. Meeting report of the 8(th) international conference on cGMP "cGMP: Generators, effectors, and therapeutic implications" at Bamberg, Germany, from June 23 to 25, 2017. *Naunyn Schmiedebergs Arch. Pharmacol.* **2017**, *390*, 1177–1188. [CrossRef] [PubMed]

76. Kraehling, J.R.; Sessa, W.C. Contemporary approaches to modulating the nitric oxide-cGMP pathway in cardiovascular disease. *Circ. Res.* **2017**, *120*, 1174–1182. [CrossRef] [PubMed]

77. Feil, R.; Kemp-Harper, B. cGMP signalling: From bench to bedside. Conference on cGMP generators, effectors and therapeutic implications. *EMBO Rep.* **2006**, *7*, 149–153. [CrossRef] [PubMed]

78. Oettrich, J.M.; Dao, V.T.; Frijhoff, J.; Kleikers, P.; Casas, A.I.; Hobbs, A.J.; Schmidt, H.H. Clinical relevance of cyclic GMP modulators: A translational success story of network pharmacology. *Clin. Pharmacol. Ther.* **2016**, *99*, 360–362. [CrossRef] [PubMed]

79. McMurray, J.J.; Packer, M.; Desai, A.S.; Gong, J.; Lefkowitz, M.P.; Rizkala, A.R.; Rouleau, J.L.; Shi, V.C.; Solomon, S.D.; Swedberg, K.; et al. Angiotensin-neprilysin inhibition versus enalapril in heart failure. *N. Engl. J. Med.* **2014**, *371*, 993–1004. [CrossRef] [PubMed]

80. Sandner, P. From molecules to patients: Exploring the therapeutic role of soluble guanylate cyclase stimulators. *Biol. Chem.* **2018**. [CrossRef] [PubMed]

81. Leineweber, K.; Moosmang, S.; Paulson, D. Genetics of NO deficiency. *Am. J. Cardiol.* **2017**, *120*, S80–S88. [CrossRef] [PubMed]

82. Ehret, G.B.; Munroe, P.B.; Rice, K.M.; Bochud, M.; Johnson, A.D.; Chasman, D.I.; Smith, A.V.; Tobin, M.D.; Verwoert, G.C.; Hwang, S.J.; et al. Genetic variants in novel pathways influence blood pressure and cardiovascular disease risk. *Nature* **2011**, *478*, 103–109. [CrossRef] [PubMed]

83. Emdin, C.A.; Khera, A.V.; Klarin, D.; Natarajan, P.; Zekavat, S.M.; Nomura, A.; Haas, M.; Aragam, K.; Ardissino, D.; Wilson, J.G.; et al. Phenotypic consequences of a genetic predisposition to enhanced nitric oxide signaling. *Circulation* **2018**, *137*, 222–232. [CrossRef] [PubMed]

84. Erdmann, J.; Stark, K.; Esslinger, U.B.; Rumpf, P.M.; Koesling, D.; de Wit, C.; Kaiser, F.J.; Braunholz, D.; Medack, A.; Fischer, M.; et al. Dysfunctional nitric oxide signalling increases risk of myocardial infarction. *Nature* **2013**, *504*, 432–436. [CrossRef] [PubMed]

85. Kessler, T.; Wobst, J.; Wolf, B.; Eckhold, J.; Vilne, B.; Hollstein, R.; von Ameln, S.; Dang, T.A.; Sager, H.B.; Moritz Rumpf, P.; et al. Functional characterization of the GUCY1A3 coronary artery disease risk locus. *Circulation* **2017**, *136*, 476–489. [CrossRef] [PubMed]

86. Maass, P.G.; Aydin, A.; Luft, F.C.; Schachterle, C.; Weise, A.; Stricker, S.; Lindschau, C.; Vaegler, M.; Qadri, F.; Toka, H.R.; et al. PDE3A mutations cause autosomal dominant hypertension with brachydactyly. *Nat. Genet.* **2015**, *47*, 647–653. [CrossRef] [PubMed]

87. Guo, D.C.; Regalado, E.; Casteel, D.E.; Santos-Cortez, R.L.; Gong, L.; Kim, J.J.; Dyack, S.; Horne, S.G.; Chang, G.; Jondeau, G.; et al. Recurrent gain-of-function mutation in prkg1 causes thoracic aortic aneurysms and acute aortic dissections. *Am. J. Hum. Genet.* **2013**, *93*, 398–404. [CrossRef] [PubMed]

88. Herve, D.; Philippi, A.; Belbouab, R.; Zerah, M.; Chabrier, S.; Collardeau-Frachon, S.; Bergametti, F.; Essongue, A.; Berrou, E.; Krivosic, V.; et al. Loss of α1β1 soluble guanylate cyclase, the major nitric oxide receptor, leads to moyamoya and achalasia. *Am. J. Hum. Genet.* **2014**, *94*, 385–394. [CrossRef] [PubMed]

89. Friebe, A.; Mergia, E.; Dangel, O.; Lange, A.; Koesling, D. Fatal gastrointestinal obstruction and hypertension in mice lacking nitric oxide-sensitive guanylyl cyclase. *Proc. Natl. Acad. Sci. USA* **2007**, *104*, 7699–7704. [CrossRef] [PubMed]

90. Feil, R. Conditional somatic mutagenesis in the mouse using site-specific recombinases. In *Conditional Mutagenesis: An Approach to Disease Models*; Feil, R., Metzger, D., Eds.; Springer: Berlin/Heidelberg, Germany, 2007; pp. 3–28.

91. Wegener, J.W.; Nawrath, H.; Wolfsgruber, W.; Kuhbandner, S.; Werner, C.; Hofmann, F.; Feil, R. cGMP-dependent protein kinase I mediates the negative inotropic effect of cGMP in the murine myocardium. *Circ. Res.* **2002**, *90*, 18–20. [CrossRef] [PubMed]

92. Chen, J.; Kuhlencordt, P.J.; Astern, J.; Gyurko, R.; Huang, P.L. Hypertension does not account for the accelerated atherosclerosis and development of aneurysms in male apolipoprotein e/endothelial nitric oxide synthase double knockout mice. *Circulation* **2001**, *104*, 2391–2394. [CrossRef] [PubMed]

93. Knowles, J.W.; Reddick, R.L.; Jennette, J.C.; Shesely, E.G.; Smithies, O.; Maeda, N. Enhanced atherosclerosis and kidney dysfunction in $eNOS^{(-/-)}Apoe^{(-/-)}$ mice are ameliorated by enalapril treatment. *J. Clin. Investig.* **2000**, *105*, 451–458. [CrossRef] [PubMed]

94. Kuhlencordt, P.J.; Gyurko, R.; Han, F.; Scherrer-Crosbie, M.; Aretz, T.H.; Hajjar, R.; Picard, M.H.; Huang, P.L. Accelerated atherosclerosis, aortic aneurysm formation, and ischemic heart disease in apolipoprotein e/endothelial nitric oxide synthase double-knockout mice. *Circulation* **2001**, *104*, 448–454. [CrossRef] [PubMed]

95. Moroi, M.; Zhang, L.; Yasuda, T.; Virmani, R.; Gold, H.K.; Fishman, M.C.; Huang, P.L. Interaction of genetic deficiency of endothelial nitric oxide, gender, and pregnancy in vascular response to injury in mice. *J. Clin. Investig.* **1998**, *101*, 1225–1232. [CrossRef] [PubMed]

96. Rudic, R.D.; Shesely, E.G.; Maeda, N.; Smithies, O.; Segal, S.S.; Sessa, W.C. Direct evidence for the importance of endothelium-derived nitric oxide in vascular remodeling. *J. Clin. Investig.* **1998**, *101*, 731–736. [CrossRef] [PubMed]

97. Yogo, K.; Shimokawa, H.; Funakoshi, H.; Kandabashi, T.; Miyata, K.; Okamoto, S.; Egashira, K.; Huang, P.; Akaike, T.; Takeshita, A. Different vasculoprotective roles of NO synthase isoforms in vascular lesion formation in mice. *Arterioscler. Thromb. Vasc. Biol.* **2000**, *20*, e96–e100. [CrossRef] [PubMed]

98. Fukumura, D.; Gohongi, T.; Kadambi, A.; Izumi, Y.; Ang, J.; Yun, C.O.; Buerk, D.G.; Huang, P.L.; Jain, R.K. Predominant role of endothelial nitric oxide synthase in vascular endothelial growth factor-induced angiogenesis and vascular permeability. *Proc. Natl. Acad. Sci. USA* **2001**, *98*, 2604–2609. [CrossRef] [PubMed]

99. Lee, P.C.; Salyapongse, A.N.; Bragdon, G.A.; Shears, L.L., 2nd; Watkins, S.C.; Edington, H.D.; Billiar, T.R. Impaired wound healing and angiogenesis in eNOS-deficient mice. *Am. J. Physiol.* **1999**, *277*, H1600–H1608. [CrossRef] [PubMed]

100. Murohara, T.; Asahara, T.; Silver, M.; Bauters, C.; Masuda, H.; Kalka, C.; Kearney, M.; Chen, D.; Symes, J.F.; Fishman, M.C.; et al. Nitric oxide synthase modulates angiogenesis in response to tissue ischemia. *J. Clin. Investig.* **1998**, *101*, 2567–2578. [CrossRef] [PubMed]

101. Kuhlencordt, P.J.; Hotten, S.; Schodel, J.; Rutzel, S.; Hu, K.; Widder, J.; Marx, A.; Huang, P.L.; Ertl, G. Atheroprotective effects of neuronal nitric oxide synthase in apolipoprotein e knockout mice. *Arterioscler. Thromb. Vasc. Biol.* **2006**, *26*, 1539–1544. [CrossRef] [PubMed]

102. Morishita, T.; Tsutsui, M.; Shimokawa, H.; Horiuchi, M.; Tanimoto, A.; Suda, O.; Tasaki, H.; Huang, P.L.; Sasaguri, Y.; Yanagihara, N.; et al. Vasculoprotective roles of neuronal nitric oxide synthase. *FASEB J.* **2002**, *16*, 1994–1996. [CrossRef] [PubMed]

103. Detmers, P.A.; Hernandez, M.; Mudgett, J.; Hassing, H.; Burton, C.; Mundt, S.; Chun, S.; Fletcher, D.; Card, D.J.; Lisnock, J.; et al. Deficiency in inducible nitric oxide synthase results in reduced atherosclerosis in apolipoprotein e-deficient mice. *J. Immunol.* **2000**, *165*, 3430–3435. [CrossRef] [PubMed]

104. Kuhlencordt, P.J.; Chen, J.; Han, F.; Astern, J.; Huang, P.L. Genetic deficiency of inducible nitric oxide synthase reduces atherosclerosis and lowers plasma lipid peroxides in apolipoprotein e-knockout mice. *Circulation* **2001**, *103*, 3099–3104. [CrossRef] [PubMed]

105. Chyu, K.Y.; Dimayuga, P.; Zhu, J.; Nilsson, J.; Kaul, S.; Shah, P.K.; Cercek, B. Decreased neointimal thickening after arterial wall injury in inducible nitric oxide synthase knockout mice. *Circ. Res.* **1999**, *85*, 1192–1198. [CrossRef] [PubMed]

106. Sennlaub, F.; Courtois, Y.; Goureau, O. Inducible nitric oxide synthase mediates the change from retinal to vitreal neovascularization in ischemic retinopathy. *J. Clin. Investig.* **2001**, *107*, 717–725. [CrossRef] [PubMed]

107. Vermeersch, P.; Buys, E.; Sips, P.; Pokreisz, P.; Marsboom, G.; Gillijns, H.; Pellens, M.; Dewerchin, M.; Bloch, K.D.; Brouckaert, P.; et al. Gender-specific modulation of the response to arterial injury by soluble guanylate cyclase alpha1. *Open Cardiovasc. Med. J.* **2009**, *3*, 98–104. [CrossRef] [PubMed]

108. Bettaga, N.; Jager, R.; Dunnes, S.; Groneberg, D.; Friebe, A. Cell-specific impact of nitric oxide-dependent guanylyl cyclase on arteriogenesis and angiogenesis in mice. *Angiogenesis* **2015**, *18*, 245–254. [CrossRef] [PubMed]

109. Aicher, A.; Heeschen, C.; Feil, S.; Hofmann, F.; Mendelsohn, M.E.; Feil, R.; Dimmeler, S. cGMP-dependent protein kinase I is crucial for angiogenesis and postnatal vasculogenesis. *PLoS ONE* **2009**, *4*, e4879. [CrossRef] [PubMed]

110. Yamahara, K.; Itoh, H.; Chun, T.H.; Ogawa, Y.; Yamashita, J.; Sawada, N.; Fukunaga, Y.; Sone, M.; Yurugi-Kobayashi, T.; Miyashita, K.; et al. Significance and therapeutic potential of the natriuretic peptides/cGMP/cGMP-dependent protein kinase pathway in vascular regeneration. *Proc. Natl. Acad. Sci. USA* **2003**, *100*, 3404–3409. [CrossRef] [PubMed]

111. Tsou, C.Y.; Chen, C.Y.; Zhao, J.F.; Su, K.H.; Lee, H.T.; Lin, S.J.; Shyue, S.K.; Hsiao, S.H.; Lee, T.S. Activation of soluble guanylyl cyclase prevents foam cell formation and atherosclerosis. *Acta Physiol.* **2014**, *210*, 799–810. [CrossRef] [PubMed]

112. Duda, D.G.; Fukumura, D.; Jain, R.K. Role of eNOS in neovascularization: NO for endothelial progenitor cells. *Trends Mol. Med.* **2004**, *10*, 143–145. [CrossRef] [PubMed]

113. Sinnaeve, P.; Chiche, J.D.; Gillijns, H.; Van Pelt, N.; Wirthlin, D.; Van De Werf, F.; Collen, D.; Bloch, K.D.; Janssens, S. Overexpression of a constitutively active protein kinase g mutant reduces neointima formation and in-stent restenosis. *Circulation* **2002**, *105*, 2911–2916. [CrossRef] [PubMed]

114. Wu, C.H.; Chang, W.C.; Chang, G.Y.; Kuo, S.C.; Teng, C.M. The inhibitory mechanism of YC-1, a benzyl indazole, on smooth muscle cell proliferation: An in vitro and in vivo study. *J. Pharmacol. Sci.* **2004**, *94*, 252–260. [CrossRef] [PubMed]

115. Tulis, D.A.; Durante, W.; Peyton, K.J.; Chapman, G.B.; Evans, A.J.; Schafer, A.I. YC-1, a benzyl indazole derivative, stimulates vascular cGMP and inhibits neointima formation. *Biochem. Biophys. Res. Commun.* **2000**, *279*, 646–652. [CrossRef] [PubMed]

116. Hirschberg, K.; Tarcea, V.; Pali, S.; Barnucz, E.; Gwanmesia, P.N.; Korkmaz, S.; Radovits, T.; Loganathan, S.; Merkely, B.; Karck, M.; et al. Cinaciguat prevents neointima formation after arterial injury by decreasing vascular smooth muscle cell migration and proliferation. *Int. J. Cardiol.* **2013**, *167*, 470–477. [CrossRef] [PubMed]

117. Hoenicka, M.; Schmid, C. Cardiovascular effects of modulators of soluble guanylyl cyclase activity. *Cardiovasc. Hematol. Agents Med. Chem.* **2008**, *6*, 287–301. [CrossRef] [PubMed]

118. Ahluwalia, A.; Foster, P.; Scotland, R.S.; McLean, P.G.; Mathur, A.; Perretti, M.; Moncada, S.; Hobbs, A.J. Antiinflammatory activity of soluble guanylate cyclase: cGMP-dependent down-regulation of p-selectin expression and leukocyte recruitment. *Proc. Natl. Acad. Sci. USA* **2004**, *101*, 1386–1391. [CrossRef] [PubMed]

119. Foster, M.W.; McMahon, T.J.; Stamler, J.S. S-nitrosylation in health and disease. *Trends Mol. Med.* **2003**, *9*, 160–168. [CrossRef]

120. Namba, T.; Koike, H.; Murakami, K.; Aoki, M.; Makino, H.; Hashiya, N.; Ogihara, T.; Kaneda, Y.; Kohno, M.; Morishita, R. Angiogenesis induced by endothelial nitric oxide synthase gene through vascular endothelial growth factor expression in a rat hindlimb ischemia model. *Circulation* **2003**, *108*, 2250–2257. [CrossRef] [PubMed]

121. Senthilkumar, A.; Smith, R.D.; Khitha, J.; Arora, N.; Veerareddy, S.; Langston, W.; Chidlow, J.H., Jr.; Barlow, S.C.; Teng, X.; Patel, R.P.; et al. Sildenafil promotes ischemia-induced angiogenesis through a PKG-dependent pathway. *Arterioscler. Thromb. Vasc. Biol.* **2007**, *27*, 1947–1954. [CrossRef] [PubMed]

122. Thunemann, M.; Fomin, N.; Krawutschke, C.; Russwurm, M.; Feil, R. Visualization of cGMP with cGi biosensors. *Methods Mol. Biol.* **2013**, *1020*, 89–120. [PubMed]

123. Nikolaev, V.O.; Lohse, M.J. Novel techniques for real-time monitoring of cGMP in living cells. In *cGMP: Generators, Effectors and Therapeutic Implications*; Schmidt, H.H.H.W., Hofmann, F., Stasch, J.-P., Eds.; Springer: Berlin/Heidelberg, Germany, 2009; pp. 229–243.

124. Russwurm, M.; Mullershausen, F.; Friebe, A.; Jager, R.; Russwurm, C.; Koesling, D. Design of fluorescence resonance energy transfer (FRET)-based cGMP indicators: A systematic approach. *Biochem. J.* **2007**, *407*, 69–77. [CrossRef] [PubMed]

125. Thunemann, M.; Wen, L.; Hillenbrand, M.; Vachaviolos, A.; Feil, S.; Ott, T.; Han, X.; Fukumura, D.; Jain, R.K.; Russwurm, M.; et al. Transgenic mice for cGMP imaging. *Circ. Res.* **2013**, *113*, 365–371. [CrossRef] [PubMed]

126. Mohrle, D.; Reimann, K.; Wolter, S.; Wolters, M.; Varakina, K.; Mergia, E.; Eichert, N.; Geisler, H.S.; Sandner, P.; Ruth, P.; et al. NO-sensitive guanylate cyclase isoforms NO-GC1 and NO-GC2 contribute to noise-induced inner hair cell synaptopathy. *Mol. Pharmacol.* **2017**, *92*, 375–388. [CrossRef] [PubMed]

127. Shuhaibar, L.C.; Egbert, J.R.; Norris, R.P.; Lampe, P.D.; Nikolaev, V.O.; Thunemann, M.; Wen, L.; Feil, R.; Jaffe, L.A. Intercellular signaling via cyclic GMP diffusion through gap junctions restarts meiosis in mouse ovarian follicles. *Proc. Natl. Acad. Sci. USA* **2015**, *112*, 5527–5532. [CrossRef] [PubMed]

128. Thunemann, M.; Schmidt, K.; de Wit, C.; Han, X.; Jain, R.K.; Fukumura, D.; Feil, R. Correlative intravital imaging of cGMP signals and vasodilation in mice. *Front. Physiol.* **2014**, *5*, 394. [CrossRef] [PubMed]

129. Schmidt, H.; Peters, S.; Frank, K.; Wen, L.; Feil, R.; Rathjen, F.G. Dorsal root ganglion axon bifurcation tolerates increased cyclic GMP levels: The role of phosphodiesterase 2A and scavenger receptor Npr3. *Eur. J. Neurosci.* **2016**, *44*, 2991–3000. [CrossRef] [PubMed]

130. Thunemann, M.; Schorg, B.F.; Feil, S.; Lin, Y.; Voelkl, J.; Golla, M.; Vachaviolos, A.; Kohlhofer, U.; Quintanilla-Martinez, L.; Olbrich, M.; et al. Cre/lox-assisted non-invasive in vivo tracking of specific cell populations by positron emission tomography. *Nat. Commun.* **2017**, *8*, 444. [CrossRef] [PubMed]

131. Das, A.; Smolenski, A.; Lohmann, S.M.; Kukreja, R.C. Cyclic GMP-dependent protein kinase ialpha attenuates necrosis and apoptosis following ischemia/reoxygenation in adult cardiomyocyte. *J. Biol. Chem.* **2006**, *281*, 38644–38652. [CrossRef] [PubMed]

132. Kato, T.; Muraski, J.; Chen, Y.; Tsujita, Y.; Wall, J.; Glembotski, C.C.; Schaefer, E.; Beckerle, M.; Sussman, M.A. Atrial natriuretic peptide promotes cardiomyocyte survival by cGMP-dependent nuclear accumulation of zyxin and Akt. *J. Clin. Investig.* **2005**, *115*, 2716–2730. [CrossRef] [PubMed]

133. Fiedler, B.; Feil, R.; Hofmann, F.; Willenbockel, C.; Drexler, H.; Smolenski, A.; Lohmann, S.M.; Wollert, K.C. cGMP-dependent protein kinase type I inhibits TAB1-p38 mitogen-activated protein kinase apoptosis signaling in cardiac myocytes. *J. Biol. Chem.* **2006**, *281*, 32831–32840. [CrossRef] [PubMed]

134. Frantz, S.; Klaiber, M.; Baba, H.A.; Oberwinkler, H.; Volker, K.; Gabetaner, B.; Bayer, B.; Abebetaer, M.; Schuh, K.; Feil, R.; et al. Stress-dependent dilated cardiomyopathy in mice with cardiomyocyte-restricted inactivation of cyclic GMP-dependent protein kinase i. *Eur. Heart J.* **2013**, *34*, 1233–1244. [CrossRef] [PubMed]

135. Kobsar, A.; Heeg, S.; Krohne, K.; Opitz, A.; Walter, U.; Bock, M.; Gambaryan, S.; Eigenthaler, M. Cyclic nucleotide-regulated proliferation and differentiation vary in human hematopoietic progenitor cells derived from healthy persons, tumor patients, and chronic myelocytic leukemia patients. *Stem Cells Dev.* **2008**, *17*, 81–91. [CrossRef] [PubMed]

136. Wong, J.C.; Fiscus, R.R. Essential roles of the nitric oxide (NO)/cGMP/protein kinase G type-Iα (PKG-Iα) signaling pathway and the atrial natriuretic peptide (ANP)/cGMP/PKG-Iα autocrine loop in promoting proliferation and cell survival of OP9 bone marrow stromal cells. *J. Cell. Biochem.* **2011**, *112*, 829–839. [CrossRef] [PubMed]

137. Foller, M.; Feil, S.; Ghoreschi, K.; Koka, S.; Gerling, A.; Thunemann, M.; Hofmann, F.; Schuler, B.; Vogel, J.; Pichler, B.; et al. Anemia and splenomegaly in cGKI-deficient mice. *Proc. Natl. Acad. Sci. USA* **2008**, *105*, 6771–6776. [CrossRef] [PubMed]

138. Rukoyatkina, N.; Walter, U.; Friebe, A.; Gambaryan, S. Differentiation of cGMP-dependent and -independent nitric oxide effects on platelet apoptosis and reactive oxygen species production using platelets lacking soluble guanylyl cyclase. *Thromb. Haemost.* **2011**, *106*, 922–933. [CrossRef] [PubMed]

139. Rangaswami, H.; Schwappacher, R.; Marathe, N.; Zhuang, S.; Casteel, D.E.; Haas, B.; Chen, Y.; Pfeifer, A.; Kato, H.; Shattil, S.; et al. Cyclic GMP and protein kinase G control a Src-containing mechanosome in osteoblasts. *Sci. Signal.* **2010**, *3*, ra91. [CrossRef] [PubMed]

140. Jaumann, M.; Dettling, J.; Gubelt, M.; Zimmermann, U.; Gerling, A.; Paquet-Durand, F.; Feil, S.; Wolpert, S.; Franz, C.; Varakina, K.; et al. cGMP-Prkg1 signaling and Pde5 inhibition shelter cochlear hair cells and hearing function. *Nat. Med.* **2012**, *18*, 252–259. [CrossRef] [PubMed]

141. Dhayade, S.; Kaesler, S.; Sinnberg, T.; Dobrowinski, H.; Peters, S.; Naumann, U.; Liu, H.; Hunger, R.E.; Thunemann, M.; Biedermann, T.; et al. Sildenafil potentiates a cGMP-dependent pathway to promote melanoma growth. *Cell Rep.* **2016**, *14*, 2599–2610. [CrossRef] [PubMed]

142. Li, W.Q.; Qureshi, A.A.; Robinson, K.C.; Han, J. Sildenafil use and increased risk of incident melanoma in US men: A prospective cohort study. *JAMA Intern. Med.* **2014**, *174*, 964–970. [CrossRef] [PubMed]

143. Loeb, S.; Folkvaljon, Y.; Lambe, M.; Robinson, D.; Garmo, H.; Ingvar, C.; Stattin, P. Use of phosphodiesterase type 5 inhibitors for erectile dysfunction and risk of malignant melanoma. *JAMA* **2015**, *313*, 2449–2455. [CrossRef] [PubMed]

144. Arozarena, I.; Sanchez-Laorden, B.; Packer, L.; Hidalgo-Carcedo, C.; Hayward, R.; Viros, A.; Sahai, E.; Marais, R. Oncogenic BRAF induces melanoma cell invasion by downregulating the cGMP-specific phosphodiesterase PDE5a. *Cancer Cell* **2011**, *19*, 45–57. [CrossRef] [PubMed]

145. Feil, R. Viagra releases the brakes on melanoma growth. *Mol. Cell. Oncol.* **2017**, *4*, e1188874. [CrossRef] [PubMed]

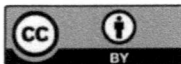

Journal of
Cardiovascular
Development and Disease

MDPI

Review

The Potential of a Novel Class of EPAC-Selective Agonists to Combat Cardiovascular Inflammation

Graeme Barker [1] , Euan Parnell [2], Boy van Basten [3], Hanna Buist [3] , David R. Adams [1] and Stephen J. Yarwood [3,*]

[1] Institute of Chemical Sciences, Heriot-Watt University, Edinburgh EH14 4AS, UK;
    Graeme.Barker@hw.ac.uk (G.B.); D.R.Adams@hw.ac.uk (D.R.A.)
[2] Department of Physiology, Feinberg School of Medicine, Northwestern University, Chicago, IL 60611, USA;
    euan.parnell@northwestern.edu
[3] Institute of Biological Chemistry, Biophysics and Bioengineering, Heriot-Watt University,
    Edinburgh EH14 4AS, UK; bv9@hw.ac.uk (B.v.B.); hkb1@hw.ac.uk (H.B.)
*   Correspondence: S.Yarwood@hw.ac.uk; Tel.: +44-(0)-131-451-3148

Received: 7 November 2017; Accepted: 30 November 2017; Published: 5 December 2017

Abstract: The cyclic $3',5'$-adenosine monophosphate (cAMP) sensor enzyme, EPAC1, is a candidate drug target in vascular endothelial cells (VECs) due to its ability to attenuate proinflammatory cytokine signalling normally associated with cardiovascular diseases (CVDs), including atherosclerosis. This is through the EPAC1-dependent induction of the suppressor of cytokine signalling gene, SOCS3, which targets inflammatory signalling proteins for ubiquitinylation and destruction by the proteosome. Given this important role for the EPAC1/SOCS3 signalling axis, we have used high throughput screening (HTS) to identify small molecule EPAC1 regulators and have recently isolated the first known non-cyclic nucleotide (NCN) EPAC1 agonist, I942. I942 therefore represents the first in class, isoform selective EPAC1 activator, with the potential to suppress pro-inflammatory cytokine signalling with a reduced risk of side effects associated with general cAMP-elevating agents that activate multiple response pathways. The development of augmented I942 analogues may therefore provide improved research tools to validate EPAC1 as a potential therapeutic target for the treatment of chronic inflammation associated with deadly CVDs.

Keywords: EPAC1; cyclic AMP; cyclic nucleotide binding domain; inflammation; endothelial cells; high-throughput screening

1. Introduction

Cyclic adenosine monophosphate (cyclic AMP) is the prototypical second messenger [1,2]; its intracellular concentration is governed by the relative expression and localization of enzymes responsible for its synthesis, adenylyl cyclases (ACs), and degradation, cyclic AMP phosphodiesterases (PDEs) [3–8]. Cyclic AMP exerts most of its effects through the activation of a range of down-stream sensors, including protein kinase A (PKA) [9–12], exchange protein directly activated by cyclic AMP proteins (EPAC) [13–15], Popeye domain-containing (POPDC) proteins [16,17] and cyclic nucleotide gated (CNG) ion channels [18]. Due to the diverse physiological responses controlled by cyclic AMP, signalling drugs have been developed to either promote cyclic AMP production, through activation of ACs [19], or inhibit its breakdown through inhibition of PDEs [7,20–23]. Both of these strategies lead to elevations in intracellular cyclic AMP, with the potential to activate all PKA, EPAC, POPDC and CNG signalling routes, depending on cell type [24]. However, such indiscriminate activation may be problematic. For example, PDE inhibitors, such as pentoxifylline, ibudilast, drotaverine and roflumilast, can cause undesirable physiological effects, including nausea, emesis, diarrhoea and cardiac arrhythmia [25], limiting their therapeutic usefulness. Similarly, the use of the di-terpene, forskolin, to activate ACs, has also been linked to various side effects, including flush syndrome and hypotension [26]. Therefore, the strategy of promoting the activation of all cyclic AMP signalling routes (e.g., PKA, EPAC, POPDC and CNG) with PDE inhibitors and forskolin may be unsuitable in therapeutic scenarios and new approaches to reduce side effects should be considered. In this regard, it may be possible to develop compounds that selectively activate EPACs, while avoiding many of the side effects associated with global cyclic AMP elevation. The focus of this review will therefore concentrate on the potential benefits of selective EPAC activation for the treatment of vascular inflammation and efforts to produce small molecule EPAC agonists to achieve this goal.

2. EPAC Proteins

EPAC proteins are cyclic AMP-regulated guanine nucleotide exchange factors (GEFs) that activate the small GTPases, Rap1 and Rap2 [27,28]. There are two main paralogues of EPAC, EPAC1 and EPAC2A [27,28], derived from distinct genes, in addition to two EPAC2A splice variants, EPAC2B and EPAC2C, which arise from differential promoter usage [29]. All EPAC isoforms consist of an N-terminal regulatory region and a C-terminal catalytic region (Figure 1) [29–32]. It is the binding of cyclic AMP to the regulatory cyclic nucleotide-binding domain (CNBD-B; Figure 1) that promotes GEF activity toward RAP1/2 [30–32] (Figure 2). The EPAC2A isoform contains an additional, N-terminal CNBD (CNBD-A; Figure 1), albeit with a much lower affinity for cyclic AMP [27,28]. It is not yet clear what the function of the second cyclic AMP binding domain is, although it has been speculated that the subcellular localization of Epac2A is, at least partly, regulated by the presence of this CNBD [33]. Other than this difference, EPAC1 and EPAC2 share similar structural motifs throughout the regulatory and catalytic domains. Indeed, the dishevelled-EGL-pleckstrin homology domain (DEP), Ras exchange motif (REM), Ras association domain (RA) and CDC25 homology GEF domains are conserved between isoforms (Figure 1) [34–36]. In the absence of cyclic AMP, EPAC is held in an inactive conformation due to intramolecular interactions between the regulatory CNBD-B and the catalytic GEF domain (Figure 2) [30,31]. Cyclic AMP binding to the phosphate binding cassette of the CNBD-B results in a local tightening and closure of the "lid" region over the cyclic AMP binding pocket (Figure 2) [32]. The conformational changes induced by binding cyclic AMP evoke an open form of EPAC that allows the GEF domain to interact with and activate Rap1 and Rap2 (Figure 2) [30,31].

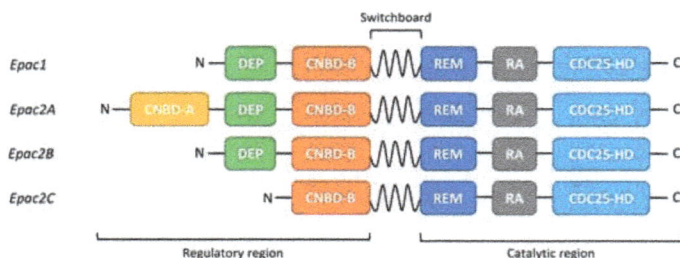

Figure 1. Primary structure of the different exchange proteins activated by cyclic AMP (EPAC) isoforms. The N-terminal regulatory region is directly connected to the C-terminal catalytic region through the switchboard region. Cyclic AMP interacts with the cyclic nucleotide-binding domain (CNBD-B), present in all EPAC isoforms, to trigger enzyme activation. Epac2A has an extra, non-functional cyclic AMP binding domain (CNBD-A). The other functional EPAC domains are indicated; DEP—Dishevelled, Egl-10, Pleckstrin domain, required for protein-protein and protein-lipid interactions; REM—Ras exchange motif, required for the stability of the CDC25-HD catalytic domain; RA—Ras association domain; allows interaction with members of the Ras-superfamily of small GTPases; CDC25-HD—CDC25 homology domain, which contains catalytic GEF activity to Rap 1/2 [14,36,37].

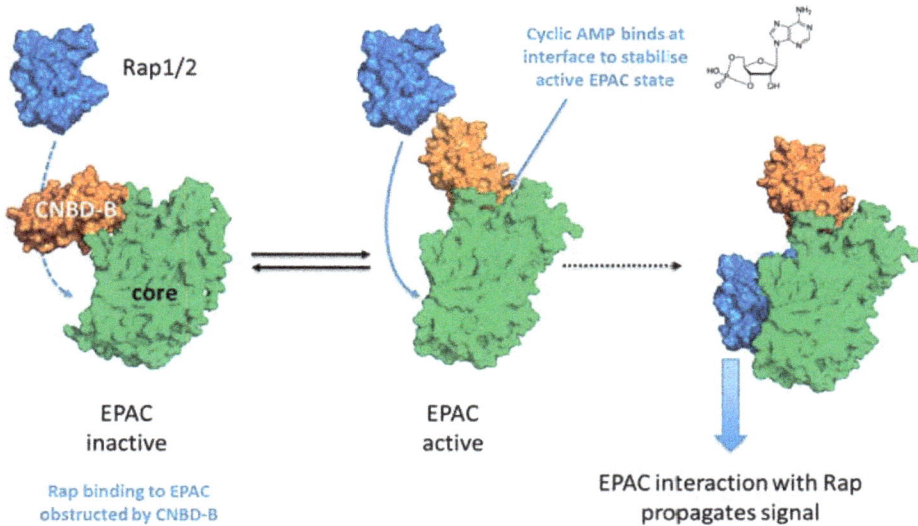

Figure 2. Activation of EPAC enzymes involves a conformational change triggered by the interaction of cyclic AMP with the EPAC CNBD-B.

3. EPAC1 Signalling and Vascular Function

A number of studies have suggested that EPAC-selective ligands may be useful for the future treatment of cardiac arrhythmia [38], obesity [39,40], diabetes [41], hypertension [42], cancer [43] and inflammatory pain [44]. Concerning inflammation, it has been suggested that selective EPAC regulators may be useful for the treatment of IL-8 driven lung inflammation associated with chronic obstructive pulmonary disorder (COPD), where EPAC2 appears to be pro-inflammatory, whereas EPAC1 suppresses lung remodelling [45–47]. Moreover, evidence is also emerging that EPAC1 is also a candidate drug target in vascular endothelial cells (VECs) due to its ability to attenuate pro-inflammatory cytokine signalling normally associated with atherosclerosis and neointimal hyperplasia (NIH), which arises from mechanical injury during angioplasty with stents [14,37]. This is because the VEC layer provides an important barrier to circulating inflammatory cytokines and leukocytes, and damage or disruption to this barrier is a key etiological precursor to various cardiovascular diseases. In addition, NIH is characterised by localised inflammation and proliferation of vascular smooth muscle cells (VSMCs) that underlie the VEC layer, thereby precipitating stent failure and myocardial infarction [48]. EPAC1 has been shown to inhibit migration of VSMCs associated with NIH [49,50], although a number of conflicting reports have been published (Table 1) and further work needs to be done in this area. Despite this, EPAC1 has emerged as an important factor in the regulation of the pro-inflammatory interleukin 6 (IL-6) trans-signalling pathway in VECs [51]. This makes EPAC1 an interesting candidate therapeutic target for the treatment of diseases in which IL-6 signalling is heavily implicated, such as atherosclerosis [52–56].

3.1. IL-6 Signalling in Vascular Endothelial Cells

IL-6 signalling is mediated by a receptor complex comprising an α chain (IL-6Rα) and a transmembrane glycoprotein (gp130) that associate on the cell surface in the presence of the cytokine to form a 2:2:2 heteromeric complex [57]. However, the pathophysiological pro-inflammatory actions of IL-6 in a variety of diseases, including atherosclerosis [56], are thought to be driven by aberrant IL-6 receptor "trans-signalling" [53]. During trans-signalling, IL-6 binds to a soluble form of the

IL-6R (sIL-6R) and this then allows IL-6 to activate gp130 on the surface of cells that are normally unresponsive to IL-6, including VECs [53]. The new signalling complex, formed of IL-6/sIL-6R/gp130, can now activate Janus tyrosine kinases (JAKs) in VECs, which then phosphorylate the cytosolic region of gp130 on key residues, including Tyr767, Tyr814, Tyr905 and Tyr915 [58]. Phosphorylation of these sites leads to the recruitment, JAK-dependent phosphorylation and activation of signal transducer and activator of transcription 3 (STAT3), which dimerizes and translocates to the nucleus (Figure 3), where it promotes transcription of pro-inflammatory genes [59], including VEGF and MCP-1.

Table 1. Effects of EPAC1 on experimental neointimal hyperplasia.

Experimental Model	Treatments	Effects
Carotid arteries and vascular smooth muscle cells (VSMCs) from wild type (WT) and EPAC1 −/− mice.	Ligation of carotid arteries and pharmacological inhibition of EPAC1	Neointima formation and VSMC proliferation were reduced in EPAC1 −/− mice. ESI09 also reduced neointima formation [60].
VSMCs from thoracic aorta explants from WT and EPAC1 −/− mice.	Injury of femoral artery	Reduced neointima formation and reduced migration of VSMCs in EPAC1 −/− mice [61].
Human saphenous vein VSMCs	Effects of pharmacological EPAC activation on VSMC migration	EPAC activation reduced VSMC migration and serum-induced vessel wall thickening [49].
Rat VSMCs from aorta explants.	Phamacological activation of EPAC and PKA	A combination of EPAC and PKA activation inhibited serum-induced VSMC proliferation [50].
VSMCs from foetal and adult rat aorta.	Pharmacological activation of EPAC and adenovirus-mediated overexpression of EPAC1	EPAC activation and overexpression of EPAC1 enhanced intimal thickening in aorta and VSMC proliferation [62].
Primary aortic VSMCs from male rats	Pharmacological activation of EPAC and PKA	PKA and EPAC work cooperatively to inhibit VSMC migration [63].

If unresolved, IL-6 trans-signalling will maintain an inflammatory condition by promoting the recruitment and activation of inflammatory cells, endothelial dysfunction and promoting VSMC proliferation and migration [64].

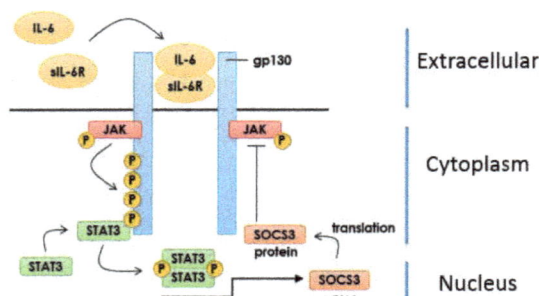

Figure 3. IL-6 Signalling and SOCS3 Induction. IL-6 binds to the soluble form of the IL-6 receptor (sIL-6R) thereby promoting the dimerization of gp130 glycoprotein and activation of receptor-associated JAKs. Activated JAKs phosphorylate STAT3, leading to its dimerization and translocation to the nucleus where it initiates gene transcription including induction of the suppressor of cytokine signalling (SOCS) 3 gene. SOCS3 protein then serves as a negative feedback regulator of JAK-STAT signalling.

Normally, IL-6 signalling is controlled through a classical negative-feedback route involving the induction of the gene encoding suppressor of cytokine signalling protein (SOCS) 3 by the same JAK-STAT3 pathways that the IL-6R activates [65] (Figure 3). Once induced SOCS3 acts by binding to

JAK-phosphorylated receptors, mediated by the SOCS3 SH2 domain, thereby inhibiting JAK activity, STAT signalling [66] and targeting JAK for proteasomal degradation [67].

3.2. Inhibition of IL-6 Signalling by SOCS3

SOCS3 is a potent inhibitor of pro-inflammatory pathways involved in atherosclerosis [68] and the development of NIH [69]. Indeed, SOCS3 expression is increased in atherosclerotic plaques [70,71] and its knockdown in apoE $-/-$ mice increases inflammatory gene expression in aorta, leading to enhanced atherogenesis [71]. Moreover, knockdown of SOCS3 promotes pro-inflammatory actions of IL-6 [72] and triggers angiogenesis in VECs [73]. In contrast, overexpression of SOCS3 suppresses JAK/STAT signalling and the development of atherosclerosis and NIH, demonstrating the importance of SOCS3 in limiting the development of cardiovascular disease [69,74,75].

3.3. Induction of SOCS3 by EPAC1 and Inhibition of IL-6 Signalling in VECs

Activation of EPAC1 in VECs leads to a down-regulation of IL-6-mediated inflammatory processes through the JAK/STAT3 pathway [51], which occurs through C/EBP transcription factor-dependent SOCS3 induction [76]. Moreover, EPAC1 exerts other cyclic AMP-dependent anti-inflammatory actions in VECs, including activation of integrins, thereby promoting adhesion of VECs to the basement membrane [77]. In addition, EPAC1 activation is able to promote endothelial barrier function [78,79] through VE-cadherin mediated cell-cell junction stability [80], in response to actin [81–85] and microtubule [86] cytoskeletal reorganisation. Thus, EPAC1 is involved in multiple anti-inflammatory processes in VECs and the links between EPAC1 and SOCS3 and the development of atherosclerosis/NIH indicate that EPAC1 regulation should be considered as a potential therapeutic avenue for the future treatment of cardiovascular disease.

4. Development of EPAC-Selective Agonists

4.1. EPAC Agonists Based on Cyclic Nucleotides

Due to the emerging potential of EPAC isoforms as drug targets, efforts have been made to develop small molecule EPAC agonists. The first of these, the cyclic AMP analogue, 8-(4-chlorophenylthio)-2'-O-methyladenosine-3',5'-cyclic monophosphate (8-pCPT-2'-O-Me-cyclic AMP; 007), and its improved cell permeable derivative (007-AM [87]; Figure 4), are able to selectively activate both EPAC1 and EPAC2 isoforms, independently of PKA [88]. The selectivity of 007 for the EPAC isoforms over PKA is due to a single amino acid difference in the CNBD cyclic AMP-binding pockets of PKA and EPACs, which are otherwise highly conserved in their amino acid composition [88]. Thus, the substitution of a key glutamic acid residue in the PKA CNBD, by a glutamine or lysine in EPAC1 or EPAC2, respectively, is responsible for the discrimination exhibited by the 2'-O-methylated nucleotide and preference for binding to the EPACs [88]. A structural understanding for the basis of this selectivity was assisted by the determination of the 3D structure of EPAC2 [30,31], and now a range of cyclic AMP analogues with varying kinetic properties have been developed that can also differentiate between EPAC1 and EPAC2 [89]. In particular, an EPAC2-selective agonist, 8-benzylthioadenosine-3',5'-cyclic monophosphorothioate (Sp-8-BnT-cAMPS; S-220; Figure 4), has been developed that exerts glucose-dependent stimulatory activity in insulin-secreting human pancreatic cells [90]. However, in vivo use of these analogues has been hampered by cardiac arrhythmia, fibrosis and cardiac hypertrophy in animal models [91,92], limiting rigorous preclinical assessment of their therapeutic benefit. These effects are likely linked to calcium signalling crosstalk within cardiomyocytes [93,94] following chronic activation of EPAC2 within the heart. These observations suggest that pharmacological exploitation of EPAC-activating compounds may need to be focused on the development of selective EPAC1 ligands, thereby avoiding these adverse effects.

Fluorescent Probe

8-NBD-cAMP

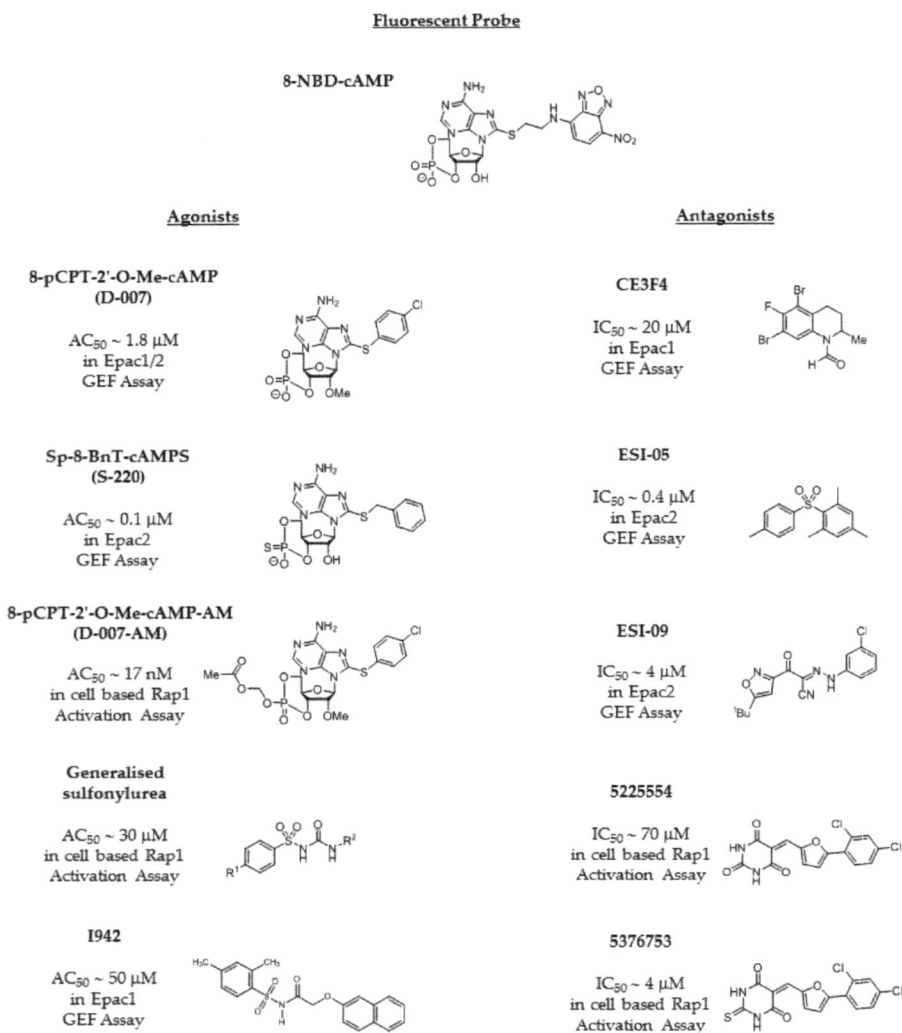

Agonists | Antagonists

8-pCPT-2'-O-Me-cAMP
(D-007)

AC₅₀ ~ 1.8 μM
in Epac1/2
GEF Assay

CE3F4

IC₅₀ ~ 20 μM
in Epac1
GEF Assay

Sp-8-BnT-cAMPS
(S-220)

AC₅₀ ~ 0.1 μM
in Epac2
GEF Assay

ESI-05

IC₅₀ ~ 0.4 μM
in Epac2
GEF Assay

8-pCPT-2'-O-Me-cAMP-AM
(D-007-AM)

AC₅₀ ~ 17 nM
in cell based Rap1
Activation Assay

ESI-09

IC₅₀ ~ 4 μM
in Epac2
GEF Assay

Generalised
sulfonylurea

AC₅₀ ~ 30 μM
in cell based Rap1
Activation Assay

5225554

IC₅₀ ~ 70 μM
in cell based Rap1
Activation Assay

I942

AC₅₀ ~ 50 μM
in Epac1
GEF Assay

5376753

IC₅₀ ~ 4 μM
in cell based Rap1
Activation Assay

Figure 4. Chemical structures of existing EPAC-selective agonists and antagonists together with the cyclic analogue AMP analogue fluorescent probe molecule, 8NBD-cAMP.

4.2. The Sulfonyl Urea Family as EPAC Agonists

After 007 and its analogues, the most studied, but controversial, group of small molecule EPAC agonists are those of the sulfonylurea (SU) family (Figure 4). SUs were originally developed as anti-diabetic drugs capable of regulating the SUR1 receptor, leading to the opening of ATP-dependent potassium channels in pancreatic β-cells, with consequent calcium release and increased insulin exocytosis [95]. Recently it has been postulated that SUs also act as isoform selective activators of EPAC2, in particular via an allosteric mechanism involving the low affinity CNBD-A of EPAC2 [96]. This idea has been challenged [97], however, and it has been shown that SUs are unable to induce GEF activity in in vitro EPAC2 activation assays [98]. Insulin secretion is known to be impaired in EPAC2 knockout mice, but the positive effect of SUs on EPAC2 activity in cellular assays may be indirect, as reports indicate that these compounds induce elevations in intracellular cyclic AMP [98].

4.3. EPAC Antagonists

Further efforts to identify small molecule EPAC regulators using high throughput screening (HTS) of compound libraries have mainly identified antagonists, both orthosteric and allosteric, rather than agonists [1,2,99,100]. Indeed, uncompetitive (CE3F4) and non-competitive EPAC1 inhibitors (5225554 and 5376753; Figure 4) have been identified using in vitro EPAC1 GEF [2] and EPAC-based bioluminescence resonance energy transfer-based [1] assays, respectively. Similarly, inhibitors for EPAC2 have been identified by HTS using a displacement assay with the cyclic AMP analogue, 8-[2-[(7-nitro-4-benzofurazanyl)aminoethyl]thio]-cyclic AMP (8-NBD-cyclic AMP; Figure 4), which fluoresces when bound within the hydrophobic environment of the cyclic AMP binding pocket [89]. Displacement of 8-NBD-cyclic AMP by competitor compounds leads to a reduction in fluorescence, allowing the identification of interacting molecules. Despite this assay being equally sensitive to agonist and antagonist molecules, so far only the EPAC2-selective competitive inhibitor, ESI-05 (4-methylphenyl-2,4,6-trimethylphenylsulfone) [101], and a non-selective EPAC1/2 inhibitor, ESI-09 (3-(5-*tert*-butylisoxazol-3-yl)-2-[(3-chlorophenyl)-hydrazonol]-3-oxopropionitrile), have been identified [99,102,103]. Subsequently, concerns were raised over the specificity of ESI-09, which is thought to display non-specific protein denaturing properties [104]. Despite this, several more potent EPAC antagonistic ESI-09 and ESI-05 analogues (Figure 4) have been developed [105–107].

4.4. Identification of Non-Cyclic Nucleotide (NCN) EPAC Agonists

HTS using 8-NBD-cAMP (Figure 4) competition assays has been limited to screens involving EPAC2, likely due to the limited fluorescence of 8-NBD-cAMP when bound to the CNBD-B of EPAC1 compared to EPAC2 [99]. This difference may be linked to structural differences between EPAC1 and EPAC2 within the CNBD-B that selectively influence the docking of ligands to the cAMP-binding pocket [90]. Moreover, the low stability of full length recombinant EPAC1 in vitro has limited its study in HTS and structural assays [89]. Although full-length EPAC1 is relatively unstable in vitro, the isolated EPAC1-CNBD-B displays superior stability and 8-NBD-cAMP has been shown to bind and fluoresce within the CNBD-B of EPAC1 [89]. Given that the CNBDs of EPAC1 and EPAC2 display structural differences [108–110], screening both CNBDs simultaneously may facilitate isoform-selective compound discovery. We have used this dual-target strategy to screen 5195 compounds from the BioAscent Compound Collection (Biocity Scotland, Newhouse, Scotland), identifying a number of ligands with varied binding affinities to the distinct isoforms [111]. Follow up characterisation of the top hit, I942 (Figure 4), using ligand observe nuclear magnetic resonance (NMR) confirmed direct interaction with both EPAC1 and EPAC2 CNBD-B [111]. However, in vitro GEF assays revealed that I942 displayed partial agonist activity toward EPAC1 (AC_{50} 10% that of cyclic AMP [111]) and no significant action towards EPAC2. Further study revealed that I942 had no effect in vitro on PKA activity as measured by phosphorylation of the transcription factor CREB, a known PKA substrate. I942 is therefore the first non-cyclic nucleotide small-molecule with selective agonist properties toward EPAC1. As a novel, NCN scaffold, the *N*-acylsulfonamide chemotype of I942 might be advantageous to nucleotide-based structures, which may require prodrug strategies for therapeutic deployment.

4.5. Putative Binding Mode of Novel EPAC Agonists

The binding mode of I942 and mechanism of EPAC1 activation remain to be experimentally determined, although in silico modelling studies have been undertaken and a plausible binding postulate developed to rationalise the compound's partial activation of EPAC1 (Figure 5). As the structure of EPAC1 has yet to be determined, homology models of EPAC1 were constructed from crystal structures (PDB: 4MH0, 4MGY, 4MGK) of EPAC2 in the nucleotide-bound, active conformation with and without an EPAC1-mimetic point mutation (K405Q) [90]. These models allowed us to explore the possible structural basis for interaction of I942 with EPAC1. Preliminary findings suggest that the acidic *N*-acylsulfonamide motif (pKa ~ 4) may occupy a similar volume to the cyclic AMP phosphate (Figure 5), engaging a key charge-pairing arginine (Arg279) within the CNBD "phosphate-binding cassette" (PBC), defined by residues 268-FGQLALVNDAPRAAT-282 of EPAC1 [32]. The PBC is strongly conserved in EPAC2 as residues 403-FGKLALVNDAPRAAS-417 in the murine constructs used for crystallography, and contains a short helix that hydrogen bonds through its N-terminus to the phosphate of cyclic AMP. The ionised *N*-acylsulfonamide is similarly predicted to cap this helix, through its carbonyl oxygen, whilst additionally engaging the PBC backbone at Ala280 and Ala281 in charge-stabilised hydrogen bonds from the nitrogen and one of the sulfonyl oxygens.

Our binding hypothesis positions the I942 *m*-xylyl group approximately coplanar with the bound nucleotide's purine in the main funnel-like opening to the binding site. However, direct overlap with the adenine bicycle is limited in this model, and I942 does not exploit the polar interactions available to the endogenous ligand through the adenine bicycle. Thus, co-crystal structures of EPAC2 constructs with bound cAMP reveal that a key lysine (Lys489) on helix-α1 of the REM domain engages the purine N-1 centre. This promotes folding of the cyclic AMP-bound CNBD onto the REM domain surface, with the helix contributing to the EPAC "lid" region that closes over the nucleotide [30]. Lys489 is conserved on the REM-α1 helix of EPAC1 as Lys353, but I942 lacks the necessary structural extension and functionality to engage it. On the other hand, our model suggests that I942 may exploit additional, hydrophobic interactions at the opposite end of the REM-α1 helix to Lys353 that are not accessible to cyclic AMP. In particular, the model invokes threading of the oxymethylene linker through a narrow passage (solvent filled in the absence of ligand; Figure 5) that leads to a second and smaller funnel opening on the opposite face of the protein surface to the adenine-binding channel. It is this second "posterior channel", we postulate, that hosts the I942 naphthyl moiety (Figure 5) and that (based on residue differences between EPAC2 and EPAC1) may be more restrictive in the case of EPAC2.

The posterior channel is heavily hydrophobic, with the side chains of several conserved CNBD residues (Leu271, Asn275, Ala277, Pro278, Ala280 and Leu314) contributing much of the putative contact surface for the ligand's naphthyloxy group. However, three residues from the REM-α1 helix of EPAC1 are also predicted to make a significant contribution to the posterior channel—namely Leu357, Ala361 and Glu360 (the latter through its side chain methylenes). Of these three residues, only the glutamic acid is conserved in EPAC2, with Leu357 and Ala361 replaced by histidine and threonine respectively. Our model suggests that packing of the napthyloxy group against these three REM-α1 residues may stabilise the closed, active state of EPAC1, albeit less effectively than cyclic AMP through its interactions in the anterior channel and perhaps with slightly altered seating of the CNBD against the EPAC core. This would account for the partial agonism, whilst the selectivity of I942 for activation of EPAC1 over EPAC2 may be explained, at least in part, by loss of the favourable surface contact with Leu357 and steric interdiction by the threonine replacement for Ala361. An implicit corollary of this "threaded model", in which the ligand binds between anterior and posterior channels, is that the mechanism of EPAC1 activation must involve stepwise binding of the ligand to the open, inactive conformation of the protein followed by hinged closure of the ligand-bound CNBD (*cf.* Figure 2). Structural studies with EPAC2 have shown that the conformation of the hinge region is sensitive to a single point mutation in the PBC, where Lys405 of EPAC2 is replaced by a glutamine, which is located at the cognate position of EPAC1 (Gln270) [90]. At present, we cannot rule out the possibility that this difference between EPAC1 and EPAC2 might also contribute to the observed selectivity of I942 by differentially modulating the seating properties of the PBC against the lid for the two EPAC isoforms. However, the model presented in Figure 5 does not invoke a direct and EPAC1-specific contact between I942 and the side chain of Q270.

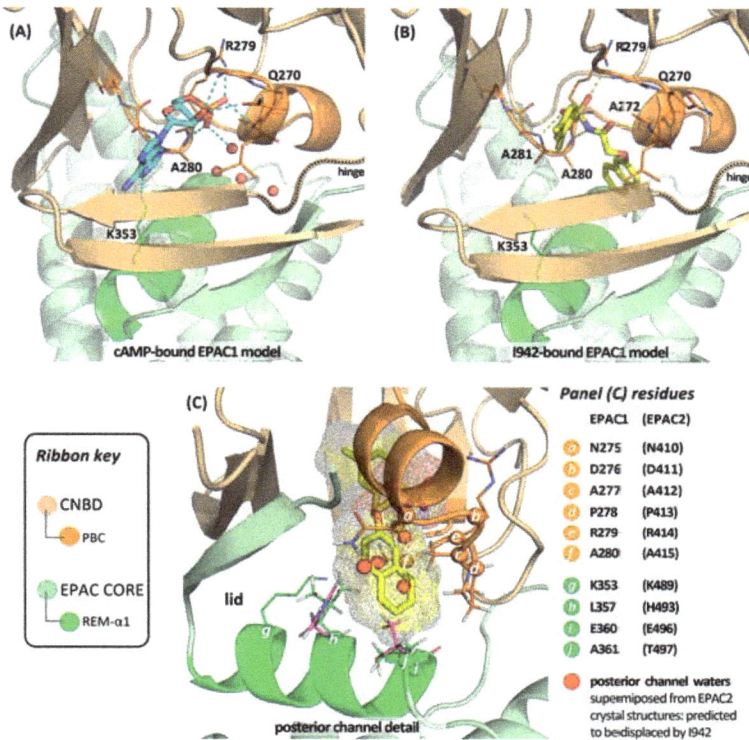

Figure 5. Modelling studies with EPAC1 homology models suggest that I942 may engage the cyclic nucleotide binding domain-B (CNBD-B) with subsequent hinged closure of the domain onto the protein core leading to a "threaded" binding mode and adoption of an active-state EPAC conformation. In this binding mode (panel (**B**)) the acidic *N*-acylsulfonamide is predicted to occupy the position of the endogenous ligand's phosphate (panel (**A**)) and form extensive phosphomimetic hydrogen bonds (dashed lines) with the protein's phosphate-binding cassette (PBC, bright orange ribbon). EPAC2 co-crystal structures show that the cyclic AMP adenine binds in a large funnel-like channel that opens on the front face of the protein as figured in panel (**A**), where the adenine N1 centre engages a lysine (conserved as K353 in EPAC1) on the REM domain's helix-α1 (bright green ribbon). An additional smaller opening, the posterior channel, communicates to the reverse face of the protein. Cyclic AMP does not directly utilise this volume, which is occupied by water molecules in available EPAC2 co-crystal structures (marked as red spheres in the panel (**A**) model). We postulate that this posterior channel, which is heavily hydrophobic, hosts the naphthyloxy group of I942, as detailed in panel (**C**). Occupancy of this channel may be entropically favoured by displacement of water (shown superimposed as red spheres in panel (**C**)), and stabilise closure of the CNBD onto the EPAC1 core by interaction of the naphthyl subunit with REM-α1 residues L357, E360 and A361 (*h*, *i* and *j* in panel (**C**)). L357 and A361 are not conserved across the EPAC isoforms, which may account for the observed selectivity of I942, as the cognate EPAC2 residues (H493, T497; magenta stick) are predicted to interdict I942 binding. In the EPAC active conformation the REM-α1 helix folds as a lid onto the ligand binding site due to reorganisation of the EPAC hinge sequence (dotted ribbon in panels (**A**,**B**)). Whilst the naphthyloxy group may favourably engage the surface of REM-α1 at the C-terminal end, it fails (in contrast to cyclic AMP) to engage K353 at the N-terminal end. This may influence equilibrium position between CNBD-B open and closed states, with weaker overall engagement of the REM-α1 lid by I942 (or/and ligand-specific domain seating penalties) accounting for the observed EPAC1 "partial agonism" relative to the endogenous ligand.

J. Cardiovasc. Dev. Dis. **2017**, *4*, 22

5. Conclusions

In summary, several cyclic nucleotide analogues have been developed as EPAC agonist tool compounds in recent years, some exhibiting discrimination between the two EPAC isoforms in addition to selectivity over PKA. To address the challenging physicochemical properties of nucleotides and enhance cell permeability, phosphate masking strategies have been used, as with the labile acetoxymethyl ester modification (007-AM; Figure 4) of the prototypical nucleotide agonist, 8-pCPT-2′-O-Me-cyclic AMP. Both nucleotide and non-nucleotide EPAC antagonists have also been reported. Very recently, we have identified a unique class of selective NCN EPAC1-activating ligand, exemplified by I942 (Figure 4). This new chemotype likely binds and stabilises the active state of EPAC1 via a previously unobserved interaction mode. Further work is required to validate the binding mode proposed for I942, but, if correct in its essentials, the model presented here suggests that there should be significant scope for optimisation of the ligand's naphthyl and m-xylyl subunits to enhance affinity and adjust efficacy with respect to the GEF activity of EPAC1. Changes to the m-xylyl group might additionally be harnessed, in principle, to modulate the pKa of the *N*-acylsulfonamide, which is a pharmacologically well-precedented moiety [112] and which we suggest serves as a cyclophosphate ester mimetic in the case of I942. We therefore propose that an integrated programme of chemical synthesis of structural analogues with concurrent assessment of bioactivity may allow the generation of a "molecular toolkit" of ligands displaying a spectrum of activity from partial to full agonism and with prospects for tractable bioavailability. The development of such a toolkit will allow a full exploration of the roles of EPAC1 in VECs, as well as in preclinical disease models of vascular dysfunction. An experimental and comprehensive structure activity relationship (SAR) study of I942 alongside confirmation of our docking models may pave the way to the development of new therapies for the treatment of cardiovascular disease.

Acknowledgments: This work and open access charges was funded by a project grant from the British Heart Foundation, awarded to S.J.Y. (grant number PG/15/15/31316).

Author Contributions: All authors contributed to the writing of this manuscript. H.B., B.v.B., G.B., E.P. and D.R.A. prepared the figures.

Conflicts of Interest: The authors declare no conflict of interest.

References

1. Brown, L.M.; Rogers, K.E.; Aroonsakool, N.; McCammon, J.A.; Insel, P.A. Allosteric inhibition of Epac: Computational modeling and experimental validation to identify allosteric sites and inhibitors. *J. Biol. Chem.* **2014**, *289*, 29148–29157. [CrossRef] [PubMed]
2. Courilleau, D.; Bisserier, M.; Jullian, J.C.; Lucas, A.; Bouyssou, P.; Fischmeister, R.; Blondeau, J.P.; Lezoualc'h, F. Identification of a tetrahydroquinoline analog as a pharmacological inhibitor of the cAMP-binding protein Epac. *J. Biol. Chem.* **2012**, *287*, 44192–44202. [CrossRef] [PubMed]
3. Dessauer, C.W.; Watts, V.J.; Ostrom, R.S.; Conti, M.; Dove, S.; Seifert, R. International union of basic and clinical pharmacology. CI. Structures and small molecule modulators of mammalian adenylyl cyclases. *Pharmacol. Rev.* **2017**, *69*, 93–139. [CrossRef] [PubMed]
4. Halls, M.L.; Cooper, D.M. Adenylyl cyclase signalling complexes—Pharmacological challenges and opportunities. *Pharmacol. Ther.* **2017**, *172*, 171–180. [CrossRef] [PubMed]
5. Nicol, X.; Gaspar, P. Routes to camp: Shaping neuronal connectivity with distinct adenylate cyclases. *Eur. J. Neurosci.* **2014**, *39*, 1742–1751. [CrossRef] [PubMed]
6. Klussmann, E. Protein-protein interactions of PDE4 family members—Functions, interactions and therapeutic value. *Cell. Signal.* **2016**, *28*, 713–718. [CrossRef] [PubMed]
7. Maurice, D.H.; Ke, H.; Ahmad, F.; Wang, Y.; Chung, J.; Manganiello, V.C. Advances in targeting cyclic nucleotide phosphodiesterases. *Nat. Rev. Drug Discov.* **2014**, *13*, 290–314. [CrossRef] [PubMed]
8. Maurice, D.H.; Wilson, L.S.; Rampersad, S.N.; Hubert, F.; Truong, T.; Kaczmarek, M.; Brzezinska, P.; Freitag, S.I.; Umana, M.B.; Wudwud, A. Cyclic nucleotide phosphodiesterases (PDEs): Coincidence

detectors acting to spatially and temporally integrate cyclic nucleotide and non-cyclic nucleotide signals. *Biochem. Soc. Trans.* **2014**, *42*, 250–256. [CrossRef] [PubMed]

9. Torres-Quesada, O.; Mayrhofer, J.E.; Stefan, E. The many faces of compartmentalized PKA signalosomes. *Cell. Signal.* **2017**, *37*, 1–11. [CrossRef] [PubMed]

10. Calejo, A.I.; Tasken, K. Targeting protein-protein interactions in complexes organized by a kinase anchoring proteins. *Front. Pharmacol.* **2015**, *6*, 192. [CrossRef] [PubMed]

11. Dema, A.; Perets, E.; Schulz, M.S.; Deak, V.A.; Klussmann, E. Pharmacological targeting of AKAP-directed compartmentalized cAMP signalling. *Cell. Signal.* **2015**, *27*, 2474–2487. [CrossRef] [PubMed]

12. Lefkimmiatis, K.; Zaccolo, M. Camp signaling in subcellular compartments. *Pharmacol. Ther.* **2014**, *143*, 295–304. [CrossRef] [PubMed]

13. Banerjee, U.; Cheng, X. Exchange protein directly activated by cAMP encoded by the mammalian rapgef3 gene: Structure, function and therapeutics. *Gene* **2015**, *570*, 157–167. [CrossRef] [PubMed]

14. Parnell, E.; Palmer, T.M.; Yarwood, S.J. The future of EPAC-targeted therapies: Agonism versus antagonism. *Trends Pharmacol. Sci.* **2015**, *36*, 203–214. [CrossRef] [PubMed]

15. Wang, P.; Liu, Z.; Chen, H.; Ye, N.; Cheng, X.; Zhou, J. Exchange proteins directly activated by cAMP (EPACs): Emerging therapeutic targets. *Bioorg. Med. Chem. Lett.* **2017**, *27*, 1633–1639. [CrossRef] [PubMed]

16. Brand, T. The popeye domain-containing gene family. *Cell Biochem. Biophys.* **2005**, *43*, 95–103. [CrossRef]

17. Schindler, R.F.; Brand, T. The popeye domain containing protein family—A novel class of camp effectors with important functions in multiple tissues. *Prog. Biophys. Mol. Biol.* **2016**, *120*, 28–36. [CrossRef] [PubMed]

18. Biel, M.; Michalakis, S. Cyclic nucleotide-gated channels. *Handb. Exp. Pharmacol.* **2009**, *191*, 111–136. [CrossRef]

19. Ammon, H.P.; Muller, A.B. Forskolin: From an ayurvedic remedy to a modern agent. *Planta Med.* **1985**, *51*, 473–477. [CrossRef] [PubMed]

20. Ahmad, F.; Murata, T.; Shimizu, K.; Degerman, E.; Maurice, D.; Manganiello, V. Cyclic nucleotide phosphodiesterases: Important signaling modulators and therapeutic targets. *Oral Dis.* **2015**, *21*, e25–e50. [CrossRef] [PubMed]

21. DeNinno, M.P. Future directions in phosphodiesterase drug discovery. *Bioorg. Med. Chem. Lett.* **2012**, *22*, 6794–6800. [CrossRef] [PubMed]

22. Knight, W.; Yan, C. Therapeutic potential of pde modulation in treating heart disease. *Future Med. Chem.* **2013**, *5*, 1607–1620. [CrossRef] [PubMed]

23. Martinez, A.; Gil, C. cAMP-specific phosphodiesterase inhibitors: Promising drugs for inflammatory and neurological diseases. *Expert Opin. Ther. Pat.* **2014**, *24*, 1311–1321. [CrossRef] [PubMed]

24. Cheng, X.; Ji, Z.; Tsalkova, T.; Mei, F. EPAC and PKA: A tale of two intracellular camp receptors. *Acta Biochim. Biophys. Sin. (Shanghai)* **2008**, *40*, 651–662. [CrossRef] [PubMed]

25. Houslay, M.D.; Conti, M.; Fancis, S.H. The cyclic nucleotides. *Handb. Exp. Pharmacol.* **2011**, *204*, v–vii.

26. Schlepper, M.; Thormann, J.; Mitrovic, V. Cardiovascular effects of forskolin and phosphodiesterase-III inhibitors. *Basic Res. Cardiol.* **1989**, *84* (Suppl. 1), 197–212. [CrossRef] [PubMed]

27. Kawasaki, H.; Springett, G.M.; Mochizuki, N.; Toki, S.; Nakaya, M.; Matsuda, M.; Housman, D.E.; Graybiel, A.M. A family of cAMP-binding proteins that directly activate Rap1. *Science* **1998**, *282*, 2275–2279. [CrossRef] [PubMed]

28. De Rooij, J.; Zwartkruis, F.J.; Verheijen, M.H.; Cool, R.H.; Nijman, S.M.; Wittinghofer, A.; Bos, J.L. EPAC is a Rap1 guanine-nucleotide-exchange factor directly activated by cyclic AMP. *Nature* **1998**, *396*, 474–477. [CrossRef] [PubMed]

29. Hoivik, E.A.; Witsoe, S.L.; Bergheim, I.R.; Xu, Y.; Jakobsson, I.; Tengholm, A.; Doskeland, S.O.; Bakke, M. DNA methylation of alternative promoters directs tissue specific expression of EPAC2 isoforms. *PLoS ONE* **2013**, *8*, e67925. [CrossRef] [PubMed]

30. Rehmann, H.; Arias-Palomo, E.; Hadders, M.A.; Schwede, F.; Llorca, O.; Bos, J.L. Structure of EPAC2 in complex with a cyclic AMP analogue and Rap1b. *Nature* **2008**, *27*, 124–127. [CrossRef] [PubMed]

31. Rehmann, H.; Das, J.; Knipscheer, P.; Wittinghofer, A.; Bos, J.L. Structure of the cyclic-AMP-responsive exchange factor EPAC2 in its auto-inhibited state. *Nature* **2006**, *439*, 625–628. [CrossRef] [PubMed]

32. Rehmann, H.; Prakash, B.; Wolf, E.; Rueppel, A.; de Rooij, J.; Bos, J.L.; Wittinghofer, A. Structure and regulation of the cAMP-binding domains of EPAC2. *Nat. Struct. Biol.* **2003**, *10*, 26–32. [CrossRef] [PubMed]

33. Parnell, E.; Smith, B.O.; Yarwood, S.J. The cAMP sensors, EPAC1 and EPAC2, display distinct subcellular distributions despite sharing a common nuclear pore localisation signal. *Cell. Signal.* **2015**, *27*, 989–996. [CrossRef] [PubMed]

34. Li, Y.; Asuri, S.; Rebhun, J.F.; Castro, A.F.; Paranavitana, N.C.; Quilliam, L.A. The Rap1 guanine nucleotide exchange factor EPAC2 couples cyclic AMP and Ras signals at the plasma membrane. *J. Biol. Chem.* **2006**, *281*, 2506–2514. [CrossRef] [PubMed]

35. Liu, C.; Takahashi, M.; Li, Y.; Dillon, T.J.; Kaech, S.; Stork, P.J. The interaction of EPAC1 and Ran promotes Rap1 activation at the nuclear envelope. *Mol. Cell. Biol.* **2010**, *30*, 3956–3969. [CrossRef] [PubMed]

36. Borland, G.; Smith, B.O.; Yarwood, S.J. EPAC proteins transduce diverse cellular actions of cAMP. *Br. J. Pharmacol.* **2009**, *158*, 70–86. [CrossRef] [PubMed]

37. Parnell, E.; Smith, B.O.; Palmer, T.M.; Terrin, A.; Zaccolo, M.; Yarwood, S.J. Regulation of the inflammatory response of vascular endothelial cells by EPAC1. *Br. J. Pharmacol.* **2012**, *166*, 434–446. [CrossRef] [PubMed]

38. Yang, Z.; Kirton, H.M.; Al-Owais, M.; Thireau, J.; Richard, S.; Peers, C.; Steele, D.S. EPAC2-Rap1 signaling regulates reactive oxygen species production and susceptibility to cardiac arrhythmias. *Antioxid. Redox Signal.* **2017**, *27*, 117–132. [CrossRef] [PubMed]

39. Edland, F.; Wergeland, A.; Kopperud, R.; Asrud, K.S.; Hoivik, E.A.; Witso, S.L.; Æsoy, R.; Madsen, L.; Kristiansen, K.; Bakke, M.; et al. Long-term consumption of an obesogenic high fat diet prior to ischemia-reperfusion mediates cardioprotection via EPAC1-dependent signaling. *Nutr. Metab.* **2016**, *13*, 87. [CrossRef] [PubMed]

40. Hwang, M.; Go, Y.; Park, J.H.; Shin, S.K.; Song, S.E.; Oh, B.C.; Im, S.S.; Hwang, I.; Jeon, Y.H.; Lee, I.K.; et al. EPAC2a-null mice exhibit obesity-prone nature more susceptible to leptin resistance. *Int. J. Obes.* **2017**, *41*, 279–288. [CrossRef] [PubMed]

41. Komai, A.M.; Musovic, S.; Peris, E.; Alrifaiy, A.; El Hachmane, M.F.; Johansson, M.; Wernstedt Asterholm, I.; Olofsson, C.S. White adipocyte adiponectin exocytosis is stimulated via beta3-adrenergic signaling and activation of EPAC1: Catecholamine resistance in obesity and type 2 diabetes. *Diabetes* **2016**, *65*, 3301–3313. [CrossRef] [PubMed]

42. Lakshmikanthan, S.; Zieba, B.J.; Ge, Z.D.; Momotani, K.; Zheng, X.; Lund, H.; Artamonov, M.V.; Maas, J.E.; Szabo, A.; Zhang, D.X.; et al. Rap1b in smooth muscle and endothelium is required for maintenance of vascular tone and normal blood pressure. *Arterioscler. Thromb. Vasc. Biol.* **2014**, *34*, 1486–1494. [CrossRef] [PubMed]

43. Sun, D.P.; Fang, C.L.; Chen, H.K.; Wen, K.S.; Hseu, Y.C.; Hung, S.T.; Uen, Y.H.; Lin, K.Y. EPAC1 overexpression is a prognostic marker and its inhibition shows promising therapeutic potential for gastric cancer. *Oncol. Rep.* **2017**, *37*, 1953–1960. [CrossRef] [PubMed]

44. Singhmar, P.; Huo, X.; Eijkelkamp, N.; Berciano, S.R.; Baameur, F.; Mei, F.C.; Zhu, Y.; Cheng, X.; Hawke, D.; Mayor, F., Jr.; et al. Critical role for Epac1 in inflammatory pain controlled by GRK2-mediated phosphorylation of Epac1. *Proc. Natl. Acad. Sci. USA* **2016**, *113*, 3036–3041. [CrossRef] [PubMed]

45. Dekkers, B.G.; Racke, K.; Schmidt, M. Distinct PKA and EPAC compartmentalization in airway function and plasticity. *Pharmacol. Ther.* **2013**, *137*, 248–265. [CrossRef] [PubMed]

46. Oldenburger, A.; Timens, W.; Bos, S.; Smit, M.; Smrcka, A.V.; Laurent, A.C.; Cao, J.; Hylkema, M.; Meurs, H.; Maarsingh, H.; et al. Epac1 and Epac2 are differentially involved in inflammatory and remodeling processes induced by cigarette smoke. *FASEB J.* **2014**, *28*, 4617–4628. [CrossRef] [PubMed]

47. Roscioni, S.S.; Prins, A.G.; Elzinga, C.R.; Menzen, M.H.; Dekkers, B.G.; Halayko, A.J.; Meurs, H.; Maarsingh, H.; Schmidt, M. Protein kinase a and the exchange protein directly activated by cAMP (Epac) modulate phenotype plasticity in human airway smooth muscle. *Br. J. Pharmacol.* **2011**, *164*, 958–969. [CrossRef] [PubMed]

48. Fanelli, C.; Aronoff, R. Restenosis following coronary angioplasty. *Am. Heart J.* **1990**, *119*, 357–368. [CrossRef]

49. McKean, J.S.; Murray, F.; Gibson, G.; Shewan, D.A.; Tucker, S.J.; Nixon, G.F. The cAMP-producing agonist beraprost inhibits human vascular smooth muscle cell migration via exchange protein directly activated by camp. *Cardiovasc. Res.* **2015**, *107*, 546–555. [CrossRef] [PubMed]

50. Hewer, R.C.; Sala-Newby, G.B.; Wu, Y.J.; Newby, A.C.; Bond, M. PKA and Epac synergistically inhibit smooth muscle cell proliferation. *J. Mol. Cell. Cardiol.* **2011**, *50*, 87–98. [CrossRef] [PubMed]

51. Sands, W.A.; Woolson, H.D.; Milne, G.R.; Rutherford, C.; Palmer, T.M. Exchange protein activated by cyclic AMP (Epac)-mediated induction of suppressor of cytokine signaling 3 (SOCS-3) in vascular endothelial cells. *Mol. Cell. Biol.* **2006**, *26*, 6333–6346. [CrossRef] [PubMed]

52. Bruunsgaard, H.; Pedersen, M.; Pedersen, B.K. Aging and proinflammatory cytokines. *Curr. Opin. Hematol.* **2001**, *8*, 131–136. [CrossRef] [PubMed]

53. Hou, T.; Tieu, B.C.; Ray, S.; Recinos, I.A.; Cui, R.; Tilton, R.G.; Brasier, A.R. Roles of IL-6-gp130 signaling in vascular inflammation. *Curr. Cardiol. Rev.* **2008**, *4*, 179–192. [CrossRef] [PubMed]

54. Kleemann, R.; Zadelaar, S.; Kooistra, T. Cytokines and atherosclerosis: A comprehensive review of studies in mice. *Cardiovasc. Res.* **2008**, *79*, 360–376. [CrossRef] [PubMed]

55. Schieffer, B.; Selle, T.; Hilfiker, A.; Hilfiker-Kleiner, D.; Grote, K.; Tietge, U.J.; Trautwein, C.; Luchtefeld, M.; Schmittkamp, C.; Heeneman, S.; et al. Impact of interleukin-6 on plaque development and morphology in experimental atherosclerosis. *Circulation* **2004**, *110*, 3493–3500. [CrossRef] [PubMed]

56. Schuett, H.; Oestreich, R.; Waetzig, G.H.; Annema, W.; Luchtefeld, M.; Hillmer, A.; Bavendiek, U.; von Felden, J.; Divchev, D.; Kempf, T.; et al. Transsignaling of interleukin-6 crucially contributes to atherosclerosis in mice. *Arterioscler* **2012**, *32*, 281–290. [CrossRef] [PubMed]

57. Heinrich, P.C.; Behrmann, I.; Haan, S.; Hermanns, H.M.; Muller-Newen, G.; Schaper, F. Principles of interleukin (IL)-6-type cytokine signalling and its regulation. *Biochem. J.* **2003**, *374*, 1–20. [CrossRef] [PubMed]

58. Schmitz, J.; Dahmen, H.; Grimm, C.; Gendo, C.; Muller-Newen, G.; Heinrich, P.C.; Schaper, F. The cytoplasmic tyrosine motifs in full-length glycoprotein 130 have different roles in IL-6 signal transduction. *J. Immunol.* **2000**, *164*, 848–854. [CrossRef] [PubMed]

59. Luo, Y.; Zheng, S.G. Hall of fame among pro-inflammatory cytokines: Interleukin-6 gene and its transcriptional regulation mechanisms. *Front. Immunol.* **2016**, *7*, 604. [CrossRef] [PubMed]

60. Wang, H.; Robichaux, W.G.; Wang, Z.; Mei, F.C.; Cai, M.; Du, G.; Chen, J.; Cheng, X. Inhibition of Epac1 suppresses mitochondrial fission and reduces neointima formation induced by vascular injury. *Sci. Rep.* **2016**, *6*, 36552. [CrossRef] [PubMed]

61. Kato, Y.; Yokoyama, U.; Yanai, C.; Ishige, R.; Kurotaki, D.; Umemura, M.; Fujita, T.; Kubota, T.; Okumura, S.; Sata, M.; et al. Epac1 deficiency attenuated vascular smooth muscle cell migration and neointimal formation. *Arterioscler. Thromb. Vasc. Biol.* **2015**, *35*, 2617–2625. [CrossRef] [PubMed]

62. Yokoyama, U.; Minamisawa, S.; Quan, H.; Akaike, T.; Jin, M.; Otsu, K.; Ulucan, C.; Wang, X.; Baljinnyam, E.; Takaoka, M.; et al. Epac1 is upregulated during neointima formation and promotes vascular smooth muscle cell migration. *Am. J. Physiol. Heart Circ. Physiol.* **2008**, *295*, H1547–H1555. [CrossRef] [PubMed]

63. Adderley, S.P.; Martin, D.N.; Tulis, D.A. Exchange protein activated by cAMP (Epac) controls migration of vascular smooth muscle cells in concentration and time-dependent manner. *Arch. Physiol.* **2015**, *2*, 2. [CrossRef]

64. Sprague, A.H.; Khalil, R.A. Inflammatory cytokines in vascular dysfunction and vascular disease. *Biochem. Pharmacol.* **2009**, *78*, 539–552. [CrossRef] [PubMed]

65. Babon, J.J.; Varghese, L.N.; Nicola, N.A. Inhibition of IL-6 family cytokines by SOCS3. *Semin. Immunol.* **2014**, *26*, 13–19. [CrossRef] [PubMed]

66. Sasaki, A.; Yasukawa, H.; Suzuki, A.; Kamizono, S.; Syoda, T.; Kinjyo, I.; Sasaki, M.; Johnston, J.A.; Yoshimura, A. Cytokine-inducible SH2 protein-3 (CIS3/SOCS3) inhibits janus tyrosine kinase by binding through the N-terminal kinase inhibitory region as well as SH2 domain. *Genes Cells* **1999**, *4*, 339–351. [CrossRef] [PubMed]

67. Williams, J.J.; Palmer, T.M. Unbiased identification of substrates for the epac1-inducible e3 ubiquitin ligase component SOCS-3. *Biochem. Soc. Trans.* **2012**, *40*, 215–218. [CrossRef] [PubMed]

68. Recio, C.; Oguiza, A.; Mallavia, B.; Lazaro, I.; Ortiz-Munoz, G.; Lopez-Franco, O.; Egido, J.; Gomez-Guerrero, C. Gene delivery of suppressors of cytokine signaling (SOCS) inhibits inflammation and atherosclerosis development in mice. *Basic Res. Cardiol.* **2015**, *110*, 8. [CrossRef] [PubMed]

69. Xiang, S.; Liu, J.; Dong, N.; Shi, J.; Xiao, Y.; Wang, Y.; Hu, X.; Gong, L.; Wang, W. Suppressor of cytokine signaling 3 is a negative regulator for neointimal hyperplasia of vein graft stenosis. *J. Vasc. Res.* **2014**, *51*, 132–143. [CrossRef] [PubMed]

70. Liang, X.; He, M.; Chen, T.; Liu, Y.; Tian, Y.L.; Wu, Y.L.; Zhao, Y.; Shen, Y.; Yuan, Z.Y. Multiple roles of SOCS proteins: Differential expression of SOCS1 and SOCS3 in atherosclerosis. *Int. J. Mol. Med.* **2013**, *31*, 1066–1074. [CrossRef] [PubMed]

71. Ortiz-Munoz, G.; Martin-Ventura, J.L.; Hernandez-Vargas, P.; Mallavia, B.; Lopez-Parra, V.; Lopez-Franco, O.; Munoz-Garcia, B.; Fernandez-Vizarra, P.; Ortega, L.; Egido, J.; et al. Suppressors of cytokine signaling modulate JAK/STAT-mediated cell responses during atherosclerosis. *Arterioscler. Thromb. Vasc. Biol.* **2009**, *29*, 525–531. [CrossRef] [PubMed]

72. Croker, B.A.; Kiu, H.; Pellegrini, M.; Toe, J.; Preston, S.; Metcalf, D.; O'Donnell, J.A.; Cengia, L.H.; McArthur, K.; Nicola, N.A.; et al. IL-6 promotes acute and chronic inflammatory disease in the absence of SOCS3. *Immunol. Cell Biol.* **2012**, *90*, 124–129. [CrossRef] [PubMed]

73. Stahl, A.; Joyal, J.S.; Chen, J.; Sapieha, P.; Juan, A.M.; Hatton, C.J.; Pei, D.T.; Hurst, C.G.; Seaward, M.R.; Krah, N.M.; et al. SOCS3 is an endogenous inhibitor of pathologic angiogenesis. *Blood* **2012**, *120*, 2925–2929. [CrossRef] [PubMed]

74. Jo, D.; Liu, D.; Yao, S.; Collins, R.D.; Hawiger, J. Intracellular protein therapy with SOCS3 inhibits inflammation and apoptosis. *Nat. Med.* **2005**, *11*, 892–898. [CrossRef] [PubMed]

75. Recio, C.; Oguiza, A.; Lazaro, I.; Mallavia, B.; Egido, J.; Gomez-Guerrero, C. Suppressor of cytokine signaling 1-derived peptide inhibits janus kinase/signal transducers and activators of transcription pathway and improves inflammation and atherosclerosis in diabetic mice. *Arterioscler. Thromb. Vasc. Biol.* **2014**, *34*, 1953–1960. [CrossRef] [PubMed]

76. Yarwood, S.J.; Borland, G.; Sands, W.A.; Palmer, T.M. Identification of CCAAT/enhancer-binding proteins as exchange protein activated by cAMP-activated transcription factors that mediate the induction of the SOCS-3 gene. *J. Biol. Chem.* **2008**, *283*, 6843–6853. [CrossRef] [PubMed]

77. Netherton, S.J.; Sutton, J.A.; Wilson, L.S.; Carter, R.L.; Maurice, D.H. Both protein kinase A and exchange protein activated by cAMP coordinate adhesion of human vascular endothelial cells. *Circ. Res.* **2007**, *101*, 768–776. [CrossRef] [PubMed]

78. Bogatcheva, N.V.; Garcia, J.G.; Verin, A.D. Role of tyrosine kinase signaling in endothelial cell barrier regulation. *Vasc. Pharmacol.* **2002**, *39*, 201–212. [CrossRef]

79. Vouret-Craviari, V.; Grall, D.; Van Obberghen-Schilling, E. Modulation of Rho GTPase activity in endothelial cells by selective proteinase-activated receptor (PAR) agonists. *J. Thromb. Haemost.* **2003**, *1*, 1103–1111. [CrossRef] [PubMed]

80. Schmidt, M.; Sand, C.; Jakobs, K.H.; Michel, M.C.; Weernink, P.A. Epac and the cardiovascular system. *Curr. Opin. Pharmacol.* **2007**, *7*, 193–200. [CrossRef] [PubMed]

81. Baumer, Y.; Drenckhahn, D.; Waschke, J. cAMP induced Rac 1-mediated cytoskeletal reorganization in microvascular endothelium. *Histochem. Cell Biol.* **2008**, *129*, 765–778. [CrossRef] [PubMed]

82. Birukova, A.A.; Zagranichnaya, T.; Fu, P.; Alekseeva, E.; Chen, W.; Jacobson, J.R.; Birukov, K.G. Prostaglandins PGE$_2$ and PGI$_2$ promote endothelial barrier enhancement via PKA- and Epac1/Rap1-dependent Rac activation. *Exp. Cell Res.* **2007**, *313*, 2504–2520. [CrossRef] [PubMed]

83. Cullere, X.; Shaw, S.K.; Andersson, L.; Hirahashi, J.; Luscinskas, F.W.; Mayadas, T.N. Regulation of vascular endothelial barrier function by Epac, a cAMP-activated exchange factor for Rap GTPase. *Blood* **2005**, *105*, 1950–1955. [CrossRef] [PubMed]

84. Fukuhara, S.; Sakurai, A.; Sano, H.; Yamagishi, A.; Somekawa, S.; Takakura, N.; Saito, Y.; Kangawa, K.; Mochizuki, N. Cyclic AMP potentiates vascular endothelial cadherin-mediated cell-cell contact to enhance endothelial barrier function through an Epac-Rap1 signaling pathway. *Mol. Cell. Biol.* **2005**, *25*, 136–146. [CrossRef] [PubMed]

85. Kooistra, M.R.; Corada, M.; Dejana, E.; Bos, J.L. Epac1 regulates integrity of endothelial cell junctions through VE-cadherin. *FEBS Lett.* **2005**, *579*, 4966–4972. [CrossRef] [PubMed]

86. Sehrawat, S.; Cullere, X.; Patel, S.; Italiano, J., Jr.; Mayadas, T.N. Role of Epac1, an exchange factor for Rap GTPases, in endothelial microtubule dynamics and barrier function. *Mol. Biol. Cell* **2008**, *19*, 1261–1270. [CrossRef] [PubMed]

87. Vliem, M.J.; Ponsioen, B.; Schwede, F.; Pannekoek, W.J.; Riedl, J.; Kooistra, M.R.; Jalink, K.; Genieser, H.G.; Bos, J.L.; Rehmann, H. 8-pCPT-2'-O-Me-cAMP-AM: An improved Epac-selective cAMP analogue. *Chembiochem Eur. J. Chem. Biol.* **2008**, *9*, 2052–2054. [CrossRef] [PubMed]

88. Enserink, J.M.; Christensen, A.E.; de Rooij, J.; van Triest, M.; Schwede, F.; Genieser, H.G.; Doskeland, S.O.; Blank, J.L.; Bos, J.L. A novel Epac-specific cAMP analogue demonstrates independent regulation of Rap1 and ERK. *Nat. Cell Biol.* **2002**, *4*, 901–906. [CrossRef] [PubMed]

89. Kraemer, A.; Rehmann, H.R.; Cool, R.H.; Theiss, C.; de Rooij, J.; Bos, J.L.; Wittinghofer, A. Dynamic interaction of cAMP with the Rap guanine-nucleotide exchange factor Epac1. *J. Mol. Biol.* **2001**, *306*, 1167–1177. [CrossRef] [PubMed]

90. Schwede, F.; Bertinetti, D.; Langerijs, C.N.; Hadders, M.A.; Wienk, H.; Ellenbroek, J.H.; de Koning, E.J.; Bos, J.L.; Herberg, F.W.; Genieser, H.G.; et al. Structure-guided design of selective Epac1 and Epac2 agonists. *PLoS Biol.* **2015**, *13*, e1002038. [CrossRef] [PubMed]

91. Metrich, M.; Berthouze, M.; Morel, E.; Crozatier, B.; Gomez, A.M.; Lezoualc'h, F. Role of the cAMP-binding protein Epac in cardiovascular physiology and pathophysiology. *Pflug. Arch. Eur. J. Physiol.* **2010**, *459*, 535–546. [CrossRef] [PubMed]

92. Hothi, S.S.; Gurung, I.S.; Heathcote, J.C.; Zhang, Y.; Booth, S.W.; Skepper, J.N.; Grace, A.A.; Huang, C.L. Epac activation, altered calcium homeostasis and ventricular arrhythmogenesis in the murine heart. *Pflug. Arch. Eur. J. Physiol.* **2008**, *457*, 253–270. [CrossRef] [PubMed]

93. Pereira, L.; Cheng, H.; Lao, D.H.; Na, L.; van Oort, R.J.; Brown, J.H.; Wehrens, X.H.; Chen, J.; Bers, D.M. Epac2 mediates cardiac β1-adrenergic-dependent sarcoplasmic reticulum Ca^{2+} leak and arrhythmia. *Circulation* **2013**, *127*, 913–922. [CrossRef] [PubMed]

94. Pereira, L.; Metrich, M.; Fernandez-Velasco, M.; Lucas, A.; Leroy, J.; Perrier, R.; Morel, E.; Fischmeister, R.; Richard, S.; Benitah, J.P.; et al. The cAMP binding protein Epac modulates Ca^{2+} sparks by a Ca^{2+}/calmodulin kinase signalling pathway in rat cardiac myocytes. *J. Physiol.* **2007**, *583*, 685–694. [CrossRef] [PubMed]

95. Zhang, C.L.; Katoh, M.; Shibasaki, T.; Minami, K.; Sunaga, Y.; Takahashi, H.; Yokoi, N.; Iwasaki, M.; Miki, T.; Seino, S. The cAMP sensor Epac2 is a direct target of antidiabetic sulfonylurea drugs. *Science* **2009**, *325*, 607–610. [CrossRef] [PubMed]

96. Herbst, K.J.; Coltharp, C.; Amzel, L.M.; Zhang, J. Direct activation of Epac by sulfonylurea is isoform selective. *Chem. Biol.* **2011**, *18*, 243–251. [CrossRef] [PubMed]

97. Rehmann, H. Epac2: A sulfonylurea receptor? *Biochem. Soc. Trans.* **2012**, *40*, 6–10. [CrossRef] [PubMed]

98. Tsalkova, T.; Gribenko, A.V.; Cheng, X. Exchange protein directly activated by cyclic AMP isoform 2 is not a direct target of sulfonylurea drugs. *Assay Drug Dev. Technol.* **2011**, *9*, 88–91. [CrossRef] [PubMed]

99. Tsalkova, T.; Mei, F.C.; Li, S.; Chepurny, O.G.; Leech, C.A.; Liu, T.; Holz, G.G.; Woods, V.L., Jr.; Cheng, X. Isoform-specific antagonists of exchange proteins directly activated by cAMP. *Proc. Natl. Acad. Sci. USA* **2012**, *109*, 18613–18618. [CrossRef] [PubMed]

100. McPhee, I.; Gibson, L.C.; Kewney, J.; Darroch, C.; Stevens, P.A.; Spinks, D.; Cooreman, A.; MacKenzie, S.J. Cyclic nucleotide signalling: A molecular approach to drug discovery for alzheimer's disease. *Biochem. Soc. Trans.* **2005**, *33*, 1330–1332. [CrossRef] [PubMed]

101. Tsalkova, T.; Mei, F.C.; Cheng, X. A fluorescence-based high-throughput assay for the discovery of exchange protein directly activated by cyclic AMP (EPAC) antagonists. *PLoS ONE* **2012**, *7*, e30441. [CrossRef] [PubMed]

102. Almahariq, M.; Tsalkova, T.; Mei, F.C.; Chen, H.; Zhou, J.; Sastry, S.K.; Schwede, F.; Cheng, X. A novel EPAC-specific inhibitor suppresses pancreatic cancer cell migration and invasion. *Mol. Pharmacol.* **2013**, *83*, 122–128. [CrossRef] [PubMed]

103. Chen, H.; Tsalkova, T.; Chepurny, O.G.; Mei, F.C.; Holz, G.G.; Cheng, X.; Zhou, J. Identification and characterization of small molecules as potent and specific EPAC2 antagonists. *J. Med. Chem.* **2013**, *56*, 952–962. [CrossRef] [PubMed]

104. Rehmann, H. Epac-inhibitors: Facts and artefacts. *Sci. Rep.* **2013**, *3*, 3032. [CrossRef] [PubMed]

105. Wild, C.T.; Zhu, Y.; Na, Y.; Mei, F.; Ynalvez, M.A.; Chen, H.; Cheng, X.; Zhou, J. Functionalized *N,N*-diphenylamines as potent and selective EPAC2 inhibitors. *ACS Med. Chem. Lett.* **2016**, *7*, 460–464. [CrossRef] [PubMed]

106. Ye, N.; Zhu, Y.; Chen, H.; Liu, Z.; Mei, F.C.; Wild, C.; Chen, H.; Cheng, X.; Zhou, J. Structure-activity relationship studies of substituted 2-(isoxazol-3-yl)-2-oxo-*N'*-phenyl-acetohydrazonoyl cyanide analogues: Identification of potent exchange proteins directly activated by cAMP (EPAC) antagonists. *J. Med. Chem.* **2015**, *58*, 6033–6047. [CrossRef] [PubMed]

107. Ye, N.; Zhu, Y.; Liu, Z.; Mei, F.C.; Chen, H.; Wang, P.; Cheng, X.; Zhou, J. Identification of novel 2-(benzo[*d*]isoxazol-3-yl)-2-oxo-*N*-phenylacetohydrazonoyl cyanide analoguesas potent epac antagonists. *Eur. J. Med. Chem.* **2017**, *134*, 62–71. [CrossRef] [PubMed]

108. Rehmann, H.; Wittinghofer, A.; Bos, J.L. Capturing cyclic nucleotides in action: Snapshots from crystallographic studies. *Nat. Rev. Mol. Cell Biol.* **2007**, *8*, 63–73. [CrossRef] [PubMed]

109. Rehmann, H. Characterization of the activation of the Rap-specific exchange factor Epac by cyclic nucleotides. *Methods Enzymol.* **2005**, *407*, 159–173.
110. Dao, K.K.; Teigen, K.; Kopperud, R.; Hodneland, E.; Schwede, F.; Christensen, A.E.; Martinez, A.; Doskeland, S.O. Epac1 and cAMP-dependent protein kinase holoenzyme have similar cAMP affinity, but their cAMP domains have distinct structural features and cyclic nucleotide recognition. *J. Biol. Chem.* **2006**, *281*, 21500–21511. [CrossRef] [PubMed]
111. Parnell, E.; McElroy, S.P.; Wiejak, J.; Baillie, G.L.; Porter, A.; Adams, D.R.; Rehmann, H.; Smith, B.O.; Yarwood, S.J. Identification of a novel, small molecule partial agonist for the cyclic AMP sensor, EPAC1. *Sci. Rep.* **2017**, *7*, 294. [CrossRef] [PubMed]
112. Ammazzalorso, A.; De Filippis, B.; Giampietro, L.; Amoroso, R. N-acylsulfonamides: Synthetic routes and biological potential in medicinal chemistry. *Chem. Biol. Drug Des.* **2017**, *90*, 1094–1105. [CrossRef] [PubMed]

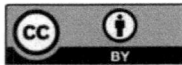

MDPI

St. Alban-Anlage 66

4052 Basel

Switzerland

Tel. +41 61 683 77 34

Fax +41 61 302 89 18

www.mdpi.com

Journal of Cardiovascular Development and Disease Editorial Office

E-mail: JCDD@mdpi.com

www.mdpi.com/journal/JCDD

www.ingramcontent.com/pod-product-compliance
Lightning Source LLC
Chambersburg PA
CBHW051717210326
41597CB00032B/5510